Editor
Marcos V. Goycoolea, M.D., M.S., Ph.D.
Minnesota Ear, Head & Neck Clinic
Minneapolis, Minnesota

Co-Editors
Michael M. Paparella, M.D.
Minnesota Ear, Head & Neck Clinic
Minneapolis, Minnesota

Rick L. Nissen, M.D.
Minnesota Ear, Head & Neck Clinic
Minneapolis, Minnesota

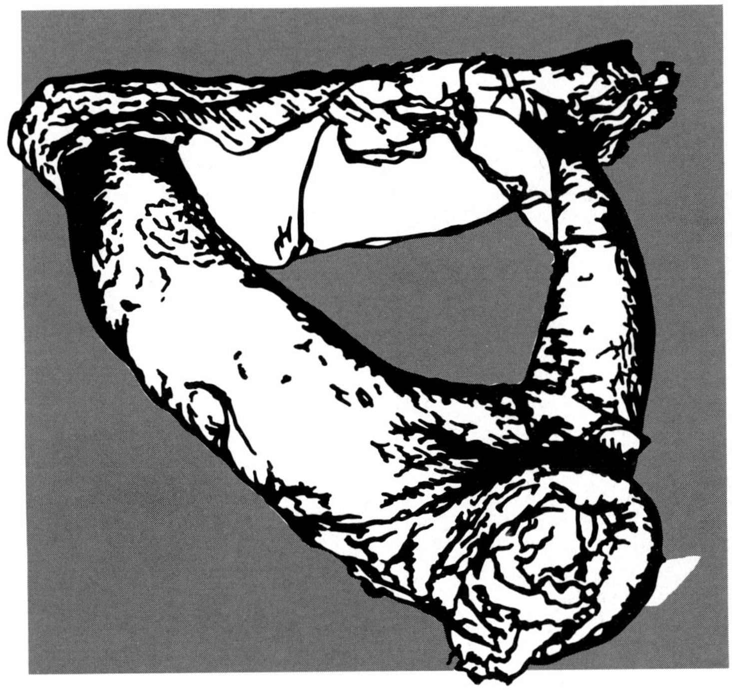

ATLAS OF Otologic Surgery

1989
W.B. SAUNDERS COMPANY
Harcourt Brace Jovanovich, Inc.
Philadelphia / London / Toronto
Montreal / Sydney / Tokyo

W. B. SAUNDERS COMPANY
Harcourt Brace Jovanovich, Inc.

The Curtis Center
Independence Square West
Philadelphia, PA 19106

Library of Congress Cataloging-in-Publication Data

Goycoolea, Marcos V.

Atlas of otologic surgery.

Bibliography: p.

1. Ear—Surgery—Atlases. I. Paparella, Michael M. II. Nissen, Rick L. III. Title. [DNLM: 1. Ear—surgery—atlases. WV 17 G724a]

RF295.G69 1989   617.8′059   88–18559

ISBN 0–7216–2337–9

Editor: W. B. Saunders Staff
Designer: Liz Schweber
Production Manager: Bill Preston
Manuscript Editor: Tom Gibbons
Illustrator: Melissa Walter
Illustration Coordinator: Walter Verbitski
Cover Designer: Michelle Maloney
Indexer: William Cole

Atlas of Otologic Surgery   ISBN 0–7216–2337–9

Last digit is the print number: 9 8 7 6 5 4 3 2 1

PURO CHILE ES TU CIELO AZULADO
PURAS BRISAS TE CRUZAN TAMBIEN
Y ESE CAMPO DE FLORES BORDADO
ES LA COPIA FELIZ DEL EDEN . . .

A TI, DULCE PATRIA . . .

(from the Chilean national anthem)

Contributors

Gwenn Afton, M.S.
Medical Illustrator, Minnesota Ear, Head and Neck Clinic and Beck Visual Communications, Minneapolis, Minnesota.

Marcos V. Goycoolea, M.D., M.S., Ph.D.
Minnesota Ear, Head and Neck Clinic. Otology Consultant, Chilean Military Hospital and Audia Chile, Santiago, Chile.

Peter Hilger, M.D., M.S.
Assistant Professor, Department of Otolaryngology, University of Minnesota. Staff Physician, St. Paul Ramsey Medical Center, St. Paul, Minnesota.

Timothy K. Jung, M.D., Ph.D.
Associate Professor, Division of Otolaryngology and Head and Neck Surgery, Loma Linda University, Loma Linda, California.

Sherry Lamey
Head technologist, Otopathology Laboratory, Department of Otolaryngology, University of Minnesota.

Alan J. Nissen, M.D.
California Ear Institute, Palo Alto, California. Clinical Instructor, Stanford University, Palo Alto, California.

Rick L. Nissen, M.D.
Minnesota Ear, Head and Neck Clinic.

Michael M. Paparella, M.D.
Minnesota Ear, Head and Neck Clinic. Chairman Emeritus, Clinical Professor, and Director of the Otopathology Laboratory, Department of Otolaryngology, University of Minnesota.

Donald Robertson, Ph.D.
Associate Professor, Department of Otolaryngology and Department of Cell Biology and Neuroanatomy, University of Minnesota.

Kurt Schellhas, M.D.
Director of Neuro-Imaging, Center for Diagnostic Imaging, St. Louis Park, Minnesota.

Robert Smith, M.D.
Chief Resident, Department of Otolaryngology, University of Minnesota.

Edward W. Szachowicz, M.D., Ph.D.
Assistant Professor, Department of Otolaryngology, University of Minnesota.
Staff Physician, St. Paul Ramsey Medical Center, St. Paul, Minnesota.

Motto

Learn to learn from everything you do
and everybody around you.

Key Words

Anatomy

Function

Pathogenesis

Research

Open mind

Common sense

Dedication

Preface

This book is written primarily for physicians in training (residents). It is my aim to make it a dialogue with you, the residents, beginning with the preface itself. The origin of this book goes back to my first year of residency in Otolaryngology. Although many good texts were available, I felt that I needed a book that went back to basics in clear and understandable language, and that would provide me with the essential concepts from which to start. It seemed to me that a complicated organ such as the ear could be made, at least at that stage, a little simpler (not simple). Over time I have been thinking of different aspects that I felt to be important and useful for this purpose, and I asked the different contributors to do the same. Accordingly, we have tried to create a book that emphasizes the basics, rather than one that shows our methods.

In the same context, this atlas is only intended to complement other texts on the subject. Because this is primarily a conceptual atlas, we have made no attempt to provide detailed discussions of evaluations and indications; such discussions are provided by the works cited in the list of selected references. This list also includes publications that describe essential concepts of anatomy and function. Because of the extent of these subjects, the works available number in the thousands; we apologize to those authors whose important publications are not cited owing to lack of space and request their understanding. We are aware that this first edition will need improvements. It is our hope that these will come from your criticisms and suggestions.

There are a number of thoughts and general philosophies that I believe are useful. I do not expect you to agree with them but to be exposed to them and think. Some of them will make sense, some will not. I hope that some of the latter will make sense to you in time.

The techniques described in this book are intended to show different approaches based on the knowledge of anatomy, function, and pathology. They are oriented more toward a way of thinking than toward a dogma of doing, in the expectation that the surgeon will think of each surgical procedure as a distinct and different act. It is my hope that this will allow the surgeon to vary an approach according to need, habit, or ability at a specific time. I believe that there is no single best technique for otologic surgery; in order to achieve a safe and efficient result, different surgeons might select different but equally valid approaches. It is easy to be rigid; it is even successful, on the whole. It is harder to tailor your approach case by case since this requires an overall concept. In the long run, however, it is much more rewarding. Research and knowledge of anatomy and pathogenesis permit proper changes and improvements. Ear surgery can be what you want it to be. If it is to be developed into an art, knowledge, creativity, dynamism, and an open mind, together with common sense, are essential. As in any discipline, there are basic principles; however, they should be regarded not as rigid rules but rather as underlying philosophies. An essential point to be remembered is that the aim of surgery is to solve problems. Patients come to you for you to solve their problem, not for the surgery itself. In the same context, solving a problem does not mean applying formulas or fitting patients into treatment classifications. Classifications and formulas are nothing more than common sense put on paper—use them as a tool, do not be "ruled by them." This may seem like a subtle concept but it makes all the difference in the world. The difference between operating and solving a problem is like the difference between passing a cloth over a table and cleaning the table.

Another important concept implied here is what I call the concept of "intent." For all actions that are to be translated into an efficient result, there must be the intention of obtaining such a result. This involves the rational use of your senses. When you look through the operating microscope you must *see*, observe, analyze, and use the information obtained. This is quite different from "glancing." You must know what you are looking at (based on anatomy) and the most likely possibilities and alternatives that can be found (based on pathogenesis).

It is also essential to understand that surgery is in the mind and the heart and not primarily in the hand. Good hands are important, but they are not enough. A mechanical task can be performed brilliantly by a moron if it is done over and over again in the same fashion. The art of surgery lies as much in the choices as in the act itself, and also in the postoperative care. The medical act begins with the first clinical visit and ends when the problem is solved.

It is always tempting to simplify our lives with what is "usual" and "customary." If you are in pursuit of excellence, avoid this temptation. A common attitude of residents (we have all been residents and I have not forgotten the experience) is to proceed as the "books say" or the "journal says." Books and journals (including this one) do not say anything; they present what different authors believe. Although important and valuable, this information should be treated as a reference, not as dogma.

On patient evaluation: Despite the fact that the amount of information available and the precision of laboratory studies have had a great impact on today's medicine, the essential process of evaluation remains unchanged. Regardless of the facilities available, the patient's history and examination are as critical as ever. Provided that they are done properly, a diagnosis is reached most of the time based on history and examination alone. For children, the parents (usually the mother) are crucial in providing information. Regardless of a mother's background, she is the one who spent the night with the sick child and provided food, clothing, cleansing, and so on. The mother will not tell you what to diagnose and do, but she will provide important clues for the diagnosis, and at times for treatment. Again, our role is to listen respectfully and learn; then, using our knowledge, diagnose and if possible teach. Laboratory studies confirm impressions, provide documented objective evidence, and rule out or detect problems or lesions not detectable otherwise. Much can be said about this; suffice it to mention that laboratory studies are ordered with specific questions in mind, and should not be ordered if the results are not oriented toward an action to be taken.

On the procedure of choice: Apart from strict physiopathology, there are other factors to consider in deciding what benefits an individual most. What is good for some may not be good for others. A procedure that requires frequent checkups might not benefit somebody who cannot be checked periodically. People and circumstances vary and so should your solutions. Although it is our duty to change attitudes for the better, it is common sense to accept that some things cannot be changed.

On the risks of surgery: it is important to reiterate that it is the patient who takes the risk, not the surgeon. How warranted a specific risk is will depend on the patient's situation and needs, and calls for common sense on the part of the surgeon. A surgeon should be conservative. Although "everybody has something that can be operated upon," the surgeon's role is to assess if the operation is indicated and really helpful. Conservatism should be a product both of knowledge and of profound respect for an individual who has trusted you; it should not come from ignorance or inability to perform what is needed. As for doing what other surgeons do successfully, again, their experience should be seen as background and reference and not as dogma. It is fine to imitate others and this should be done by all means, provided that what is imitated is understood, agreed upon, and applicable to your patients. It is important to evaluate and rationalize what the leading surgeons do; behind each of the true leading surgeons are many hours of study and hard work. Question positively their methods and rationale. Ask yourself what is intended by a specific method and why. Is it reasonable? Is it the best way? "Trendy" procedures and "state of the art" instruments also require thorough knowledge and understanding. They usually have good reasons behind them; you must understand and agree with those reasons. If all you need to do is kill a fly, use a 50-cent fly swatter; do not buy a $50,000 electronic fly killer because it is "state of the art." Trends come and trends go. Use common sense when investing.

Otologic surgery, like medicine itself, is a never-ending learning process. You are never too good to learn from everybody else. Seeking advice is a sign not of weakness but of maturity. Learn to use your senses; observe and listen to other surgeons and specialists, the operating team, your patients, and others. Learn positively from those who want to help you *and* from those who want to harm or use you. Learn to learn from everything you do and everybody around you. Each surgical case is different. When placing pressure-equalizing tubes, study the ear canals and their contents, the tympanic membrane, the middle ear mucosa, characteristics of the effusion, and so on. Relate them to one another, to the laboratory studies, and to the clinical history. This simple process will enrich you and you will learn what you never thought you would. A difficult task is to learn how to accept reality and our lack of true knowledge. As hard as it is to deal with success, it is harder and demands more stamina to deal with failure. Complications and unwanted results do happen, even if you seemingly have done your job properly. Objective self-assessment and complete revision of the subject should follow every failure, even if it "was bound to happen." You may easily forget 200 successful stapedectomies and never forget one case of hearing loss due to a reparative granuloma. You must also learn to accept that in many cases in otology, surgery does not turn back the disease process, and that different individuals have different responses to similar surgical procedures and different healing capabilities. From this standpoint alone, the results of tympanoplasty may vary from 60% to 100%. A 60% success in a population with poor nutritional background can be better than 90% in one with optimal nutrition. Percentages are relative; your own and those of others should be analyzed in their full context. There are many other points and ideas that I would have liked to discuss here. Some of them are discussed in the text.

A few words on the contributors to this atlas:

Gwenn Afton, the illustrator, has an MS in Medical Illustration from the Medical College of Georgia. I had the privilege of writing the temporal bone dissection manual that she illustrated as her master's thesis. At the time she not only performed such dissections herself but requested direct supervision and explanations. In spite of her being by far the youngest member of this team, her professionalism, dedication, interest, and talents are what I would have expected from an experienced and famed medical illustrator. I worked directly with her on each and every drawing (in all chapters) in this atlas. However, it must be mentioned that the designs for Chapter 1 (Pertinent Anatomy) were selected by Donald Robertson; for the discussions of neuro-otology (in Chapters 5, 17, 18, and 19) by Rick Nissen; and for Chapter 14 (Lasers in Otologic Surgery) by Alan Nissen. We have been asked to lend many of the illustrations (only those designed by Gwenn and me) to Michael Paparella for the otology volume of his forthcoming text. I have no doubt that with the appearance of this atlas we are also witnessing the emergence of an artist who will be a significant contributor to medical illustration in the coming years.

Timothy Jung is my former fellow resident at Minnesota. Tim oriented his research toward biochemistry of the ear and has remained working in this area while practicing primarily clinical otolaryngology. He has contributed directly to the discussions of the Thiersch graft (in Chapter 7) and mastoid obliteration and surgery for complications of suppurative otitis media (in Chapter 10), and is wholly responsible for Chapter 8 (External Ear Canal Procedures). His clinical and surgical experience, coupled with his approach toward ear disease based on anatomy and pathogenesis, made him a natural contributor to this book.

Sherry Lamey has headed the Otopathology Laboratory at the University of Minnesota for 20 years. She is, in my opinion, directly responsible for transforming this laboratory into one of the best, if not the best, of its kind in the world. Many generations of residents (including mine) and research fellows have benefited from her knowledge and expertise. The histology and histopathology slides in this atlas, as well as Chapter 4 (Temporal Bone Removal), are all products of her work.

In order to include a solid discussion of the use of lasers in otologic surgery (Chapter 14), we asked Alan Nissen to be a contributor. Alan trained at the University of Nebraska and took a postdoctoral fellowship with Dr. Michael Glasscock in Tennessee. He is currently a member of the California Ear Institute in Palo Alto, where he has developed expertise in the use of lasers.

Rick Nissen is a member of our team at the Minnesota Ear Head and Neck Clinic, where he directs the Neuro-otology division. Rick did his residency at the University of Nebraska and had his postdoctoral training in Neuro-otology at the House Ear Institute in Los Angeles. He started as a contributor to this atlas, but his interest, efficiency, and understanding of the spirit of the book were such that he also became a co-editor of the chapters dealing wholly or in part with neuro-otology (Chapters 5, 17, 18, and 19). This section is the product of his work.

Michael Paparella was Professor and Chairman of the Department of Otolaryngology at the University of Minnesota for 17 years. Under his leadership, the department became one of the primary otology centers in the world, both clinically and in research. His contributions to our specialty in the last two decades have been among the most significant by any single individual, and his name has a well-deserved place of honor in the history of otology. In addition, he had the vision and openness to train specialists from all over the world. The results of his teachings and philosophies are becoming more evident every year as his former students gradually reach the highest academic positions both in the United States and abroad. After his retirement as active chairman, he developed the Minnesota Ear, Head and Neck Clinic. Clinically more active than ever, he has continued doing research as Clinical Professor and Director of the Otopathology Laboratory at the University of Minnesota. I originally trained with him in Minnesota and have rejoined him at the Minnesota Ear, Head and Neck Clinic. When I came from Chile to train with him, he opened the doors of the department and of his friendship to me. He has undoubtedly had a direct influence on my training; at the same time, he has trained many of the contributors to this work. It was a privilege for me to have Michael as a co-editor of this atlas.

Donald Robertson has headed the anatomy course for medical and graduate students in the Department of Cell Biology and Neuroanatomy (formerly Department of Anatomy), and the yearly course in Head and Neck Anatomy for otolaryngology residents for 17 years at the University of Minnesota. Having been his student both as a resident and as a graduate in anatomy, I have appreciated the value of his experience and his teaching. It has been a privilege for me to have him contribute Chapter 1 (Pertinent Anatomy).

Kurt Schellhas has contributed Chapter 3 (Pertinent Concepts in High Resolution Temporal Bone Imaging). Kurt went to medical school, did his residency, and took his neuroradiology fellowship at the University of Minnesota. His experience with and clarification of concepts in diagnostic imaging in otology have been instrumental in this short but conceptual chapter.

Chapter 20 (Plastic Surgery of the Pinna) was written by Ed Szachowicz, Peter Hilger, and Robert Smith. Ed and Peter trained in Otolaryngology under Michael Paparella. Ed had postdoctoral training in Plastic Surgery with Drs. William Wright and Russell Kridel in Houston and Dr. Clyde Litton in Washington, DC. Peter had his postdoctoral training in Plastic Surgery at Harvard Medical School and Massachusetts Eye and Ear Infirmary under Dr. Richard Webster. Robert is currently a Chief Resident at the Department of Otolaryngology at the University of Minnesota.

Other contributors to this atlas are Dr. Hammed Sajjadi, formerly a Fellow in our clinic (1986–1987), who assisted with Chapter 6 (Operating Room Principles and General Concepts), and Drs. Michael Morris and Richard Fox, currently otology Fellows, who served as reviewers and critics. Professor A. Rosales from Santa Cruz, Bolivia, provided me with the diagrams and design of his consistently successful piston wire prosthesis. David Muchow took the scanning electron micrograph of the stapes used on the cover, and Jodi Nielsen, the radiology and vestibular technologist and medical photographer at the Minnesota Ear, Head and Neck Clinic, took the photographs in Chapter 6. The "patients" in this chapter are my children Marcos and Hortensia, and the nurse is Joanne Epley, RN, head nurse at our institution. Kay Emery typed and edited the manuscript and Joyce Hansen assisted in typing. Gail E. Mowen assisted Alan Nissen with his chapter.

The contributions of grants No. 5P-50-NS-14538 from the National Institute of Neurological and Communicative Disorders and No. NS-19433-04 from the Deafness Research Foundation, as well as a grant from the 3M Company of Minnesota, are acknowledged.

A final note: The opinions in this preface, as well as the selection of the dedication, key words, and motto, are my own and do not necessarily represent the opinions and choices of the contributors to this atlas.

MARCOS V. GOYCOOLEA, M.D.

Contents

SECTION I

Basic Anatomic Concepts

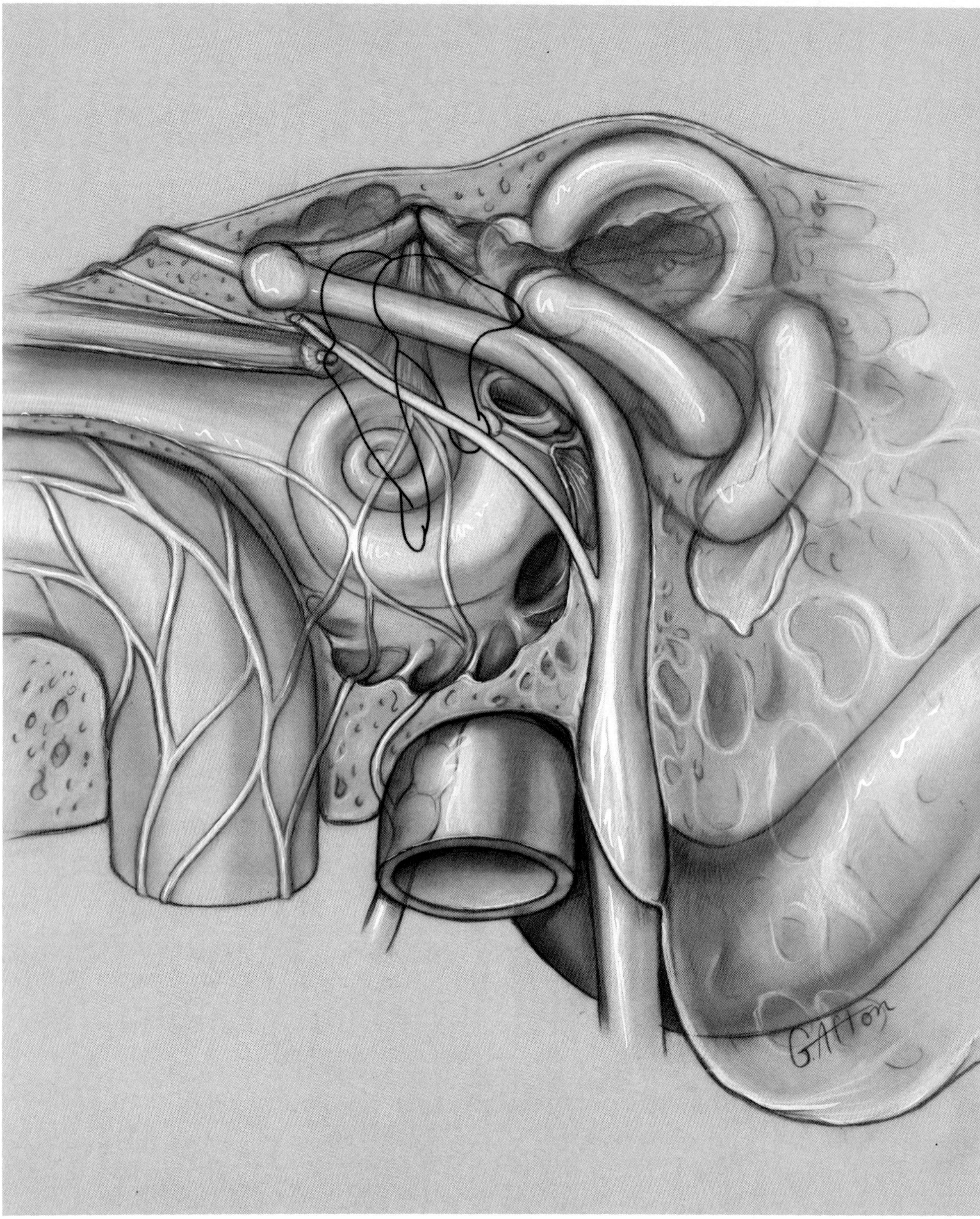
G.Alton

CHAPTER 1

Pertinent Anatomy

For descriptive purposes the ear is divided into three parts: (1) the external ear, consisting of the auricle, the external acoustic meatus, and the tympanic membrane; (2) the middle ear (tympanic cavity) and the associated ossicles and muscles; and (3) the inner ear, containing the organs of equilibration and hearing.

The External Ear

Bony Features and Relationships

The bony components of the external ear (Fig. 1–1) are all part of the temporal bone. They include the following:

1. The *squamous portion*, forming a small, superiorly located part of the bony external auditory meatus and the anterolateral portion of the mastoid process. Extending laterally and anteriorly from the inferior part of the squamous portion of the temporal bone is the *zygomatic process*, which has three roots. The *anterior root* extends medially to become confluent with the articular tubercle; the *medial root* forms the posterior wall of the mandibular fossa; and the *posterior root* curves slightly downward onto the mastoid process. This root bears the small *suprameatal spine* (of Henle) on its dorsal extremity. Hence, the upper portion of the external acoustic meatus is located between the middle and posterior roots. The crest of the posterior root and the posterosuperior portion of the bony meatus are joined by an imaginary line to form the *suprameatal triangle*, marking the site of access to the antrum of the middle ear.

2. The *tympanic portion*, forming most of the bony meatus. The greatest part of this component develops after birth, and the alteration in form as it develops brings about a shift in the depth of the external meatus as well as in the orientation of the tympanic membrane. In the newborn it is a slight bone ring that is imperfect superiorly. With subsequent growth, small projections of bone arising from its anterior and posterior crura extend into the lumen of the ring, eventually fusing to divide the annulus into the superiorly located acoustic meatus proper and a small, inferiorly situated aperture. Although the latter usually closes with continued development, it may on occasion persist to form what is designated the *foramen of Huschke*. The superiorly located discontinuity in the tympanic ring persists into adult life as the *tympanic notch* (of Rivinus).

Posteriorly the tympanic ring forms, in conjunction with both the squamous and petrous portions of the mastoid process, the *tympanomastoid* and *petrotympanic* sutures (frequently designated collectively the tympanomastoid suture). Anteriorly the ring participates in the formation of the *squamotympanic* and *petrotympanic* sutures. It is in the latter suture that the foramen transmitting the chorda tympani nerve (the iter chordae anterius) is found. It should be appreciated that the tympanic ring, with its growth, forms a portion of the posterior wall of the mandibular fossa.

3. The *petrous portion*, forming the tip and posterior portion of the mastoid process.

The Auricle

The auricular component of the external ear consists of a single cartilaginous plate with its covering skin. This cartilage framework is responsible for the shape of the auricle, and determines all of the various

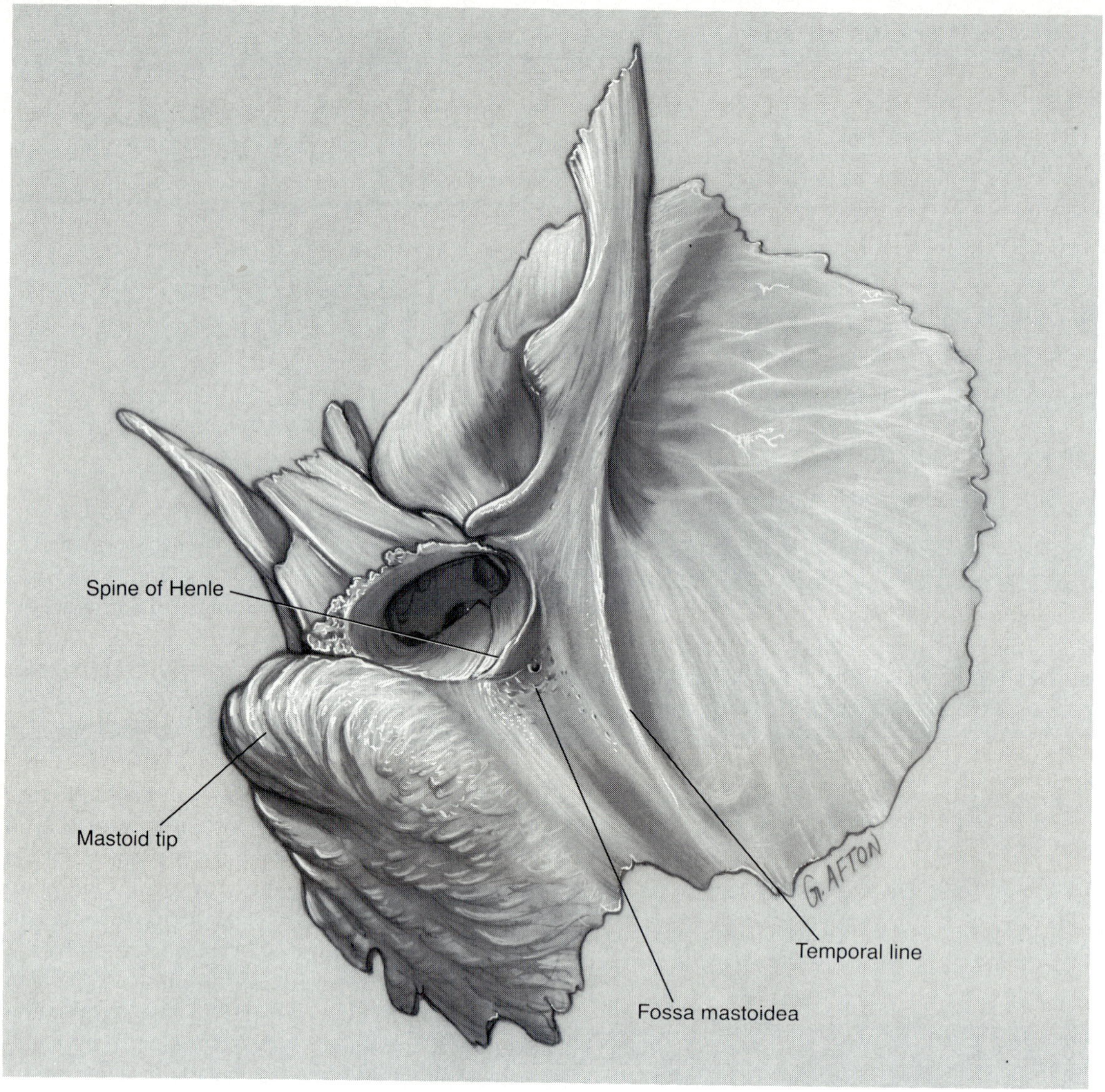

FIGURE 1–1.
Bony components of the external ear.

prominences and depressions seen on the ear, with the exception of the lobule.

In addition to the features that are superficially discernible, the cartilage plate contains other features that become evident upon removal of overlying skin. These include the following (Fig. 1–2*A*):

1. The *spine of the helix*, projecting anteriorly from the helix, near the crus.

2. The *tail of the helix* (cauda helix), the terminal portion of the helix, located at the posteroinferior margin of the auricle.

3. The *isthmus*, the point of continuity between the auricular and meatal cartilages, located immediately posterior to the entrance of the external meatus.

4. The *terminal incisure*, between the isthmus and the tragal lamina of the auricular cartilage. Its inferior extremity is the opening of the external meatus. Superiorly it is marked by the anterior incisure.

The auricle is attached to the side of the head by the following features:

1. Its continuity with the cartilaginous portion of the external acoustic meatus.
2. The skin covering the ear and continuing onto the skull. The skin of the auricle is tightly bound to the perichondrium of the lateral aspect of the ear but is somewhat freer on the medial surface. There is very little fat in the subcutaneous tissue of the ear. Except in the tragal and antitragal regions, the hair of the auricle is rudimentary. Sebaceous

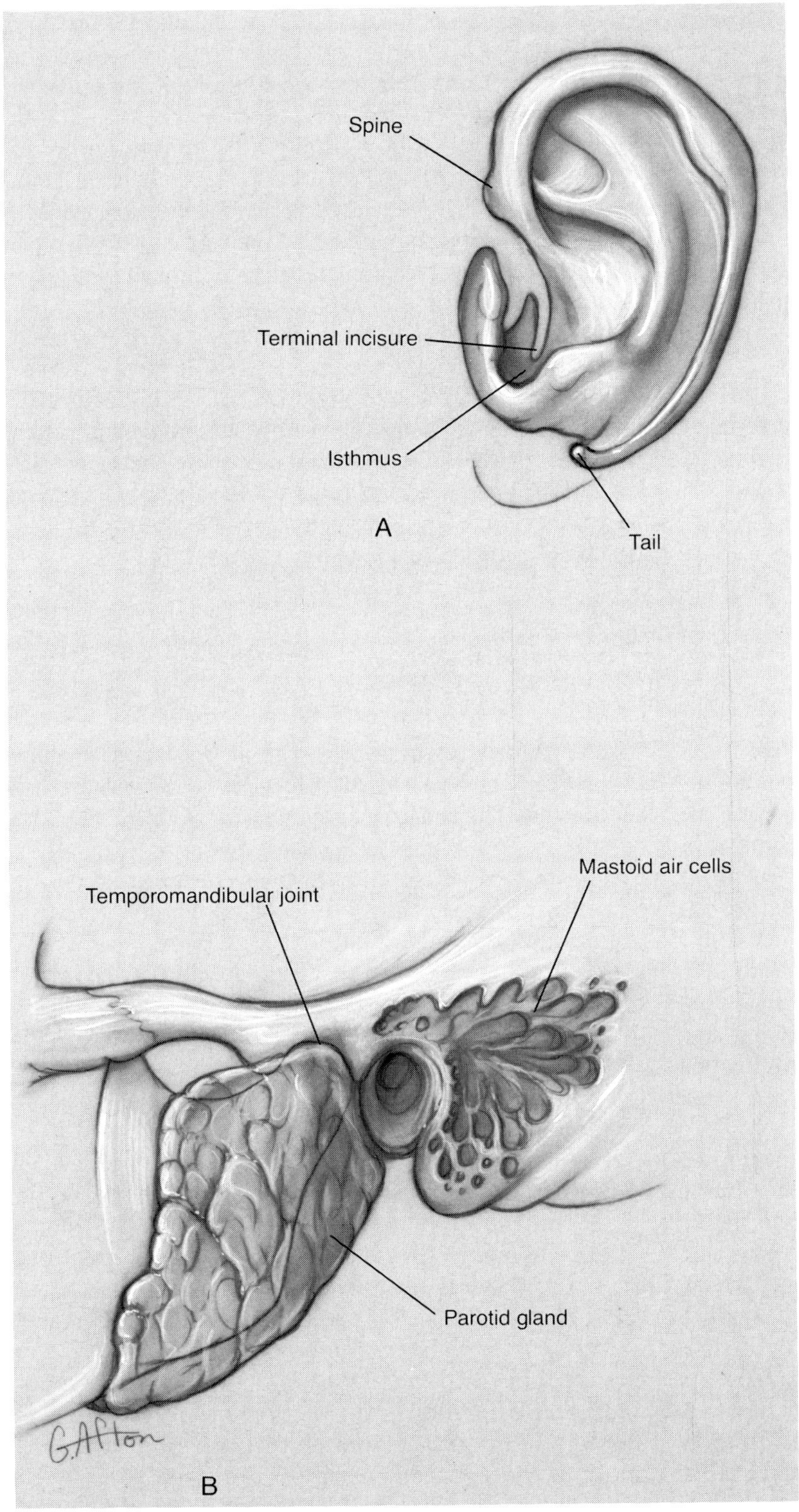

FIGURE 1–2.
A, Major relationships of the auricular cartilage. *B*, External acoustic meatus.

glands are present on both surfaces and are particularly numerous in the concha and triangular fossa.

3. Three *extrinsic ligaments*. These include:
   A. The *anterior ligament*, extending from the zygoma to the helix and the tragus.
   B. The *superior ligament*, extending from the superior margin of the bony meatus to the spine of the helix.
   C. The *posterior ligament*, extending from the mastoid process to the concha of the auricle.
4. Muscles, consisting of the following:
   A. An *extrinsic* group, formed of three small muscles (anterior, superior, and posterior) belonging to the facial group of muscles and supplied by the facial nerve.
   B. An *intrinsic* group of six small muscles, which are extremely variable in their development and have no functional significance in humans.

The External Acoustic Meatus

The external acoustic meatus is a bony-cartilaginous canal extending from the concha of the auricle to the tympanic membrane. In its adult configuration it describes a slight S-shape, with the lateral cartilaginous portion somewhat concave anteriorly and inferiorly and the medial bony portion slightly concave posteriorly and superiorly. Owing to the obliquity of the tympanic membrane, the posterosuperior wall of the meatus is slightly shorter than the anteroinferior wall (approximately 25 mm and 31 mm, respectively). Slightly more than half of the external meatus is entirely bony (medially), with the anterior wall, floor, and lower posterior wall formed by the tympanic portion of the temporal bone. Its roof and the upper part of the posterior wall are formed by the squamous portion.

The cartilaginous (lateral) portion of the external meatus forms a trough-shaped structure that is open superiorly and posteriorly. This canal is completed in the latter quadrants by the squamous portion of the temporal bone. In addition to being slightly curved, it is somewhat broader in its lateral aspect where it makes up approximately two thirds of the circumference of the meatus. Medially it makes up roughly one third of the meatal wall. At its lateral extremity the cartilage of the meatus is continuous with that of the auricle through the isthmus; medially, it articulates with the bony portion of the meatus. The anterior wall is characterized by the presence of two fissures (incisures of the cartilaginous meatus or fissures of Santorini), which assist in imparting a limited mobility to the auricle.

The major relationships of the meatus are the following (Fig. 1–2*B*):

1. Anteriorly and laterally, the parotid gland. The more medial and anterior relationships include the mandibular fossa and the condyle of the mandible.
2. Inferiorly, the parotid gland.
3. Superiorly and medially, the epitympanic recess of the middle ear.
4. Posteriorly, the mastoid air cells.

The skin lining the external meatus is continuous with that of the auricle, and also forms the external layer of the tympanic membrane. It varies considerably in thickness, being much heavier in the cartilaginous portion of the meatus where there is a population of large sebaceous glands and numerous fine hairs. The skin of the bony meatus, which is much thinner, is firmly bound to the periosteum of the underlying bone and contains a rather sparse population of glands and hair cells, located predominately on the superoposterior wall.

The Tympanic Membrane

The tympanic membrane (Fig. 1–3*A*) is a thin, elliptically shaped membrane situated between the medial end of the external meatus and the middle ear cavity. Its vertical axis measures approximately 9 to 10 mm; its horizontal axis measures approximately 8 to 9 mm. In its final adult position the tympanic membrane slopes medially from superior to inferior and from posterior to anterior, so that its external (meatal) surface faces somewhat inferiorly and anterolaterally. In the newborn the membrane is situated much more horizontally, but gradually shifts to the adult position with development of the tympanic portion of the temporal bone.

The major features of the tympanic membrane, as viewed from the lateral aspect, include the following:

1. The *umbo*, which is the center of the slight lateral concavity. It marks the point of attachment of the tip of the manubrium of the malleus.

2. The *malleal stria*, extending superiorly and slightly anteriorly from the umbo. It is formed by the manubrium of the malleus. The stria and a perpendicular line extending through the umbo divide the membrane into quadrants (anterosuperior, anteroinferior, posterosuperior, and posteroinferior).

3. The *mallear prominence*, marking the attachment of the lateral process of the malleus to the membrane. Extending from the prominence in anteroinferior and

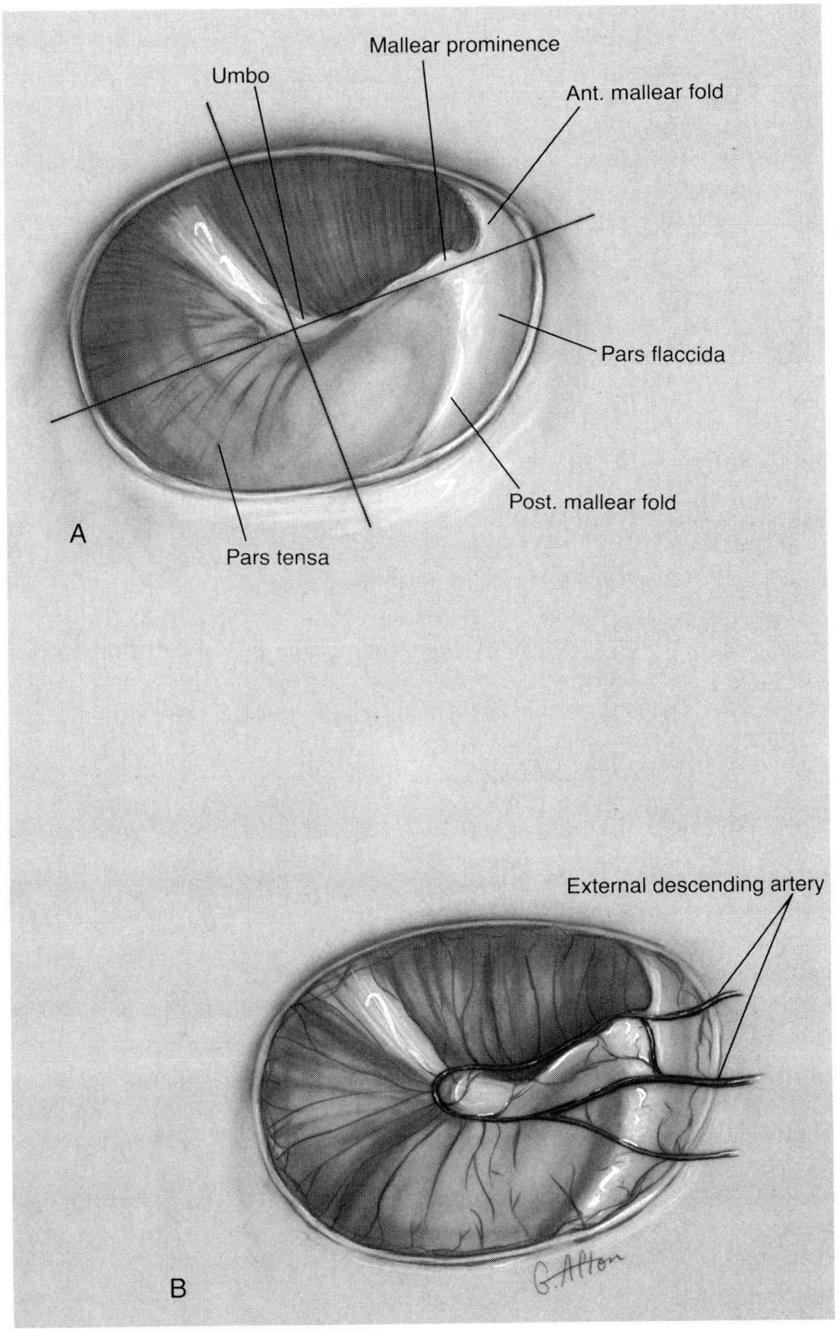

FIGURE 1–3.
A, Tympanic membrane. *B,* Vascular supply of the tympanic membrane.

posteroinferior directions are, respectively, the *anterior* and *posterior mallear folds.*

4. The *pars tensa,* that portion of the membrane lying below the mallear prominence and the mallear folds and making up the greatest part of the membrane.

5. The *pars flaccida,* that portion of the membrane lying above the mallear prominence and the mallear folds. It is named for its characteristic laxity.

Structurally, the membrane consists of three layers approximately 0.1 mm thick (combined). These include:

1. An outer cutaneous layer of thin skin, which is continuous with the skin of the external meatus.
2. A middle layer of connective tissue consisting of the following:
   A. The radiate fibrous layer, made up of fibers radiating peripherally from the umbo and manubrium of the malleus.
   B. The circular fibrous layer, made up of concen-

trically arranged fibers that are most prominent peripherally, where they thicken to form a fibrocartilage ring or annulus, attaching the membrane to the tympanic sulcus of the temporal bone.

3. An inner layer of mucous membrane continuous with that of the middle ear cavity.

Vascular Supply of the External Ear

The arteries of the external ear originate from several sources. The auricle has an abundant blood supply, which is derived primarily from the *posterior auricular branch of the external carotid artery* and the *auricular rami* arising from the superficial temporal artery. These are shared by the meatus, which also receives the *deep auricular branch of the maxillary artery*. This artery passes through the parotid gland to enter either the cartilaginous or bony part of the meatus.

The tympanic membrane is supplied on both its lateral and medial surfaces. Laterally, the deep auricular artery forms a small peripheral vascular ring from which small branches radiate onto the membrane. Superiorly, a large vessel, the *external descending artery*, arises from the vascular ring to descend to the region of the umbo, with a course more or less parallel to the manubrium (Fig. 1–3*B*). Internally, a second peripheral vascular ring is formed primarily by the *stylomastoid branch of the posterior auricular artery* and the *anterior tympanic branch of the maxillary artery*. The largest of the vessels arising from this inner vascular ring is the *internal descending artery*, which descends on the inner surface of the membrane in a course parallel to that of its external counterpart.

The venous channels draining the structures of the external ear roughly correspond to the arteries of supply. Those draining the auricle and the external meatus are the *anterior auricular* tributaries of the superficial temporal veins and the *auricular* tributaries of the posterior auricular vein. Drainage of the tympanic membrane is both external (via vessels communicating with veins of the external meatus) and internal (via branches paralleling the arteries).

Innervation of the External Ear

The external ear is a region of transition between skin originally overlying the branchial area and the postbranchial region. For this reason, both the cranial nerves supplying the branchial arches (V, VII, IX, and X) and the cervical nerves may be represented by sensory components. Although there is considerable variation, the approximate sensory distribution is as follows (Fig. 1–4):

1. The cervical plexus of nerves (C2–3), via the *great auricular* nerve, supplies most of the lateral surface of the auricle (except for the upper anterior portion). The lesser occipital nerve from the plexus supplies much of the medial surface of the auricle.
2. The mandibular division of the trigeminal nerve, via its *auriculotemporal* branch, supplies the upper anterior portion of the auricle, the upper and anterior walls of the external meatus, and the upper anterior part of the lateral surface of the tympanic membrane.
3. The *auricular branch* of the vagus supplies approximately half of the external meatus and lateral surface of the tympanic membrane. Although this nerve is typically described as being of vagal origin, it should be appreciated that branches of VII and IX may join it and contribute to the sensory innervation of the external ear. It is impossible to differentiate between the distribution of the components; clinical studies of herpes zoster indicate that all three may participate.

The distribution of nerves supplying the tympanic membrane is very much like that of the arteries—small, peripheral contributions supplying the margins of the membrane while the primary nerves descend from the superior aspect of the membrane and parallel the course of the external descending artery, tending to lie slightly posterior to the vessel. The pars tensa of the membrane is not particularly well supplied with sensory nerves; in contrast, the pars flaccida has an extremely rich innervation.

The Middle Ear

Morphology

The middle ear, or tympanic cavity, is an irregularly shaped chamber lying within the temporal bone, bounded laterally by the squamous and tympanic portions and medially by the petrous portion. Its greatest dimensions are in the anteroposterior and vertical planes, which measure approximately 15 mm each, while the transverse diameter (between the medial and lateral walls) varies with location and ranges from 2 to 6 mm. It is not a confined space but communicates anteriorly with the nasopharynx

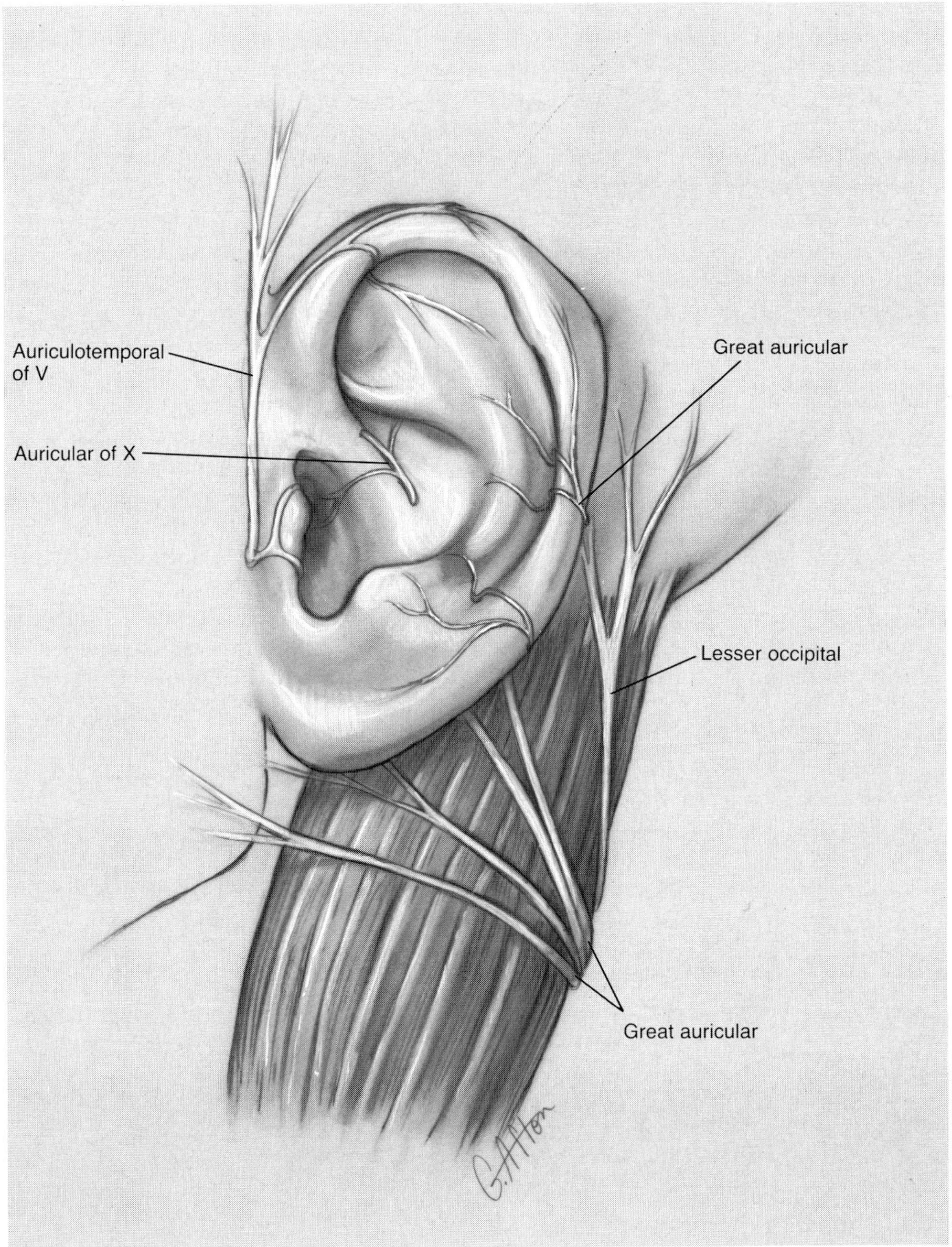

FIGURE 1–4.
Innervation of the external ear.

through the auditory tube and posteriorly with the mastoid antrum and air cells.

The middle ear can be divided into the *tympanic cavity proper*, which is that portion situated medial to the tympanic membrane, and the *epitympanic recess*, the upward extension of the tympanic cavity proper above the level of the tympanic membrane.

The *lateral wall* (membranous wall) of the middle ear is formed for the most part by the tympanic membrane. Superiorly, within the epitympanic recess this wall is formed by a plate of bone (the *scutum*) derived from the squamous portion of the temporal bone. The head of the malleus and the body and short process of the incus lie in the epitympanic recess.

The *roof* (tegmental wall) of the middle ear consists of a thin plate of bone, the *tegmen tympani*, which separates the epitympanic recess from the cranial cavity. It is traversed by the petrosquamous suture, which persists into adult life in approximately 50% of the population, and by small foramina that transmit nerves and arteries.

The *floor* (jugular wall) is a very narrow, irregular surface lying slightly below the level of the meatus, and is formed by a plate of bone separating the cavity from the bulb of the internal jugular vein. If the bulb of the vein is small, the floor may be as much as 8 to 10 mm thick and may contain hypotympanic air cells. In contrast, a large bulb may cause the floor to bulge upward into the middle ear. In such cases the floor may be imperfect, and the vessel and cavity are separated only by the mucosa of the middle ear.

The *anterior wall* (carotid wall) is a very thin, bony septum separating the middle ear from the carotid canal. Perforations in the plate allow the transmission of nerves and vessels from the canal to the middle ear. Above this is the site of the opening of the *semicanal for the tensor tympani muscle,* and immediately inferior to this is the *tympanic ostium of the auditory tube,* through which the middle ear communicates with the nasopharynx.

The *posterior wall* (mastoid wall) (Fig. 1–5*A*) is somewhat triangular, with the narrowest portion situated inferiorly where it is related to a number of tympanic air cells. Superiorly, at the level of the epitympanic recess, the posterior wall is deficient and forms the *aditus,* through which the middle ear communicates with the mastoid antrum. Salient features of the posterior wall include the following:

1. The *pyramidal eminence,* located just below the aditus. At the apex of the eminence is a small aperture that transmits the tendon of the stapedius muscle.
2. The *iter chordae tympani posterior,* a small foramen immediately lateral to the pyramidal eminence. Through this foramen the chorda tympani nerve enters the middle ear.
3. The *posterior sinus,* a small fossa just above the pyramidal eminence.
4. The *fossa of the incus,* situated just above the posterior sinus. This marks the point of attachment of the posterior ligament of the incus.

The *medial wall* (labyrinthine wall), which separates the middle ear cavity from the inner ear, is the most complex of the middle ear boundaries. Its major features are shown in Figure 1–5*B*:

1. The *promontory,* a slight elevation formed by the basal turn of the cochlea of the inner ear. Extending inferiorly and posteriorly from the promontory is a slight ridge, the *subiculum.* More superiorly, running from the posterior aspect of the promontory toward the pyramidal eminence, is a second ridge, the *ponticulus.* The subiculum and the ponticulus create three small depressions on the posterior part of the medial wall.
2. The *fossula fenestrae cochleae* (cochlear fossa or round window niche), which is posteroinferior to the promontory. The lowest of the three depressions of the medial wall, it is bounded superiorly by the subiculum and is the site of the *cochlear window* (round window), in which the *secondary tympanic membrane* (round window membrane) resides. The round window and associated membrane may or may not be visible, depending upon the size and configuration of the promontory and subiculum.
3. The *tympanic sinus,* occupying the middle depression formed by the subiculum and ponticulus at the junction of the posterior and medial walls. The extent of the sinus is variable; it may extend far enough into the petrous portion of the temporal bone to bring it into close relationship to the ampullary end of the posterior semicircular canal and the posterior end of the lateral canal.
4. The *fossula fenestrae vestibuli* (fossa of the oval window or "stapes niche"), lying in the superior depression above the ponticulus. It contains the vestibular (oval) window, which is closed by the footplate of the stapes and the associated annular ligament.
5. A slight bony ridge, *the prominence of the lateral semicircular canal,* which lies high on the posterior aspect of the medial wall in the region of the aditus and marks the anterior end of that component of the inner ear.
6. The *prominence of the facial canal,* lying above the posterior edge of the promontory and the oval window, immediately below and parallel to the prominence of the lateral semicircular canal. It runs almost horizontally across the posterior half of the medial wall, then turns to enter the posterior wall. The facial nerve courses through this canal.
7. The *cochleariform process,* located anterosuperiorly on the medial wall. It represents the curved end of the bony semicanal of the tensor tympani muscle.

The Ossicles

The ossicles form an articulated bony chain that extends across the middle ear and connects the tympanic membrane with the vestibular window. This chain acts as a bent lever to convert the vibrations of the tympanic membrane into intensified thrusts of the stapes against the perilymph.

Developmentally, the ossicles arise from three different sources. The first branchial arch of the embryo (mandibular arch) gives rise to the head of the malleus and the long and short process of the incus; the second arch (facial arch), to the long process of the incus and the stapes. The anterior process of the malleus develops independent of the branchial arches as a membranous bone.

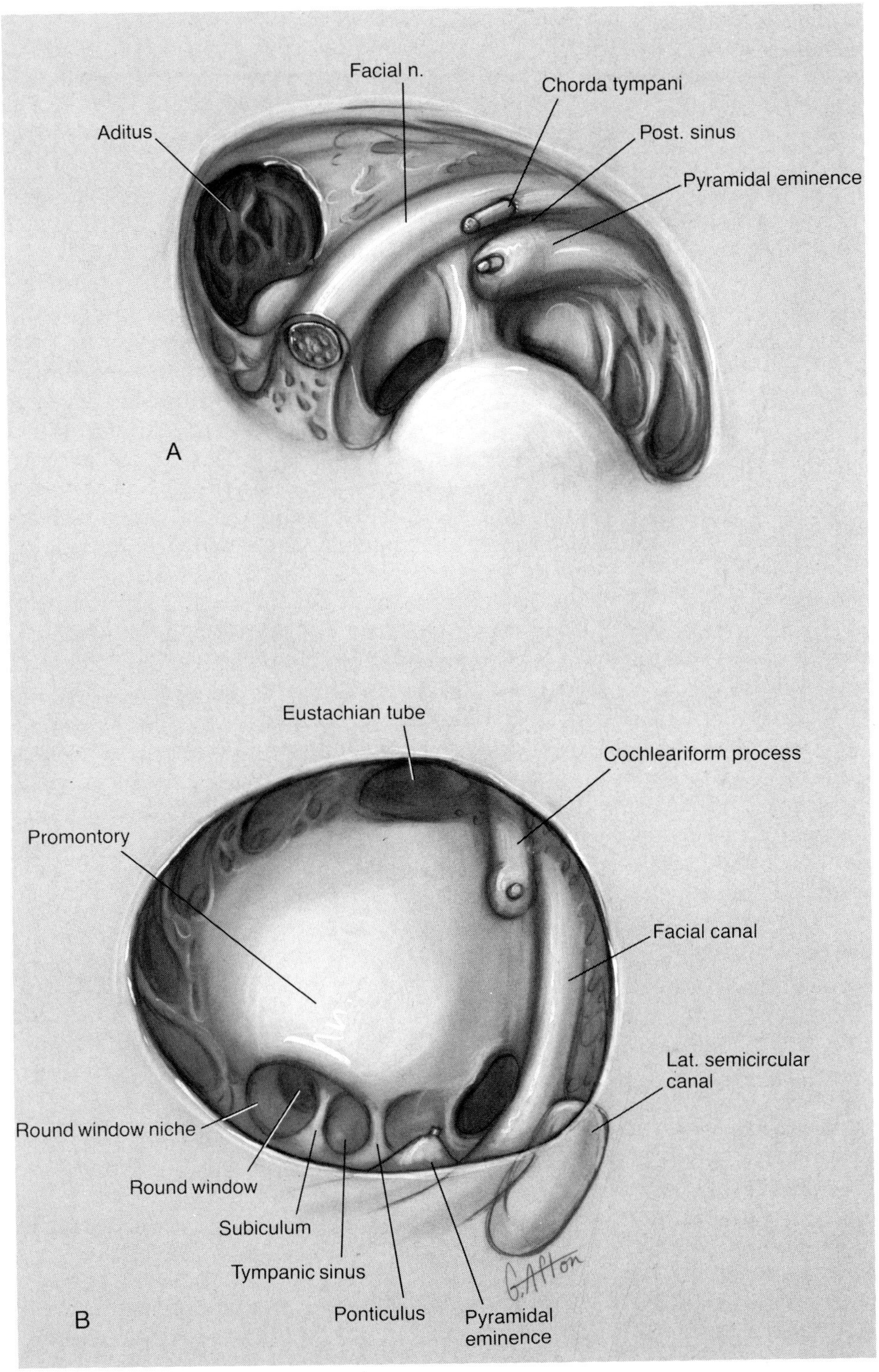

FIGURE 1–5.
A, Posterior wall of the middle ear.
B, Medial wall.

The major features of the malleus include the following (Fig. 1–6*A*):

1. A relatively large and heavy *head* lying within the epitympanic recess, which bears on its surface a small facet for articulation with the incus.
2. A short, somewhat constricted *neck* from which three processes arise, including:
   A. The long and prominent *manubrium*, the largest of the mallear processes. It is attached to the tympanic membrane and in turn is the site of insertion of the tensor tympani muscle.
   B. The *lateral process*, which creates the mallear prominence of the tympanic membrane.
   C. The *anterior (long) process*, a long and delicate bony projection in the fetal malleus. In the adult it is a small bony stump that is the site of attachment of the anterior ligament of the malleus.

The malleus is suspended by three small ligaments (Fig. 1–6*B*), which include the *anterior mallear ligament*, extending from the anterior process to the tympanosquamous fissure; the *superior mallear ligament*, extending from the top of the head to the roof of the epitympanic recess; and the *lateral mallear ligament*, which runs from the lateral process to the margin of the tympanic notch.

Also associated with the malleus is the *tensor tympani* muscle. This muscle arises from the cartilaginous part of the auditory tube, the adjacent sphenoid bone, and the semicanal situated directly above the osseous portion of the auditory tube. Its tendon of insertion passes through the cochleariform process, turns sharply lateral, and inserts on the manubrium of the malleus, close to the neck. The muscle acts to draw the manubrium medially, tensing the tympanic membrane, and thus serves a protective function. The tensor tympani is innervated by a branch of the mandibular division of the trigeminal nerve.

The *incus* (Fig. 1–6C) is characterized by the following features:

1. A relatively large *body* that is deeply indented anteriorly to form an articular facet.
2. Two bone processes. These include:
   A. The *short process*, which extends posteriorly from the body.
   B. The slender *long process*, extending inferiorly from the body and paralleling the manubrium of the malleus. On the medial side of the very distal extremity of the long process is the small *lenticular process*, through which the incus articulates with the stapes.

Like the malleus, the incus is suspended by small ligaments (Fig. 1–6*D*). These are the *posterior ligament*, which acts to hold the short process in the fossa of the incus, and the *superior ligament*, which extends from the body to the roof of the epitympanic recess.

The *stapes* (Fig. 1–6*E*) consists of the following:

1. A small, cylindrical *head*, which articulates with the lenticular process of the incus.

2. Two *crura* (anterior and posterior), which extend from the head. The anterior crus is somewhat shorter and straighter than the posterior.

3. A thin *base* (footplate), a flattened plate of bone attached on its end to the distal extremities of the crura. It fits into the vestibular window and, like that structure, has a straight inferior border and a curved superior border.

The ligamentous support of the stapes is through the elastic *annular ligament*, which attaches to the margins of the footplate and the vestibular window and allows movement of the stapes. Such movement is greatest at the anterior end and upper border of the footplate and very slight posteroinferiorly. It has been stated that loud tones change the normal pattern of movement to a rocking motion; this would result in a net decrease in the displacement of perilymph, thereby protecting the inner ear. This change presumably is brought about by contraction of the *stapedius muscle* (Fig. 1–6*F*), which inserts onto the posterior crus. As mentioned above, this muscle serves a protective function by preventing excessive excursion of the footplate; it does not move the ossicle unless the ossicular chain is broken. It is innervated by a branch of the seventh nerve.

The joints of the ossicular chain are true synovial (diarthrodial) joints with characteristic articular capsules. There are two such joints within the chain. The first is the *incudomalleal*, between the head of the malleus and the body of the incus. This is a relatively lax joint that allows the movement of the incus to lag behind that of the malleus; as a result, the amplitude of the movement of the bony process of the incus is less than that of the manubrium. The second joint is the *incudostapedial*, between the lenticular process of the incus and the head of the stapes.

The Auditory (Pharyngotympanic or Eustachian) Tube

The auditory tube extends from its tympanic ostium within the anterior wall of the middle ear cavity to its pharyngeal ostium within the nasopharynx. The latter is situated just posterior to the dorsal end of the inferior nasal concha. In the adult the tube is between 30 and 40 mm in length, and has a slight S-shaped configuration as it passes obliquely down-

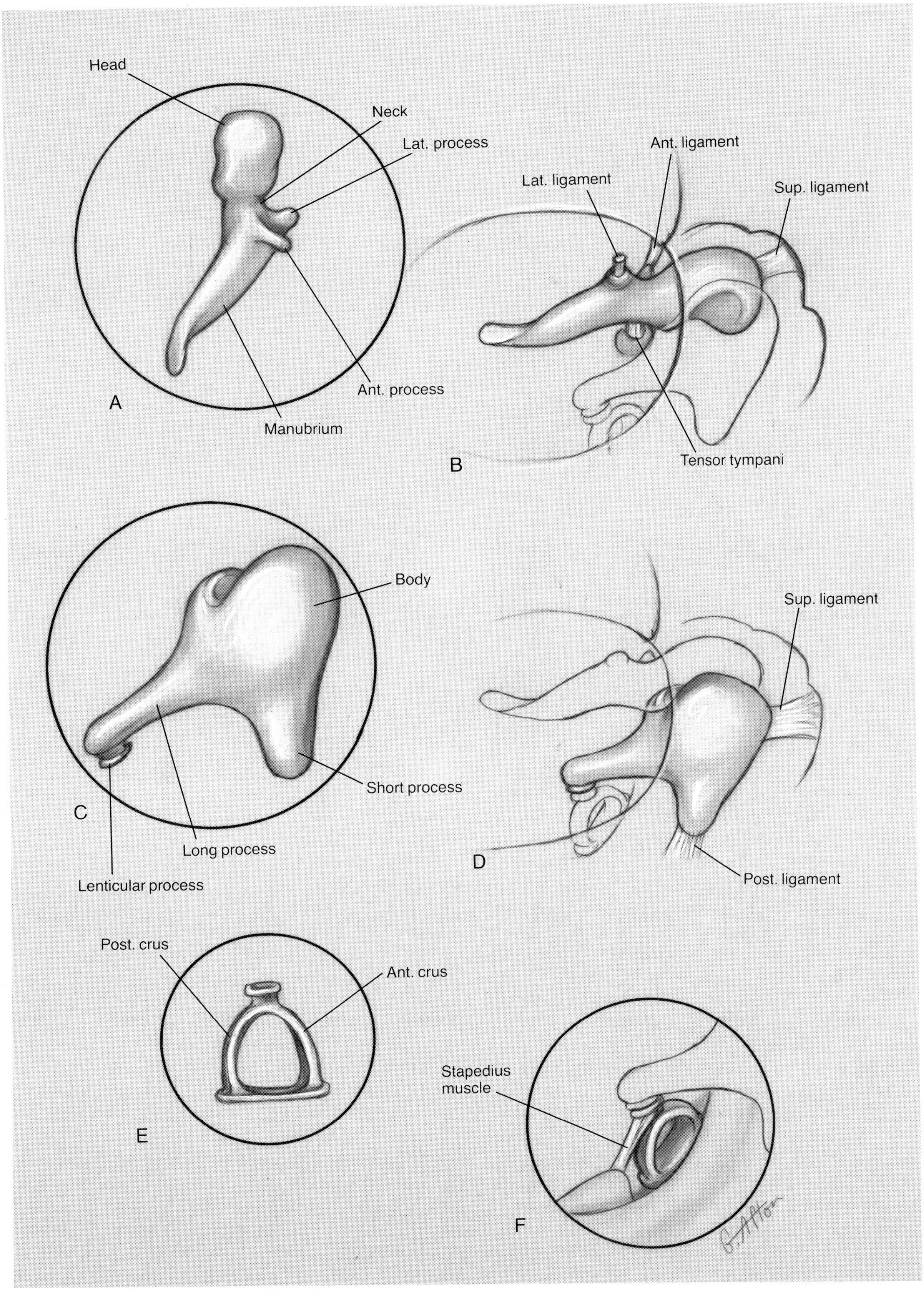

FIGURE 1–6.
A–B, Malleus. *C–D*, Incus. *E–F*, Stapes.

ward, medial, and anterior from the middle ear to the pharynx. The tympanic ostium is roughly 25 mm higher than the pharyngeal ostium in the adult. There are some basic and significant morphologic differences between the auditory tube of the child and that of the adult; in the child the tube is shorter and relatively wider and more horizontally situated.

Structurally, the auditory tube consists of both cartilaginous and bony components. The bony portion makes up approximately two thirds of the tube; it is widest at the tympanic orifice and gradually narrows throughout its length, with its anterior extremity (the isthmus) the most constricted portion of the entire tube. In its course the bony tube is lateral to the carotid canal, superior to the jugular fossa. The cartilaginous portion of the tube extends from the isthumus to the nasopharynx. It is not totally cartilaginous, however; its lower lateral and inferior walls consist of fibrous connective tissue overlying the tensor and levator veli palatini muscles.

The lumen of the auditory tube, in the resting state, is a closed, slitlike cavity. The pharyngeal end of the tube strongly resists passage of air from the pharynx to the middle ear. Passage from the tympanic cavity to the pharynx is much easier.

The Mucosal Lining of the Middle Ear

The tympanic cavity is lined throughout by a thin, transparent, vascular membrane that is continuous with that of the auditory tube anteriorly and the tympanic antrum and mastoid cells posteriorly. The membrane is tightly bound to the periosteum and also invests the ossicles and their associated ligaments. In reflecting from the walls of the cavity to the ossicles and their ligaments, the mucous lining forms various folds and pouches; the most important of these are the *superior pouch* (Prussak's pouch), situated medial to the pars flaccida of the tympanic membrane, and the *anterior* and *posterior pouches* (of Tröltsch), which are related to the anterior and posterior mallear ligaments respectively.

Vascular Elements of the Middle Ear

The middle ear receives blood via a number of small arteries (Fig. 1–7*A*,*B*), which with one exception are derived from the external carotid or its branches. They include:

1. The *anterior tympanic*, a branch of the maxillary artery. It is distributed to the anterior part of the cavity, including the medial surface of the tympanic membrane, and enters the middle ear by passing through the petrotympanic fissure.
2. The *stylomastoid branch* of either the *posterior auricular* or *occipital* artery. This artery enters the facial canal and gives rise to the *posterior tympanic artery*, which then enters the middle ear in company with the chorda tympani nerve.
3. The *inferior tympanic artery*, derived from the ascending pharyngeal branch of the external carotid. It accompanies the tympanic branch of nerve IX through the tympanic canaliculus to gain the middle ear cavity.
4. The *superficial petrosal* and *superior tympanic* arteries, which are both branches of the middle meningeal artery. The former runs through the facial canal for a short distance, then pierces the tegmen tympani to enter the middle ear; the latter enters through the petrosquamous fissure.
5. The *caroticotympanic arteries* arise from the internal carotid as it passes through the carotid canal and enter the middle ear by passing through the thin bony lamina separating the carotid canal from the middle ear.

The veins of the middle ear parallel the arteries. They are tributary to the superior petrosal dural sinus and the pterygoid plexus of veins.

Nerves of the Middle Ear
(Fig. 1–8)

The major nerve of the middle ear is the *tympanic branch of the glossopharyngeal nerve* (Jacobson's nerve). Arising from the inferior ganglion of the parent trunk, the tympanic nerve enters the tympanic canaliculus through a small foramen located on the crest of the thin plate of bone separating the jugular foramen and the external orifice of the carotid canal. Once in the middle ear, the nerve forms the *tympanic plexus* within the mucosa overlying the promontory. There are two modalities represented in the tympanic nerve/plexus. The greatest portion of the fibers are sensory; these are distributed to the mucosa of the middle ear, the mastoid air cells, and the auditory tube. The remaining fibers are parasympathetic and have no function in the middle ear. Instead, they emerge from the upper border of the plexus to pierce the tegmen tympani and run forward on the floor of

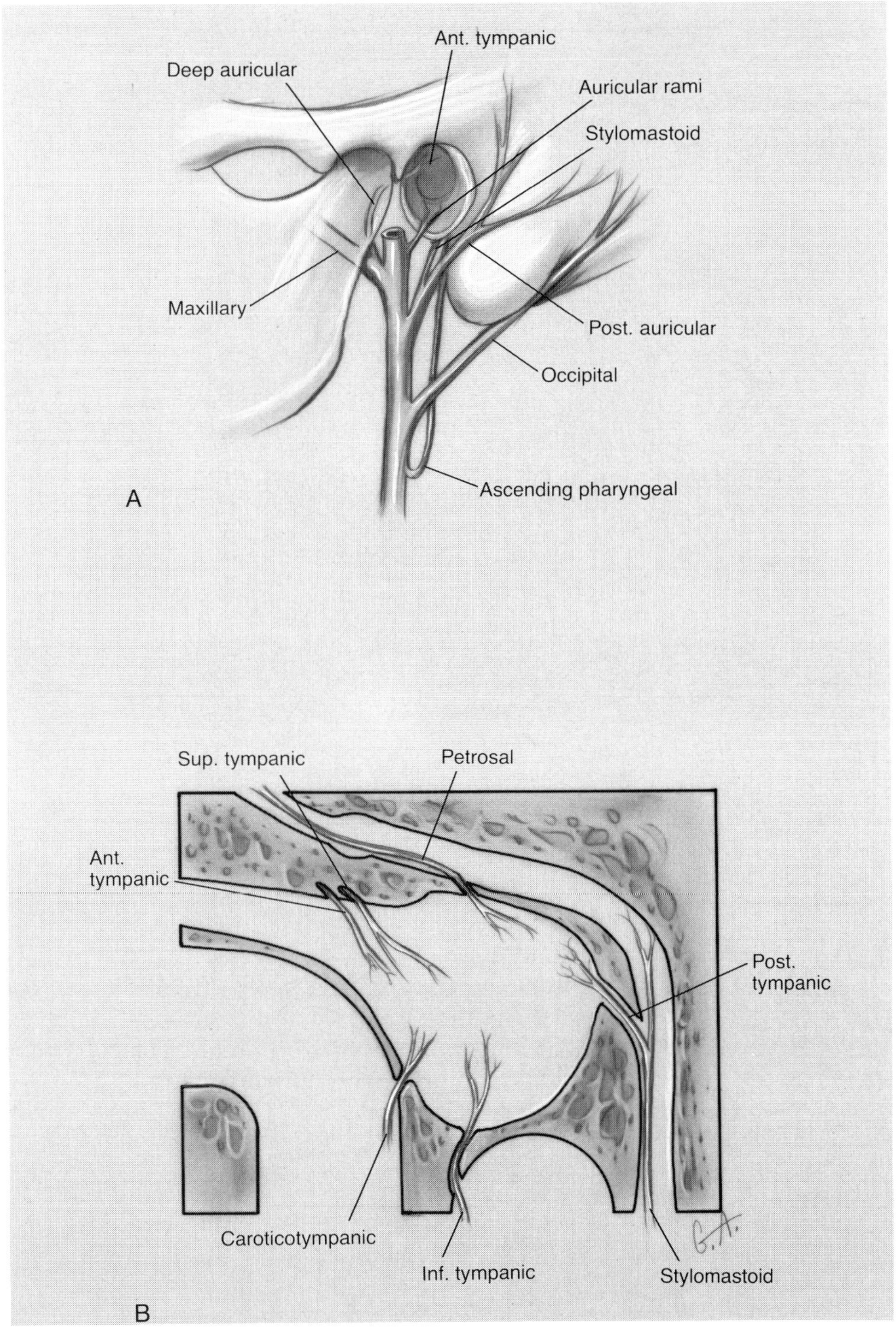

FIGURE 1–7.
A–B, Arteries of the middle ear.

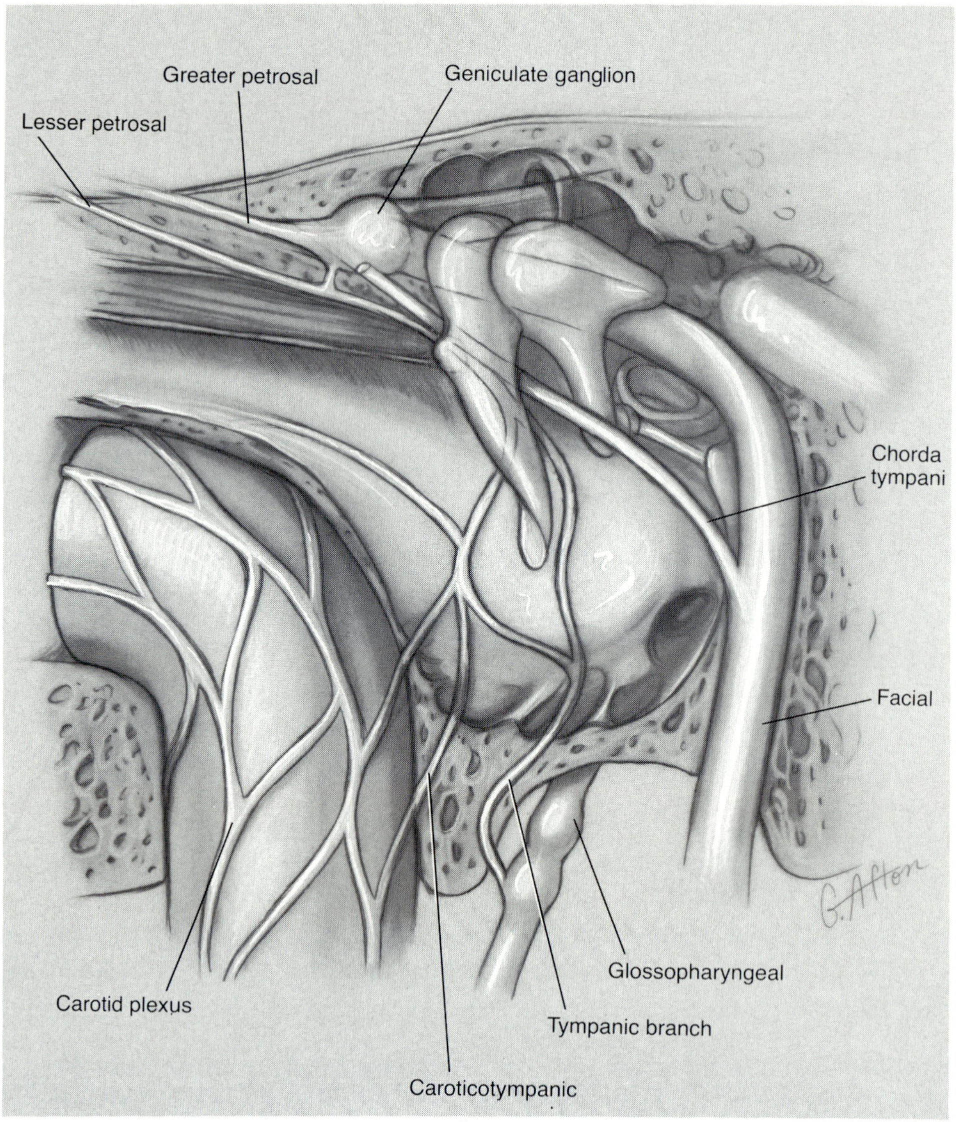

FIGURE 1–8.
Nerves of the middle ear.

the middle cranial fossa as the *lesser petrosal nerve;* ultimately they leave the skull to run with the auriculotemporal branch of V3 and supply the parotid gland.

The middle ear receives sympathetic fibers derived from the internal carotid plexus. These fibers, which enter the middle ear along with the caroticotympanic arteries, are primarily associated with the vessels of the cavity and have a vasoconstrictive effect.

The *chorda tympani* branch of the facial nerve enters the middle ear through the iter chordae posterius, passes forward and down between the manubrium of the malleus and the long process of the incus, then leaves the cavity by passing through the petrotympanic suture. The chorda tympani has no function in the middle ear. It contains both parasympathetic fibers supplying the submandibular and sublingual glands and taste fibers for the anterior two thirds of the tongue. After leaving the middle ear it joins the lingual branch of V3 to be distributed with that nerve.

Although they do not enter the middle ear, the nerves to the muscles associated with the ossicles must be mentioned since they are vital to normal function. The nerve to the stapedius muscle is a branch of the facial nerve, and arises from the parent trunk as it descends through the vertical portion of the osseous facial canal. The nerve to the tensor tympani is a branch of the mandibular division of the trigeminal nerve.

Pneumatization of the Temporal Bone

The temporal bone exhibits varying degrees of pneumatization. Because of the intimate relationship of the middle ear to these areas, a basic appreciation of the location and extent of pneumatized areas is desirable.

Since the mastoid process develops from both petrous and squamous portions of the temporal bone, there is a sutural line between the two components that normally is obliterated with growth. Occasionally, however, a heavy plate of bone persists between the two portions, forming what has been designated Körner's septum or the "false bottom." The existence of this septum can cause confusion in surgical approaches through the mastoid process.

The mastoid process is rather consistently pneumatized (80%), the process usually being completed by the third or fourth year. There is, however, considerable variation both in its extent and in the arrangement of the air cells. Because of this variation, several types are described, including the pneumatized, in which the entire process is occupied by air cells; the diploic, in which the process is occupied by bone marrow instead of air cells; the mixed type, consisting of a combination of the pneumatized and diploic types; and the sclerotic or nonpneumatized/nondiploic process. Owing to the considerable variation in the extent and location of the mastoid cells, several terminologies have been used. The position of the sigmoid sinus in the posterior cranial fossa will influence markedly the position or occurrence of all types.

Mastoid air cells may invade adjacent areas of the temporal bone. Some of the more frequent extensions form the *hypotympanic* cells, which lie in the plate of bone separating the middle ear cavity from the jugular bulb, and the *epitympanic* cells, which are extensions into the roof of the middle ear. The latter group may be extensive enough to include cells that will invade the root of the zygomatic arch and the squamous portion of the temporal bone.

The petrous apex of the temporal bone (i.e., that part of the petrous portion anterior to the labyrinth) may also be pneumatized, particularly by outgrowths from the tympanic cavity. These cells, the *petrous apex cells*, are necessarily related to the auditory tube and the carotid canal.

The Facial Nerve in the Temporal Bone

After traversing the internal acoustic meatus and passing through the lateral end of that structure, the facial nerve enters the bony *facial canal* (fallopian canal). This canal continues laterally for a short distance and brings the facial nerve to just above the base of the cochlea, where it makes a sharp turn (the *external genu*) to run posteriorly. The genu is also the site of the *geniculate ganglion* of the nerve, which contains the cell bodies of the nerve's sensory components. The genu and the ganglion are anterolateral to the superior semicircular canal and between the vestibule of the inner ear and the cochlea, and can be easily localized from the middle ear as a point situated just medial to the tip of the cochleariform process. Continuing posteriorly with a slight inferolateral inclination, the bony canal forms the prominence of the facial canal on the medial wall of the middle ear. This prominence may be large enough to partially cover the oval window and the base of the stapes. The lateral wall of the canal in this part is extremely thin and may be dehiscent. Behind the base of the pyramidal eminence the canal makes a broad turn to descend vertically and somewhat laterally through the mastoid process. In this descending or vertical portion the nerve may have a slight anterior concavity. Relative to the exterior of the skull, the canal normally lies deep to the sutural groove between the tympanic and mastoid portions of the temporal bone. It should be remembered that there may be marked deviation from this "normal" position, in which case the canal is usually situated more posteriorly.

In its course from the brainstem through the facial canal the facial nerve is supplied with blood by small arteries derived from the anteroinferior cerebellar branch of the basilar artery, the stylomastoid or occipital branches of the external carotid, and the petrosal arteries. There are apparently no anastomoses between the labyrinthine blood supply and these arteries, which seem to anastomose freely with one another. Insufficiency of the vascular supply to the facial nerve, from whatever cause, is regarded by some as one of the primary causes of Bell's palsy.

The Inner Ear

The inner ear containing the essential cochlear and vestibular mechanisms, lies within the petrous portion of the temporal bone. The labyrinth of the inner ear is surrounded by the bony otic capsule, which is a unique structure for several reasons. It is formed from 14 separate centers of ossification that fuse, leaving no sutural lines. These centers, though formed from cartilage, retain no areas of chondral growth. In addition, the bone of the capsule retains its fetal character, that is, typical haversian systems

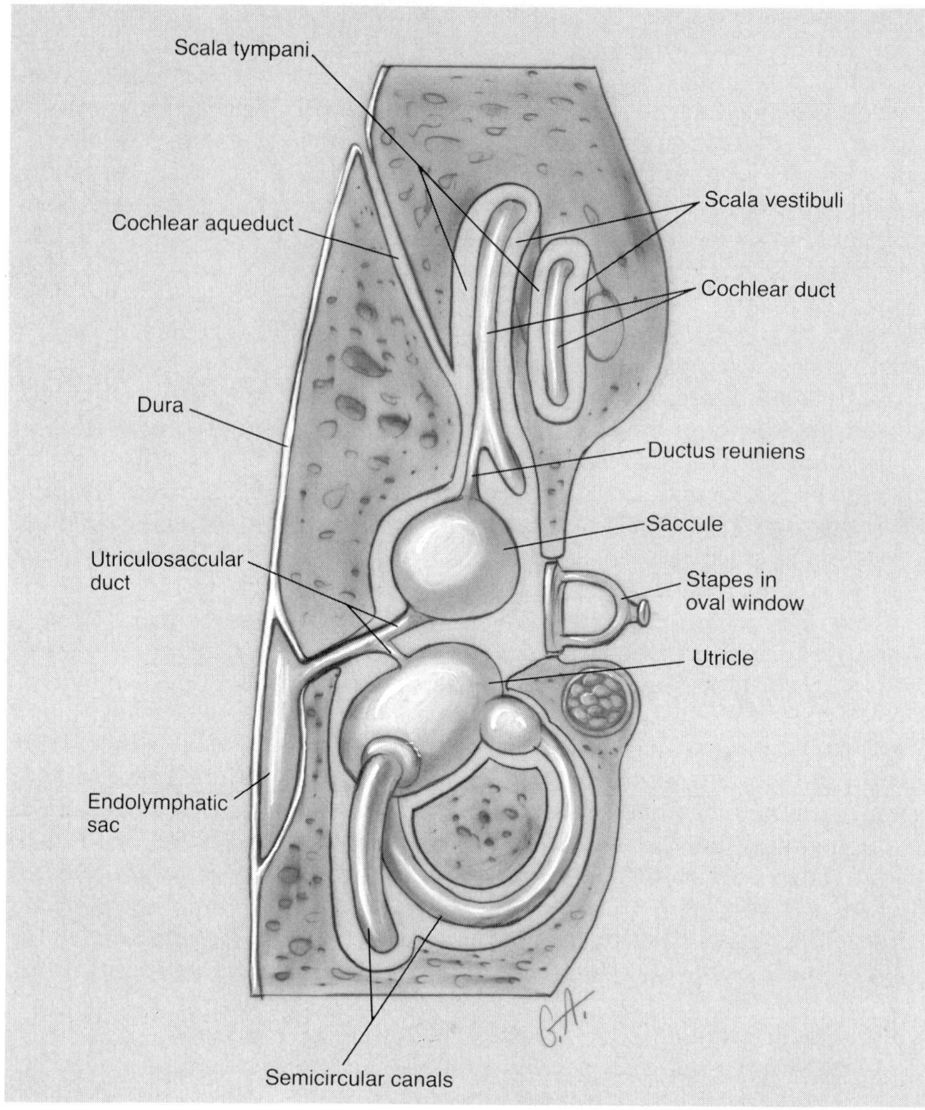

FIGURE 1–9.
Diagram of the membranous labyrinth.

never develop. Finally, the capsule's maximum dimensions are attained by the fifth week of intrauterine life.

The labyrinth of the inner ear is divided into osseous and membranous components. The *osseous labyrinth*, a system of bony canals within the otic capsule, consists of three parts:

1. The *vestibule*, which forms the central portion of the labyrinth; it is a relatively large, ovoid space approximately 4 mm in diameter. Its characteristic features include the following:
   A. The *elliptical recess*, located on the floor of the vestibule. It receives the anterior end of the utricular portion of the membranous labyrinth.
   B. The *spherical recess*, located anterior and slightly inferior to the elliptical recess. It is the site of the saccular portion of the membranous labyrinth.
   C. The *vestibular window*, within the lateral wall of the vestibule.
   D. Small orifices for the passage of nerves to the vestibular portion of the inner ear. These are found on the medial wall and adjacent floor, where the vestibule abuts on the lateral end of the internal acoustic meatus.
2. The *semicircular canals*, which are continuous with the vestibule. The *anterior* (superior) canal forms the arcuate eminence on the bony floor of the middle cranial fossa. The *posterior* canal has no externally located landmarks associated with it. The *lateral* canal, as mentioned above, creates a prominence in the region of the aditus of the middle ear. All of the semicircular canals communicate with the vestibule through both of their crura. There are only five openings into the vestibule, however, since the posterior crus of the

anterior canal and the superior crus of the posterior canal unite to form a single crus.

The canals have very definite planes of orientation. The anterior is situated in the vertical plane at an angle of 45 degrees with respect to the sagittal plane of the skull, the posterior crura being more medial. The posterior canal is also in the vertical plane, at 45 degrees with respect to the sagittal plane of the skull (that is, at 90 degrees with respect to the plane of the anterior canal). The lateral canal forms an angle of approximately 30 degrees with the horizontal plane, its anterior end being highest, and is situated in the angle between the anterior and posterior canals.

3. The *cochlea*, a cone-shaped, hollow, bony spiral of about two and three quarters turns with a relatively broad base and a pointed apex or cupula. Its base lies against the anteromedial surface of the vestibule and the lateral end of the internal auditory meatus. Part of the basal turn of the cochlea forms the promontory of the middle ear. From its base the axis of the cochlea is directed anterolaterally and slightly upward.

The central bony core of the cochlea is the *modiolus*, through which nerves and vessels travel to attain the structures of the cochlea. From the outer surface of the modiolus the *osseous spiral lamina* projects into the cavity of the cochlea, partially subdividing the duct. It terminates at the cupular end of the cochlea by projecting slightly beyond the apex of the modiolus. This projecting bony process of the lamina is the *hamulus*.

By convention, and for ease of reference and description, the cochlea is described as if it were sitting on its base with the apex pointing directly up. Viewed in this orientation, it can be seen that the spiral lamina is initiating the division of the cochlear duct into an upper chamber, the *scala vestibuli*, and a lower chamber, the *scala tympani*. Only the scala vestibuli communicates with the vestibule of the inner ear; it also communicates with the scala tympani at the apex of the duct. The scala tympani ends blindly at the round window (secondary tympanic membrane) of the middle ear.

The osseous labyrinth is not a closed chamber; there are several areas of communication with the exterior. These include the following:

1. The *vestibular aqueduct*, extending through the otic capsule from the vestibule to the posterior cranial fossa. Its cranial end lies lateral to the internal acoustic meatus on the posterior surface of the petrous portion of the temporal bone, where it is usually overlaid by a scale of bone. This aqueduct transmits the endolymphatic duct and an accompanying vein.

2. The *cochlear aqueduct*, which begins in the scala tympani of the basal coil of the cochlea near the round window. This small canal terminates on the inferior surface of the petrous pyramid, between the jugular fossa and the external orifice of the carotid canal. In the human it is not patent, being filled with connective tissue.

3. The *oval window*, which is closed by the footplate of the stapes and the associated annular ligament.

4. The *round window*, closed by the secondary tympanic membrane.

5. The *fissula ante fenestram* and the *fossula post fenestram*, small clefts related to the vestibular window of the lateral wall. The fissula ante fenestram usually extends completely through the bony lateral wall of the vestibule, while the fossula does so in only about 25% of all individuals. Both normally are filled with connective tissue. The fissula is important because of its predilection for otosclerotic bone formation.

6. The orifices of the nerves and vessels attaining the inner ear.

Lining the entire osseous labyrinth is a layer of periosteum or *endosteum*, which is continuous with the periosteum of the cranium through the various apertures and lies in close apposition to the walls of the osseous labyrinth. The areas of modification that merit further description occur within the cochlea. At the free edge of the osseous spiral lamina the endosteum is thickened to form the *limbus*, which then divides into vestibular and tympanic lips separated by a groove, the *internal spiral sulcus*. The vestibular lip is confluent with the vestibular membrane. The tympanic lip extends from the edge of the osseous spiral lamina across the lumen of the cochlea to the opposing peripheral wall, forming the fibrous *basilar membrane*. It attaches peripherally to the crest of the *spiral ligament*, which in turn is an area of thickened, modified endosteum overlying the lateral wall of the cochlea. While the basilar membrane divides the lumen of the cochlea, it does not extend all the way to the cupula but terminates just before it, leaving a small area of communication termed the *helicotrema* between the scala vestibuli and the scala tympani.

The *membranous labyrinth* is a system of delicate, epithelium-lined channels surrounded by connective tissue and lying within the osseous labyrinth (Fig. 1–9). Like its osseous counterpart, the membranous labyrinth has vestibular, semicircular, and cochlear components that communicate with one another. The membranous labyrinth exhibits certain general features:

1. Its luminal capacity is much less than that of the osseous labyrinth.

2. The membranous labyrinth tends to be placed peripherally within the osseous labyrinth; it is surrounded by the perilymphatic space (and perilymph). In most locations this space is traversed by numerous delicate trabeculae extending from the endosteum to the membranous labyrinth. The exception to this is in the cochlea, where the trabeculae are very much reduced or absent.

3. The membranous labyrinth contains the receptors for hearing and equilibration.

4. It is a self-contained system with no patent communication with other areas.

5. The membranous labyrinth contains endolymph.

Individual Components of the Membranous Labyrinth

The vestibular portion of the membranous labyrinth is characterized by two large dilatations, the *utricle* and *saccule*. The utricle, located in the posterior portion of the osseous vestibule, receives the crura of the three membranous semicircular canals. From its anterior end arises the minute *utricular duct* through which it communicates with both the endolymphatic duct and the saccule. Situated within the utricle on its floor and lower lateral wall is the *macula*, one of the receptor sites of the vestibular system. The saccule is located anteromedial to the utricle within the osseous vestibule. From its posterior aspect arises the small *saccular duct* that is continuous with the utricular duct (hence, *utriculosaccular*) and the endolymphatic duct. Anteriorly the saccule is continuous with the cochlear duct through the extremely small *ductus reuniens*. The saccule has a macula located on its lateral wall.

The *endolymphatic duct* arises from the union of the utricular and saccular ducts and passes through the vestibular aqueduct to terminate in a blind dilatation, the *endolymphatic sac*, within a dural cleft on the medial surface of the petrous portion of the temporal bone. Within the sac are extensive folds of epithelium with cores of vascular connective tissue, which would seem to indicate that this particular site is the region of greatest physiologic activity.

The *membranous semicircular canals* conform closely to the configuration of their osseous counterparts. At the anterior ends of the anterior and lateral canals and at the posterior (inferior) end of the posterior canal are prominent dilatations or *ampullae*, which house the receptor sites (cristae).

The cochlear portion of the membranous labyrinth is the most highly modified. Situated within the bony cochlea, where it lies upon the upper surface of the basilar membrane, it is a triangular duct extending the full length of the basilar membrane (but not to the apex of the cochlea). Basally it is continuous with the saccule through the ductus reuniens. The three basic structural components of the cochlear duct include the following:

1. The *vestibular membrane*, which forms the roof of the cochlear duct and separates the endolymphatic space of the duct from the perilymphatic space of the scala vestibuli. It is an extremely thin membrane (approximately 0.003 mm).

2. The lateral wall, consisting of the *stria vascularis*, a highly vascular region situated on the inner surface of the spiral ligament. As its name implies, it is characterized by its highly vascular nature and is generally believed to be the source of endolymph.

3. The floor, consisting of the organ of Corti, which is the sensory organ for hearing.

The Sensory Receptors of the Inner Ear

Within the vestibular portion of the inner ear the receptors consist of the following:

1. The *cristae*, located within the ampullae of the membranous semicircular canals. They consist of thickened epithelium containing neuroepithelial hair cells. Overlying the epithelium and extending to the opposite wall of the ampulla is the gelatinous *cupula*. The cilia of the hair cells project into the base of the cupula.

2. The *maculae*, which are located in the utricle and saccule and have similar structures. The hair cells of the neuroepithelium are stiff, nonmotile projections embedded in an overlying gelatinous membrane, the *statoconic* or *otolithic membrane*. This membrane is unique in that it contains numerous crystals termed *otoliths*.

The sensory portion of the cochlear duct, the *organ of Corti* or *spiral organ*, has the same basic structure as the cristae and maculae. It lies upon the basilar membrane and consists of supporting cells and hair cells overlaid by a gelatinous *tectorial membrane*. The supporting cells are of several different types; however, all contain fibrils within their cytoplasm, and their free edges form a reticular membrane against which the tectorial membrane rests. The most important of the supporting cells are the *phalangeal cells*, arranged in a single inner row, and an outer group consisting of three to five rows depending on the level of the cochlea under consideration, there being more rows apically than basally. The inner row is associated with a single row of hair cells, while the outer group has phalangeal cells alternating with rows of hair cells. Between the inner and outer group of phalangeal cells is an intercellular space extending the entire length of the spiral organ and termed the tunnel, inner tunnel, or *canal of Corti.* It is bounded by special supporting cells designated the inner and outer pillars (Corti's rods). Together the pillars and the canal form Corti's arch. Peripheral to the phalangeal cells are other supportive elements, the tall cells of Hensen and the shorter, more peripherally located cells of Claudius.

The hair cells of the spiral organ have numerous "hairs" projecting from their reticular surface (40 to 100 per cell). The innermost of these cells are long and are thought to be the least sensitive to sound. In contrast, the outer hair cells are short, being wedged between the apical portions of the phalangeal cells.

Vascular Supply of the Inner Ear

The primary source of blood to the inner ear is the *labyrinthine* (internal auditory) *artery.* While this vessel is usually described as originating from the basilar artery, it probably arises more frequently from the anterior inferior cerebellar artery. In addition, it may be duplicated by terminal branches that arise independently to enter the internal acoustic meatus.

In its course the labyrinthine artery accompanies nerves VII and VIII through the internal acoustic meatus. Its main branches run in the endosteum of the labyrinth, and small branches traverse the trabeculae to gain the membranous labyrinth. Apparently there are no functional anastomoses between these two areas of distribution.

The most common first branch of the labyrinthine artery is that which is distributed to the utricle, part of the saccule, and the anterior ends of the anterior and lateral semicircular canals. This branch has been called both the *anterior vestibular* and *vestibular artery.* When there is an apparent doubling of the labyrinthine artery, it is this branch that most frequently arises independently. The other two common branches of the labyrinthine artery are the *vestibulocochlear* (posterior vestibular) artery, which is distributed to the saccule, the posterior semicircular canal and parts of the anterior and lateral canals, part of the utricle, and the entire basal coil of the cochlea; and the *cochlear artery,* which is distributed to the remaining portion of the cochlea. There is considerable variation in the pattern of branching of the labyrinthine artery. Any one of the normal branches may be missing or may arise via a common trunk with another branch.

Descriptions of the venous drainage of the inner ear conflict. In all probability most are accurate, reflecting a considerable but normal variation. The described patterns include the following:

1. A *vein of the vestibular aqueduct,* draining most of the semicircular canals and emptying into either the sigmoid or the inferior petrosal dural sinus.
2. A *vein of the cochlear aqueduct,* draining the entire cochlea and vestibule. It runs in a long canal paralleling the cochlear aqueduct to enter the superior bulb of the internal jugular vein or the inferior petrosal dural sinus.
3. A *labyrinthine vein,* which seems to be inconsistent. When present, it drains the apical and middle coils of the cochlea and traverses the internal acoustic meatus to become tributary to the inferior petrosal dural sinus.

Nerves of the Inner Ear

Before describing the innervation of the inner ear we will consider the fundus of the internal acoustic meatus. The fundus is divided into superior and inferior portions by a horizontal bony ridge termed the *transverse crest.* Located posteriorly within the smaller superior depression are a number of small foramina that transmit the nerves to the utricle and the ampullae of the anterior and lateral semicircular canals. This is the *superior vestibular area.* Anteriorly within the upper depression is a relatively large foramen that transmits the facial nerve. In the larger inferior depression, immediately under the posterior end of the transverse crest, is the *inferior vestibular area,* which contains small foramina transmitting the nerves to the saccule. Below and slightly posterior to the inferior vestibular area is the *foramen singulare,* through which nerves pass to gain the ampulla of the posterior semicircular duct. Anteriorly the inferior depression is occupied by the *foraminiferous spiral tract,* a series of minute foramina arranged in spiral fashion that appose the base of the cochlea and the modiolus. At the center of the spiral is the somewhat larger *orifice of the modiolar canal.*

The nerve of the inner ear is the *vestibulocochlear* (statoacoustic, acoustic, or auditory) *nerve.* Functionally, it consists of two divisions:

1. The *vestibular division,* containing fibers arising from the *vestibular ganglion,* a sensory ganglion situated at the lateral end of the internal acoustic meatus.

These sensory fibers form the *superior* and *inferior vestibular nerves*. The superior vestibular nerve supplies the ampullae of the anterior and lateral semicircular canals plus the maculae of the utricle and saccule. Hence, it is this nerve that enters the inner ear through the superior vestibular area of the fundus of the meatus. The inferior vestibular nerve supplies the ampulla of the posterior semicircular canal and the macula of the saccule. It is associated with the inferior vestibular area and the foramen singulare of the meatal fundus.

2. The *cochlear division*, consisting of fibers arising from the *spiral ganglion*, which is situated in the coils of the modiolus at the base of the osseous spiral lamina. These fibers pass through the lamina to gain the organ of Corti. Within the internal meatus these fibers are associated with the foraminiferous spiral tract and orifice of the modiolar canal.

Associated with the nerves of the inner ear is the *bundle of Oort*, a small number of efferent fibers arising from the superior olive of the brainstem. These fibers run from the brainstem to the inner ear within the inferior vestibular nerve, then pass over to join the cochlear nerve. Although it is assumed that these fibers are distributed primarily to the cochlea, where they may play a part in some sort of feedback mechanism, their exact function has yet to be determined.

CHAPTER 2

Pertinent Histology

This short chapter presents four photomicrographs of horizontal temporal bone sections at different levels. The sole purpose is to provide a general orientation in terms of temporal bone anatomy; these sections are useful in achieving the three-dimensional visualization necessary for temporal bone surgery. A detailed description of horizontal temporal bone sections is beyond the purpose of this atlas. The horizontal sections are also to be used as references for the pertinent histopathologic slides described in this book, which for practical reasons are included in their specific chapters rather than grouped together here.

When describing horizontal sections of temporal bones, "superior" means cephalad; "inferior" is caudad; "anterior" is ventral; "posterior" is dorsal; "lateral" is toward the external ear canal; and "medial" is away from the external ear canal.

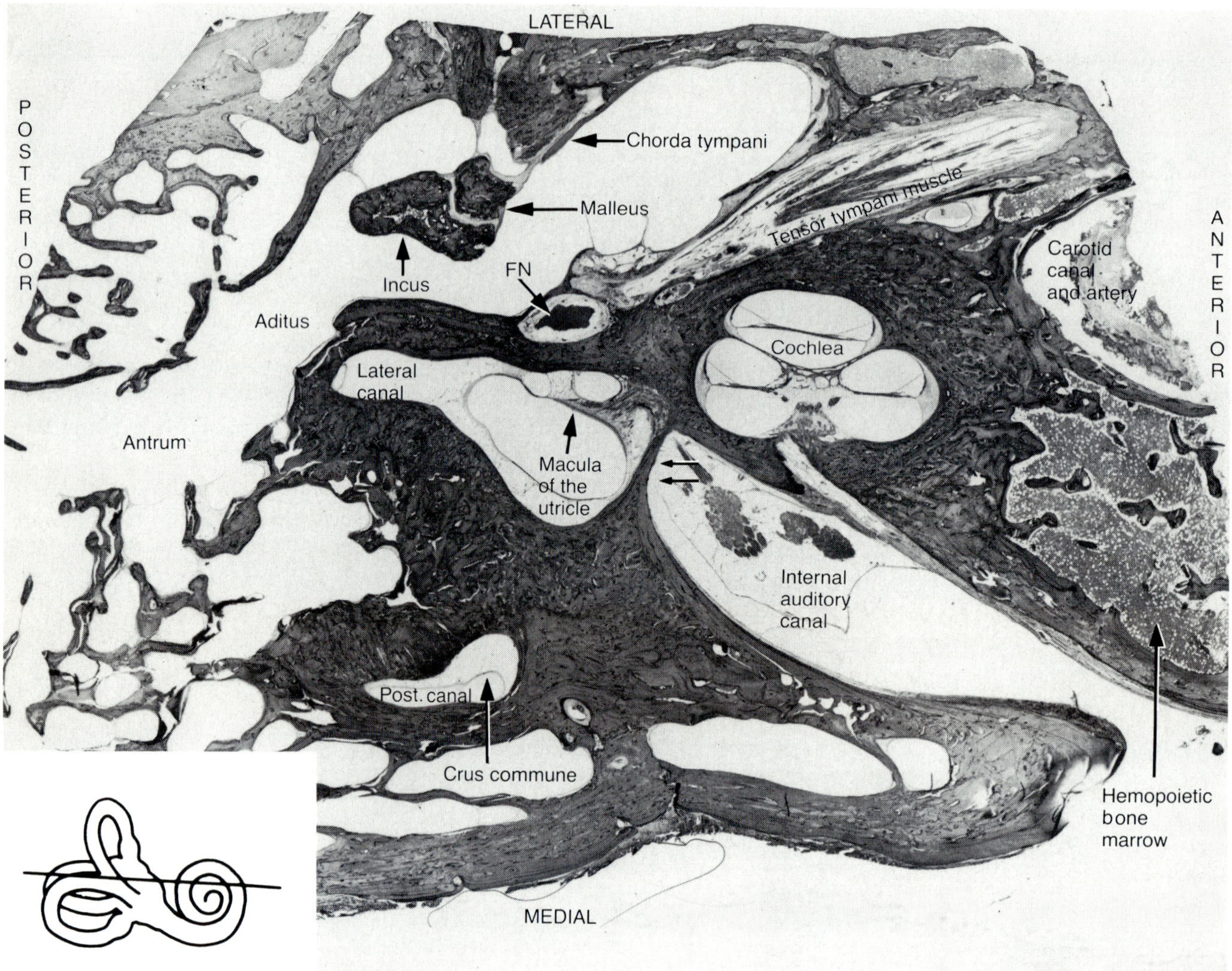

FIGURE 2–1

This section is in the area of the epitympanum. It is important to remember that the middle ear cavity extends superiorly above the tympanic membrane. It is at this level that the malleus can be laterally fixed (not shown in this section). The wide communication between the middle ear and mastoid can be observed, as can the close proximity of the incus and horizontal (lateral) semicircular canal to the aditus and antrum. At this high level the tensor tympani occupies the anterior wall and is in close proximity to the facial nerve (FN), which is surrounded by a thin plate of bone that is sometimes dehiscent. It is also important to recognize the thinness of the bone plate separating the vestibule from the internal auditory canal (*parallel arrows*). This must be kept in mind when doing a labyrinthectomy, since it is very easy to accidentally create a fistula with subsequent cerebrospinal fluid leak during this procedure. Note in these sections the air space that exists in the normal mastoid cavity, compared with that in temporal bones with otitis media (see Chapter 10).

At this higher level, the nerves of the internal auditory canal are the facial nerve anteriorly and the superior division of the vestibular nerve posteriorly.

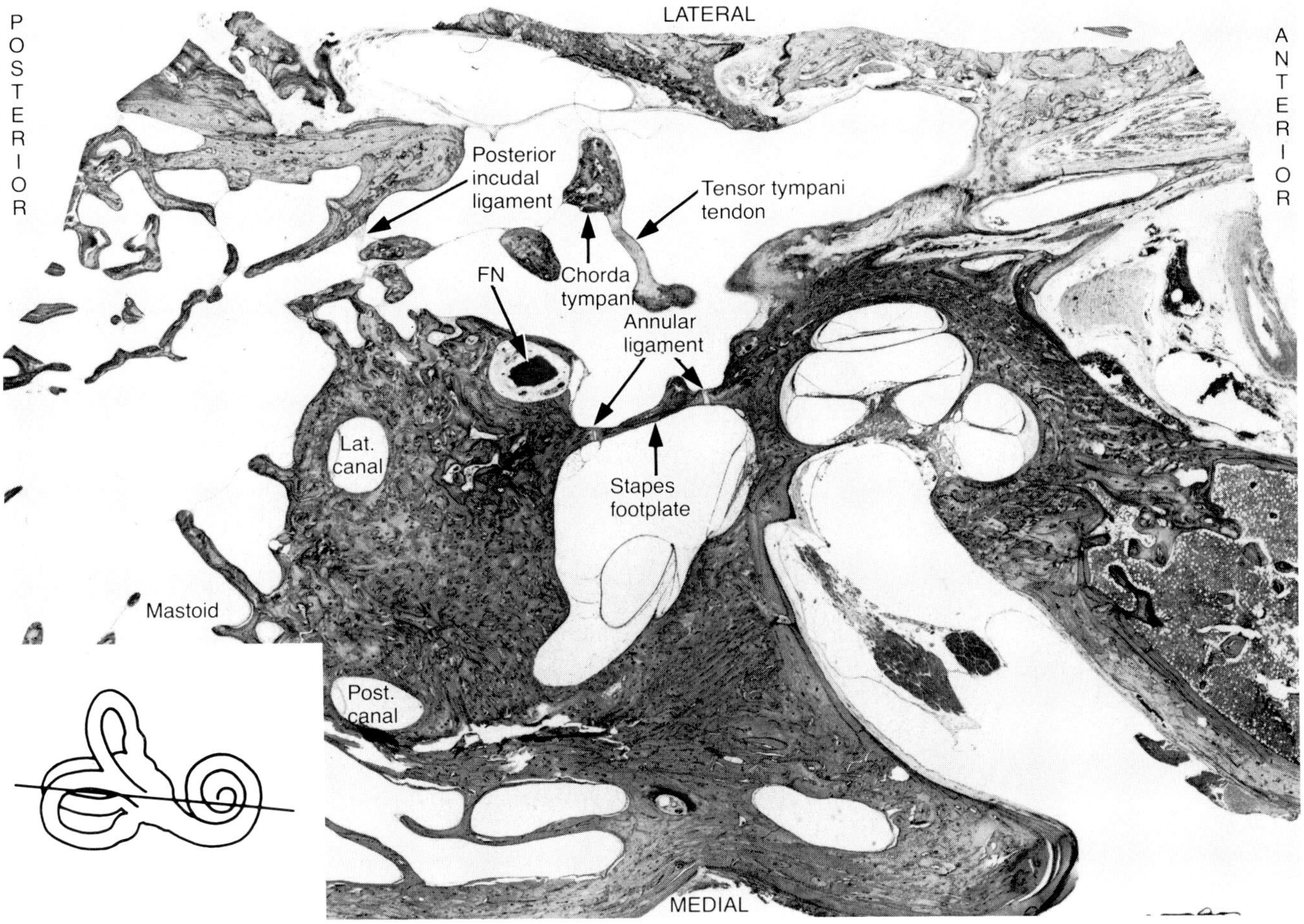

FIGURE 2–2

This section is at the level of the stapes footplate, which is bound to the oval window by the annular ligament. The short distance from the footplate to the contents of the vestibule (utricle and saccule) should be noted. There is very little room (1.5 to 2.0 mm) to work with a Hough hoe (or similar instrument) when removing the footplate without touching vestibular structures. At this level the FN is located posterior to the oval window; dehiscence (sometimes bulging) is not uncommon at this site. This should be remembered when working in this area.

This section also provides guidance for placing tubes in the superior quadrants of the tympanic membrane. The risk of damaging the incus or leaving it directly exposed to the exterior by placing a tube in the posterior superior quadrant is obvious in this section; the safe placement in the anterosuperior quadrant is more evident in Figure 2–3.

The tendon of the tensor tympani can be observed inserting laterally over the anteromedial surface of the manubrium of the malleus. It is here that the tendon of the tensor tympani is sectioned (when this procedure is needed). The body of the incus is reduced in diameter at this level to form the body of the descending long crus (long process of the incus). The posterior incudal ligament can be observed as it attaches at the fossa of the incus (fossa incudis). At this level the nerves of the internal auditory canal are the cochlear nerve anteriorly and the inferior division of the vestibular nerve posteriorly.

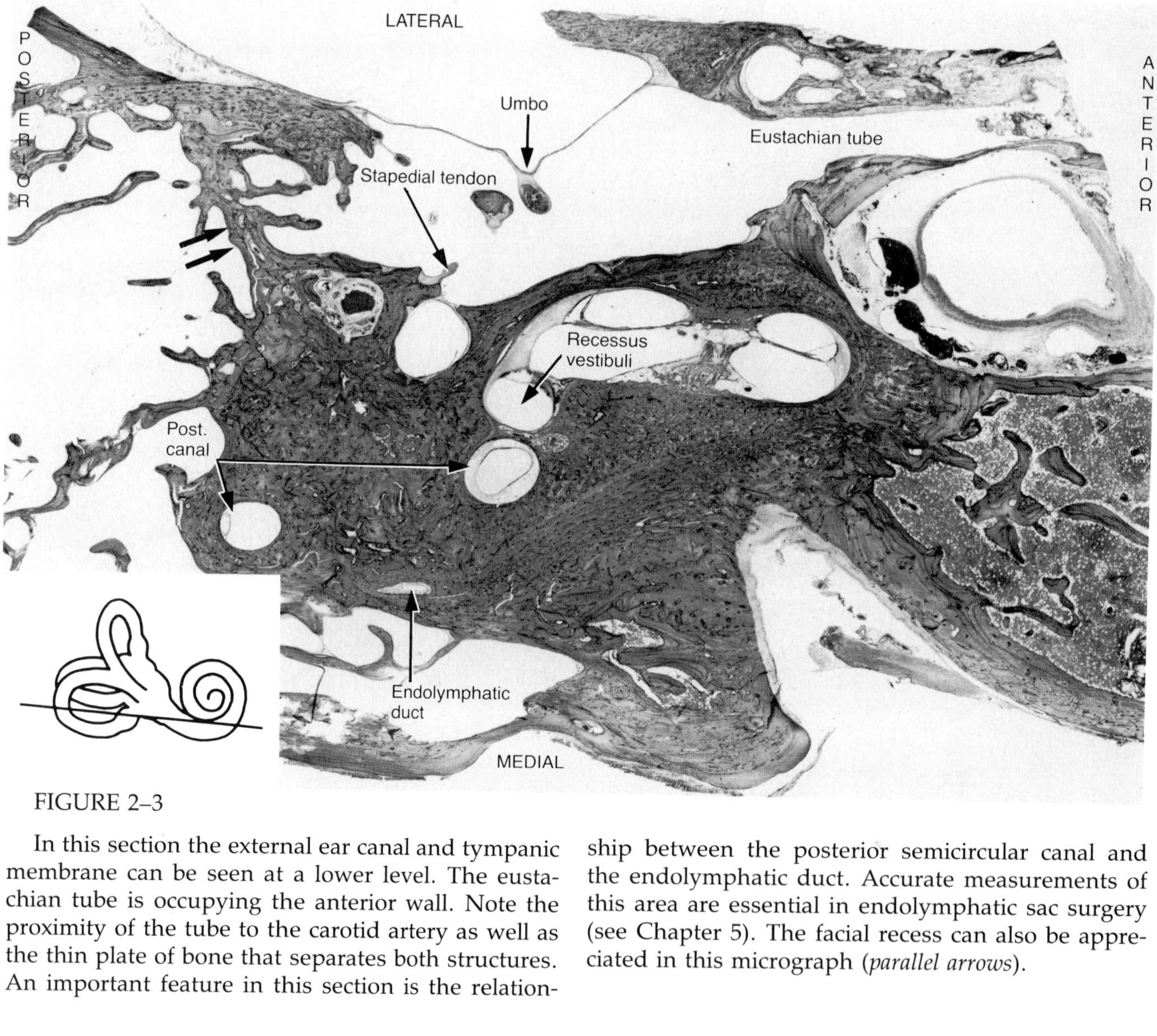

FIGURE 2–3

In this section the external ear canal and tympanic membrane can be seen at a lower level. The eustachian tube is occupying the anterior wall. Note the proximity of the tube to the carotid artery as well as the thin plate of bone that separates both structures. An important feature in this section is the relationship between the posterior semicircular canal and the endolymphatic duct. Accurate measurements of this area are essential in endolymphatic sac surgery (see Chapter 5). The facial recess can also be appreciated in this micrograph (*parallel arrows*).

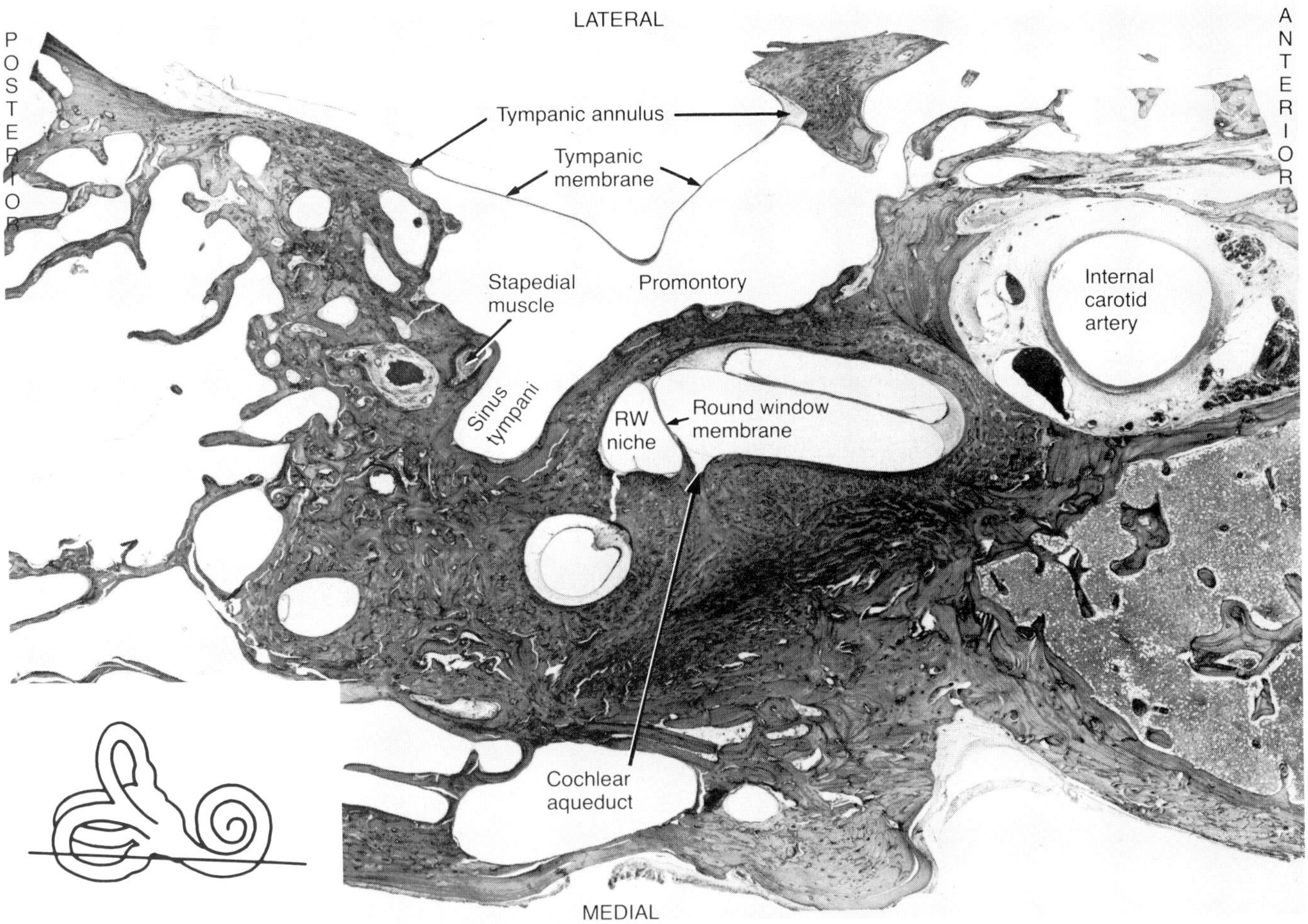

FIGURE 2–4

At this lower level in the mesotympanum the promontory is clearly apparent, as is the tympanic membrane in its full horizontal extent. This section provides a clear image of the middle ear space anteriorly and posteriorly for placement of tubes in the inferior quadrants. The sinus tympani can be observed and the difficulty of cleansing it adequately if it is involved with chronic disease can be seen. In these four figures the thinness of the mucoperiosteum should be noted as a reference for comparison with the pathologic slides shown in specific chapters.

CHAPTER 3

Pertinent Concepts in High Resolution Temporal Bone Imaging

Computed Tomography and Magnetic Resonance Imaging

High resolution computed tomography (CT) and magnetic resonance (MR) imaging have dramatically enhanced the field of temporal bone imaging. Thin section axial and coronal CT provides detailed views of the ossicles, bony labyrinth, cochlea, and mastoid air cells (Figs. 3–1 to 3–5*A*). MR provides superior soft tissue contrast resolution over CT and often eliminates the need for invasive procedures such as arteriography and pneumocisternography (Figs. 3–5*B* to 3–9). The multiplanar characteristics of MR permit demonstration of soft tissue anatomy in any desired plane of projection, and imaging parameters may be adjusted to fit each particular case. Thin section CT is recommended whenever bony structures need to be viewed in detail. Temporal bone injuries, developmental anomalies, otosclerosis, and inflammatory middle ear or mastoid lesions are best studied with CT, but MR is the procedure of choice for evaluation of internal auditory canal mass lesions.

Vascular Ultrasound for Atherosclerosis Screening

High resolution real-time duplex ultrasound with Doppler and spectral analysis is a useful and cost-effective screening procedure for cervical carotid atherosclerosis. Real-time ultrasound provides direct visualization of the cervical carotid arteries (Figs. 3–10, 3–11). Doppler and spectral analysis define flow patterns and velocity. These noninvasive screening procedures are easily performed upon patients with common complaints such as "dizziness" or "lightheadedness," precluding the need for arteriography in most circumstances. MR shows immense promise for noninvasive study of the intracranial vessels (see Fig. 3–7*B*, *C*).

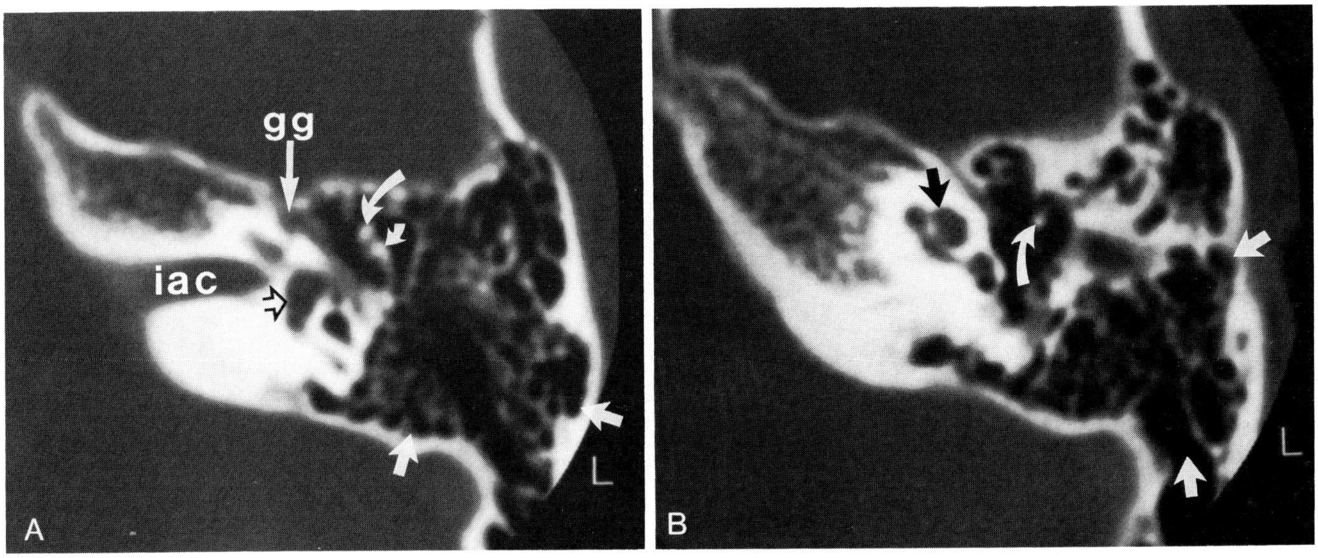

FIGURE 3–1.
Normal temporal bone (1.5 mm thick axial CT images, GE 9800). *A,* Internal auditory canal (iac); vestibule *(open arrow).* The geniculate ganglion (gg) lies within the anterosuperior aspect of the temporal bone. The normal malleus head *(large curved arrow)* and incus body *(small curved arrow)* are sharply delineated. *Arrows* denote normal mastoid air cells. *B* (3 mm below *A*), Normal cochlea *(black arrow);* handle of malleus *(curved arrow);* normal mastoid air cells *(white arrows).*

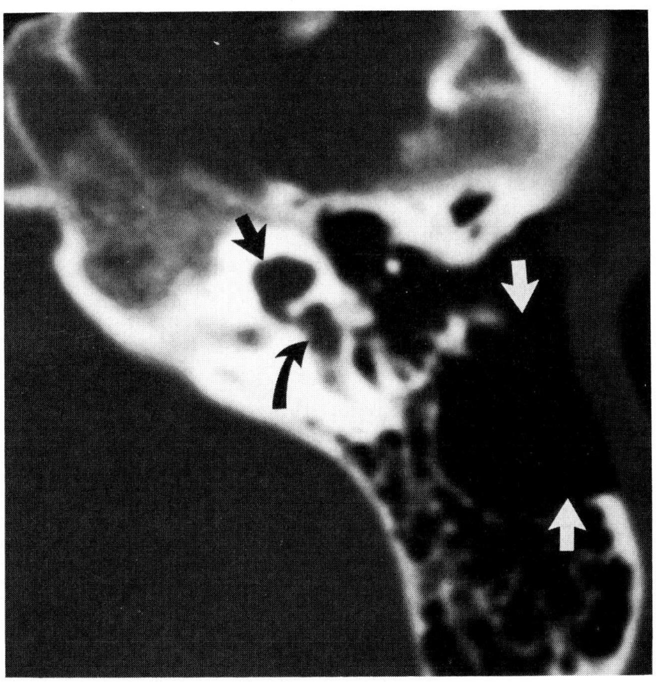

FIGURE 3–2.
Mondini deformity in a child with congenital deafness. The deformed cochlea *(arrow)* is globular in configuration and is continuous with the deformed vestibule *(curved arrow).* Note an operative defect *(white arrows)* from previous exploratory surgery.

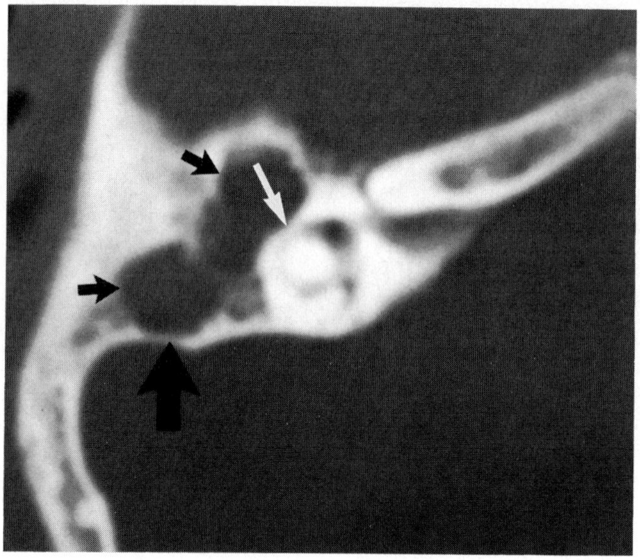

FIGURE 3–3.
Cholesteatoma in an 18-year-old woman with bilateral disease and a history of chronic, recurrent otitis media and tympanic membrane perforations. Attic expansion and air cell destruction *(black arrows)* caused by cholesteatoma. At surgery, focal erosion of the lateral semicircular canal was found *(white arrow)*.

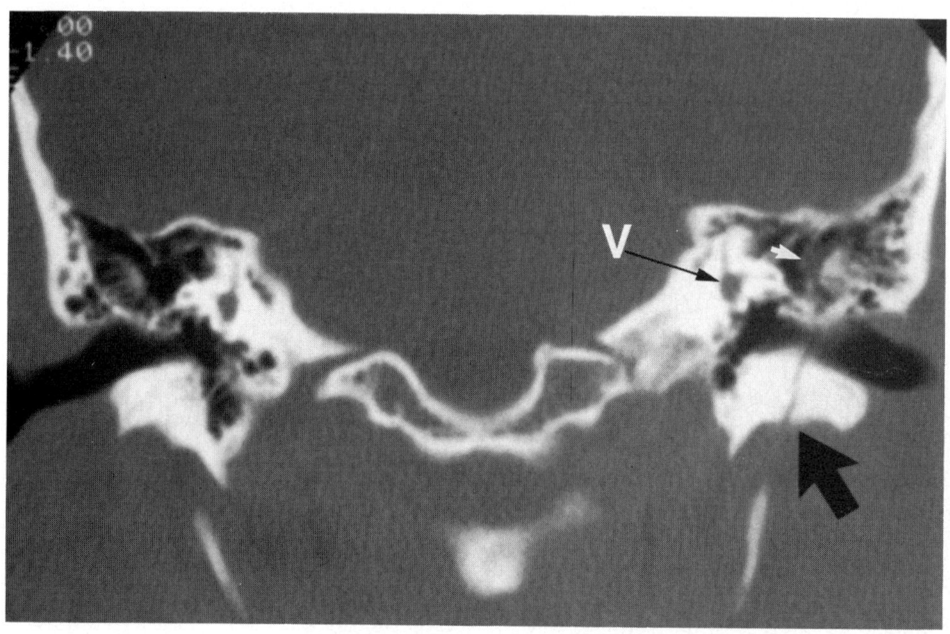

FIGURE 3–4.
A tympanic plate fracture (1.5 mm thick coronal CT scan) resulting in seventh nerve paresis in a 27-year-old man. A vertical tympanic fracture *(large arrow)* involves the temporal bone near the descending facial nerve. Note hematoma *(arrow)* within mastoid air cells. Normal vestibule (V).

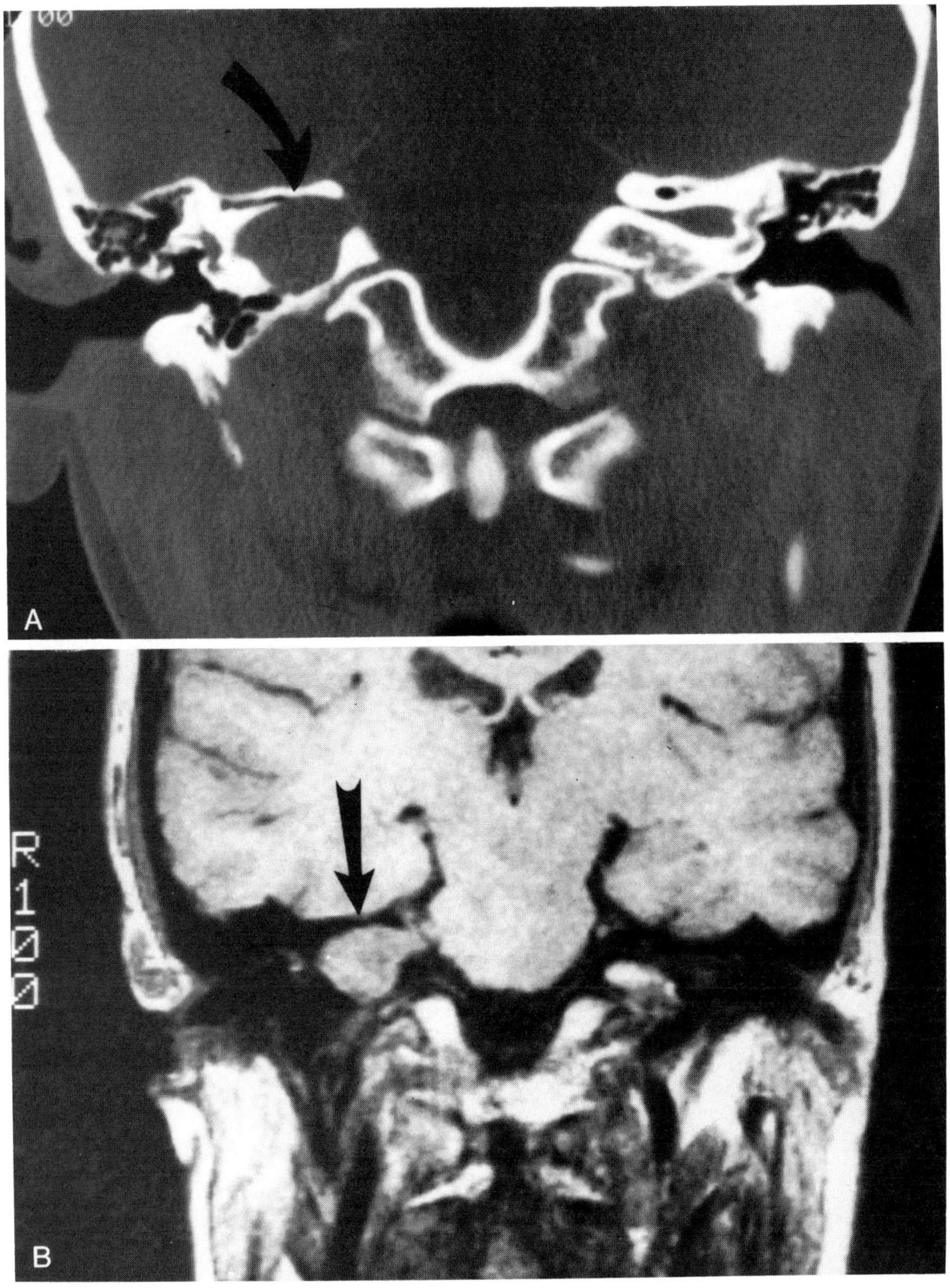

FIGURE 3–5.
Intracanalicular acoustic schwannoma shown with coronal CT *(A)* and MRI *(B)*. *A,* There is marked expansion of the right internal auditory canal *(arrow)*. *B,* Expansile mass *(arrow)* is isointense with brain (TR = 800, TE = 20).

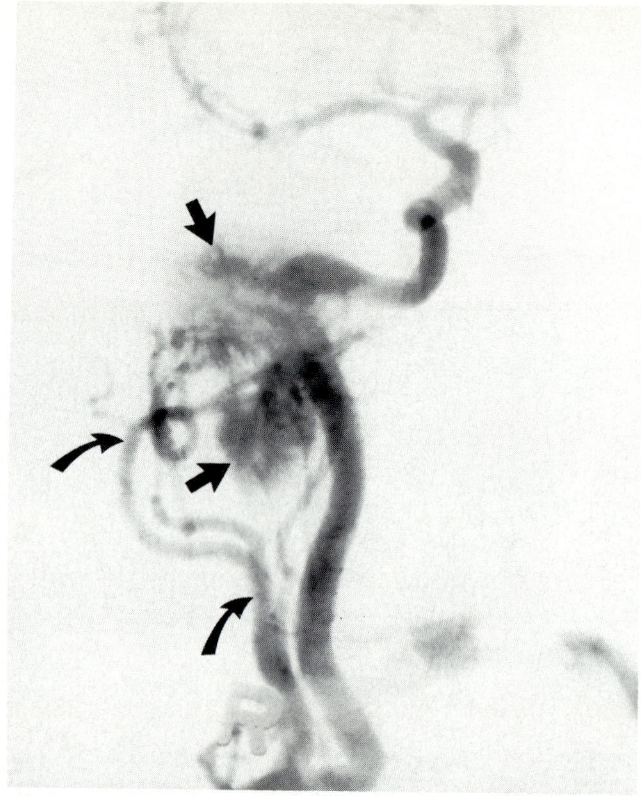

FIGURE 3–6.
Paraganglioma of the temporal bone demonstrated with carotid arteriography (frontal projection). An intense tumor blush *(large arrows)* is seen within the temporal bone on this common carotid injection. Note enlarged external carotid artery branches *(curved arrows)* leading into the tumor. Internal carotid artery also is shown.

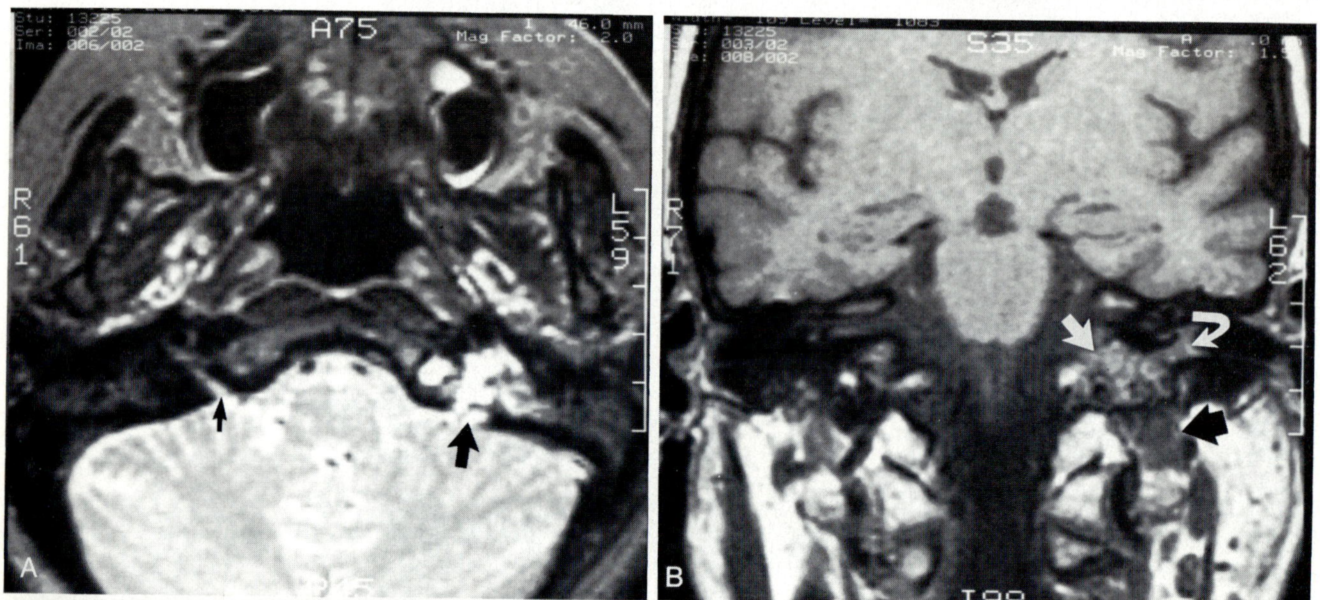

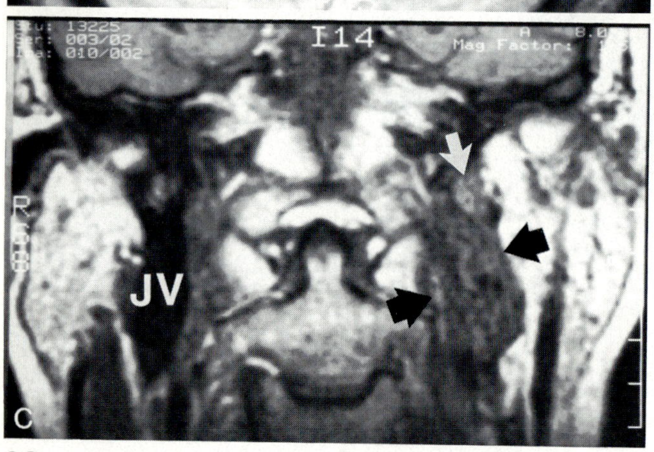

FIGURE 3–7.
Non-chromaffin paraganglioma (chemodectoma) of jugular foramen causing tinnitus, hearing loss, and paresis of cranial nerves 10 to 12. *A*, Axial 3-mm thick image shows signal-intense mass *(large arrow)* in inferomedial temporal bone (TR = 2300, TE = 30). *Small arrow* shows normal cochlear aqueduct. *B, C*, Coronal 3-mm images show hypointense mass *(straight white arrows)* with occluded internal jugular vein *(black arrows)* (TR = 800, TE = 20). JV denotes normal opposite internal jugular vein. *Curved arrow* in *B* shows fluid in the middle ear caused by a tumor obstructing the eustachian tube.

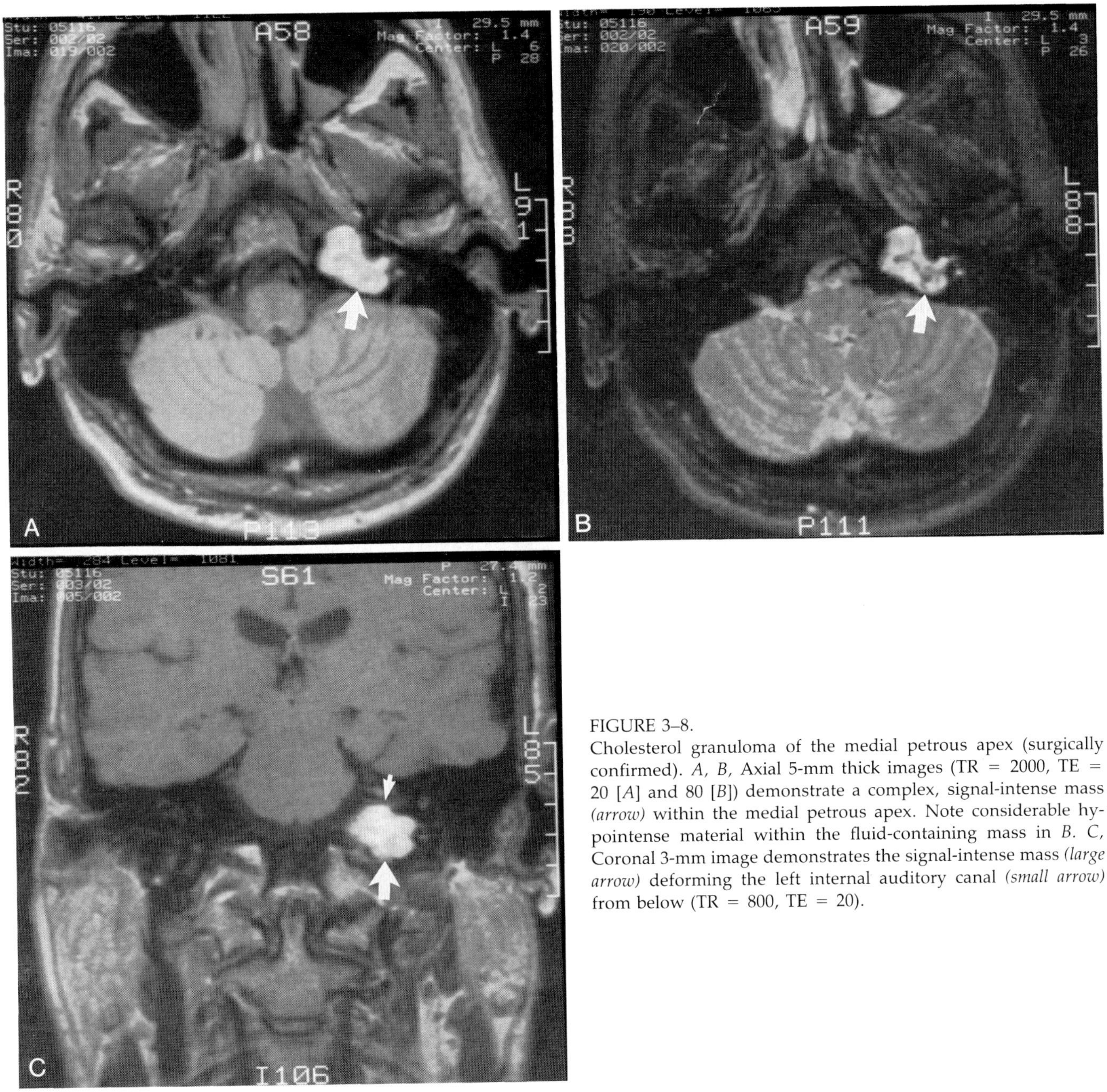

FIGURE 3–8.
Cholesterol granuloma of the medial petrous apex (surgically confirmed). *A, B,* Axial 5-mm thick images (TR = 2000, TE = 20 [*A*] and 80 [*B*]) demonstrate a complex, signal-intense mass *(arrow)* within the medial petrous apex. Note considerable hypointense material within the fluid-containing mass in *B*. *C,* Coronal 3-mm image demonstrates the signal-intense mass *(large arrow)* deforming the left internal auditory canal *(small arrow)* from below (TR = 800, TE = 20).

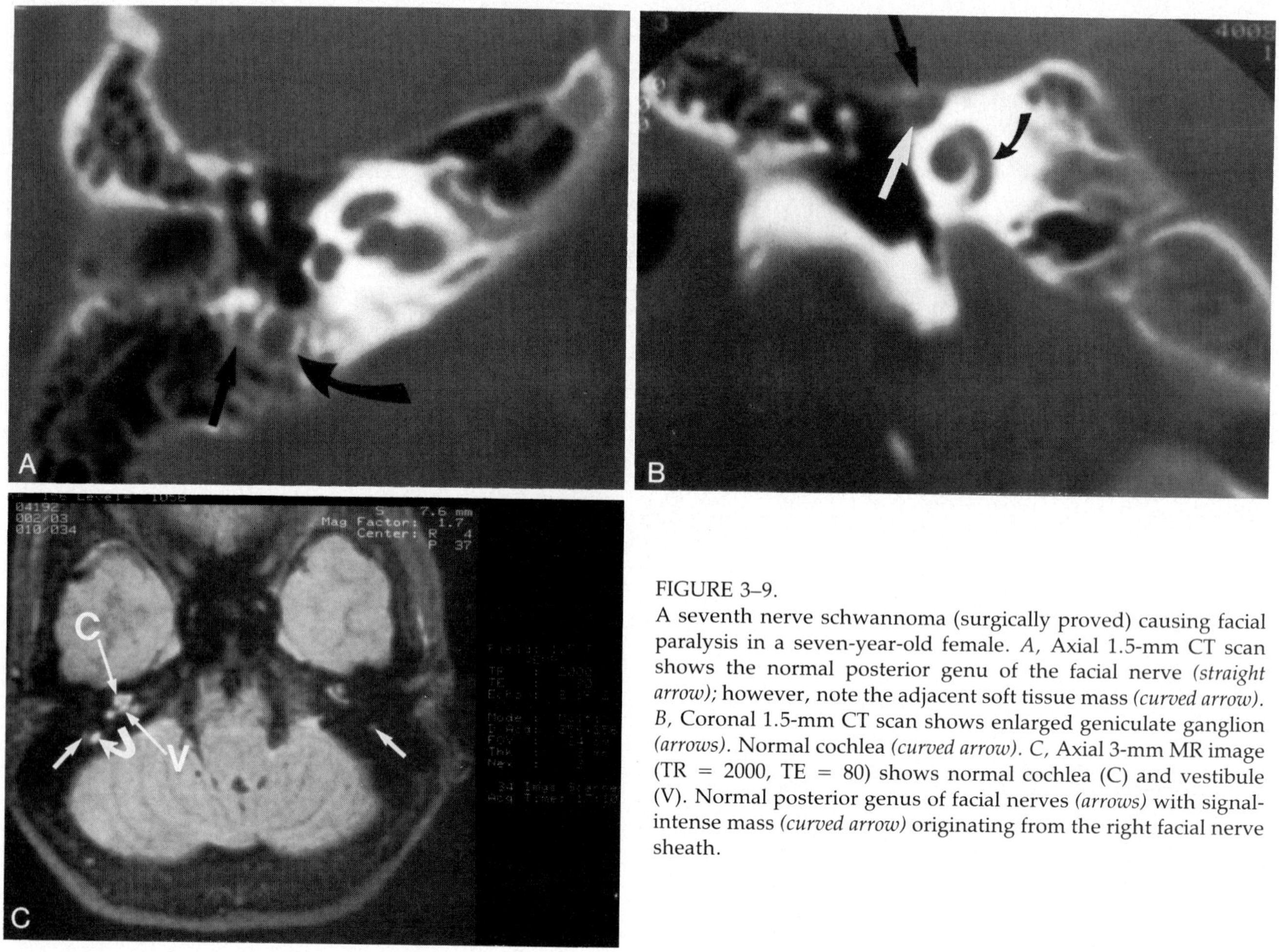

FIGURE 3–9.
A seventh nerve schwannoma (surgically proved) causing facial paralysis in a seven-year-old female. *A,* Axial 1.5-mm CT scan shows the normal posterior genu of the facial nerve *(straight arrow);* however, note the adjacent soft tissue mass *(curved arrow). B,* Coronal 1.5-mm CT scan shows enlarged geniculate ganglion *(arrows).* Normal cochlea *(curved arrow). C,* Axial 3-mm MR image (TR = 2000, TE = 80) shows normal cochlea (C) and vestibule (V). Normal posterior genus of facial nerves *(arrows)* with signal-intense mass *(curved arrow)* originating from the right facial nerve sheath.

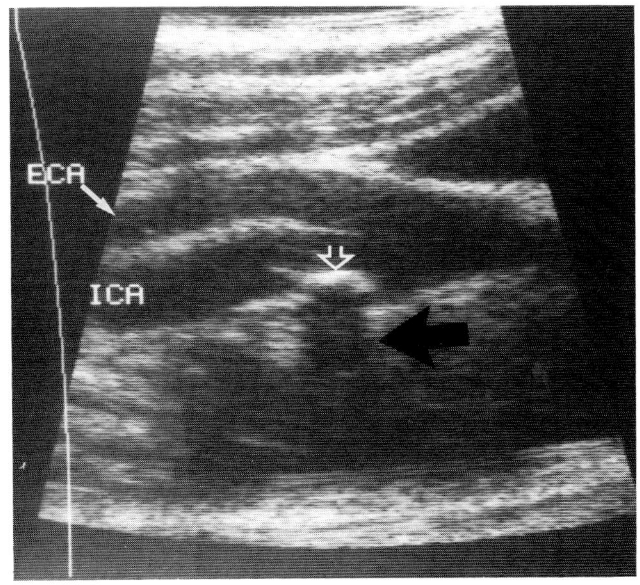

FIGURE 3–10.
A longitudinal ultrasound image of the carotid bifurcation (10 MHz transducer). An irregular, calcific plaque *(open arrow)* at the origin of the internal carotid artery (ICA) causes moderate narrowing of the proximal vessel lumen. Normal external carotid artery (ECA). Note the acoustic shadow *(arrow)* caused by calcium within the plaque.

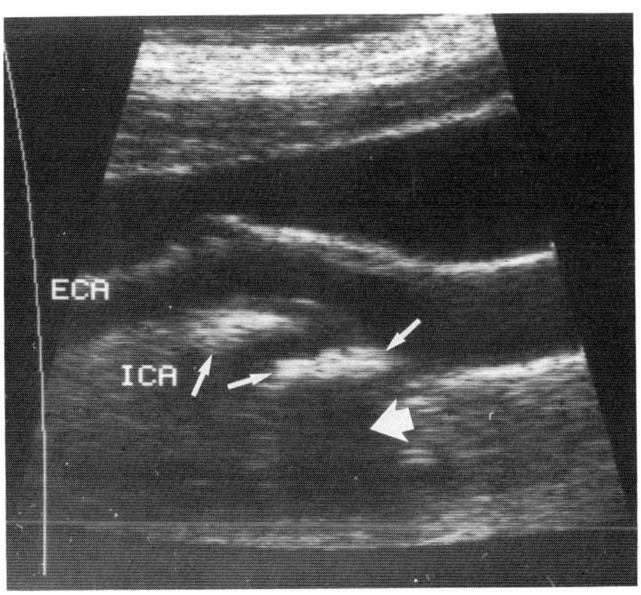

FIGURE 3–11.
Advanced carotid atherosclerosis with internal carotid artery (ICA) stenosis. A large, circumferential calcific plaque *(arrows)* causes stenosis of the proximal internal carotid artery. Normal external carotid artery (ECA). Note the acoustic shadow *(large arrow)* from heavily calcified plaque.

SECTION II

Temporal Bone Dissection

CHAPTER 4

Temporal Bone Removal

Knowledge of the human temporal bone is essential for the study of anatomy, histology, and pathology, and for the practice of microscopic surgical dissection. This knowledge helps provide a solid basis for medical and surgical treatment, and allows rational innovations and progress. It is useful for the surgeon to learn how to remove a temporal bone adequately. The specimen removed should contain the external auditory canal, middle ear, mastoid, inner ear structures, and surrounding petrous pyramid.

Technique

The calvarium is opened and the brain is exposed. The brain is then removed, care being taken to section cranial nerves VII and VIII sharply at the surface of the internal auditory meatus (Fig. 4–1*A*). Thus the nerve trunks remain with the temporal bone specimen. The two most common methods of removal are (1) the block method and (2) the bone plug method.

Block Method (Fig. 4–1*B*)

A motor-driven saw or, preferably, a Stryker saw* (rocker-type oscillating saw) is used. Four saw cuts are made. The first (1) is made at a right angle, as close to the apex of the petrous bone as the regional anatomy will allow. If the cut is made further anterior the eustachian tube can be removed. The second cut (2) is made parallel to the first, through the mastoid process and as close to the lateral wall as possible. The third cut (3) is made approximately 2.5 cm anterior and parallel to the petrous ridge in the floor of the middle cranial fossa. It includes the bony external ear canal. The fourth cut (4) is made in the horizontal plane, close to the floor of the posterior cranial fossa. This undermining cut severs the bone from its inferior attachments. The temporal bone is still not loose, and great care must be taken to avoid fracturing it.

A "lion-jawed" forceps is used to grasp the specimen, and the remaining bony connections are loosened by a gentle rocking motion that will free the specimen for further dissection. A sharp chisel, knife, or scissors is used to cut the remaining ligamentous, fibrous, and bony attachments.

Whether the temporal bone is removed by the block method or the bone plug method, the carotid artery should be ligated and a suture placed in the external auditory canal to prevent any leakage of fluid.

Bone Plug Method (Schuknecht's)

This technique requires the use of a specially designed oscillating bone plug saw attached to the conventional Stryker apparatus. The procedure is simple and provides an adequate specimen. For the adult skull, a 1.5-in diameter saw adjusted to a depth of 1.5 in is used; a 1-in diameter saw adjusted to a depth of 1 in is used for smaller skulls.

The saw should be centered over the arcuate eminence (superior semicircular canal prominence or the superior surface) (Fig. 4–2*A*) and directed to the floor of the middle cranial fossa. The skull is held by an assistant, and a stream of water is directed at the

*Available from the Orthopedic Frame Company, Kalamazoo, MI.

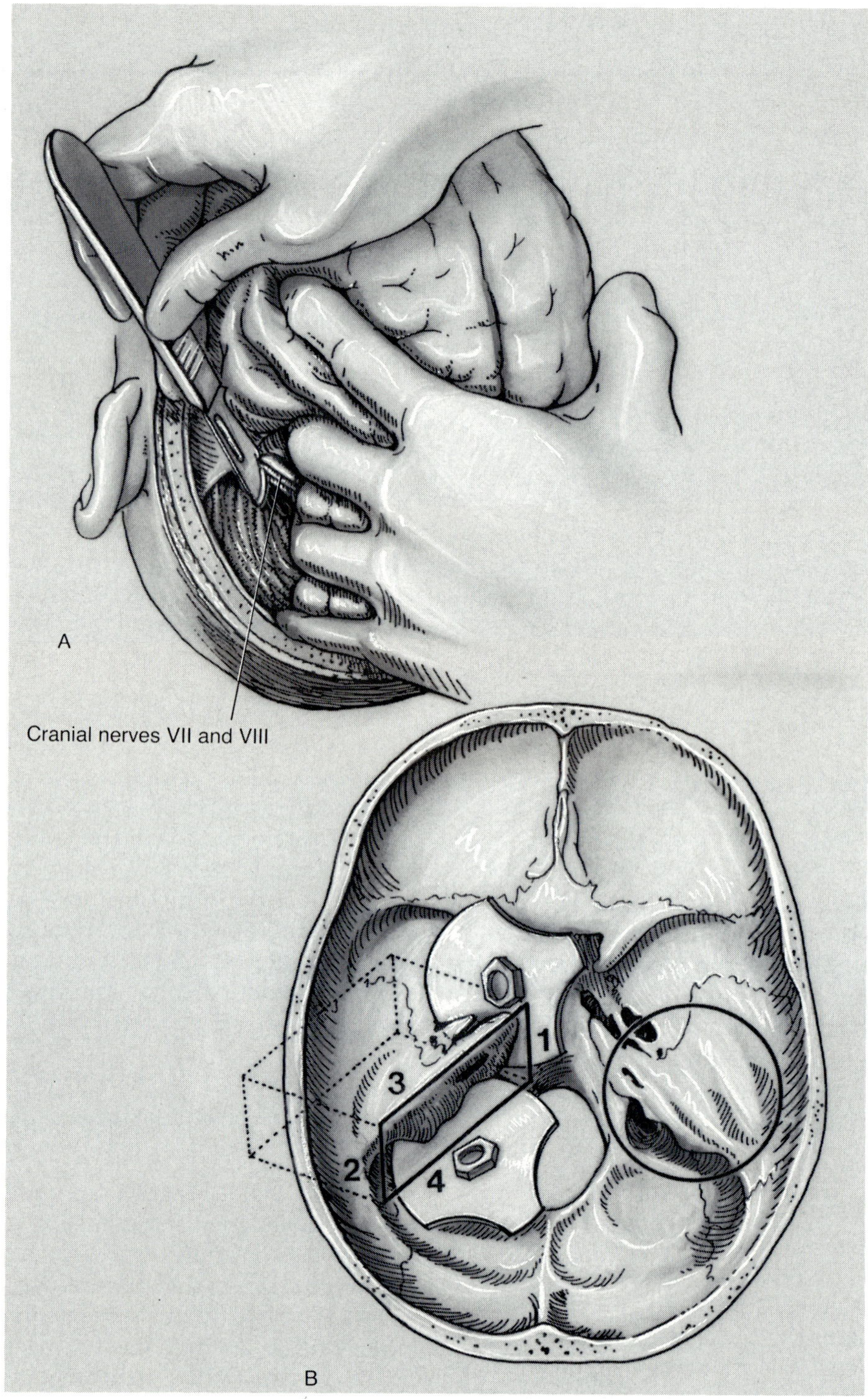

FIGURE 4–1.

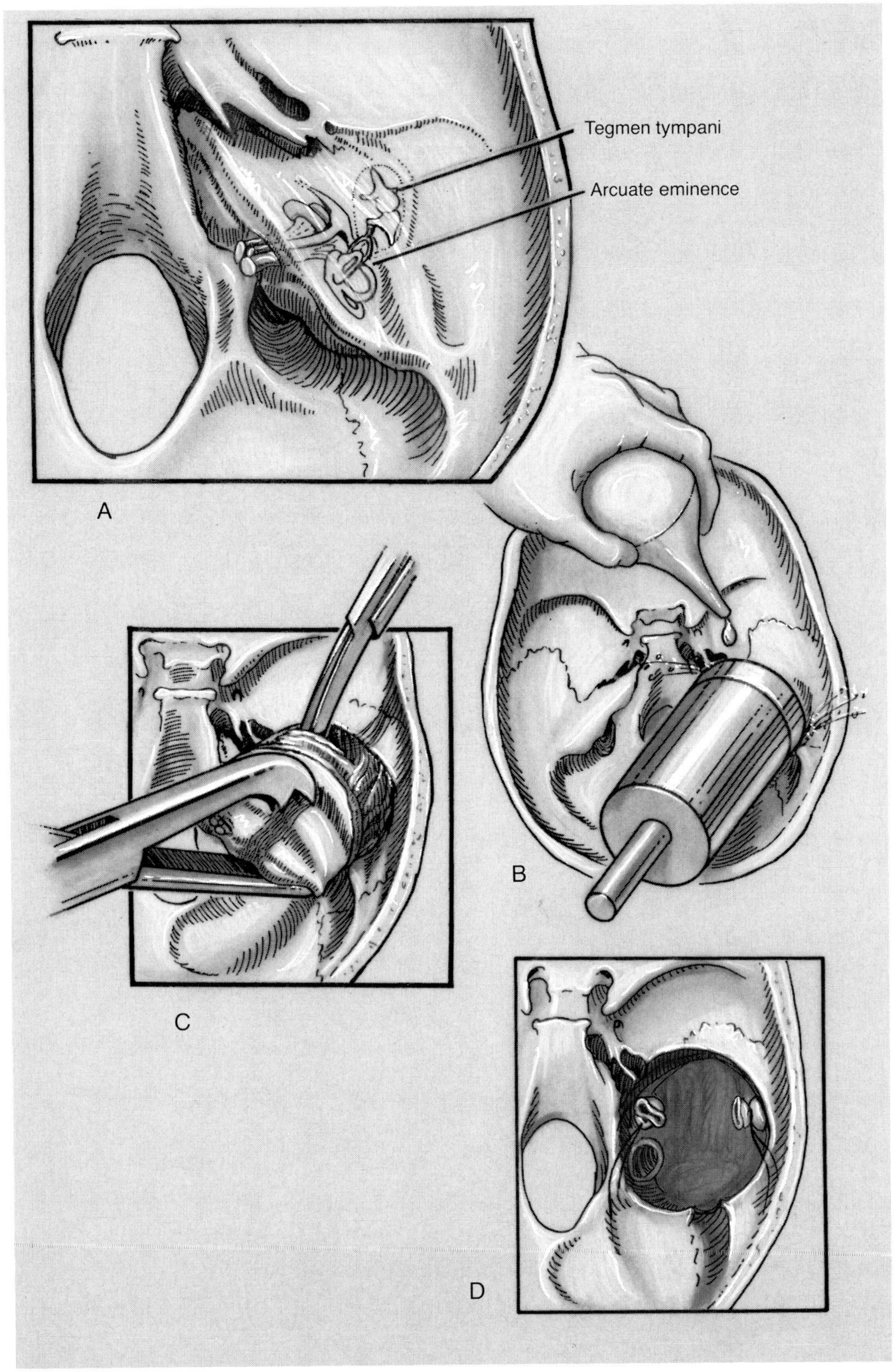

FIGURE 4–2.

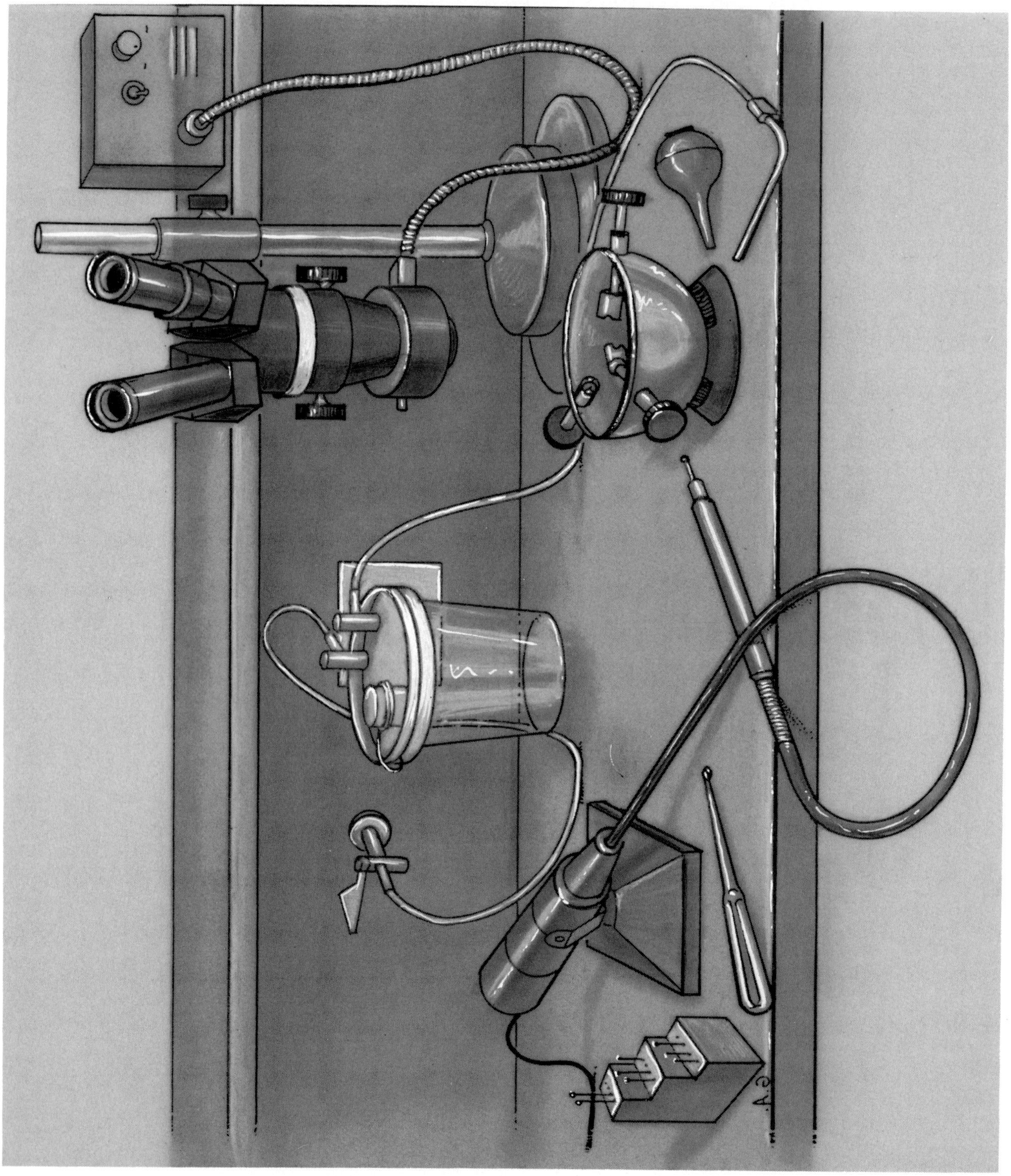

FIGURE 4–3.

blade for lubrication (Fig. 4–2*B*). Cutting is completed when a loss of resistance is felt, indicating penetration through the base of the skull. An improved cutting action is obtained by slight rotation of the saw. The plug is then grasped with the "lion-jawed" forceps (Fig. 4–2*C*), and the bone is rotated, permitting visualization of the internal carotid artery on its inferior surface. The artery is ligated. Additional attachments are sectioned with a knife, scissors, or osteotome.

Fresh temporal bones can be wrapped in water-sealed cotton or placed in Teflon bags; the air is expelled and the bones are frozen. This helps to preserve the soft tissues for later use.

General Setup and Equipment

A temporal bone dissection station (Fig. 4–3) should be arranged to simulate actual operating room conditions as closely as possible. Essential items of equipment include a proper table, a comfortable chair, an operating microscope, a motor-driven drill or other otologic drill, suction apparatus, an assortment of otologic instruments, and a temporal bone holder. A list of suggested instruments appears below.

In general, two types of temporal bone holders are most commonly used: one that embeds and fixes the temporal bone in a medium such as plaster of Paris, and another that secures the temporal bone specimen with specially designed screw holders, allowing study of all surfaces and relationships of the bone during dissection.

List of Instruments and Materials

- Operating microscope
- Drill with a set of cutting burs
- Bulb syringe
- Suction
- Suction tips No. 1 and No. 5
- Stapes curets
- Straight canal knife
- Sickle knife
- Joint knife
- Straight pick
- Stapes bending die
- Hough hoe
- Whirlybird
- Small alligator forceps
- Fenestrometer
- Scalpel
- 4-0 silk (mounted on curved needle)
- 0.05-mm stainless steel wire
- Silastic sheeting
- Gelfoam
- TORP, PORP, PE tube
- Scissors (small plastic)
- Ossicle holder
- Measuring rod

Residents with imagination can obviate many of these instruments and materials by adapting broken instruments and selecting similar, cheaper materials than those suggested.

CHAPTER 5

Surgical Procedures

The guidelines in this chapter have been designed for the practical purpose of being read and followed as the dissection proceeds. They are intended to serve as a dialogue between the instructor and the surgeon dissecting the temporal bone. Aims, highlights, pitfalls, pertinent anatomy, and surgical steps are discussed during the dissection in an attempt to simulate a rational procedure.

The authors encourage dissection of temporal bones as an essential prerequisite for otologic training in residency programs or for otolaryngologists who wish to practice specific techniques. This practice, plus a knowledge of anatomy and histopathology, is essential for developing rational and not merely imitative means of surgical treatment.

The succession of procedures has been organized for the fullest utilization of the bones. Four "wet" temporal bones are needed for full completion of these guidelines.

When describing or discussing a temporal bone dissection procedure, "superior" means toward the temporal line (cephalad); "inferior" is toward the mastoid tip (caudad); "anterior" is toward the external auditory canal (ventral); "posterior" is away from the external auditory canal (dorsal); "lateral" is toward the mastoid cortex (superficial); and "medial" is away from the mastoid cortex (deep).

Simple Mastoidectomy

Aim

Exenteration (removal) of all mastoid air cells while maintaining the integrity of the posterior canal.

Highlights

1. Use the microscope at all times.
2. Drill under direct vision, avoiding "holes" (drill evenly).
3. When in doubt, identify landmarks and use a mastoid curet.
4. Develop a gradual, step-by-step procedure.
5. Think anatomically and three-dimensionally. Look for structures; do not "find them."
6. Keep anatomic aberrations in mind (high sigmoid sinus, anterior sigmoid sinus, Körner's septum, etc.).

Pitfalls

1. Failing to identify the antrum.
   A. Körner's septum.
   B. Insufficient thinning of the tegmen and/or posterior osseous canal.
2. Injuring a high sigmoid sinus.
3. Injuring the facial nerve by going
   A. Deep to the horizontal semicircular canal.
   B. Too far anterior in the digastric ridge.
4. Dislocating the incus by drilling blindly into the antrum area.

Surgical Steps

Assess External Anatomy (Fig. 5–1). Place the temporal bone in surgical position (simulating its normal anatomic location for surgery). Visualize and study

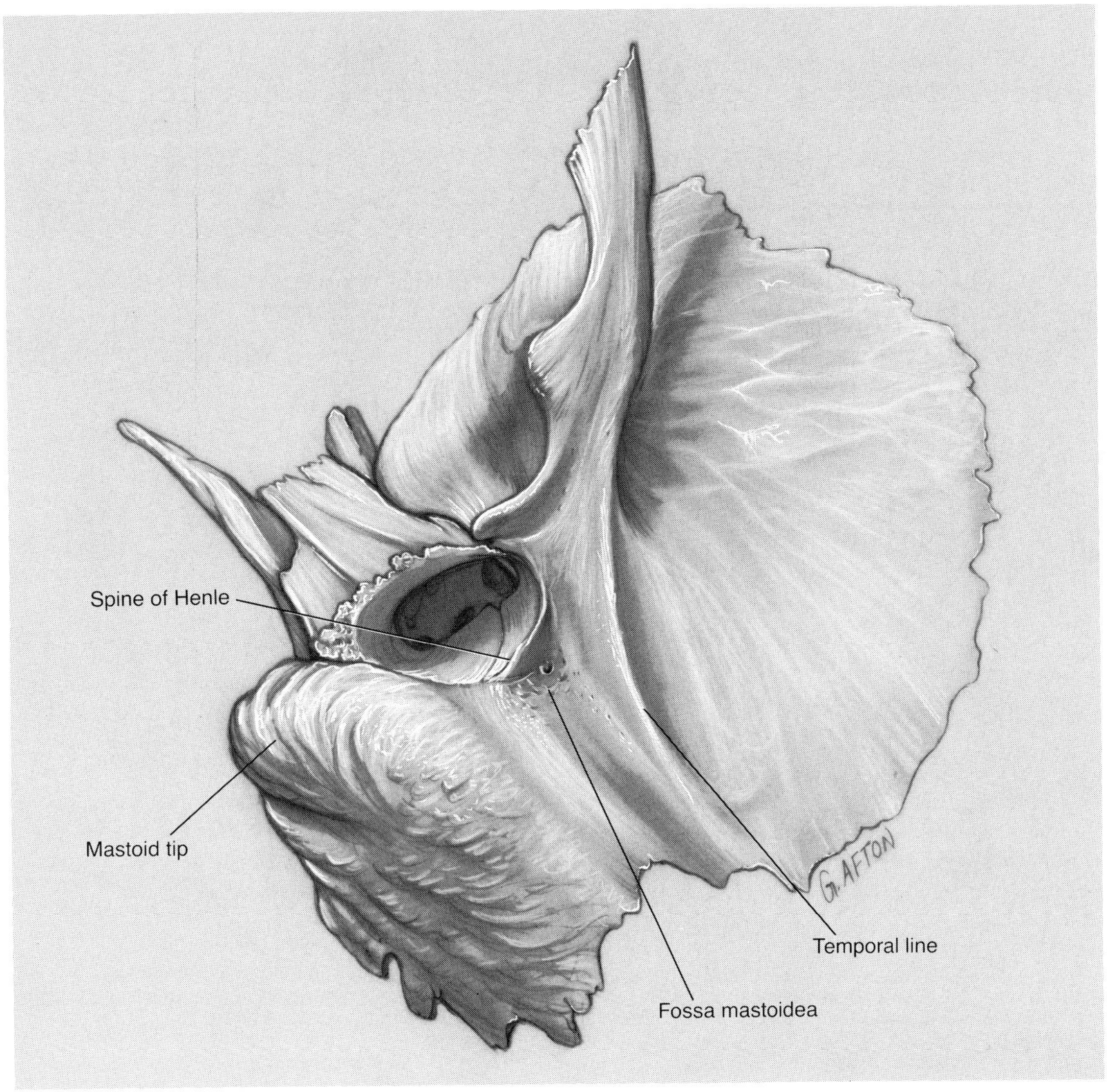

FIGURE 5–1.

the lateral surface (cortex) in its entirety from the temporal line (linea temporalis) superiorly to the mastoid tip inferiorly. Identify the posterior aspect of the osseous canal anteriorly. Note the presence of the suprameatal spine (spine of Henle) immediately posterior to the osseous canal. Review the imaginary lines that overlie the mastoid antrum, that is, between the temporal line and spine of Henle (fossa mastoidea or Macewen's triangle). Imagine the inner structures of the mastoid cavity in a three-dimensional fashion and trace your surgical plan.

Initiate Drilling (Use Large Burs, Saucerize). Employing the microscope, use a large bur and start saucerizing in an even fashion, beginning at the fossa mastoidea until air cells appear (Fig. 5–2*A*). Make a wide cortical removal, including thinning of the posterior canal. As you go deeper, keep thinking of your future landmarks to orient yourself toward the antrum. Your superior limit is the tegmen mastoideum (level of temporal line), superior to which lies the dura of the middle cranial fossa. Thin the tegmen down, being careful to keep it intact; this is important if adequate access to the antrum is intended. The posterior canal wall should be thinned down as well for the same purpose. Again, drilling should remain even at all times, not straight but oriented anteriorly toward the nose of our imaginary patient. Our anterosuperior limit is the root of the zygomatic process. This should be opened without opening the epitympanum.

Identify the Lateral Sinus (Sigmoid Sinus). In drilling posteriorly you will encounter the sigmoid sinus (lateral sinus) (Fig. 5–2*B*). It is identified in surgery by its bluish color and smooth bony plate. (In this

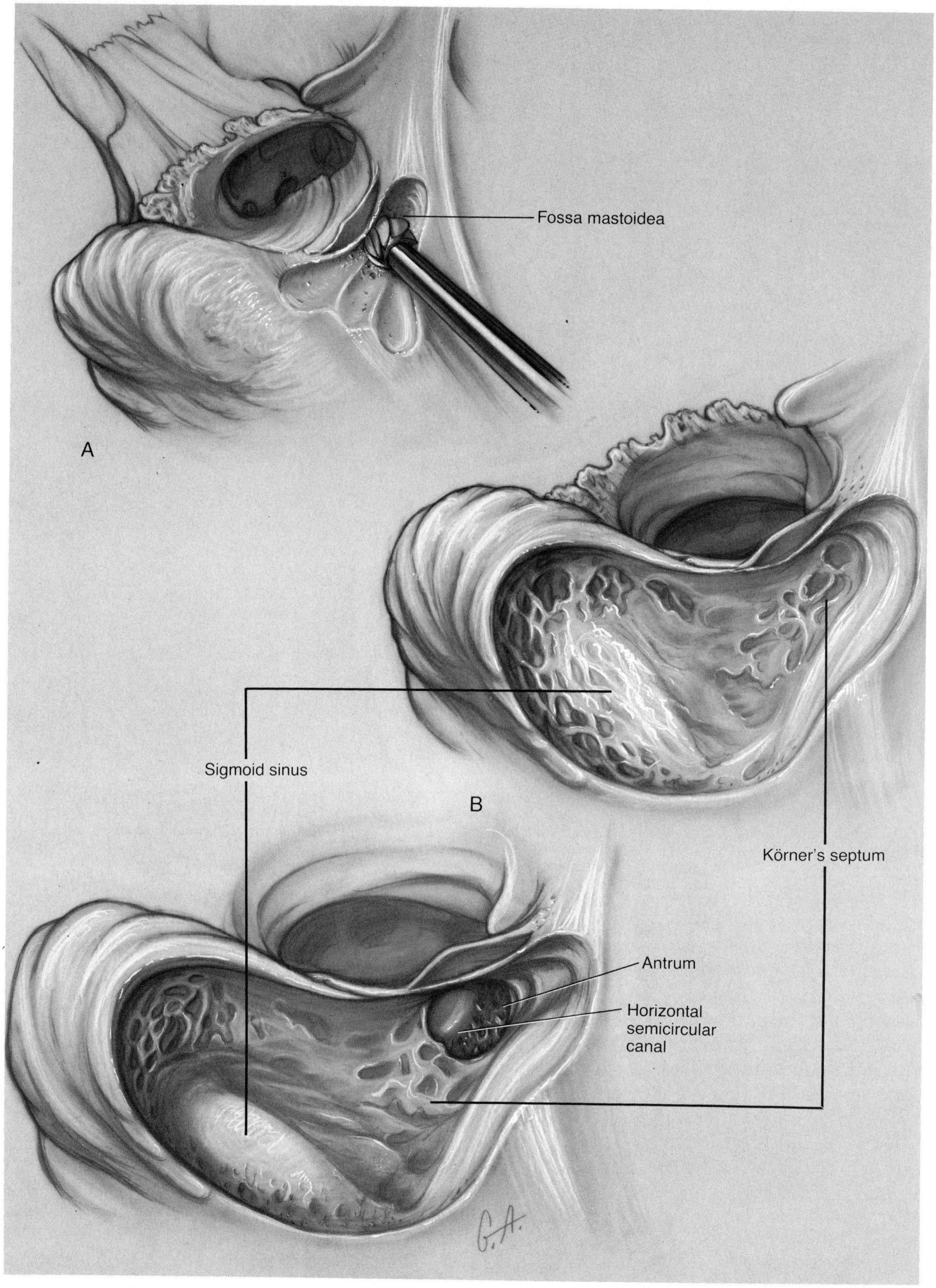
Fossa mastoidea
A
Sigmoid sinus
B
Körner's septum
Antrum
Horizontal
semicircular
canal

FIGURE 5–2.

dissection we are looking for the smooth bony plate.) These characteristics are the best guides to the sigmoid sinus. A change in the sound of the burs is a helpful hint but does not suffice as a guide; visualization far outweighs sensation in temporal bone surgery. It must be remembered that the sigmoid sinus does not have a uniform anatomy; it can be high (lateral) or low (medial/deep). The surgeon should be cautious with the use of the drill. Inferiorly, toward the mastoid tip, the air cells are to be drilled evenly with the level of drilling superiorly. Little by little, a typical kidney-shaped mastoid cavity becomes evident.

Identify Körner's Septum and Antrum. In proceeding medially (deeper down), occasionally one may encounter a thick plate of bone that may give the impression of having reached the antrum. This is Körner's septum, a solid plate that represents the fusion of the squamous and petrous portions of the temporal bone. When in doubt, go back to your previously identified landmarks and structures, verify your location, and imagine the bone three-dimensionally along with the suspected area of the antrum. Using mastoid curet, curet superiorly and posteriorly until identifying the "true antrum." The antrum is posterosuperior to the osseous canal. A common error is to go too far below the temporal line owing to lack of thinning of the plate. An important guideline is that the antrum should be reached or entered from above if damage is to be avoided. Once the antrum is identified, avoid uncovering the incus; identify the horizontal semicircular canal, which is one of the most important landmarks. At that point, you know that you are definitely in the antrum and that you are superior to the facial nerve. If you are unable to see the incus, work anteriorly just inferior to the dura of the tegmen; this is the widest distance between the ossicles and epitympanum.

Identify and Define the Sinodural Angle, Hard Angle, and Facial Nerve (Fig. 5–3). Drill posteriorly, thinning the sigmoid sinus, and between the sinus and the tegmen plate until they meet in a sharp angle (sinodural angle or Citelli's angle). Continue drilling inferiorly toward the mastoid tip, exenterating cells from the digastric ridge area. Keep in mind that the facial nerve and its point of exit from the stylomastoid foramen are immediately anterior to the digastric ridge. At this point, we are left with an intact area in the so-called "hard angle" (an area containing the posterior semicircular canal in the plate that overlies the posterior cranial fossa, and an unidentified facial nerve). It is important to remain above the area of the horizontal semicircular canal. The location of the horizontal canal allows exposure of the fossa incudis (and short process of the incus) inferolaterally to the antrum and the horizontal canal, the epitympanum, and also the external genu of the facial nerve, which is medial to the horizontal semicircular canal.

Using a fenestrometer, measure an imaginary triangle 10 mm from the tip of the short process of the incus or fossa incudis, along the axis of the horizontal semicircular canal (30 degrees from the tegmen), and 12 mm from the fossa incudis at an angle of 45 degrees from the tegmen. This area identifies and isolates the hard angle (containing the posterior semicircular canal) (Fig. 5–3*C*). Immediately inferior to it and anterior to the sigmoid (lateral sinus) is the plate of bone that overlies the dura of the posterior cranial fossa, where the endolymphatic sac is found. Now identify Trautmann's triangle (Fig. 5–3*D*), bordered by the lateral sinus (sigmoid sinus), tegmen, and semicircular canals. This triangle identifies the location of the posterior cranial fossa.

The facial nerve is identified but not unroofed. We will come back to it further in the dissection. The simple mastoidectomy is now completed, that is, all air cells have been removed (except those in the petrous apex). Reidentify all anatomic structures, landmarks, triangles, and angles.

Endolymphatic Sac Surgery

Aim

To identify and expose the endolymphatic sac overlying the dura mater of the posterior cranial fossa.

Highlights and Surgical Steps

1. Complete simple mastoidectomy (already performed).
2. Drill to, but not below, the dome of the horizontal semicircular canal.
3. Identify, preserve, and measure the hard angle containing the posterior semicircular canal.
4. Identify the position of the sigmoid sinus and its relationship to Trautmann's triangle.
5. Decompress the lateral sinus and dissect the infralabyrinthine cell tract.
6. Incise the endolymphatic sac, probe its lumen, and place Silastic sheeting.

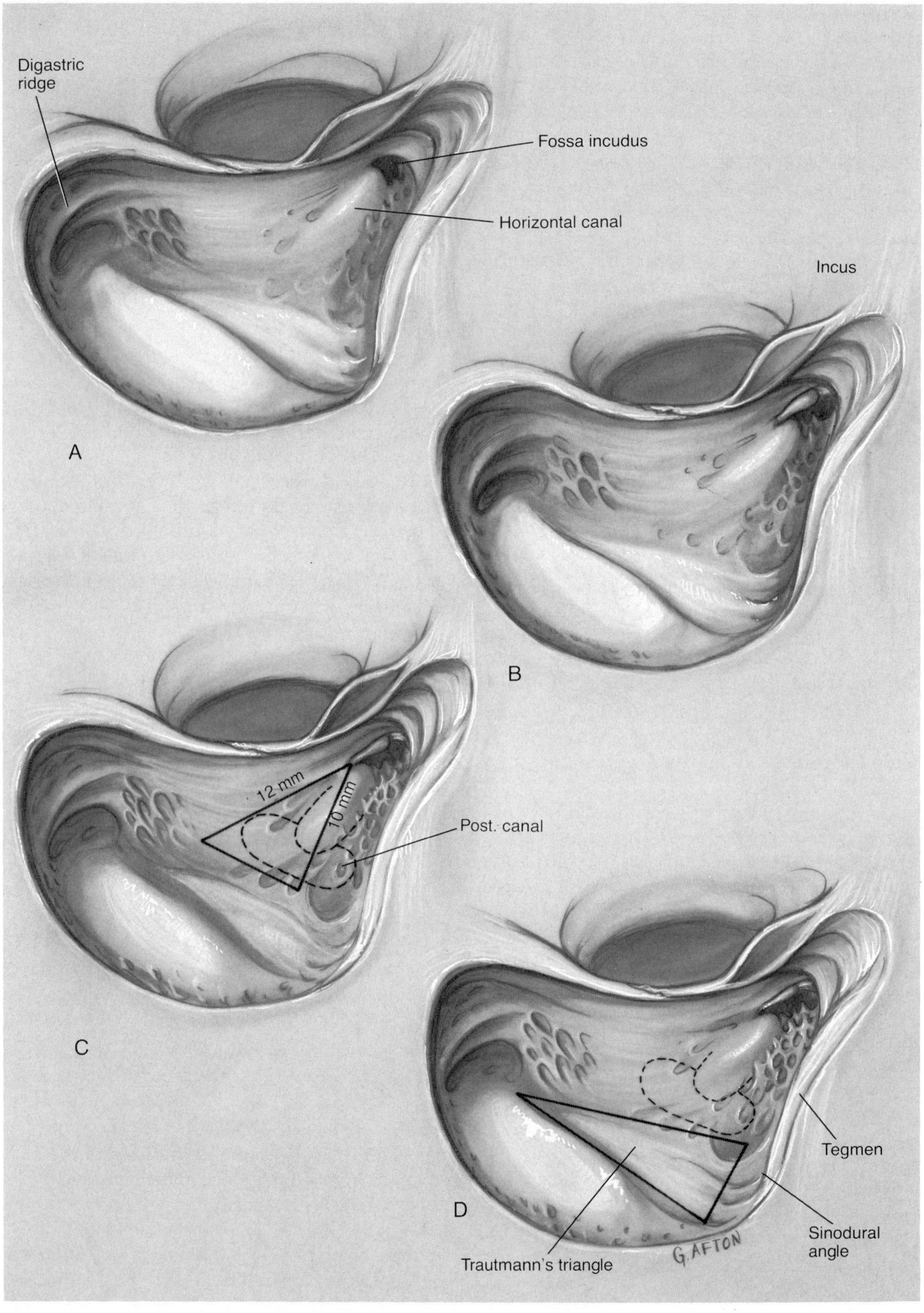
Digastric ridge
Fossa incudus
Horizontal canal
A
Incus
B
12 mm
10 mm
Post. canal
C
Tegmen
D
Sinodural angle
Trautmann's triangle
G. AFTON

FIGURE 5–3.

Pitfalls

1. Skeletonizing or damaging the posterior semicircular canal.
2. Insufficient unroofing of the dural plate.
3. Failing to identify the endolymphatic sac and its lumen.
4. Damaging the incus.
5. Depositing debris in the middle ear.
6. Lateral sinus bleeding.

Procedure

In endolymphatic sac surgery, the authors advocate a thorough simple mastoidectomy (which has already been done). In our dissection, we have already identified the bone plate overlying the posterior cranial fossa dura. Redefine Trautmann's triangle, identify the hard bone containing the posterior semicircular canal, and measure the distances again (Fig. 5–4*B*): 10 mm from the tip of the short process of the incus or fossa incudis, along the axis of the horizontal semicircular canal (30 degrees from the tegmen); 12 mm from the fossa incudis at an angle of 45 degrees from the tegmen. Drill into the infralabyrinthine cell tract to help expose the sac location. Pay special attention to the position of the sigmoid sinus. On occasion it partially overlies the dural plate, reducing the size of Trautmann's triangle. The plate is thinned down to eggshell thickness, then gently elevated and separated from the underlying dura with a duckbill elevator. The sac is identifiable as a thickened white area of the dura over the thin surrounding dura (Fig. 5–5). The posterior semicircular canal shoud *not* be thinned or skeletonized. Drilling is done immediately inferior to this area. The sac comes toward the dura from the direction of the posterior semicircular canal. If the lateral sinus is in such a position that it tends to partially cover the dura or make access to it difficult, first recheck the position of the bone; the "head" might be bent too far forward. If the sinus is still prominent after repositioning of the "head," it should be decompressed by removing part of its bony covering facing the dura. Infralabyrinthine cells might have to be drilled (leading toward the jugular bulb). The sac is incised gently with a sickle knife and the lumen probed with a Whirlybird.

Facial Recess Approach, Posterior Tympanotomy

Aim

Removal of air cells immediately lateral to the facial nerve at the external genu (facial recess collection of air cells).

Highlights

1. Define the landmarks clearly.
2. Thin the posterior canal wall.
3. Drill parallel to facial nerve fibers.
4. If the approach is troublesome, combine transmastoid and transcanal visualization.

Pitfalls

1. Damaging the facial nerve.
2. Perforating the bony external ear canal.
3. Perforating the tympanic membrane.
4. Those of a simple mastoidectomy.

Procedure

Define your landmarks (Fig. 5–6*A*). The external genu of the facial nerve is medial; the fossa incudis is superior. Thin the posterior canal wall. Identify the facial nerve by its pearly white color underneath the thin layer of bone. The bone is still too thick; thin it down very carefully by drilling parallel to the direction of the facial nerve fibers (Fig. 5–6*B*). Small cutting burs should be used since the recess is quite small. Inferiorly, identify the chorda tympani (which is to be preserved) as it leaves the facial nerve in an anterosuperior direction; it then takes a lateral direction toward the annulus (Fig. 5–7*A*). On occasion, the facial recess is quite small and the procedure difficult. Rather than insisting on taking unnecessary risks, use a combined transcanal-transmastoid approach.

Text continued on page 54

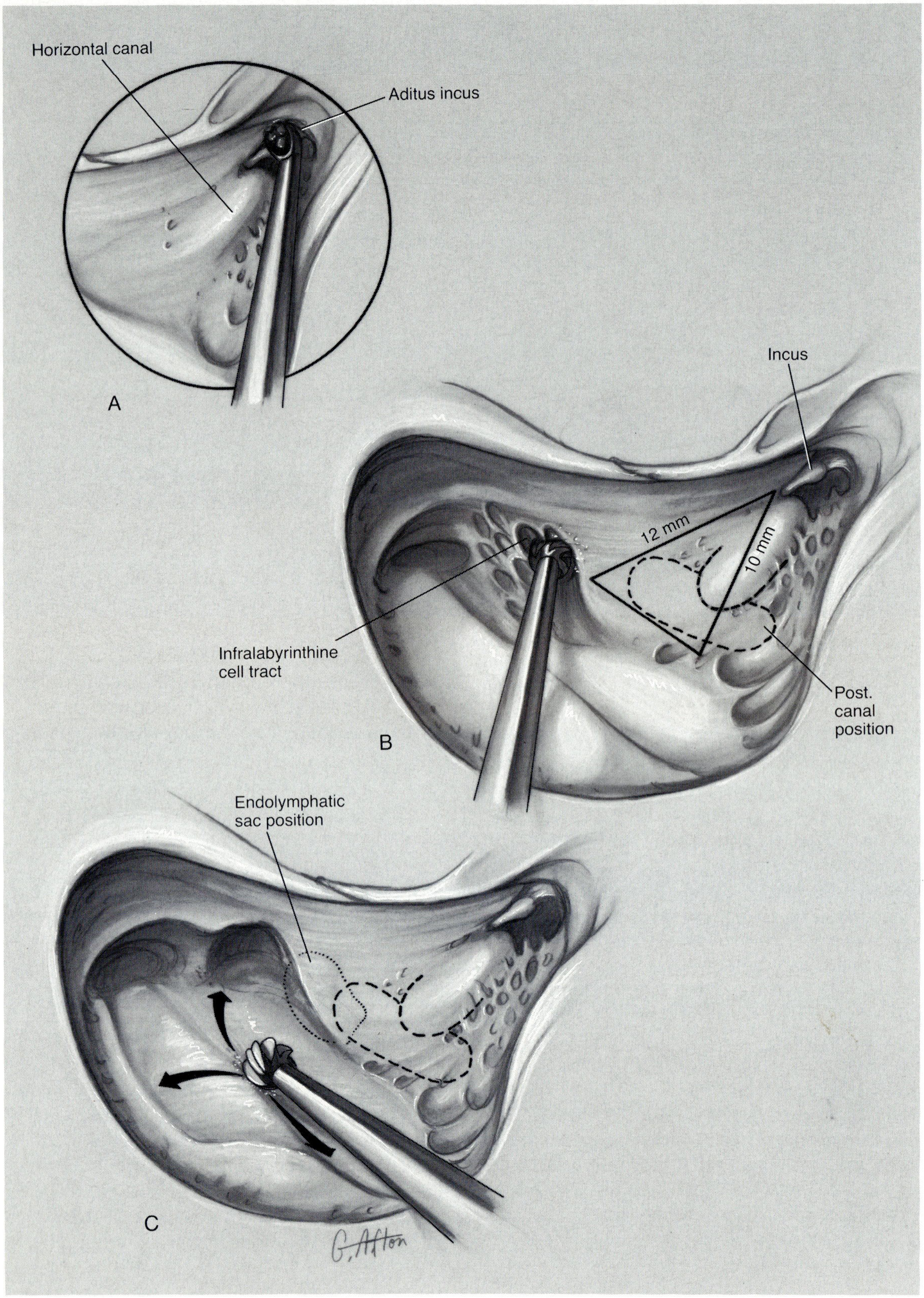
Horizontal canal
Aditus incus
A
Incus
12 mm
10 mm
Infralabyrinthine cell tract
Post. canal position
B
Endolymphatic sac position
C
G. Afton

FIGURE 5–4.

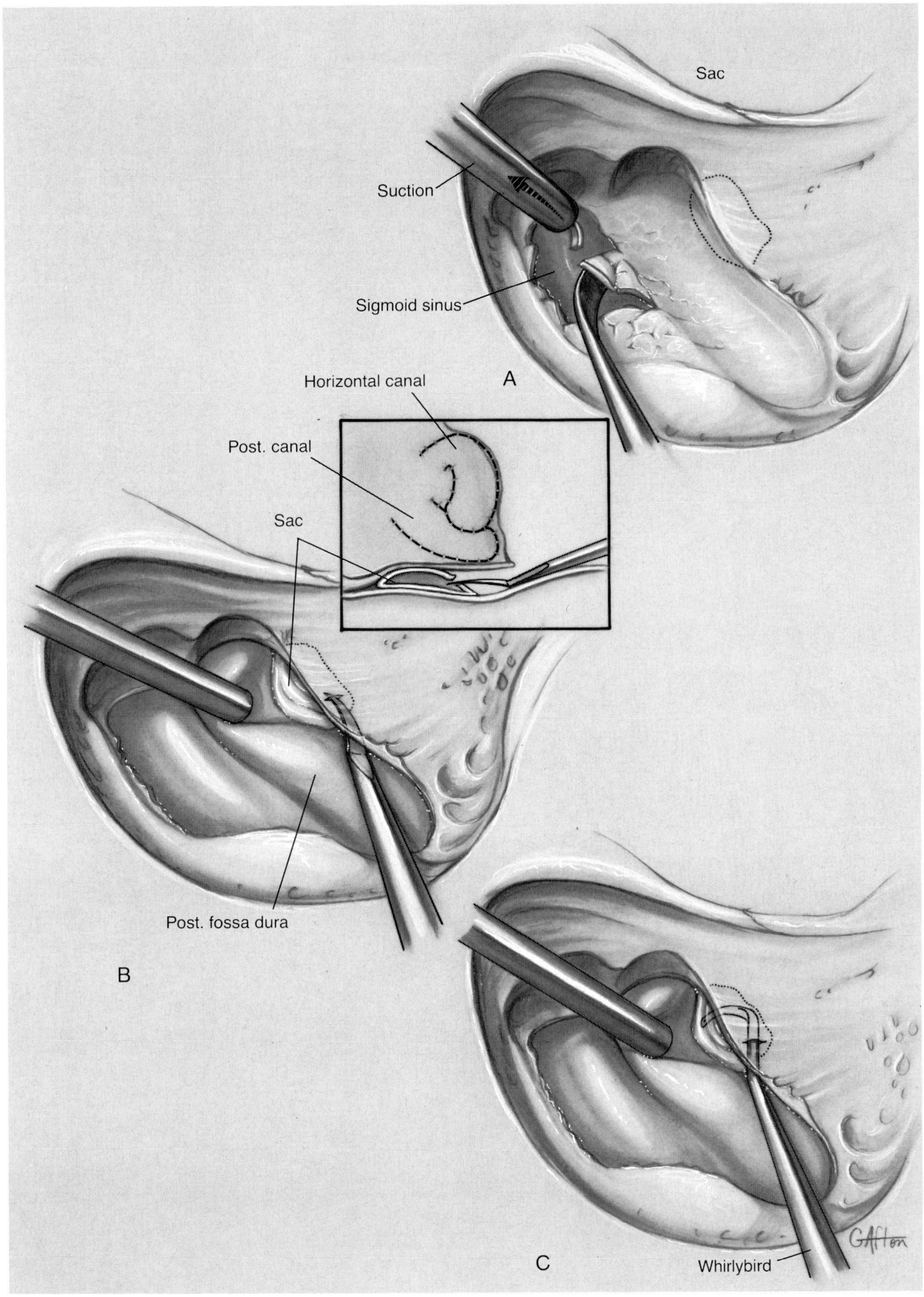
Sac
Suction
Sigmoid sinus
Horizontal canal
A
Post. canal
Sac
Post. fossa dura
B
C
Whirlybird
GAlton

FIGURE 5–5.

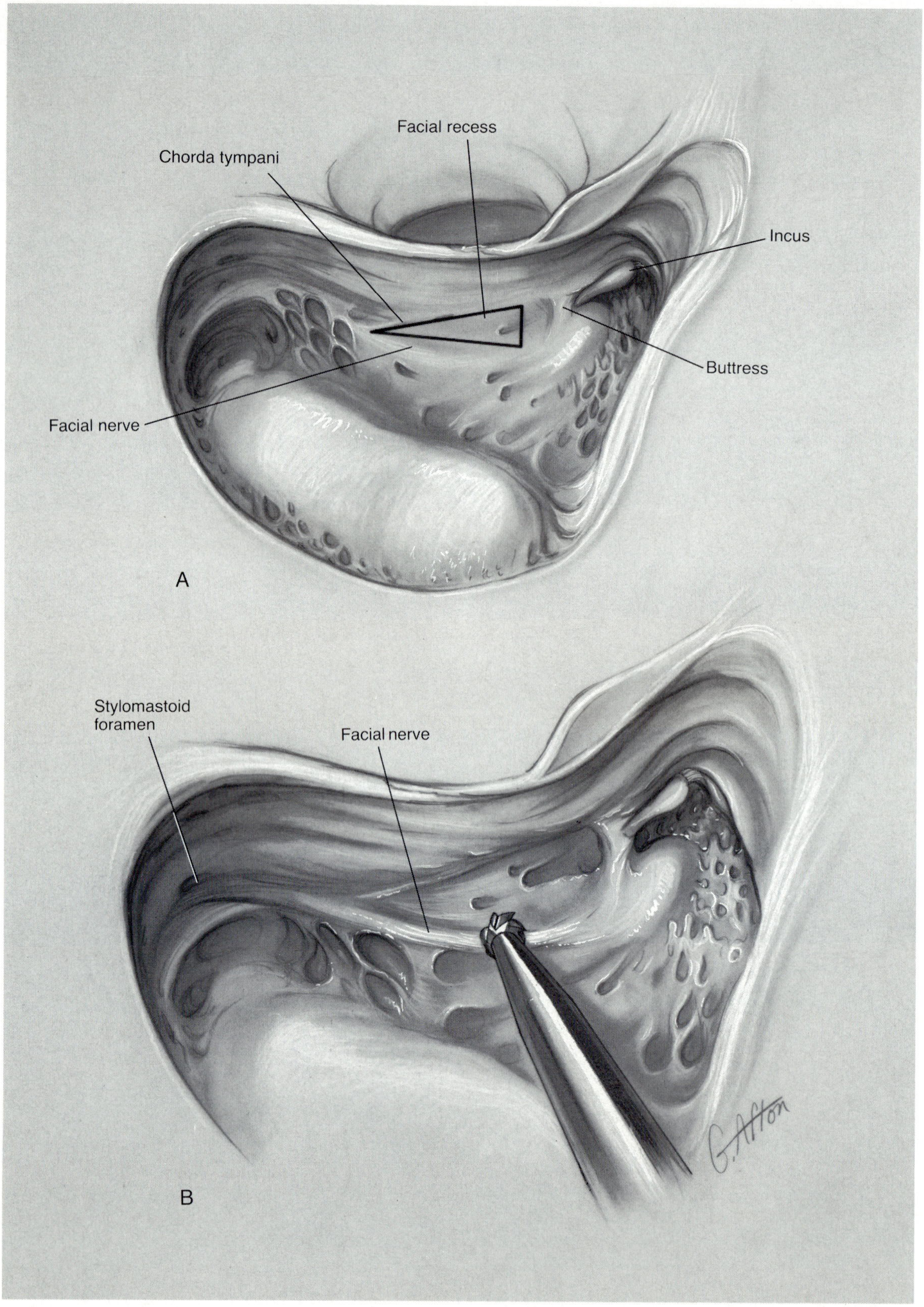
Facial recess
Chorda tympani
Incus
Buttress
Facial nerve
A
Stylomastoid
foramen
Facial nerve
B
G. Afton

FIGURE 5–6.

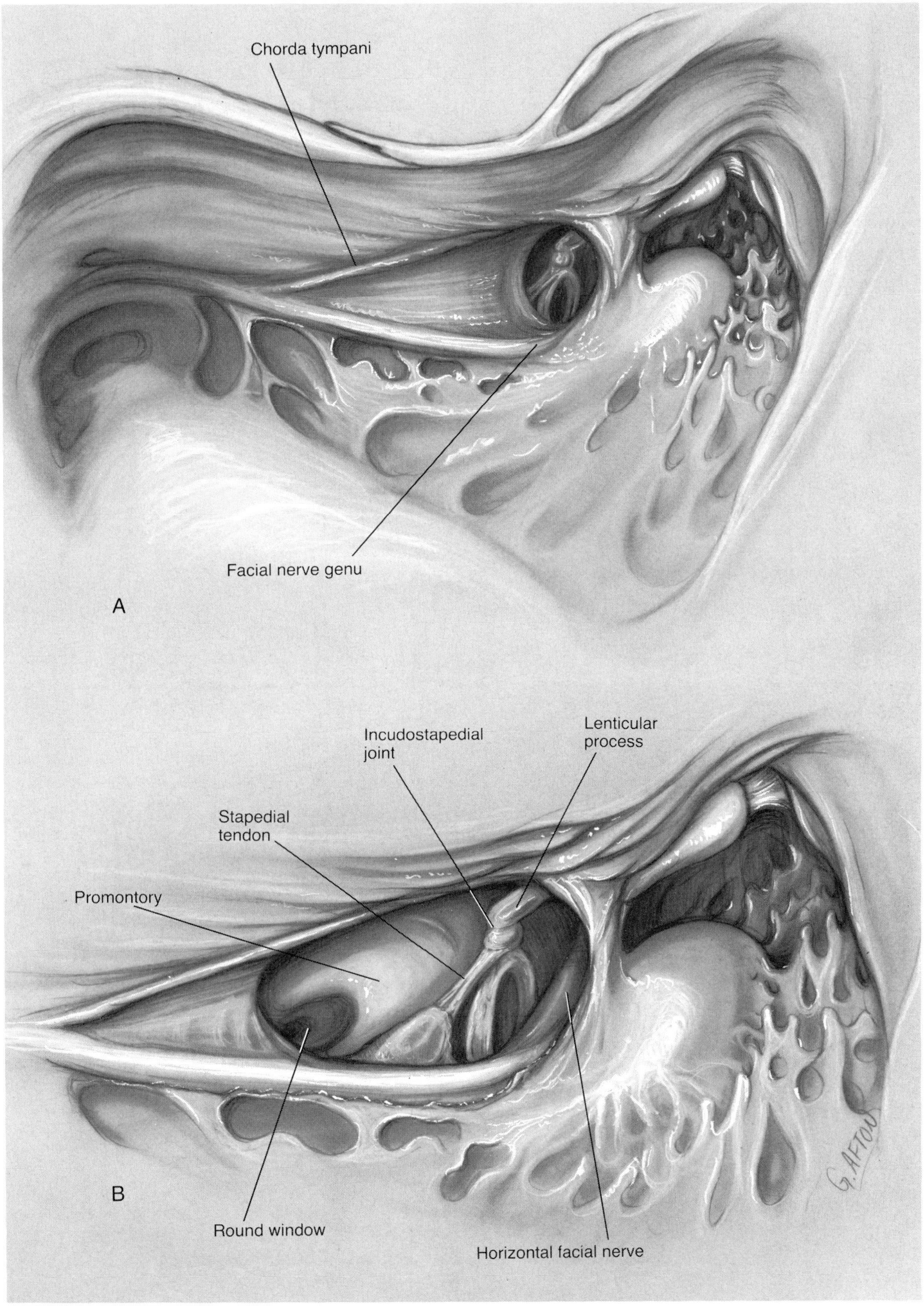
Chorda tympani
Facial nerve genu
A
Incudostapedial joint
Lenticular process
Stapedial tendon
Promontory
B
Round window
Horizontal facial nerve
G. AFTON

FIGURE 5–7.

Once the recess is opened, the landmarks are reidentified: the external genu of the facial nerve is medial; the fossa incudis is superior; the chorda tympani is inferolateral and posterior; and the tympanic membrane is anterolateral.

Now observe the following structures (Fig. 5–7*B*): the horizontal portion of the facial nerve, the lenticular process of the incus, the incudostapedial joint, the capitulum of the stapes, and the stapedial tendon. Next identify the promontory, and inferomedially the round window niche.

Cochlear Implant (Facial Recess Approach)

Aim

To place an electrode into the cochlea by sliding it through the round window. (We will deal only with intracochlear electrode placement and with electrodes that are placed far into the interior of the cochlea.)

Highlights

1. Ensure good visualization via an adequate facial recess approach.
2. Clearly identify the round window niche and round window membrane.

Pitfalls

1. Those of the facial recess approach itself.
2. Inadequate visualization of the round window, with the electrode unable to be passed beyond the hook.

Surgical Steps

1. Those of a simple mastoidectomy and facial recess approach.
2. Prepare a seat for the internal receiver.
3. Insert the intracochlear electrode.

Procedure

At this point in the dissection, the main drilling for the procedure has been done. You are left with inserting the electrode through the round window and drilling a seat for the internal receiver posterosuperior to the mastoid cavity. Locate a position for the internal receiver; it should be immediately posterior to the posterior limit of the drilled mastoid cavity, with its anterior (toward the ear canal) border no further than where the border of the imaginary pinna (auricle) would be if it were pushed posterior (that is, immediately posterior to the posterior border of the pinna). Superiorly, the border should not be above the superior border of the pinna. Drill a seat, using as a guideline the circumference of the internal receiver of your practice electrode (Fig. 5–8). If a practice electrode is not available, drill a seat into which a nickel-sized coin would fit. Drilling can be done carefully with a regular bur, or it can be done with either a butterfly bur or a bur specially designed by one of the cochlear implant manufacturers. If a screw type of internal receiver is to be used, drill four holes in the corresponding openings of the base of the pedestal to a maximum depth of 2 mm.

Regardless of the type of internal receiver, with a small bur drill two small holes immediately superior and inferior to the location of your already drilled seat, that is, two holes superiorly and two holes inferiorly (Fig. 5–9*A*). Bring the small holes together very carefully. Then pass 2-0 silk through these openings (Fig. 5–9*B*); this will be used to cross over the internal receiver and seat it in place. Do not place your internal receiver yet.

Our attention is now turned back to the active electrode. Again, visualize the round window niche. If visualization is not adequate, a transcanal approach can be made. Verify the opening of the round window niche. On occasion, it is necessary or useful to gently drill the anterior border of the niche (Fig. 5–9*D*). This will provide a slightly larger opening with beter visualization, and at the same time will present a "straight shot" at the cochlea, skipping the hook portion that sometimes is difficult to bypass. Position the electrode in the opening of the window and then gently push it in, using a blunt pick or wire guide or one of the special electrode guides provided by the implant manufacturers (Fig. 5–10). If there is some resistance, it is likely that the electrode is caught up in the hook. Retract the electrode gently and try to rotate it, while imagining the direction of the cochlea. On the left, for example, turn gently toward the right (clockwise); on the right, turn gently toward the left

Text continued on page 59

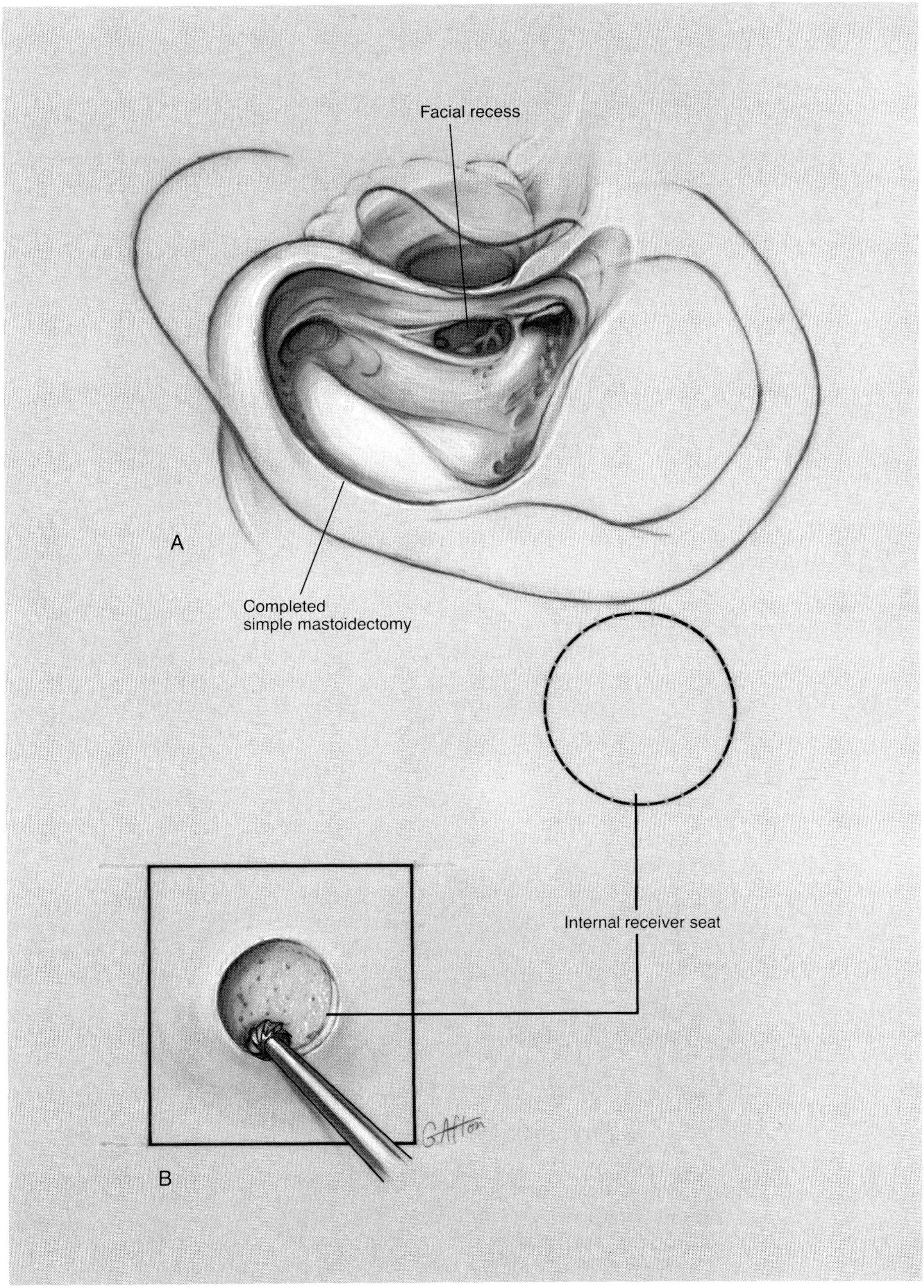
Facial recess
A
Completed
simple mastoidectomy
Internal receiver seat
B

FIGURE 5–8.

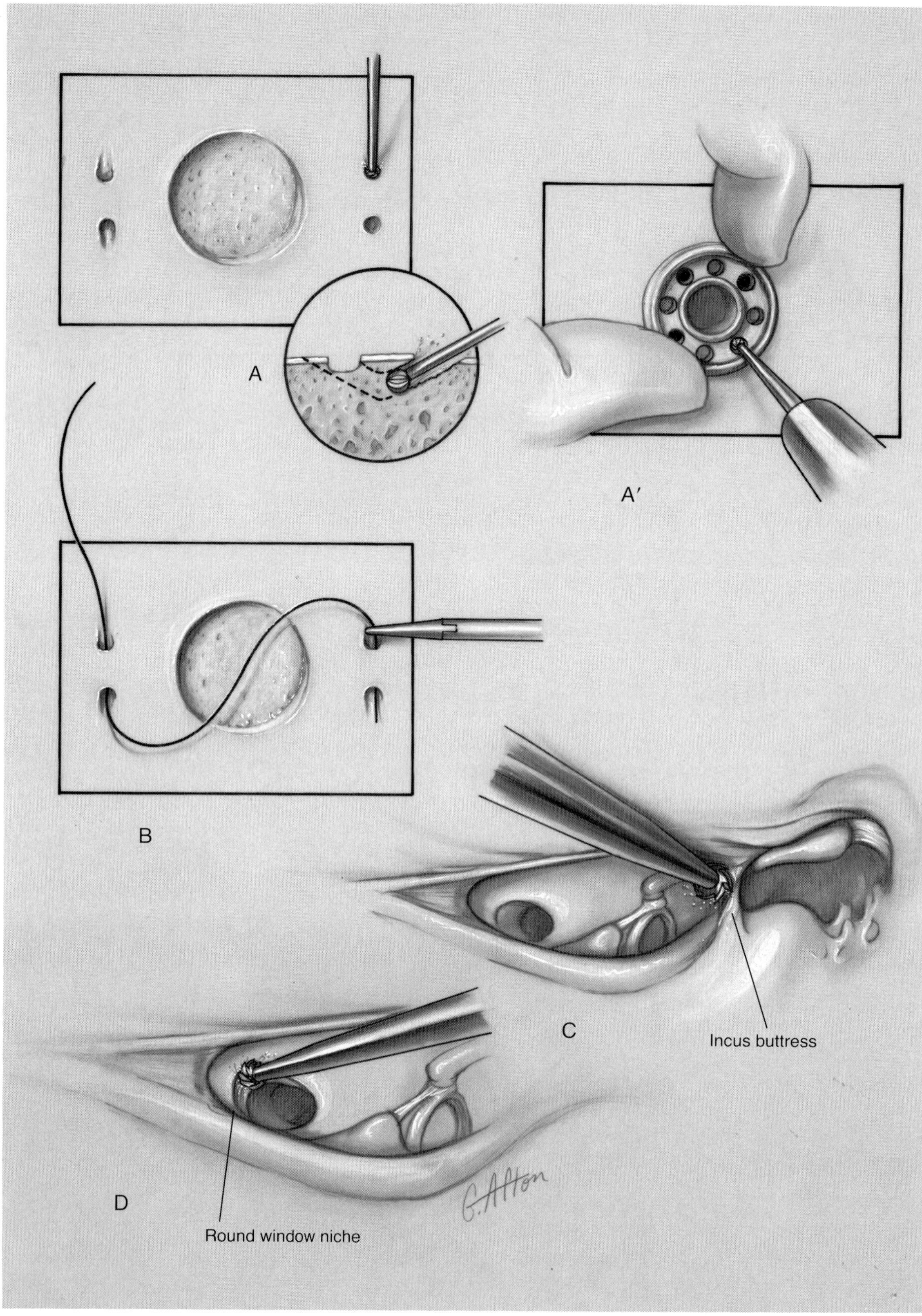

FIGURE 5–9.

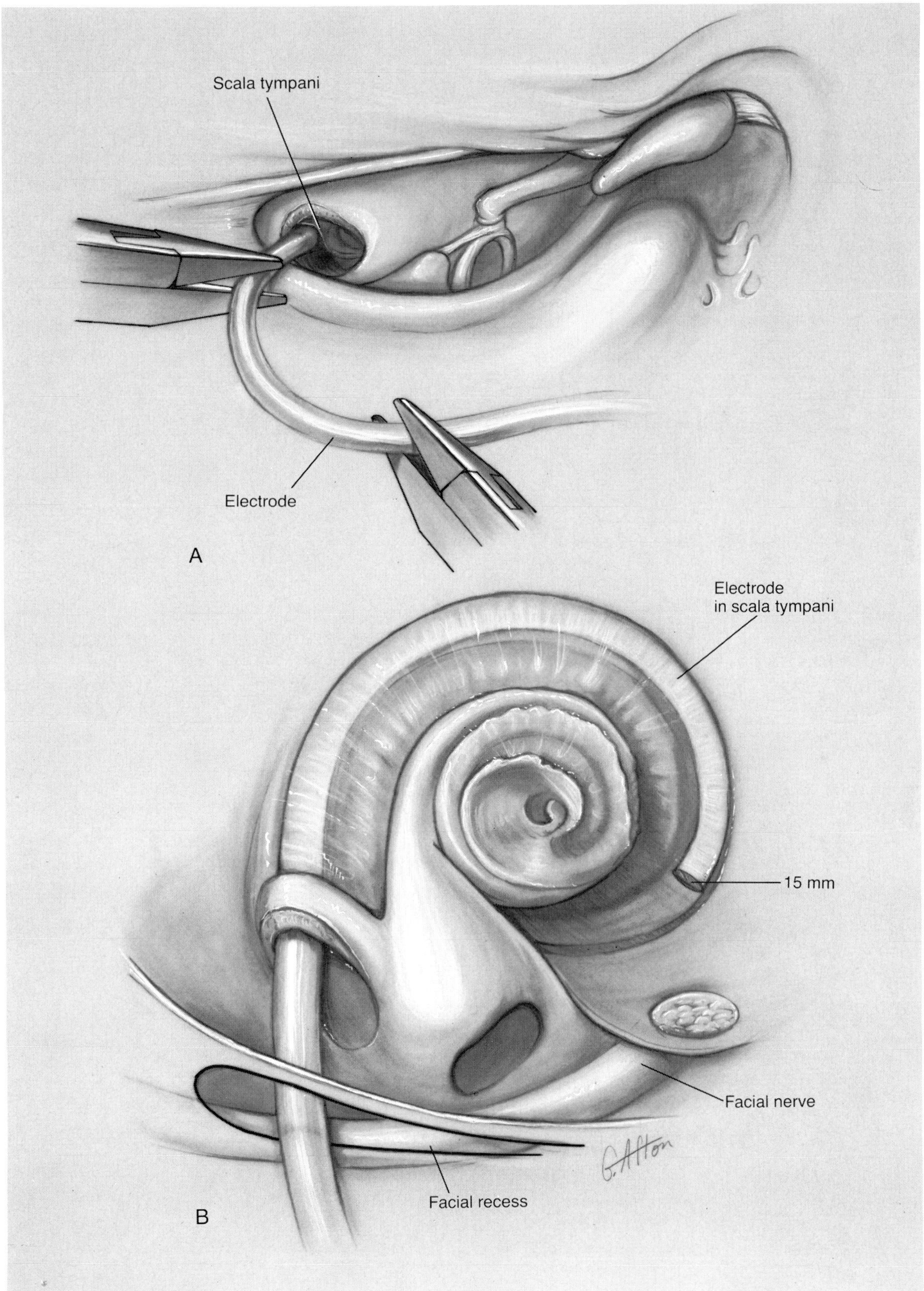
Scala tympani
Electrode
A
Electrode
in scala tympani
15 mm
Facial nerve
Facial recess
B
G. Alton

FIGURE 5–10.

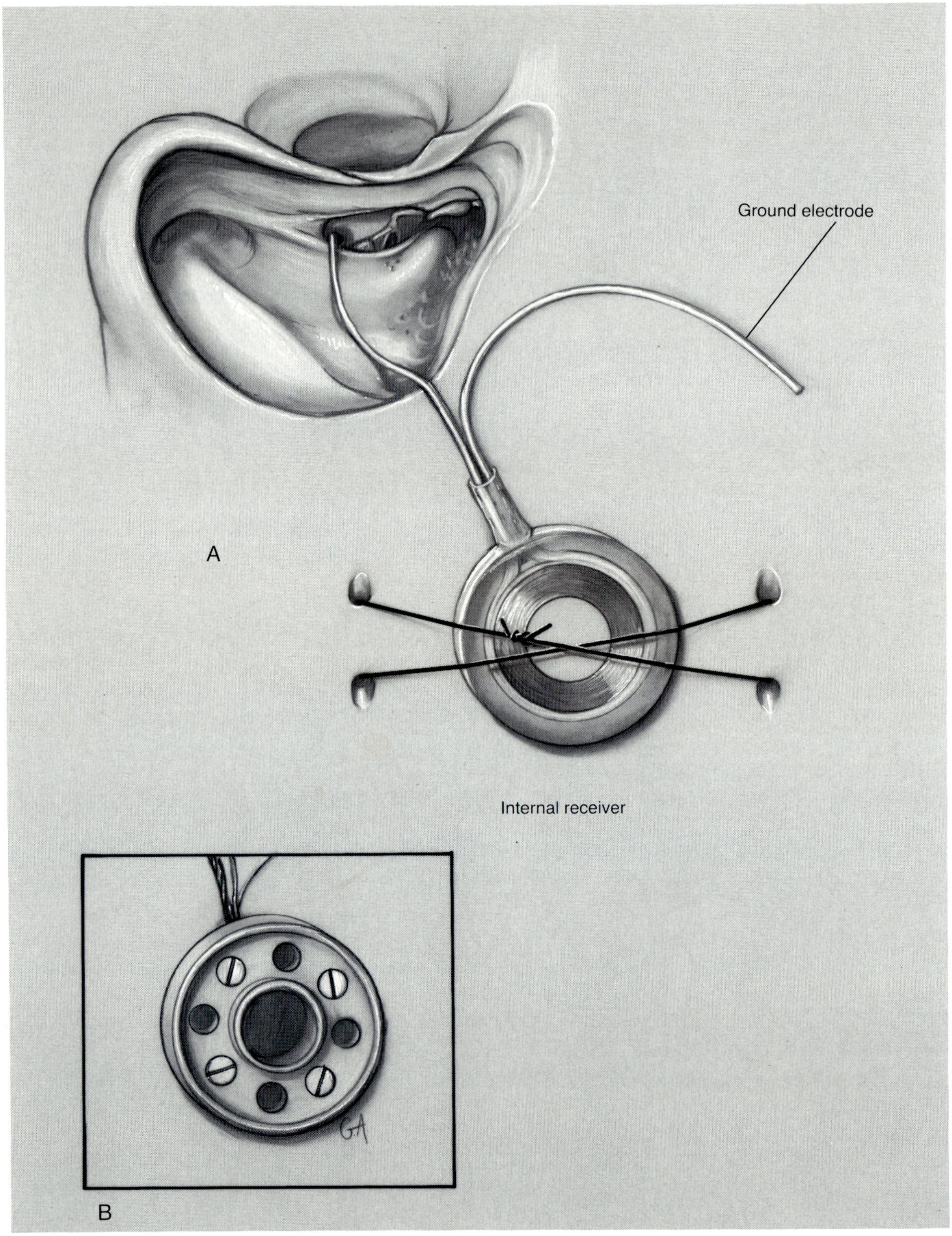

FIGURE 5–11.

(counterclockwise). Place the electrode and then secure the internal receiver with either screws or sutures (Fig. 5–11).

Transmastoid Facial Nerve Decompression

Highlights and pitfalls are discussed in the text.

Surgical Steps

1. Those of a simple mastoidectomy.
2. Identify the different segments of the facial nerve, and skeletonize the fallopian canal.
3. Fracture and remove any bony covering.
4. Open the sheath of the facial canal.

Procedure

In the course of the complete simple mastoidectomy, the vertical portion and external genu of the facial nerve were fairly well delineated. For practical surgical purposes the facial nerve can be divided into three segments: (1) that within the internal auditory canal; (2) the tympanic segment (horizontal/middle ear); and (3) the vertical segment (mastoid). We will deal now with the vertical and horizontal segments, in that order.

From the external genu, the nerve proceeds vertically to the stylomastoid foramen at the level of the anterior edge of the digastric ridge (Fig. 5–12). It is important to visualize its anatomy and, if possible, compare it with other bones, since there is considerable variation. The nerve is lateral to the horizontal canal; however, it may have a posterior projection at the genu, lending itself to potential damage. It is useful to visualize the nerve anterior to the digastric ridge and to appreciate how lateral it becomes as it reaches the mastoid tip. Its tympanic or middle ear segment appears in the region of the cochleariform process at the geniculate ganglion, then runs posteriorly towards the oval window (stapes) to a point just inferior and usually medial (deep) to the horizontal semicircular canal.

The vertical segment can be dissected from the level of the fossa incudis or from the digastric ridge. From the ridge it can be followed superiorly to the external genu; however, this is not a reliable landmark. Although this approach is perfectly acceptable, the authors tend to follow nerves peripherally rather than centrally, which seems both safer and simpler.

After visualization of the genu, the canal is skeletonized all the way down to the stylomastoid foramen. Drilling is done in strokes parallel to the direction of the nerve (superior to inferior or vice versa). Exposure of the tympanic segment is helped by enlarging the aditus ad antrum. This dissection, plus enlargement of the facial recess approach, allows visualization anteriorly toward the cochleariform process. Visualize the segment at the level of the oval window and the pyramidal eminence. This is a very useful image to keep in mind. If necessary, adequate visualization can be obtained by a combined approach. Visualize the tympanic segment through the canal. It is also possible to obtain adequate visualization by removing the incus (Fig. 5–13*A*). Before disarticulating the incus, try to drill under it without damaging or dislocating it, using the smallest possible burs. Now try to remove and replace the incus. If drilling toward the geniculate ganglion was incomplete, drill now without the incus in place. (The incus should be left in place for use in the next procedure; however, practice placing and replacing the incus to become familiar with its normal anatomic position.) Once the entire facial canal has been thinned to eggshell consistency, fracture it with a pick and lift the bone fragments gently with a Whirlybird *without using the facial nerve as a fulcrum* (Fig. 5–13*B*). The sheath is then opened with a sharp sickle knife (Fig. 5–13C).

Canalplasty (Fig. 5–14)

Aim

Enlargement of the bony canal and visualization of the entire fibrous and bony annulus.

Pitfalls

Excessive drilling of the anterior wall and entrance into the temporomandibular joint space.

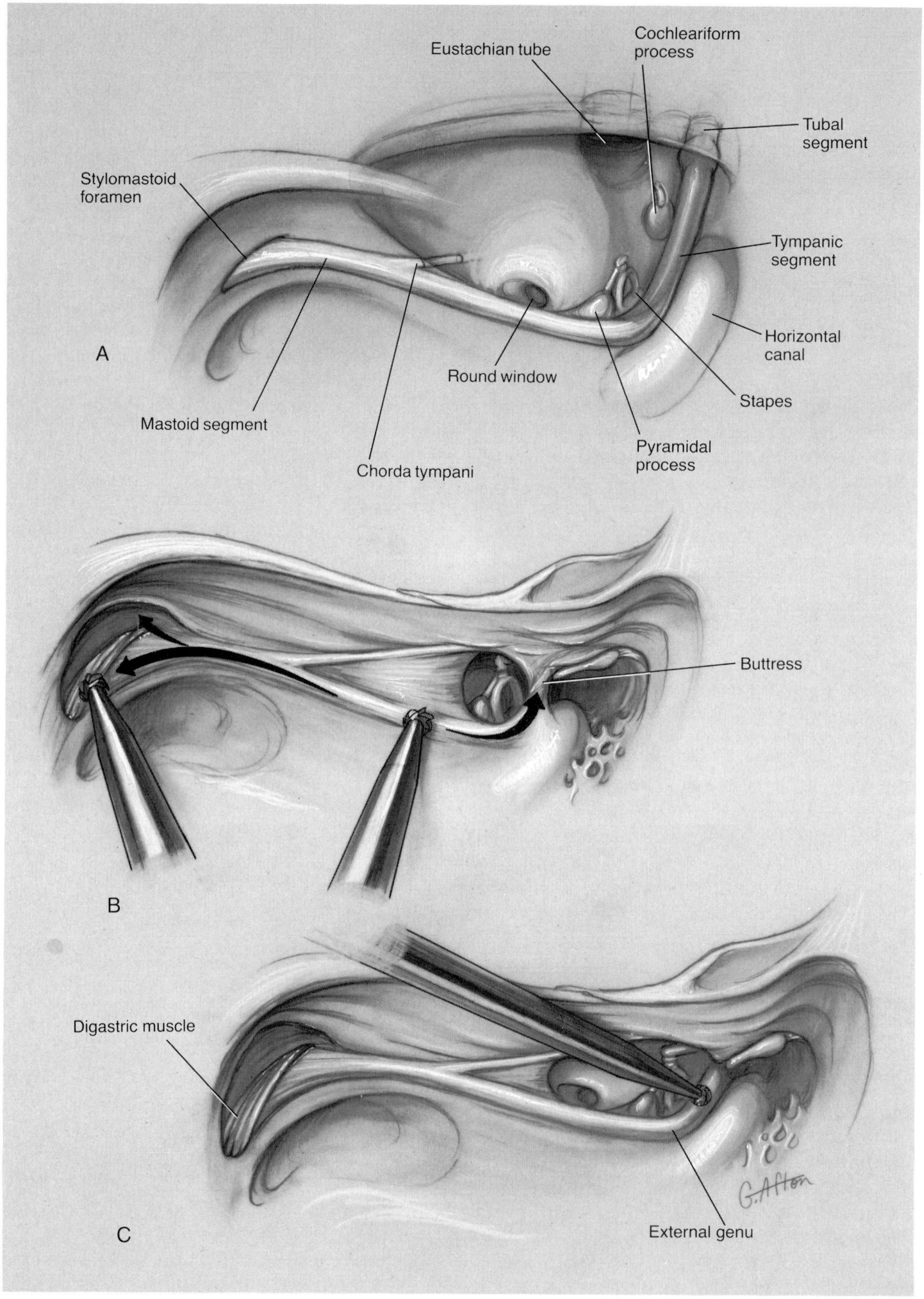

Eustachian tube
Cochleariform process
Tubal segment
Stylomastoid foramen
Tympanic segment
Horizontal canal
A
Round window
Stapes
Mastoid segment
Pyramidal process
Chorda tympani
Buttress
B
Digastric muscle
C
External genu
G. Afton

FIGURE 5–12.

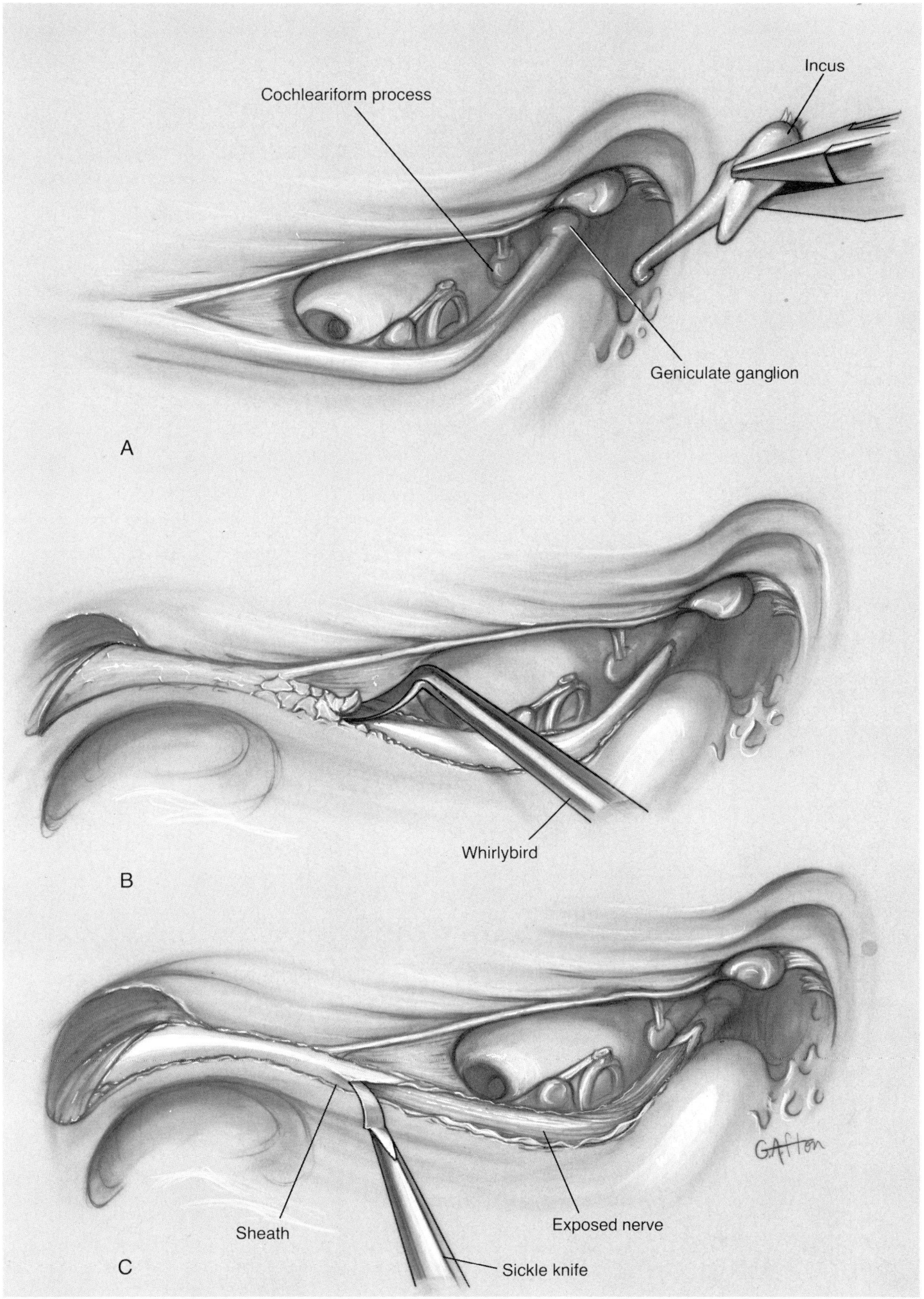
Incus
Cochleariform process
Geniculate ganglion
A
Whirlybird
B
Sheath
Exposed nerve
Sickle knife
C
GAfton

FIGURE 5–13.

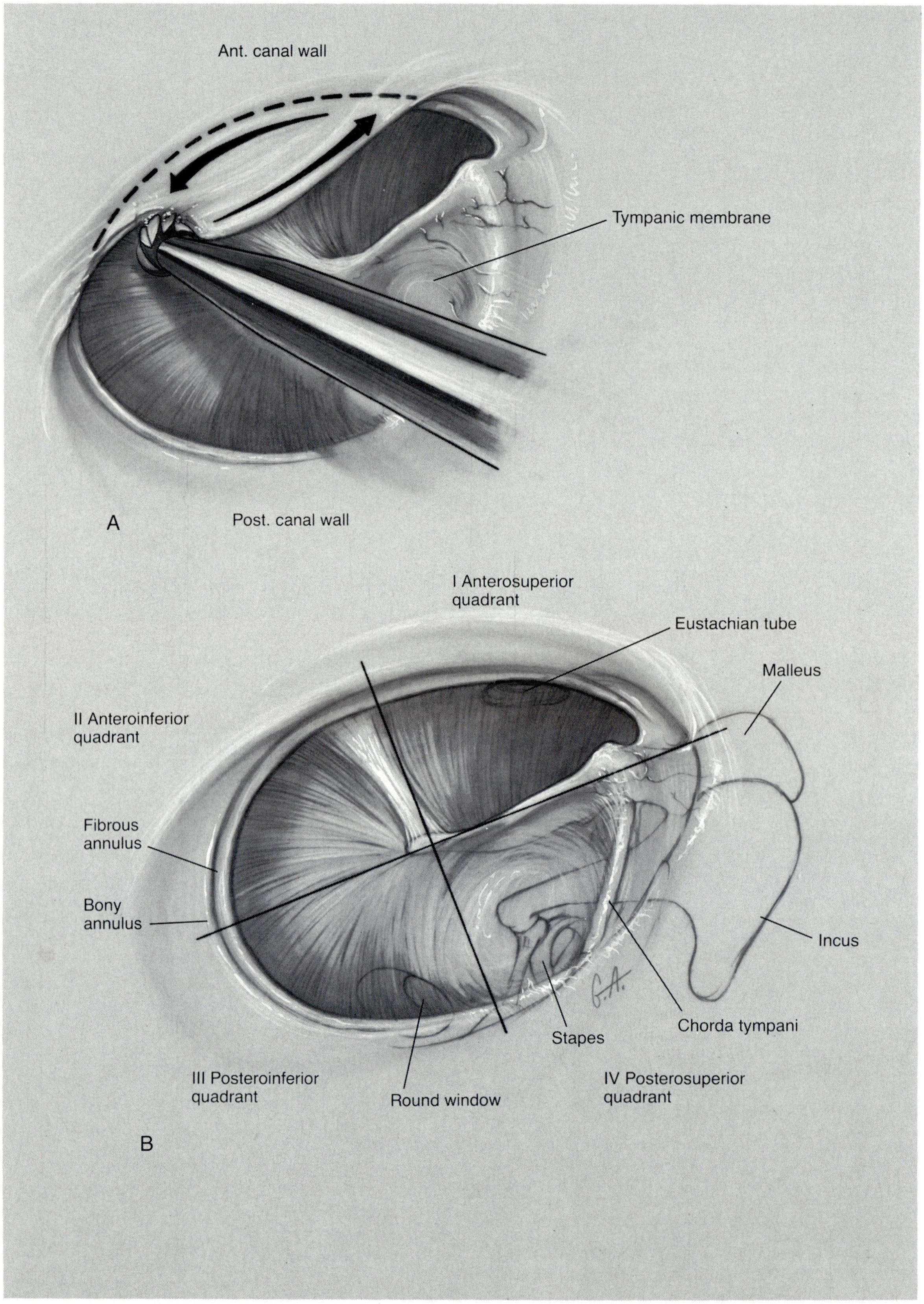
Ant. canal wall
Tympanic membrane
A
Post. canal wall
I Anterosuperior quadrant
Eustachian tube
Malleus
II Anteroinferior quadrant
Fibrous annulus
Bony annulus
Incus
Stapes
Chorda tympani
III Posteroinferior quadrant
Round window
IV Posterosuperior quadrant
B

FIGURE 5–14.

Procedure

Using a large bur, drill the canal wall evenly until visualization of the entire fibrous annulus is achieved (Fig. 5–14*A*). Do not drill in one spot, but "sweep" the bur gently with even pressure and go one step at a time. (Skin procedures will not be dealt with, since the skin is thick, tight, and difficult to elevate adequately for these purposes in harvested temporal bones.)

Underlay Graft of the Tympanic Membrane

Aim

Placement of a graft under the tympanic membrane, covering all edges of the perforation.

Procedure

Visualize the tympanic membrane. Imagine it in four quadrants (Fig. 5–14*B*). Using a straight pick and a sickle knife, make a central perforation (Fig. 5–15*A*). Fill the middle ear space with Gelfoam (Fig. 5–15*B*). Obtain a piece of fascia (or paper) that exceeds the size of the perforation by at least 30%. Scarify the undersurface of the tympanic membrane around the perforation, using a Hough hoe. Now place the graft over the perforation and position it medially by using the Hough hoe (Fig. 5–15*C*, *D*).

Ossiculoplasty (Incus Procedures)

Aim

Restoration of ossicular chain continuity (in this case, where incus problems are the cause of the loss).

Procedure

Remove the "graft," the entire tympanic membrane, and the Gelfoam filling the cavity. Now visualize the cavity and what is found beneath the different quadrants (see Fig. 5–14*B*). Familiarize yourself with the anatomy. Mobilize the temporal bone and learn what areas can be seen best at different angles. Palpate the ossicles with a blunt pick, and observe the round window niche area, the opening of the eustachian tube, the stapedial tendon, and other features. Compare the views of the middle ear cavity with the transcanal and posterior tympanotomy approaches. The incus is already loose.

Clip the distalmost portion of the long process of the incus ("necrosis of the lenticular process") (Fig. 5–16*A*). Since the mastoidectomy has been done already, remove a piece of "cortical bone" posterior to the mastoid cavity opening. Using a small bur, delineate a square of bone and remove it. Shape this piece of bone in order to restore continuity. Drill a small acetabulum for the head of the stapes and a groove for the remaining long process of the incus (Fig 5–16*B–E*).

Remove the entire incus. Restoration of ossicular continuity in this case can be achieved in a number of ways (Fig. 5–17). We will use a sculptured incus, a sculptured cortical bone and, if available, a partial ossicular replacement prosthesis (PORP). Clip the short process of the incus and drill an acetabulum in the remaining long process, for fitting over the head of the stapes. Then drill a groove over the remaining body for fitting under the malleus. Now try to sculpture a piece of cortical bone in this same shape. Avoid contact of the incus graft with the promontory. Try a PORP as well, if available.

Intact Bridge Mastoidectomy (IBM), Modified Radical Mastoidectomy, and Radical Mastoidectomy

Aims

Exteriorization of the disease process within the epitympanum, antrum, and mastoid to the meatus.

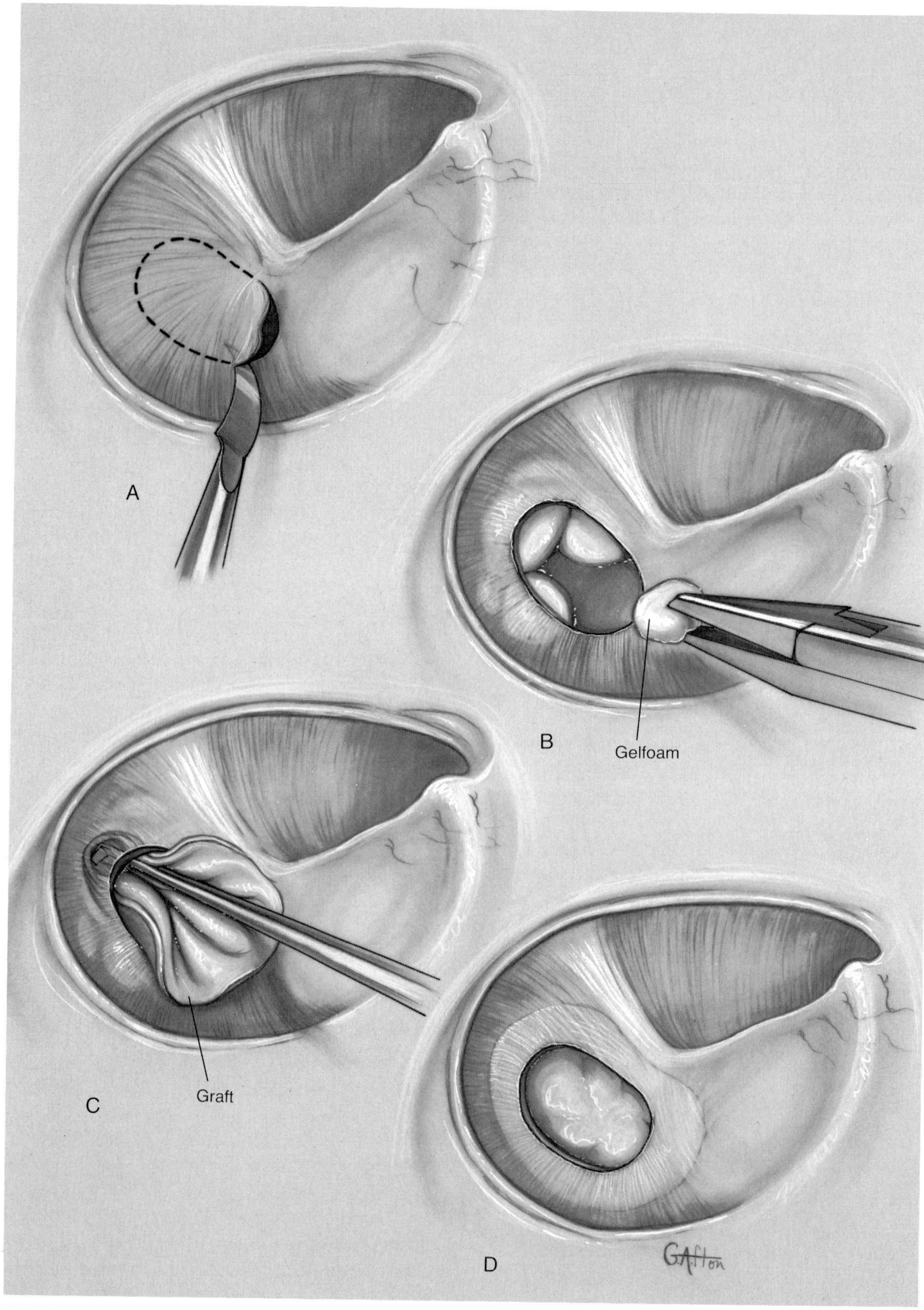

FIGURE 5–15.

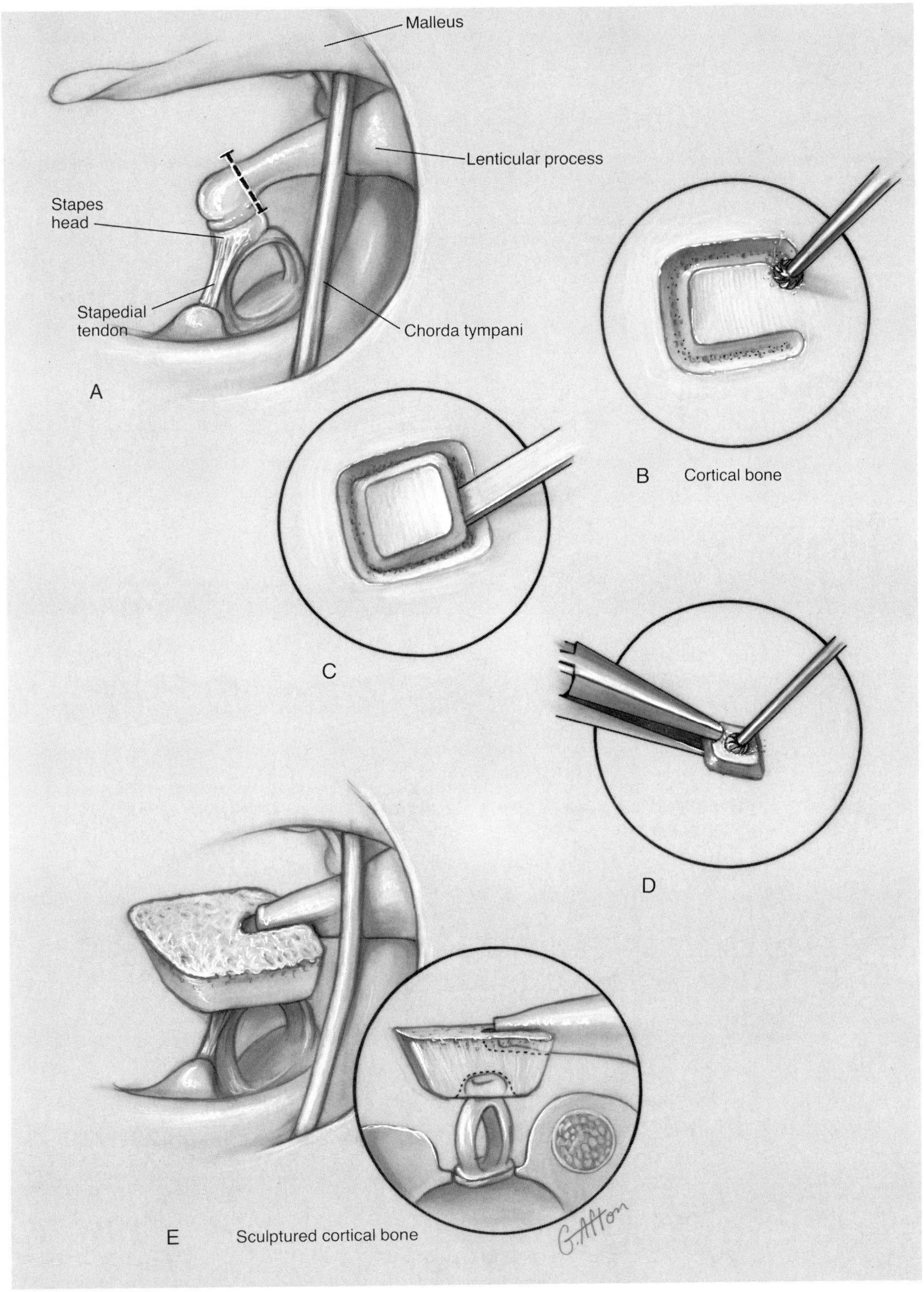
Malleus
Lenticular process
Stapes head
Stapedial tendon
Chorda tympani
A
B Cortical bone
C
D
E Sculptured cortical bone
G. Alton

FIGURE 5–16.

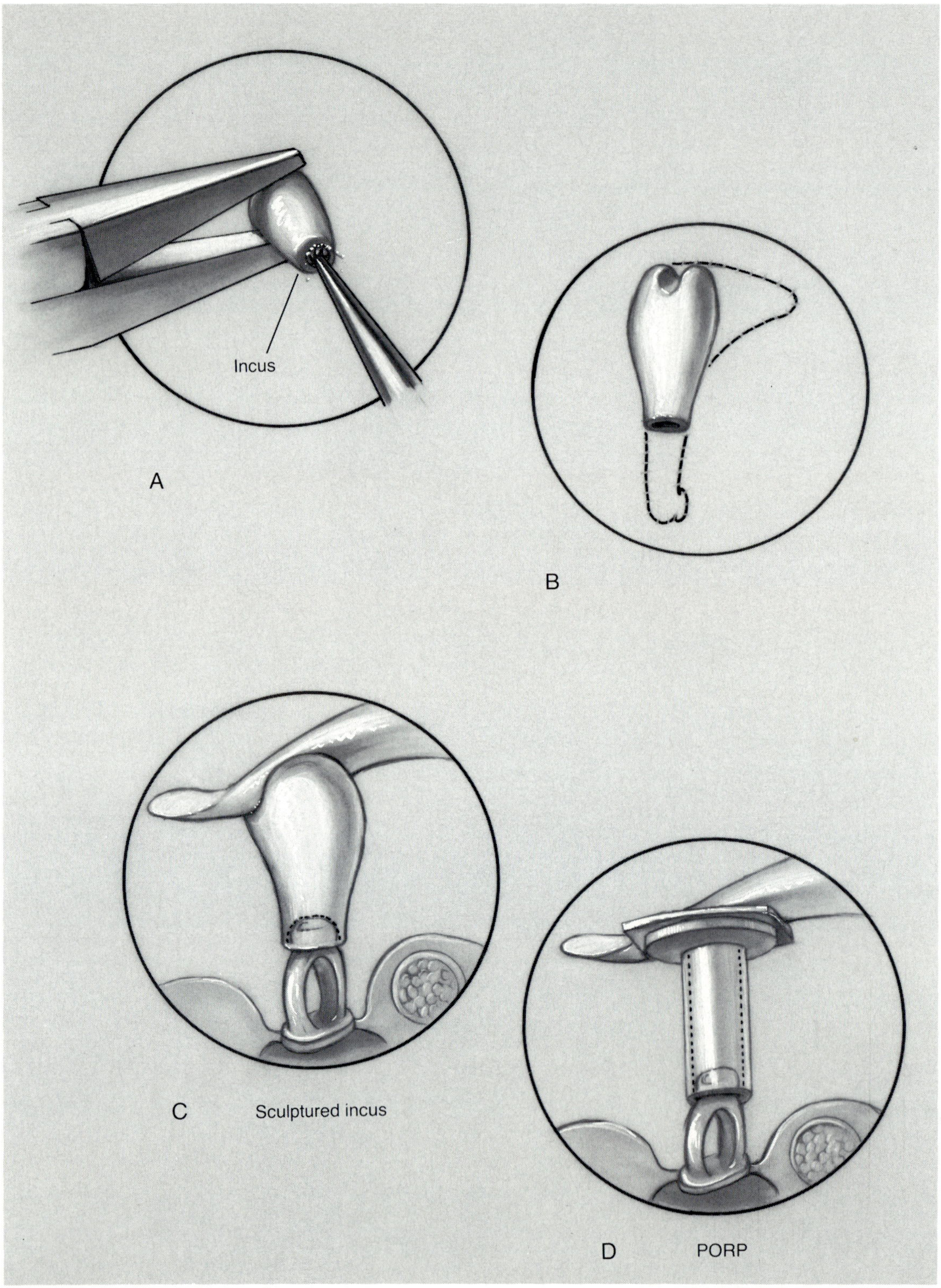

FIGURE 5–17.

The IBM is a version of modified radical mastoidectomy with bridge preservation, allowing tympanoplasty repairs.

Highlights

1. Enlarging the anterior canal wall without opening the temporomandibular joint, and visualizing the entire fibrous and bony annulus.
2. Large meatoplasty is crucial for the success of the procedure.

Pitfalls

1. Incomplete removal of the posterior meatal wall.
2. Poor meatoplasty.

Surgical Steps

1. Meatoplasty.
2. Canalplasty.
3. Saucerize the mastoid circumferentially.
4. Enlarge the aditus and sculpture the bridge to widen the mesotympanum.
5. Remove all disease.
6. Preserve when possible the anterior tympanic membrane and manubrium.
7. Use a ventilation tube.
8. Ossiculoplasty, tympanoplasty.
9. Obliterate the aditus with periosteum or cartilage.
10. Obliterate the mastoid (usually not necessary).
11. Thiersch graft (at the primary procedure or 3–4 weeks postoperatively).

Procedure

These procedures involve removal of the posterior meatal wall. The original Bondy modified radical mastoidectomy implies this step; however, in the Bondy procedure the middle ear cavity is not entered. Both the IBM and the modified radical mastoidectomy imply entering the middle ear.

Intact Bridge Mastoidectomy

The "bridge" is the most medial portion of the posterosuperior meatal wall; it is literally the bridge that crosses the attic toward the tegmental area. It has both anterior and posterior buttresses. The anterior buttress is the superior portion where the posterior bony canal meets the tegmen. The posterior buttress is the inferior portion where the posterior bony canal meets the floor of the external auditory canal, lateral to the facial nerve. Drill the anterior canal wall, enlarging it until clearly visualizing the entire fibrous and bony annulus but without entering the temporomandibular joint space (Fig. 5–18*A*). Lower the posterior canal wall, leaving the bridge intact (Fig. 5–18*B*). Normally the facial recess is not drilled open, but in our bone this has already been done. Visualize and section the tensor tympanic tendon (this maneuver lateralizes the manubrium) (Fig. 5–18C). At this point in a clinical case, you would place a tube in the tympanic membrane remnant and perform an ossiculoplasty, place a graft, and obliterate the aditus with either periosteum or cartilage.

Modified Radical Mastoidectomy

For practical purposes, a modified radical mastoidectomy has already been performed, except that the bridge is still intact. Removing the bridge will complete the modified radical mastoidectomy.

There are two approaches for the modified radical mastoidectomy: the "inside-out" or atticotomy approach, and the "outside-in" or atticoantrotomy approach. We have already performed, step by step, an outside-in approach in this bone. In our next bone, which will be used for middle ear dissection, the inside-out modified radical mastoidectomy approach will be used.

Drilling is started in the epitympanum and followed posteriorly into the antrum. In doing this, the bridge is removed. The antrum is identified, as well as the dome of the horizontal canal (Fig. 5–19*A*). With this landmark under direct vision, mastoidectomy is performed and the posterior bony wall is lowered to the level of the facial ridge (Fig. 5–19*B*). This method is easier and safer than the outside-in approach in a sclerotic mastoid.

Radical Mastoidectomy (Fig. 5–20)

The purpose of this procedure is to create an exteriorized cavity that includes the mastoid, antrum,

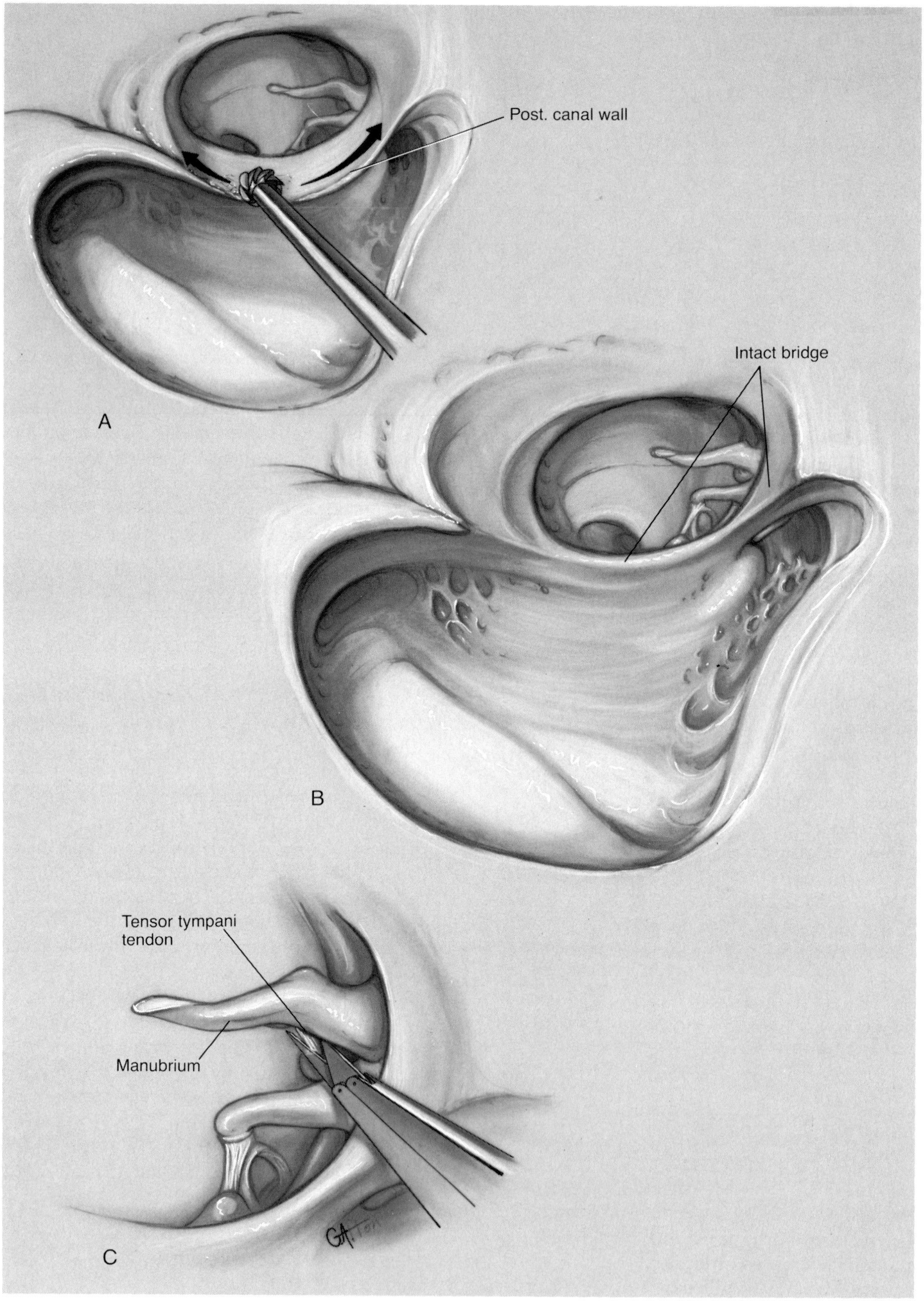
Post. canal wall
A
Intact bridge
B
Tensor tympani tendon
Manubrium
C

FIGURE 5–18.

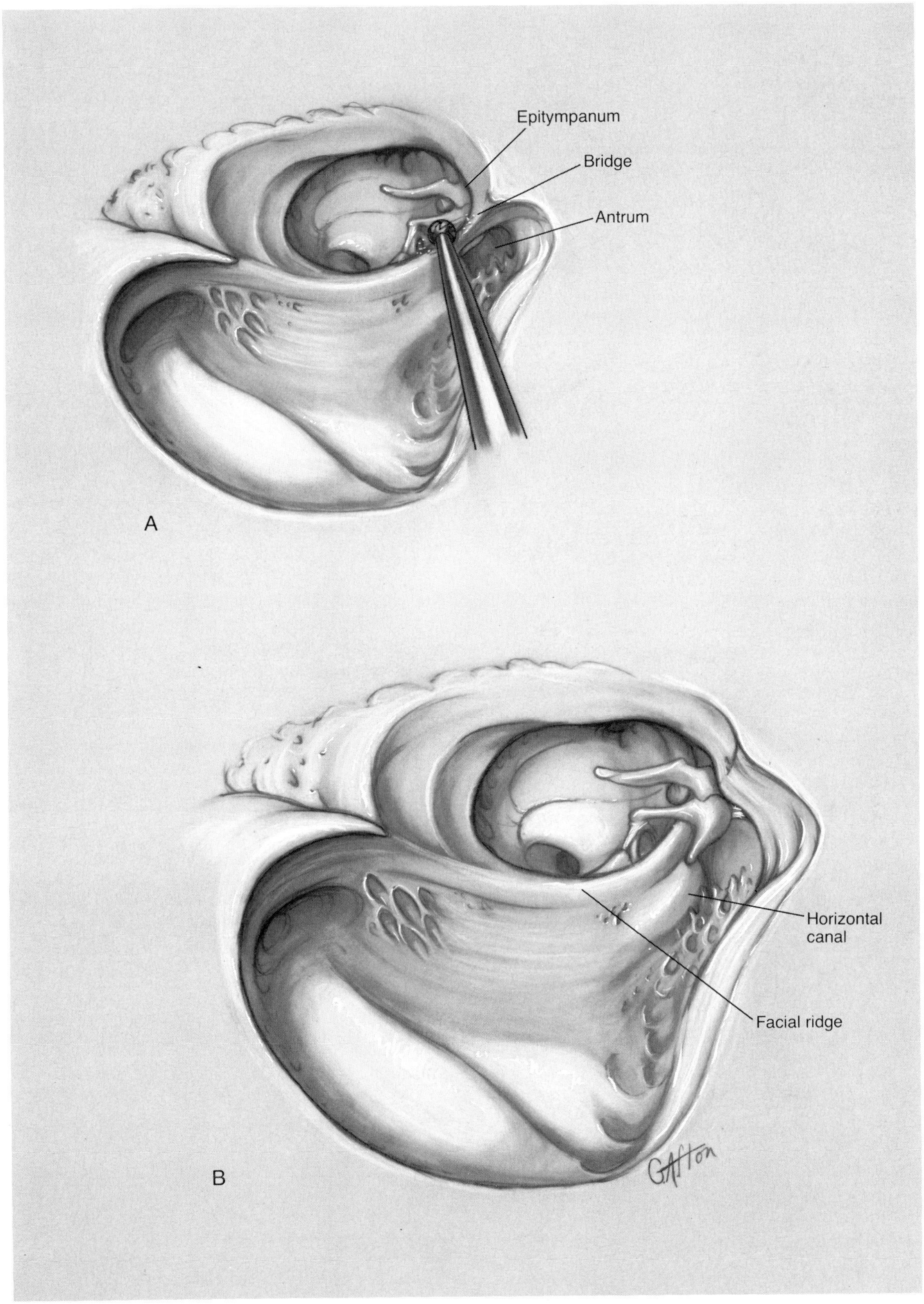

Epitympanum
Bridge
Antrum
A
Horizontal canal
Facial ridge
B

FIGURE 5–19.

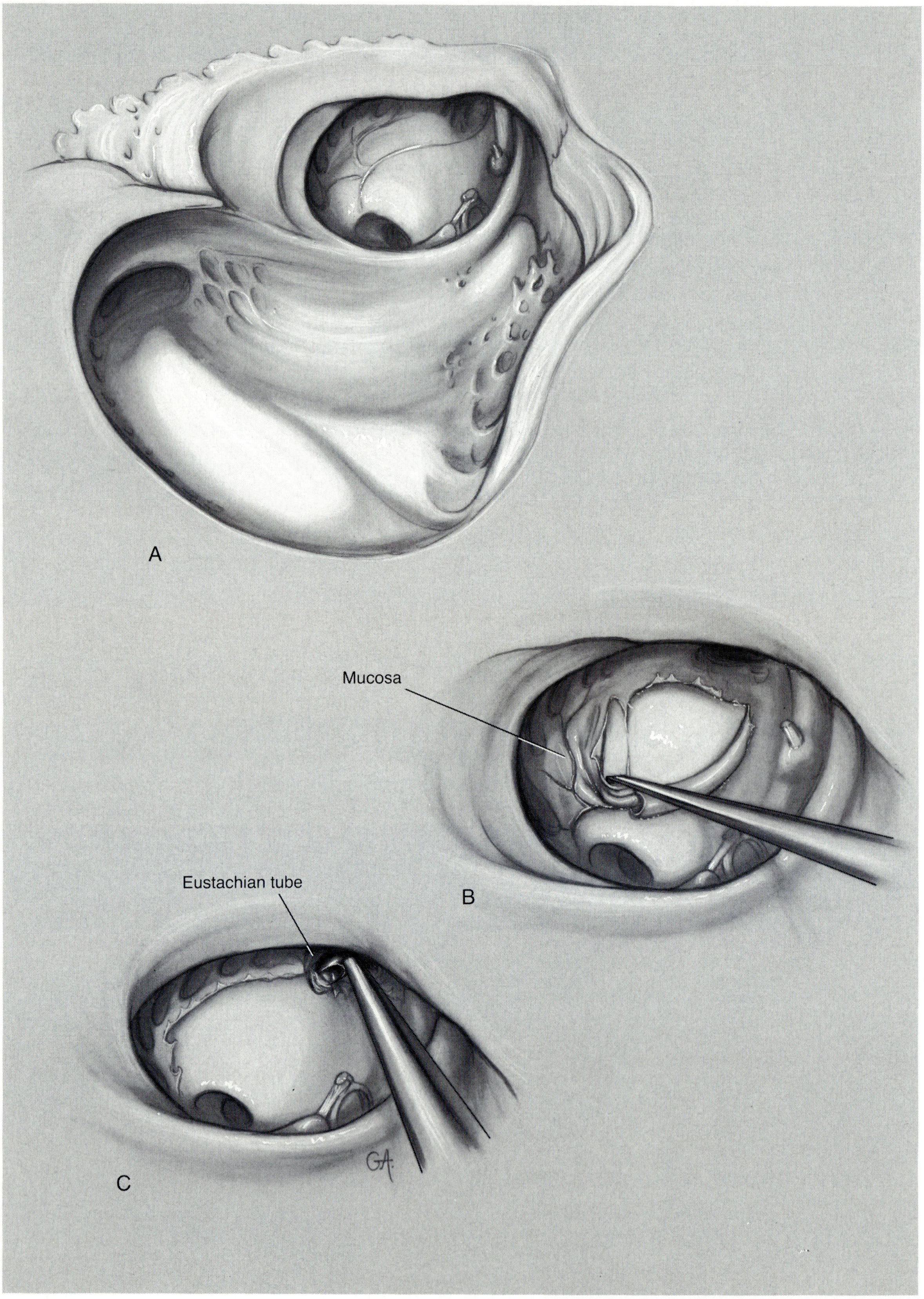

FIGURE 5–20.

epitympanum, and mesotympanum, leaving a dry epithelialized cavity continuous with the external meatus. The procedure involves removing the malleus and incus while leaving the stapes intact. The mucosa of the middle ear is removed as well.

Petrous Drainage

Aim

Exenteration (removal) of petrous apex air cells while maintaining the integrity of the inner ear structures.

The petrous apex (petrous pyramid) has two major groups of air cells, the anterior and the posterior. The posterior group (Fig. 5–21*A*) includes cell tracts superior, posterior, and inferior to the semicircular canals; the anterior group (Fig. 5–21*B*) includes cell tracts in the superomedial aspect of the eustachian tube orifice, where the carotid artery is located. In order to reach these anterior cell tracts, a radical mastoidectomy (described above) must be done. Hypotympanic air cells also are present adjacent to the round window niche.

Posterior Cell Tract

For this dissection, skeletonization of the sigmoid sinus, the posterior fossa dura, and the facial nerve is required. This has already been done. Our next step is to carefully skeletonize the semicircular canals (Fig. 5–21C). Use small burs (3-0 or 4-0 size). Four areas or tracts, which may or may not be present, should be looked for. The first tract is through the arch of the superior semicircular canal. The second tract is anterosuperior to the semicircular canal, leading into the supracochlear air cells; visualize this tract and its relationship to the facial nerve. The third tract is posterior to the superior canal and runs between the tegmen mastoideum and common crus of the membranous labyrinth toward the internal auditory canal. Do not expose the common crus—this is to be done later. The intention here is to obtain a better visualization of this anatomic relationship. The fourth or retrolabyrinthine cell tract is inferior to the posterior semicircular canal, medial to the vertical segment of the facial nerve, and superior to the jugular bulb.

Anterior Cell Tract

A radical mastoidectomy has already been done. The tegmen should be skeletonized and the anterior wall thinned; both of these procedures have already been performed. The cells of the anterior tract are found in the "peritubal" and carotid areas in the bony wall just medial to the eustachian tube orifice anterior to the promontory. These cells are closely associated with the tegmen mastoideum; therefore, dissection must be done very carefully. The authors prefer to use small curets at this level.

Labyrinthectomy (Transmastoid Labyrinthine Dissection)

Aim

Complete removal of the semicircular canals and soft tissue of the vestibule

Highlights

1. The sinodural angle must be completely thinned for adequate exposure of the vestibule.
2. The tegmen must be thinned for adequate visualization of the superior aspect of the semicircular canals.

Procedure

The three semicircular canals are skeletonized until the membranous labyrinth is visible through the bone as a thin blue line (Fig. 5–22*A*). Note the relationship of the facial nerve to the horizontal semicircular canal (Fig. 5–22*B*). Fenestrate the horizontal canal. Unroof the posterior and anterior portions of the superior semicircular canal. Follow the superior semicircular canal until it reaches its common crus with the posterior semicircular canal. The arcuate artery penetrates the hard labyrinth in the center of the arch of the superior semicircular canal. Go back to the superior semicircular canal, identify the superior vestibular nerve, and follow it into the internal auditory meatus (Fig. 5–22C). Visualize the common crus. Now identify the endolymphatic duct as it enters the posterosuperior end of the vestibule. Verify its presence and its direction toward the endolymphatic sac; this is a useful anatomic relationship to keep in mind, since this area is not visualized in endolymphatic sac enhancement procedures. Bone is now removed from

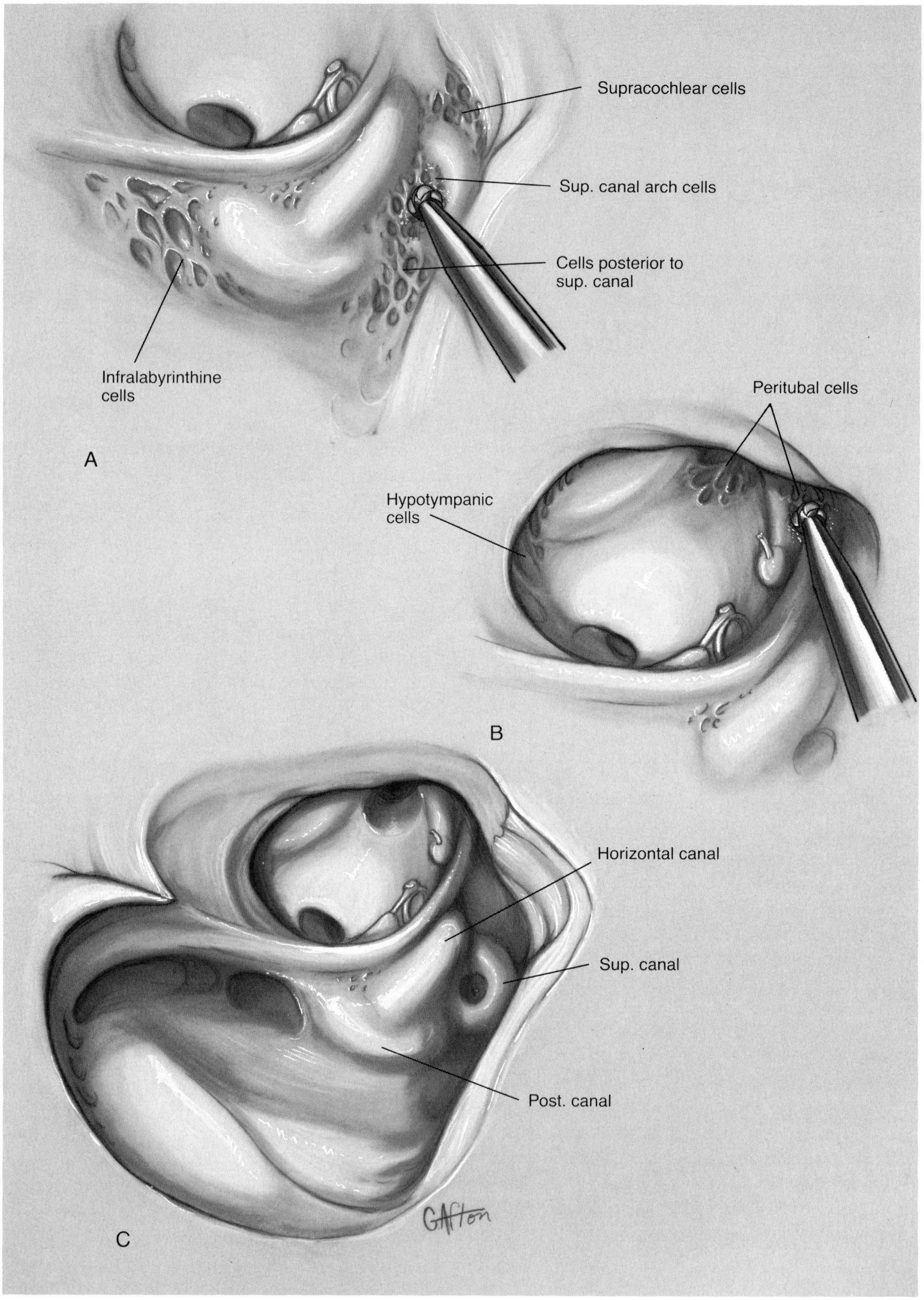
Supracochlear cells
Sup. canal arch cells
Cells posterior to sup. canal
Infralabyrinthine cells
A
Peritubal cells
Hypotympanic cells
B
Horizontal canal
Sup. canal
Post. canal
C
GAlton

FIGURE 5–21.

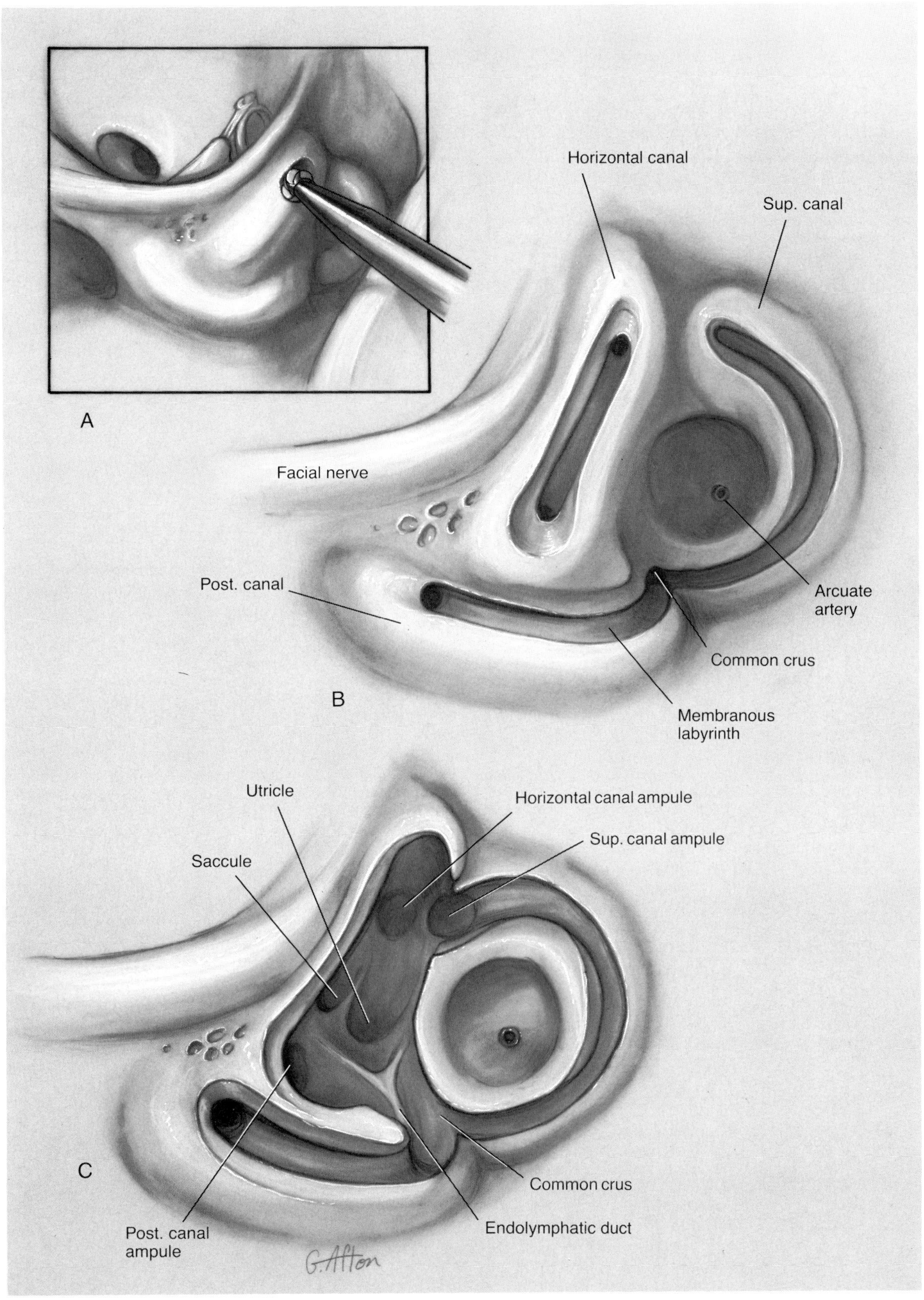
A
Horizontal canal
Sup. canal
Facial nerve
Post. canal
Arcuate artery
Common crus
B
Membranous labyrinth
Utricle
Horizontal canal ampule
Sup. canal ampule
Saccule
C
Common crus
Endolymphatic duct
Post. canal ampule
G. Afton

FIGURE 5–22.

the floor of the vestibule where the inferior vestibular nerve is encountered.

Follow the common crus anteriorly into the vestibule. Open it widely and try to identify the membrane of the utricle and saccule. Notice the relationships and distances between the footplate, saccule, and utricle. Now skeletonize the round window, since two additional observations can be made in this area. First, drill carefully at the inferior margin of the round window and identify the singular nerve (Fig. 5–23*A*). Second, drill this area and identify the hook of the basal turn of the cochlea (Fig. 5–23*B*). Cochlear electrodes may be obstructed in this area when being inserted into the cochlea. Visualize its

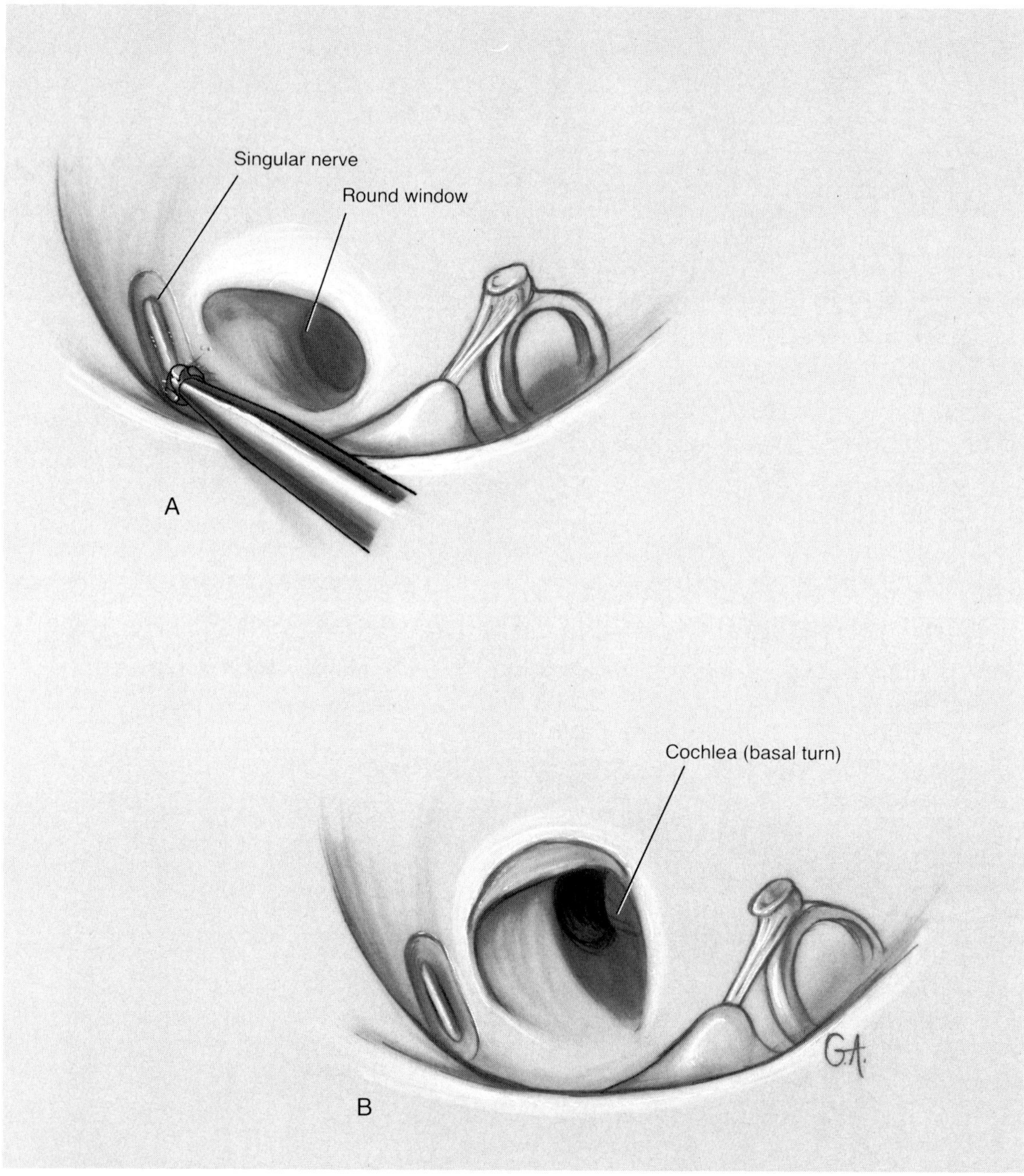

FIGURE 5–23.

anatomy in order to see the direction in which the electrode should be pointed and the amount of bone that should be drilled to bypass the hook.

Middle Ear Dissection

Procedure

This procedure is started with a new wet bone. Skin procedures will not be dealt with since the skin is thick, tight, and difficult to elevate adequately for these purposes. Identify the walls of the ear canal. Visualize the tympanic membrane; imagine it in four quadrants (Fig. 5–24*A*). Make openings in the anterosuperior, anteroinferior, posteroinferior, and posterosuperior quadrants. Now gently elevate the tympanic membrane and identify the areas and structures beneath the four openings. Visualize what is found beneath the posterosuperior quadrant opening. Now bend the tympanic membrane forward; if it is too brittle, remove it. Visualize the middle ear (Fig. 5–24*B*). Palpate the ossicles, Jacobson's nerve, the round window niche area, and the opening of the eustachian tube, and identify the tensor tympani.

Remove the skin, leaving the annulus intact. Identify the tympanosquamous suture superiorly and the tympanomastoid suture posteriorly. Between the sutures is the vascular strip. Identify the anterior wall and carefully drill the anterior bony overhang without entering the temporomandibular joint space. Enlarge the canal until the entire tympanic membrane annulus is clearly visualized (Fig. 5–24C).

Using a large stapes curet, curet the scutum from superior to inferior, thus avoiding injury to the ossicles (Fig. 5–25). Visualize the stapedial tendon. Make sure it is clearly in sight. At this point you are ready for a stapedectomy. Instead of sectioning the stapedial tendon (which can be done, as well), try to lift it along with its periosteum with the incudostapedial joint knife, leaving it attached to the periosteum of the long process of the incus (Fig. 5–26*A*). This is not a simple procedure. Using the incudostapedial joint knife, separate the joint very gently. Fracture the footplate in the middle with a straight pick (Fig. 5–26*B*). Mobilize the stapes, using superior-to-inferior and inferior-to-superior movements, and remove it, hooking the joint knife to the area immediately inferior to the capitulum (Fig. 5–26C). The remaining footplate portions are lifted gently with a Hough hoe (Fig. 5–26*D*). Using the wire bending die 0.005 stainless steel and Gelfoam, make the prosthesis as described in Figure 5–27. Place it over the long process of the incus and gently crimp—not too tightly, not too loosely—allowing it some mobility since excessive tightness might result in necrosis of the long process of the incus. Make a Teflon piston (Rosales technique) as described in Figure 5–28. Place this piston prosthesis over the long process of the incus and gently crimp it.

Now remove the incus. Try to make a longer prosthesis of stainless steel wire and Gelfoam to extend from the malleus to the oval window (Fig. 5–29). Use the incus to make a strut for use between the malleus and the stapes. Section the short process of the incus and drill an acetabulum over the body so that it will fit under the malleus. Use a small graft to cover the oval window.

At this point, with the use of a curet or very small bur, curet or drill the attic in order to perform an atticotomy. Use a Whirlybird to probe the antrum.

Cochlear Implant (Mastoidotomy-Tympanotomy Approach)

Aim

To place an electrode into the cochlea by sliding it through the round window.

Highlights and Surgical Steps

1. Achieve good visualization of the middle ear and round window niche via an endaural approach (Lempert I incision).
2. Perform an atticotomy.
3. Remove the incus.
4. Expose the mastoid cortex and drill a mastoidotomy (Lempert II incision).
5. Perform a small postauricular incision and drill a seat for the internal receiver.
6. Tunnel the electrode from the postauricular incision to the mastoidotomy into the antrum, middle ear, and round window niche.
7. Secure the internal receiver in place.

Text continued on page 82

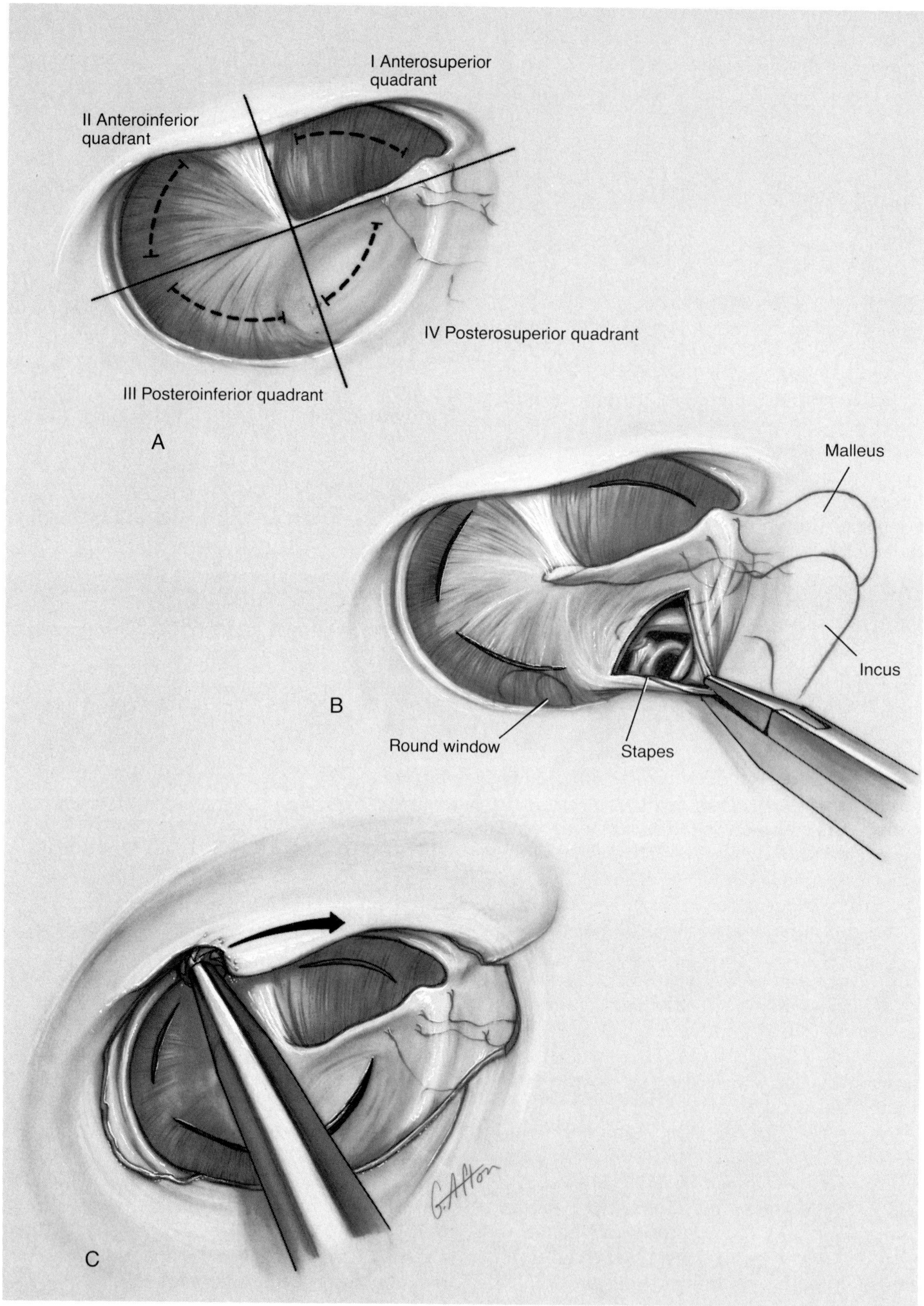
I Anterosuperior quadrant
II Anteroinferior quadrant
IV Posterosuperior quadrant
III Posteroinferior quadrant
A
Malleus
Incus
B
Round window
Stapes
C

FIGURE 5–24.

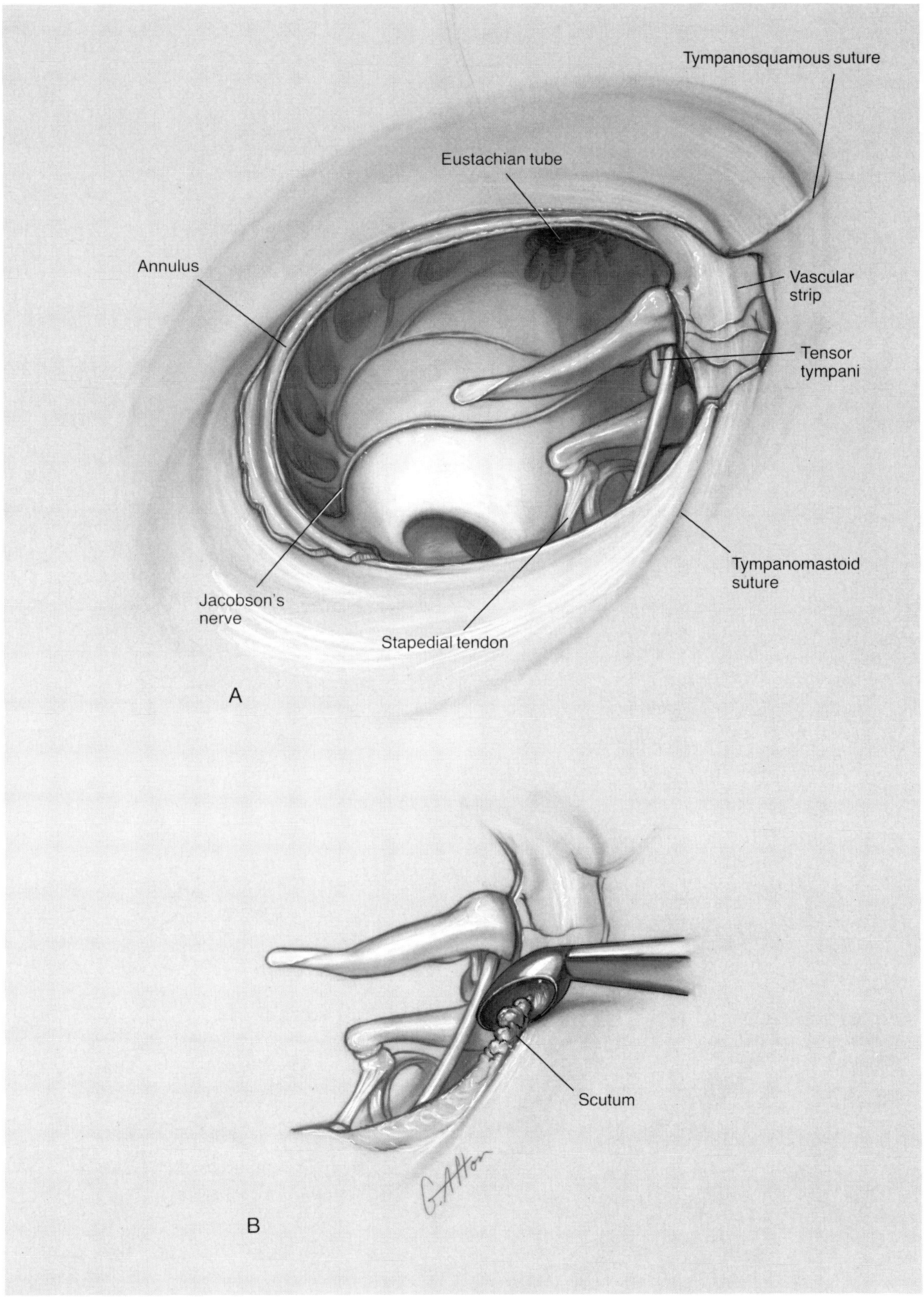
Tympanosquamous suture
Eustachian tube
Annulus
Vascular strip
Tensor tympani
Tympanomastoid suture
Jacobson's nerve
Stapedial tendon
A
Scutum
B

FIGURE 5–25.

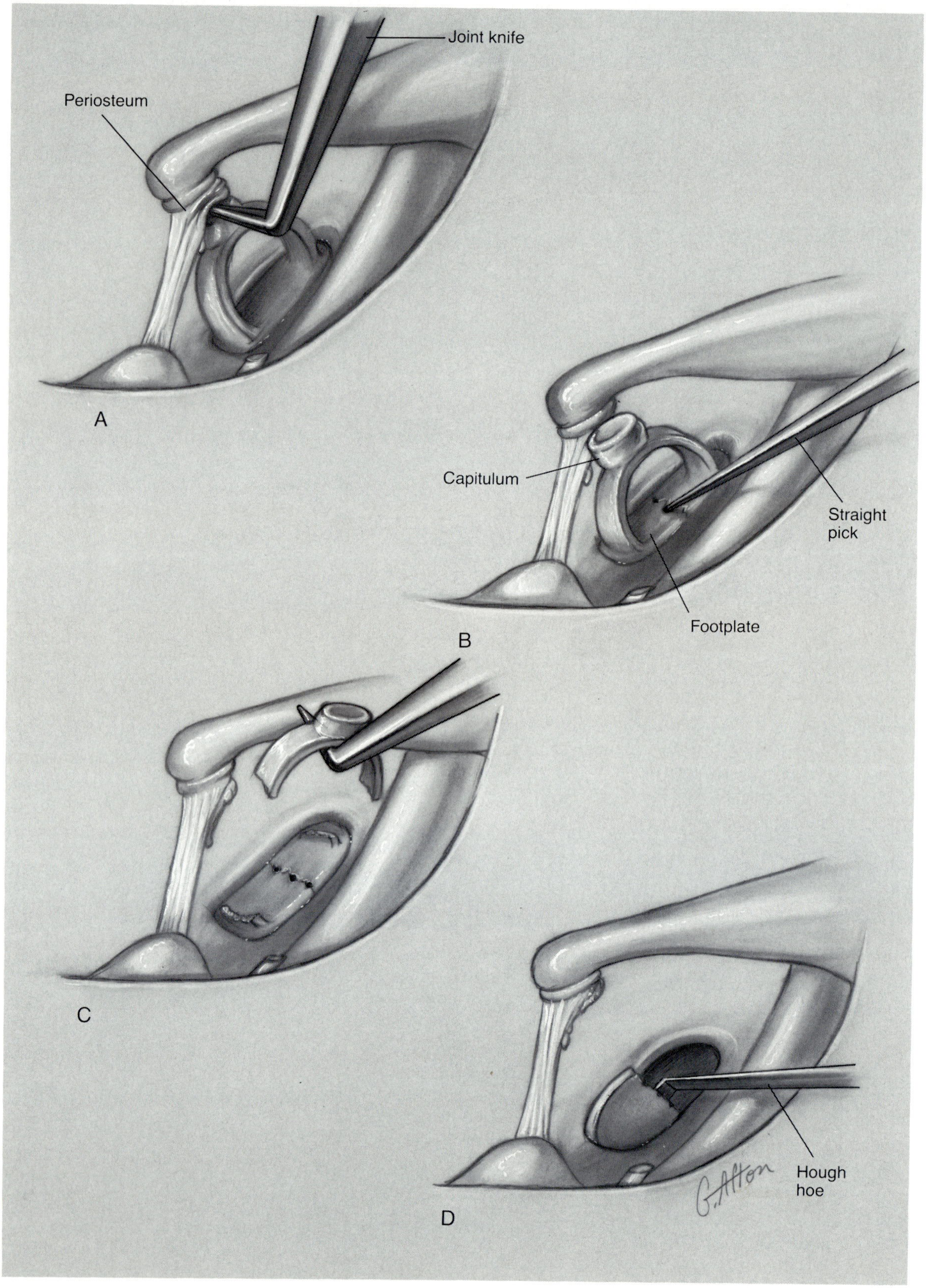
Joint knife
Periosteum
A
Capitulum
Straight pick
Footplate
B
C
Hough hoe
D
G. Alton

FIGURE 5–26.

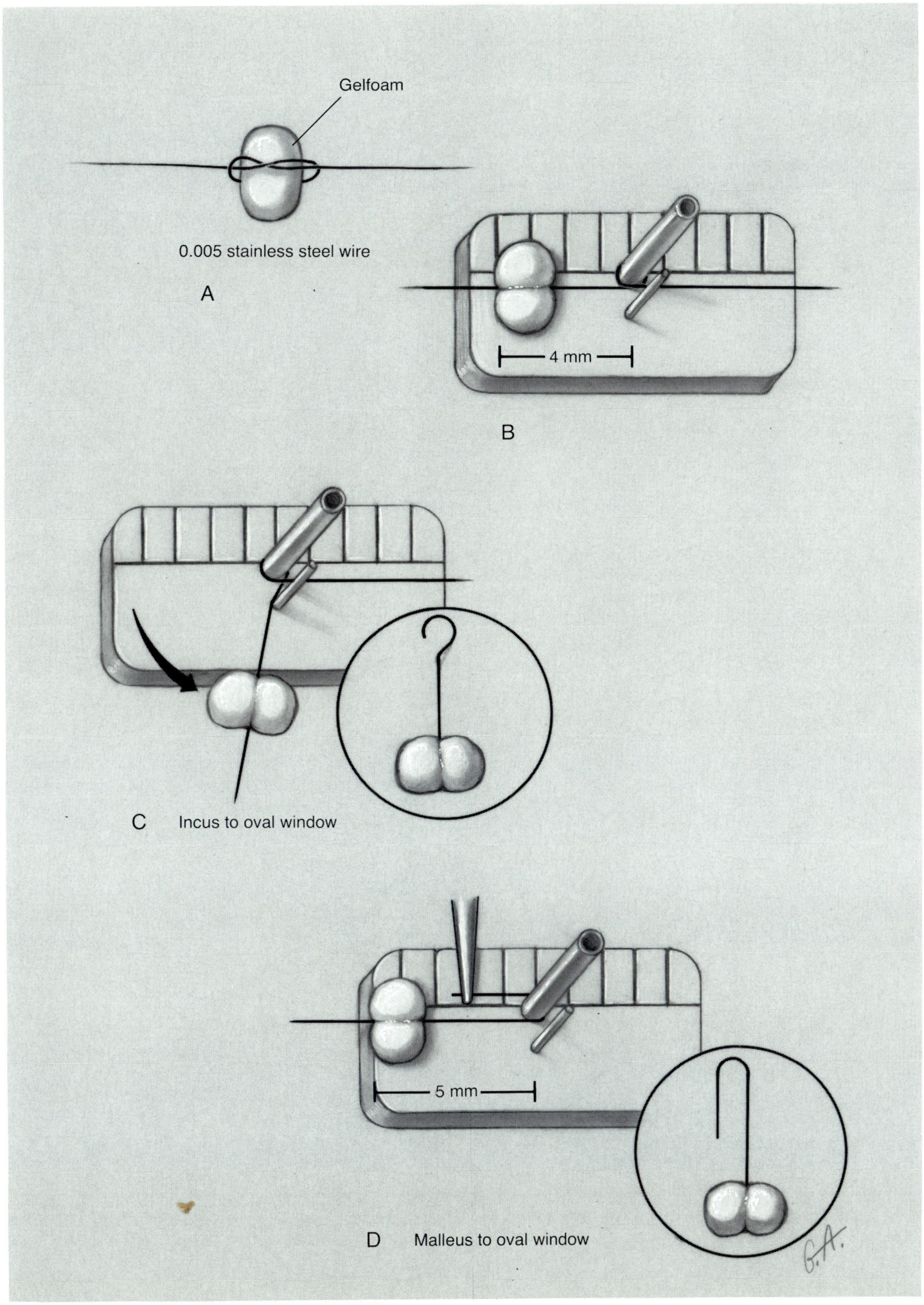
Gelfoam
0.005 stainless steel wire
A
4 mm
B
C Incus to oval window
5 mm
D Malleus to oval window

FIGURE 5–27.

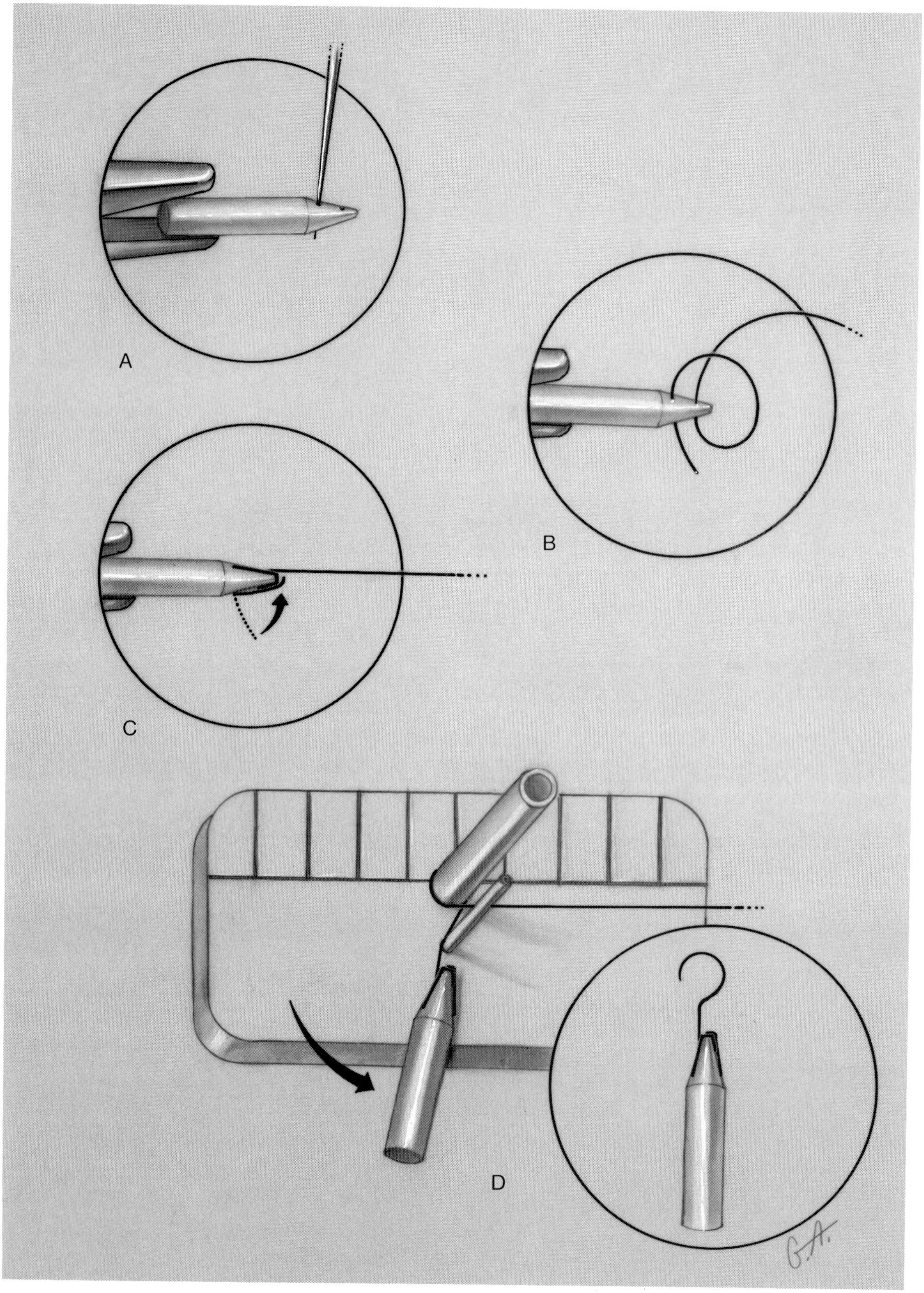

FIGURE 5–28.

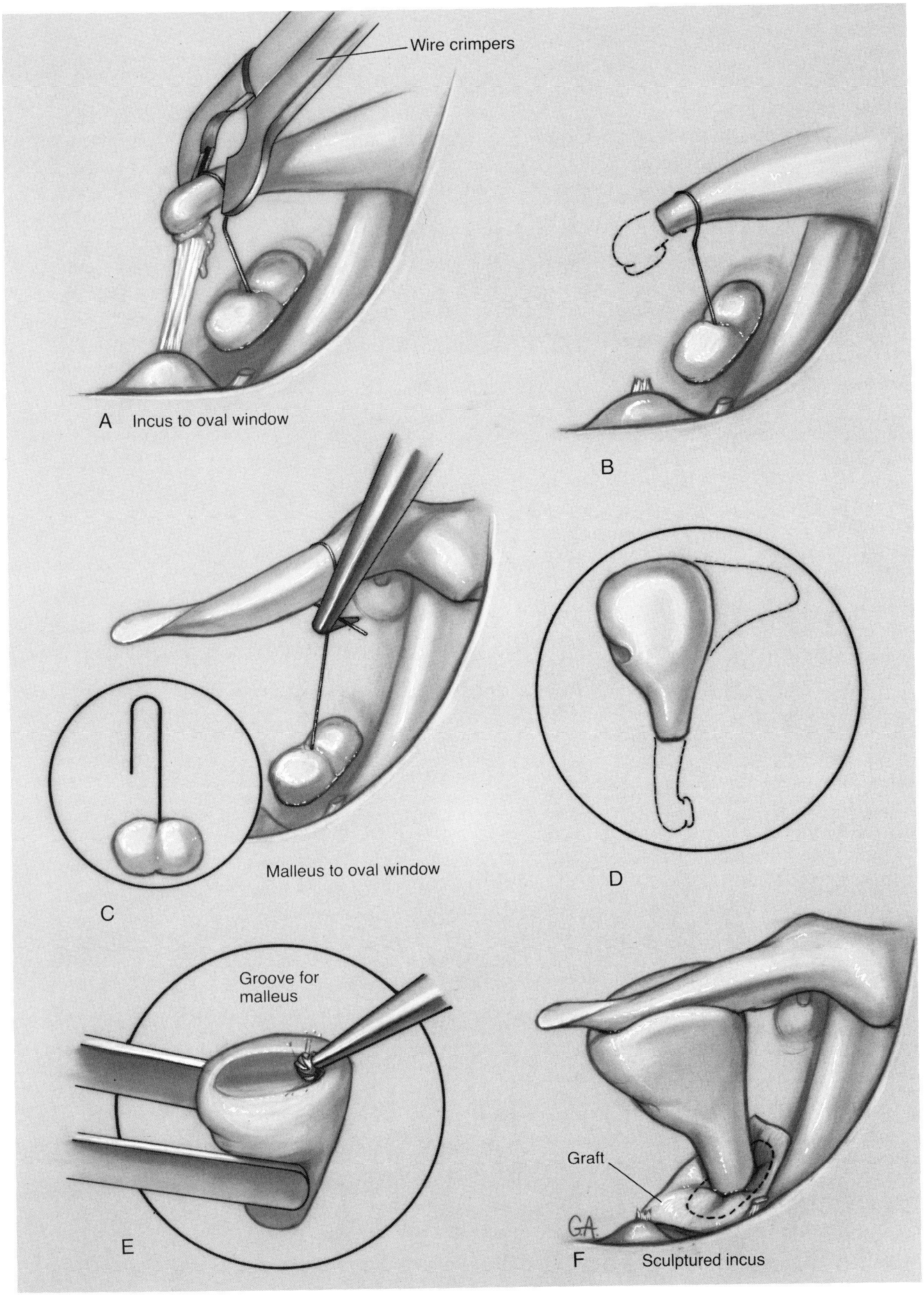
Wire crimpers
A Incus to oval window
B
Malleus to oval window
C
D
Groove for malleus
E
Graft
F Sculptured incus

FIGURE 5–29.

Procedure

This procedure implies an endaural approach, exposing both the middle ear and mastoid cortex. Once the round window niche is clearly exposed and defined, an atticotomy (Fig. 5–30*A*) is done and the incus is removed. A small mastoidotomy is performed (Fig. 5–30*C*). This opening will allow passage of the electrode into the middle ear through the antrum (Fig. 5–30*E*). The receiver is placed as in the posterior tympanotomy approach; however, only a small postauricular incision is needed, and the electrode is tunneled anteriorly toward the mastoidotomy.

Since this is a temporal bone dissection, an attempt can be made to place the receiver, performing a mastoidotomy and passing the electrode through the antrum and into the round window (Fig. 5–31). The incus must be removed (which has already been done). A mastoidotomy is the creation of an opening in the fossa mastoidea without performing a complete cortical mastoidectomy. The bone is drilled in the direction of the antrum by visualizing the attic area directly through the middle ear. In order to ascertain the location of the antrum, a Whirlybird can be used for direct probing. Even if a mastoidotomy is not precisely a cortical mastoidectomy, the opening should be large enough; a blind, small opening is dangerous. The mastoidotomy itself is a useful exploratory tool for the antrum when blockage is suspected or improved aeration of the middle ear is desired. Insertion of the electrode through the round window is the same as in the posterior tympanotomy approach; the electrode is passed through the opening into the cochlea.

Transcanal Labyrinthectomy

Procedure

Visualize the middle ear cavity (Fig. 5–32). Identify the oval and round windows and promontory, as well as the facial nerve. The purpose of this procedure is to destroy the labyrinth. The stapes footplate has been removed, and the vestibule containing the saccule and utricle is exposed. By the use of a hook or Hough hoe, the saccule can be destroyed (Fig. 5–33*A*). Using this same route, the ampule of the superior semicircular canal can be reached above and in front of the facial nerve, that of the posterior canal below and behind the nerve, and the ampule of the horizontal canal inferiorly beneath the nerve (Fig. 5–33*A*, *B*). In this process, the utricle is destroyed as well. It is important to stay within the bony confines and to destroy only the "membranous labyrinth." Immediately inferior to the vestibule is the internal auditory canal, where the bony plate is quite thin. The facial nerve also can be injured. To complete the procedure, drill the promontory and join the oval and round windows, exposing the beginning of the basal turn of the cochlea (Fig. 5–33*C*). Additional drilling can be done at this point for purposes of orientation to the cochlear anatomy. Placing an electrode via the basal turn can give the surgeon a clearer grasp of this procedure and its anatomic location.

At this point, an inside-out modified radical mastoidectomy (atticotomy) can be performed, as described earlier in this chapter.

After this procedure, it will be possible to repeat some of the operative procedures done with the first wet bone. For the next procedures two wet bones are recommended: one for the middle fossa approach and one for the remaining approaches.

Retrolabyrinthine Approach to the Cerebellopontine Angle

Aim

To obtain surgical access to the cerebellopontine angle and preserve integrity of the labyrinth.

Highlights

1. Complete removal of bone up to the posterior semicircular canal.
2. Skeletonization and mobilization of the sigmoid sinus to allow posterior retraction.
3. Complete removal of bone from the posterior fossa dura, sinodural angle, and posterior portion of the tegmen.
4. Removal of bone over the posterior fossa dura posterior to the sigmoid sinus.

Before beginning this approach, a small segment of IV tubing or red rubber catheter should be placed in the internal auditory canal to simulate cranial nerves VII and VIII. Bone wax or glue will hold it in position.

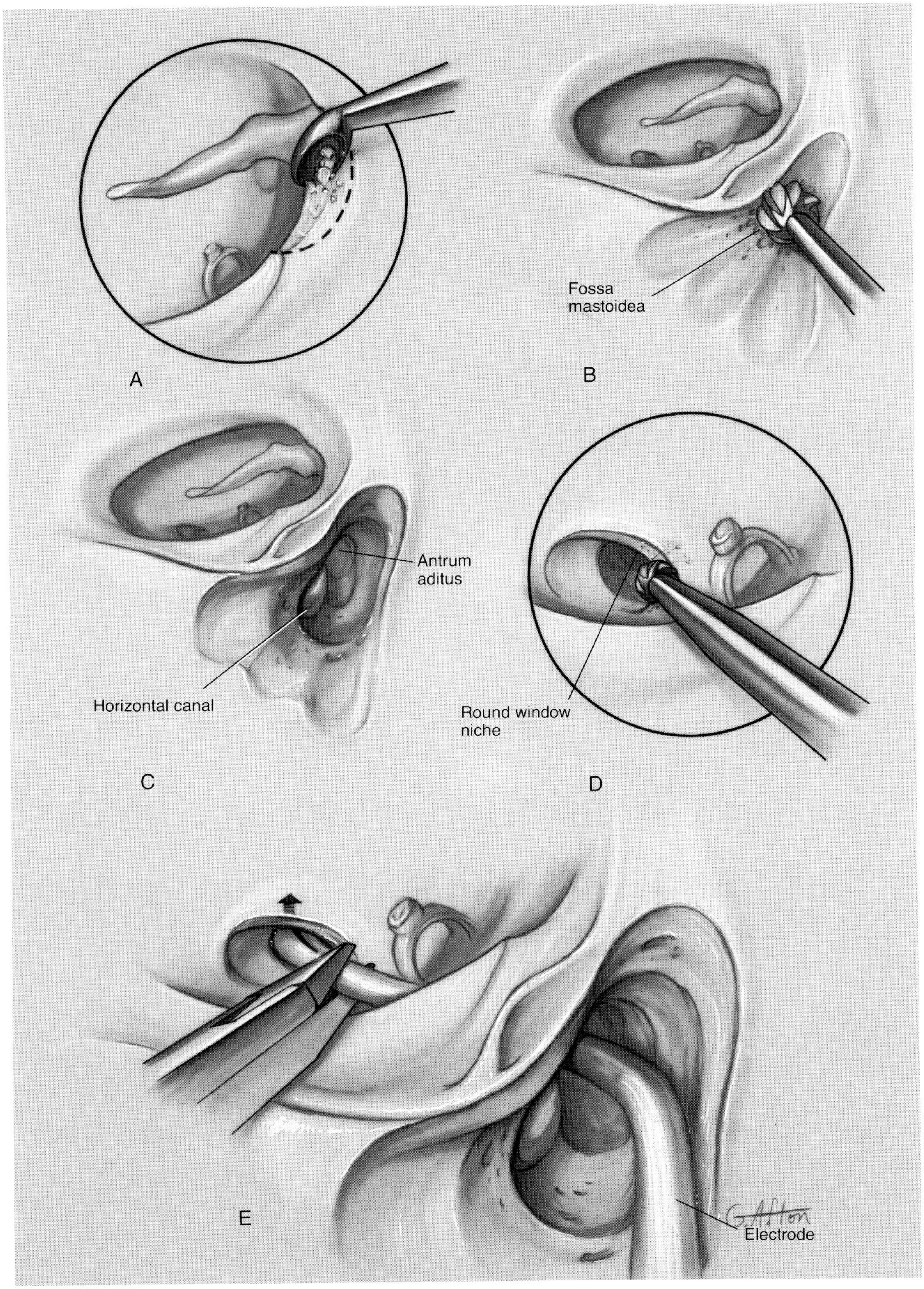
A
Fossa
mastoidea
B
Antrum
aditus
Horizontal canal
C
Round window
niche
D
E
G. Afton
Electrode

FIGURE 5–30.

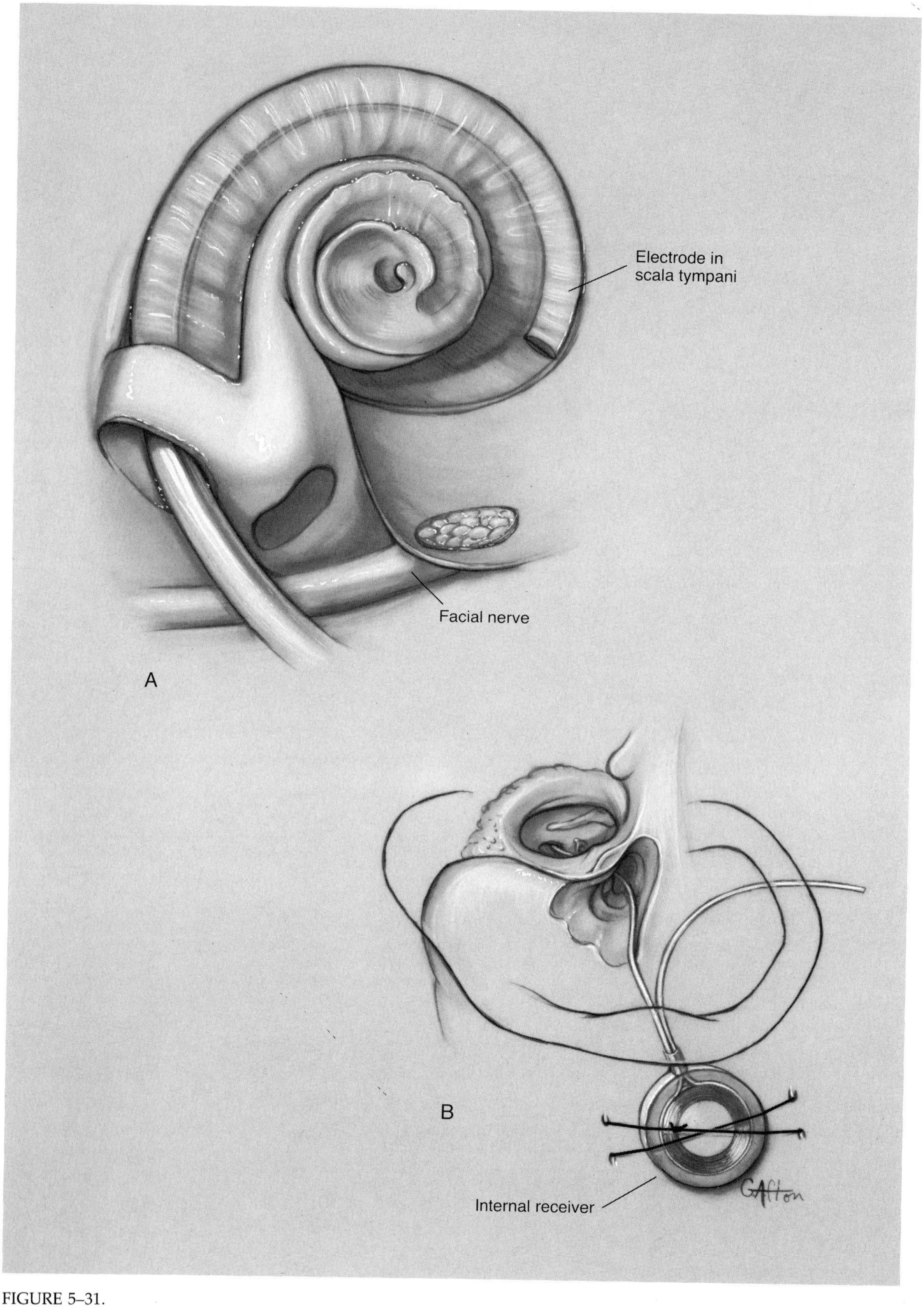
Electrode in
scala tympani
Facial nerve
A
B
Internal receiver

FIGURE 5–31.

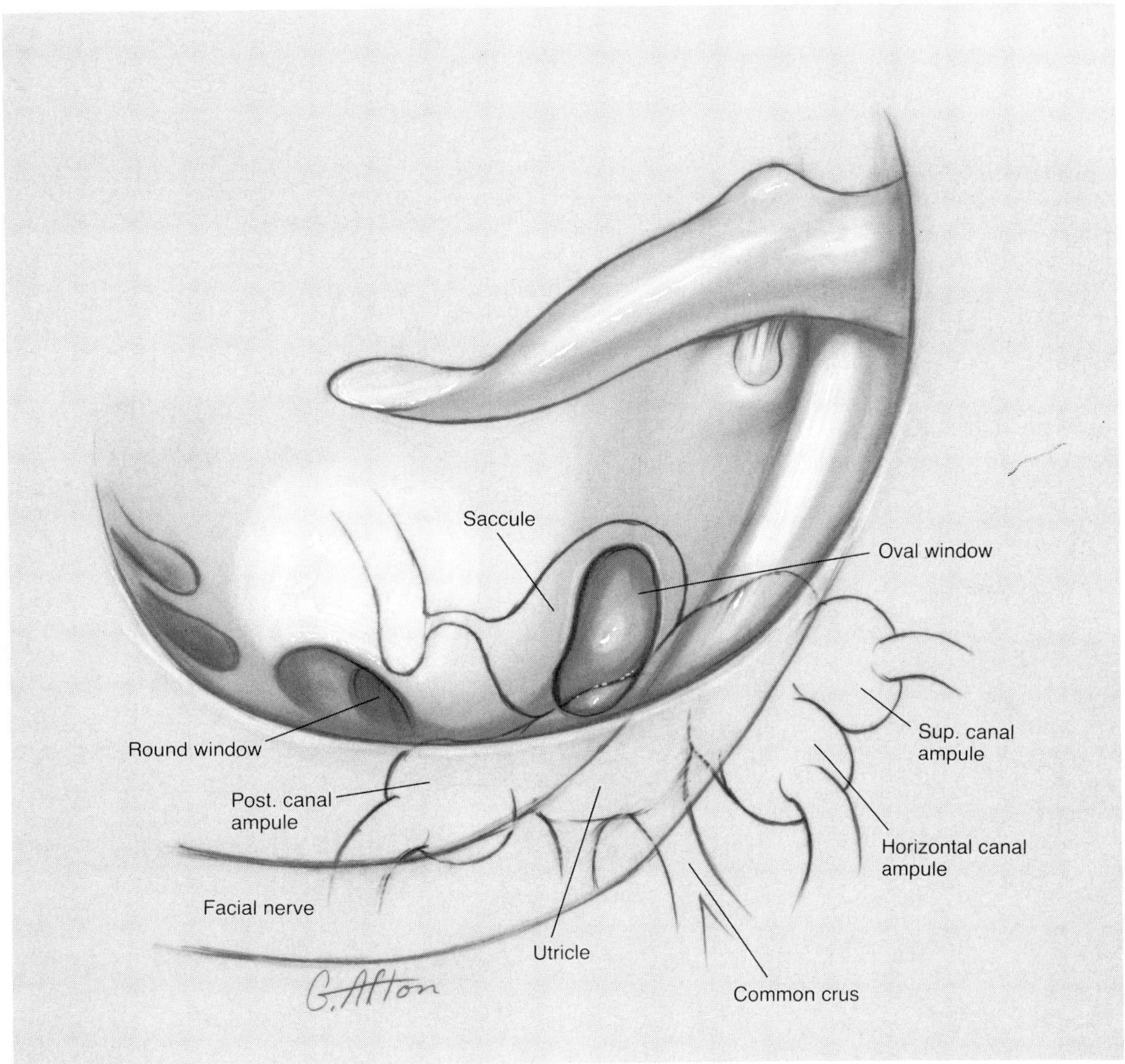

FIGURE 5–32.

Procedure

The initial step in the retrolabyrinthine approach is a thorough simple mastoidectomy as described earlier in this chapter. Clear identification of the posterior semicircular canal is essential, as this is the anterior limit of the dissection and exposure. Hence, it is important to remove bone up to the canal. Exposure also is enhanced by adequate removal of bone in the infralabyrinthine cell tract. The sigmoid sinus is skeletonized and mobilized, if this has not already been completed. The authors prefer to leave an island of bone on the sinus (Bill's island) to protect it from accidental rupture with a shaft of the bur or during retraction; bone can be completely removed from the sinus if so desired. Bone can be either completely removed with the diamond drill or thinned to eggshell thickness and removed with a blunt instrument.

Following mobilization of the sigmoid sinus, the bone over the posterior fossa dura and sinodural angle is removed in the same way. Dura is very fragile in prepared bone, and care must be taken not to tear it. It is important to remember that the superior petrosal sinus runs in the sinodural angle; bleeding in this area must be prevented. Removal of bone is continued up to the posterior semicircular canal. Exposure is enhanced with bone removal continued a short distance into the tegmen.

It should be remembered that the posterior fossa dura must also be exposed posterior to the sigmoid

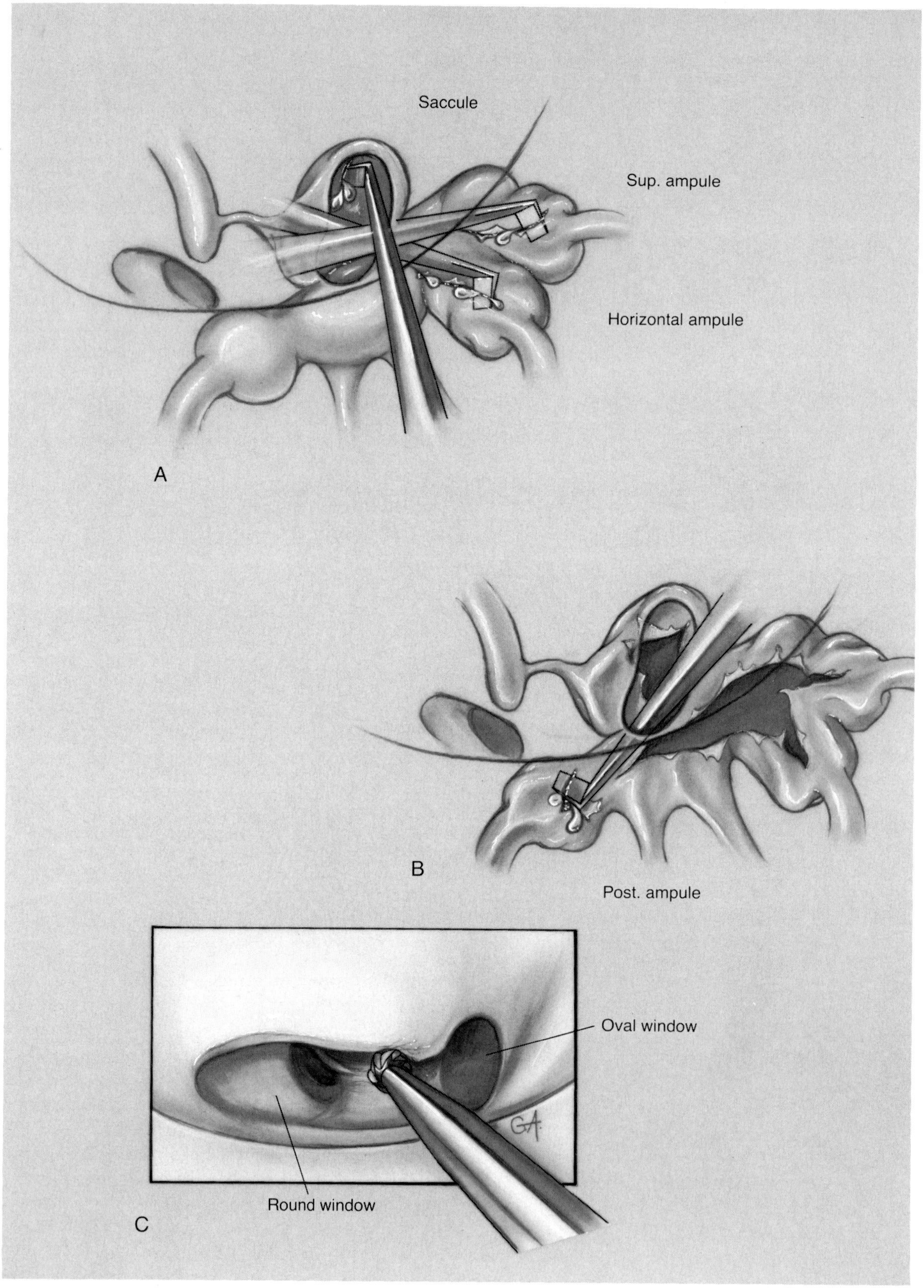
Saccule
Sup. ampule
Horizontal ampule
A
B
Post. ampule
Oval window
Round window
C

FIGURE 5–33.

sinus to allow for better retraction. This is usually not possible in temporal bone specimens, as this bone is needed to hold bone in position.

Following decompression of the dura and sinus, the dura is opened with a sickle knife and Malis scissors. The incision lines are depicted in Figure 5–34*A*. The lateral incision parallels the sigmoid sinus, running from superior to inferior, and runs just lateral to the endolymphatic sac in its inferior aspect. The second incision runs from lateral to medial and parallels the superior petrosal sinus. The dura is hinged at the posterior semicircular canal; the dura flap is draped over the canal. With retraction of the cerebellum (not present in specimen) and angling of the microscope anteriorly, good visualization of the cerebellopontine angle and cranial nerves V, VII, VIII, IX, X, and XI is afforded (Fig. 5–34*B*). For this demonstration, identification of the internal auditory canal marker should be accomplished.

Translabyrinthine Approach to the Internal Auditory Canal

Aim

To expose and open the internal auditory canal and identify the four cranial nerves contained within.

Highlights

1. Complete mastoidectomy and labyrinthectomy.
2. Identifying and outlining the internal auditory canal.
3. Opening into the internal auditory canal; identifying Bill's bar and the transverse crest.
4. Identifying the superior and inferior vestibular nerves, the cochlear nerve, and the facial nerve.

Procedure

The initial step in the translabyrinthine approach is the complete mastoidectomy and labyrinthectomy (described earlier). To help in later identification of the superior vestibular nerve, the medial wall of the ampulla of the semicircular canal is often preserved. It is helpful to visualize the internal auditory canal as it traverses the temporal bone.

Several points should be remembered. The internal auditory canal, as it runs anterior to posterior, starts away from the dissection; hence, at the posterior fossa dura it will be deeper or more medial than at the vestibule. There is a common wall between the vestibule and internal auditory canal. In other words, the medial wall of the vestibule represents the lateral wall of the internal auditory canal. A reference for the direction in which the canal runs is from the external genu to the sinodural angle.

Bone removal is continued medially following the labyrinthectomy. Again, it is important to remember that the canal becomes more medial (or deeper) as it approaches the posterior fossa dura. As the canal is approached a dark blue color will be seen, as in the blue lining of any hollow structure. Diamond burs are used at this point to decrease the risk of damage to important structures. It is important to skeletonize the internal auditory canal 180 degrees to allow adequate exposure and prevent bony overhangs.

Superiorly, the middle fossa dura is identified and followed medially. A thin layer of bone is left over the internal auditory canal. The "trench" that is developed extends from the facial nerve anteriorly to the posterior fossa dura posteriorly. It is important to remember that the superior petrosal sinus runs posterior superiorly in the sinodural angle; careful bone removal is required here. The inferior border of the internal auditory canal is now delineated. It is extremely important to be aware of and alert for the jugular bulb as soon as the posterior semicircular canal is removed in the labyrinthectomy. While usually positioned low in the mastoid tip, the bulb may present as high as the posterior semicircular canal (Fig. 5–35*A*). Again, the internal auditory canal has a blue lining, and a trench is developed inferior to the canal. The inferior margin of this canal will be the jugular bulb. It is safest to begin at the posterior fossa junction and proceed medially and anteriorly. As the incision continues anteriorly, a small white discoloration in the bone will appear. This represents the cochlear aqueduct, which is an important landmark. Extreme diligence is needed to identify this structure. Cerebrospinal fluid often is released when the aqueduct is entered. Anterior to this lie cranial nerves IX, X, and XI. Again, bone should be removed for 180 degrees around the internal auditory canal. The bone overlying the canal is thinned to eggshell thickness; it can then be carefully cracked with a blunt instrument and removed in one piece. The dura is best opened inferiorly to protect the facial nerve.

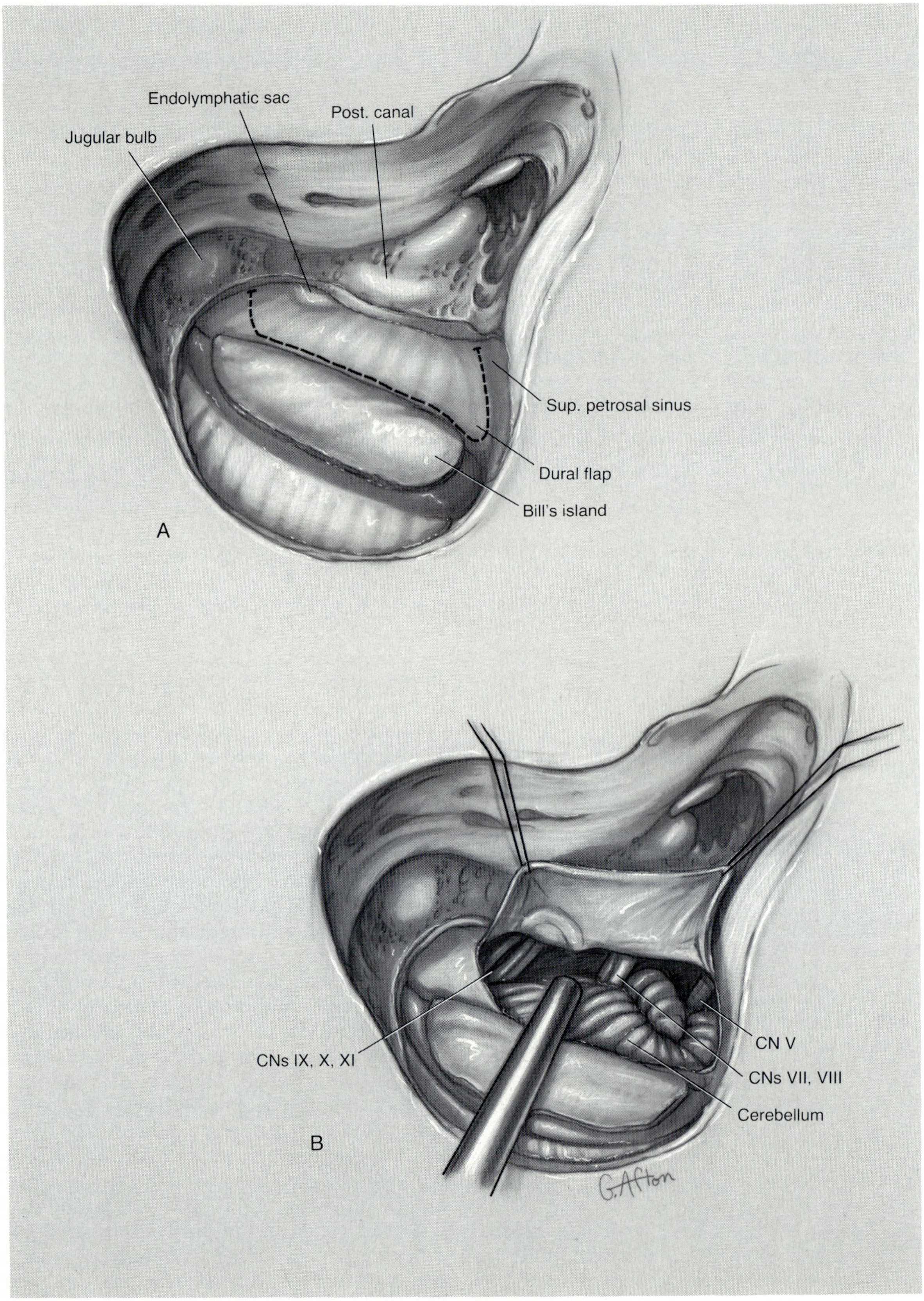
Endolymphatic sac
Post. canal
Jugular bulb
Sup. petrosal sinus
Dural flap
Bill's island
A
CNs IX, X, XI
CN V
CNs VII, VIII
Cerebellum
B
G.Afton

FIGURE 5–34.

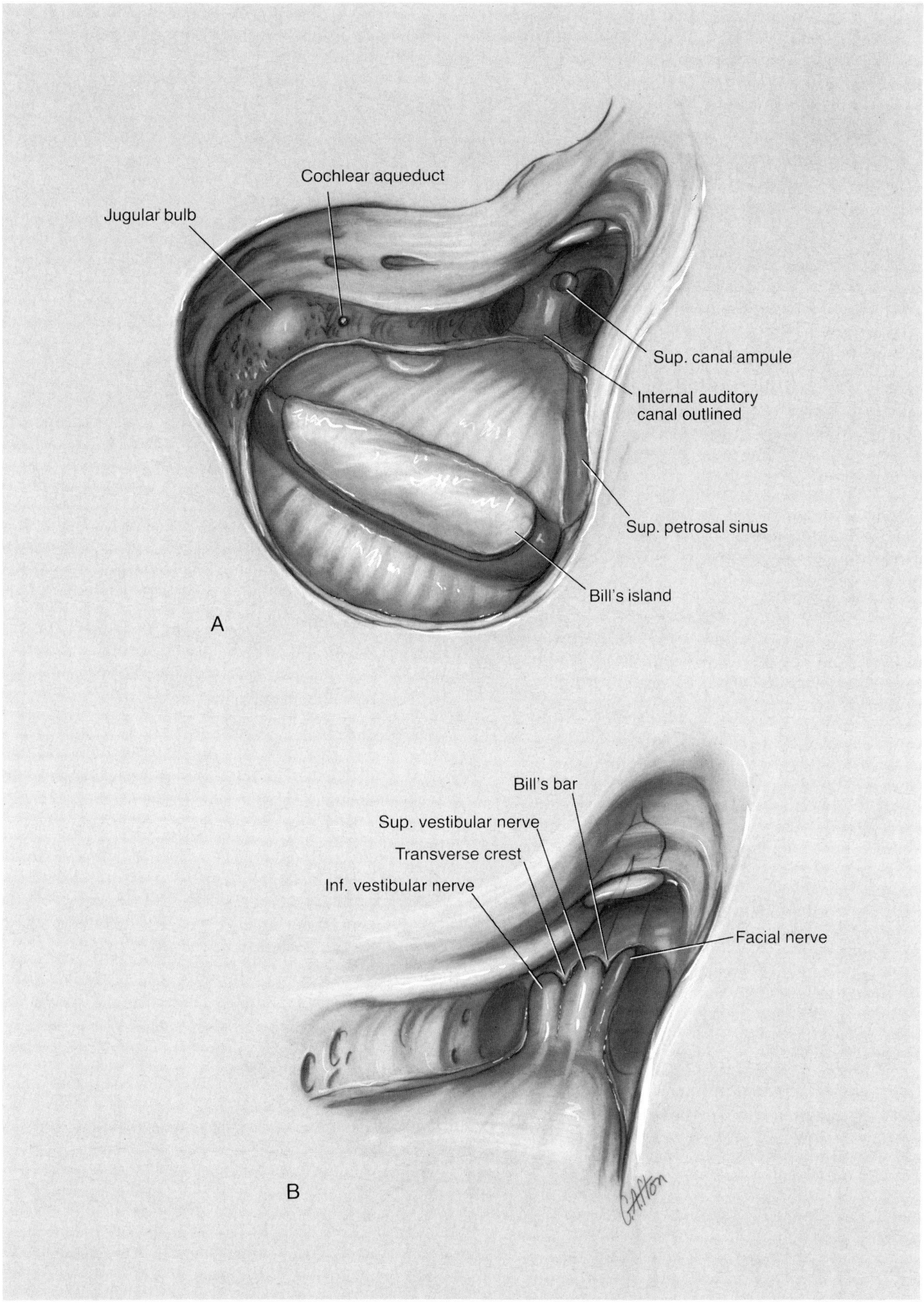
Cochlear aqueduct
Jugular bulb
Sup. canal ampule
Internal auditory canal outlined
Sup. petrosal sinus
Bill's island
A
Bill's bar
Sup. vestibular nerve
Transverse crest
Inf. vestibular nerve
Facial nerve
B

FIGURE 5–35.

To locate the various nerves in the internal auditory canal, the facial nerve must first be identified as it runs through its labyrinthine course (Fig. 5–35*B*). With the use of small diamond burs, the facial nerve can be skeletonized (blue-lined) from the area of the superior semicircular canal ampulla to the first genu. Again, a trench can be developed between the nerve and tegmen. The superior semicircular canal ampulla helps to identify the superior vestibular nerve; its medial wall represents the last remaining bone over the superior vestibular nerve at its termination in the ampulla. Upon removal of this bone, the superior vestibular nerve is identified. A 1-mm hook can be used to perforate Bill's bar, which is the ridge of bone separating the facial and superior vestibular nerves. To prevent damage to the facial nerve, the hook should never be inserted into the fallopian canal. The superior vestibular nerve is then avulsed (Fig. 5–36*A*). After proper identification of Bill's bar, it is safe to remove everything lateral to this ridge of bone.

Next, the transverse crest should be identified. A bony prominence that lies inferior to the superior vestibular and facial nerves, it divides the internal auditory canal into superior and inferior portions. Immediately inferior to the transverse crest is the inferior vestibular nerve. Medial to this lies the cochlear nerve (Fig. 5–36*B*). This completes the exposure and identification of the internal auditory canal.

Transcochlear Approach to the Skull Bone

Aim

To gain access to the cerebellopontine angle medial to the porus acusticus and/or anterior to the brainstem. Access to this area is limited with a conventional suboccipital approach by the cerebellum and brainstem; in the translabyrinthine approach it is limited by the facial nerve in the tympanum and mastoid.

Highlights

1. Complete mastoidectomy and labyrinthectomy.
2. Mobilization of the facial nerve within the entire fallopian canal.
3. Transposition of the facial nerve posteriorly.
4. Removal of the fallopian canal at all turns of the cochlea.
5. Anterior limit becomes the internal carotid artery.

Procedure

The transcochlear approach is an anterior extension of the translabyrinthine approach to the cerebellopontine angle. Again, the initial steps are a complete mastoidectomy and labyrinthectomy, as described earlier. The internal auditory canal is then outlined, and the facial nerve is identified as it enters the labyrinthine segment of the fallopian canal. This is found by using the ampulla of the superior semicircular canal as a landmark for the superior vestibular nerve. With a small diamond bur, the tegmen is followed medially in this area to develop the superior aspect of the internal auditory canal. The facial nerve will be blue-lined as it leaves the internal auditory canal and begins its course in the labyrinthine segment of the fallopian canal (Fig. 5–37*A*).

The next step is to completely skeletonize the facial nerve from the stylomastoid foramen to the internal auditory canal. An extended facial recess opening is made (Fig. 5–37*B*). After adequate thinning of the posterior external auditory canal, a cutting or diamond bur is used to enlarge an area immediately inferor to the fossa incudis and lateral to the facial nerve at the beginning of its mastoid segment. It is important to use as large a drill as possible to prevent tunneling and poor visualization. In a true facial recess, care must be taken not to disrupt the chorda tympani (lateral limit) and the tympanic membrane. These structures will be removed in this approach so that dissection may be accomplished more swiftly. After the opening is made into the middle ear, the incudostapedial joint is visualized and separated. The incus is removed through the attic. The facial recess is then enlarged superiorly through to the fossa incudus and inferiorly to the level of the floor of the tympanum.

The external auditory canal is then removed with a rongeur to improve visualization of the facial nerve. The anterior buttress is drilled to the level of the middle fossa tegmen and inferiorly as a smooth transition to the floor of the tympanum is accomplished. With the diamond drill, the facial nerve is then skeletonized completely within the temporal bone. The chorda tympani has already been sacrificed. When the bone has been completely removed,

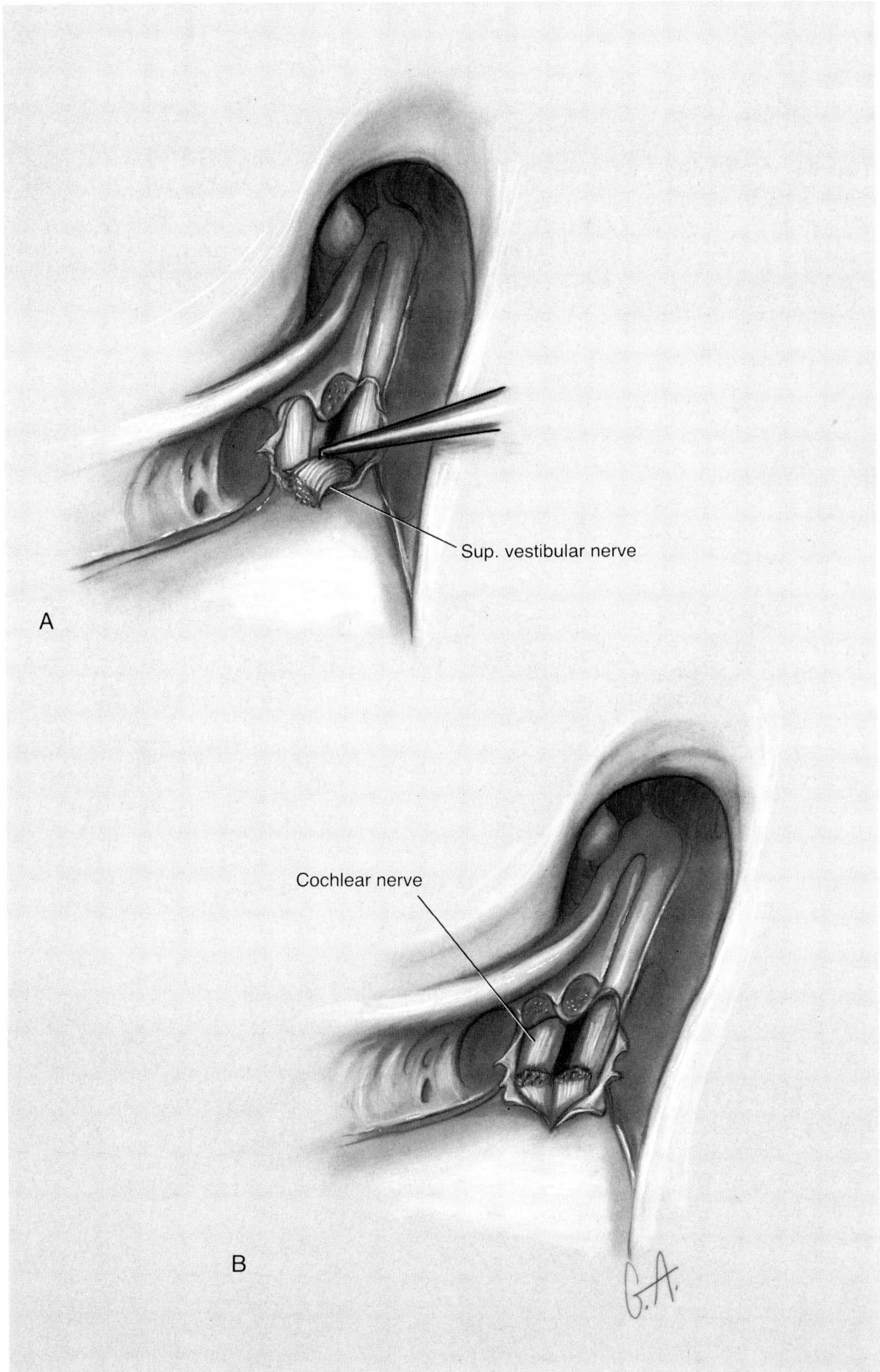

FIGURE 5–36.

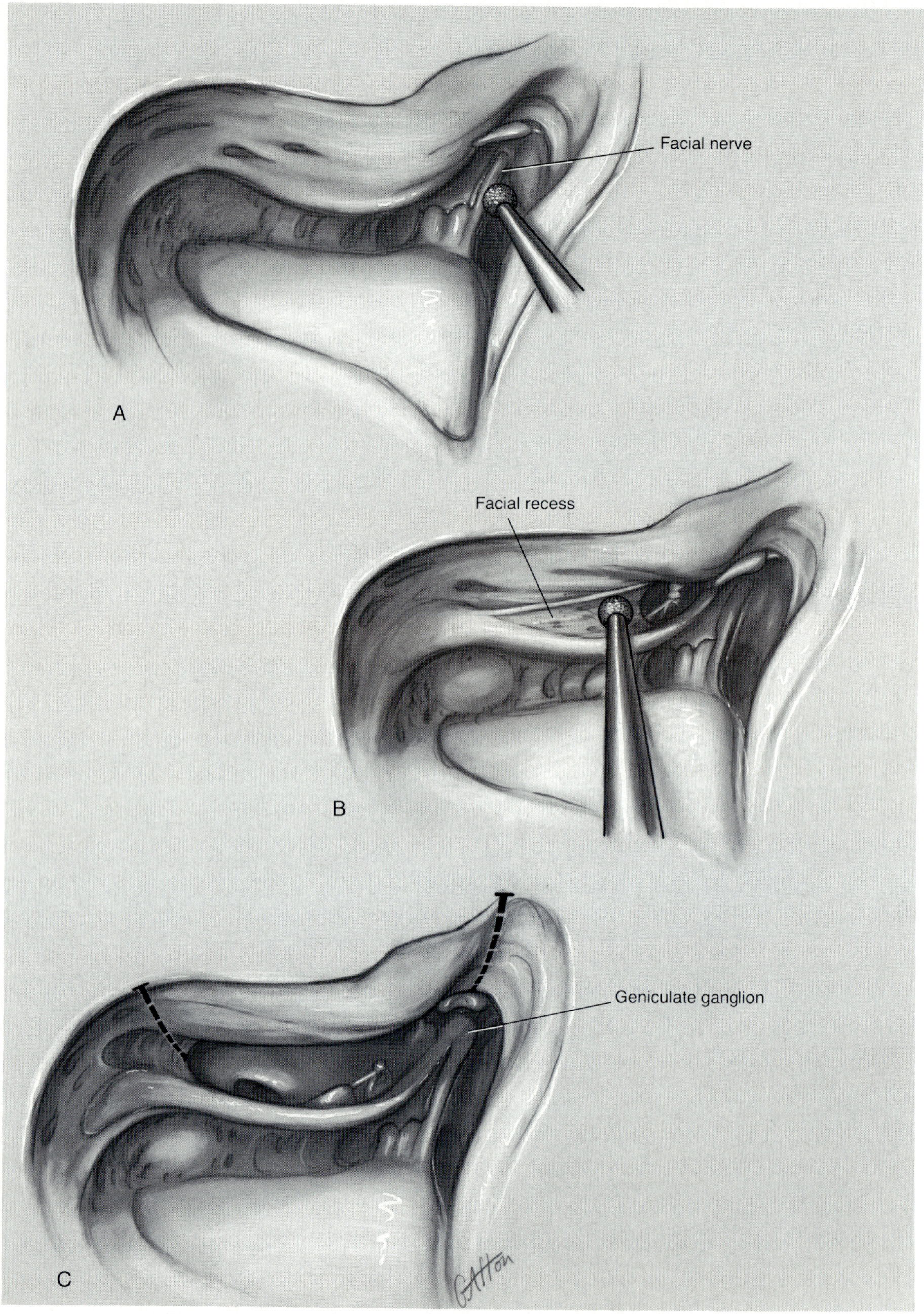

FIGURE 5–37.

the greater superficial petrosal nerve is cut at its origin from the geniculate ganglion (Fig. 5–37C). This frees the facial nerve from all attachments in the temporal bone. It is then carefully reflected posteriorly out of its bony bed.

Any remaining tympanic membrane is now removed, as well as any skin remaining on the anterior part of the external auditory canal. The anterior external auditory canal and any bony overhang are drilled to the level of the temporomandibular joint. The stapes is also removed at this point. Starting with the basal coil, the cochlea is completely drilled out, as well as the remnant of the fallopian canal (Fig. 5–38*B*). (It is good practice to follow the cochlea's coils to gain a better understanding of its anatomy.) Bone removal is carried forward to the septum that lies between the internal carotid artery and anterior wall of the basal coil. The internal carotid artery can be blue-lined with the diamond drill, much as the jugular bulb is blue-lined in the translabyrinthine approach. Inferiorly, bone removal extends to the inferior petrosal sinus and jugular bulb. Superiorly, the superior petrosal sinus and tegmen are followed medially to Meckel's cave (Fig. 5–38C). Medially, removal of bone continues to the lateral clivus. When bone removal has been completed, a large window covered by dura (bounded superiorly by the superior petrosal sinus and inferiorly by the jugular bulb and inferior petrosal sinus, with its apex just below Meckel's cave and the internal carotid artery located anteriorly) is created into the skull bone. If the dura is still intact, this window can be opened posterior to the internal auditory canal and extended as far forward as needed for exposure. Cuts may run medially, anteriorly, and parallel to the superior petrosal sinus and jugular bulb.

In an actual procedure, the dural defect is packed with abdominal fat and the external ear canal is sewn shut to prevent postoperative leakage of cerebrospinal fluid.

Middle Fossa Approach to the Internal Auditory Canal

Aim

To expose the floor of the middle cranial fossa and identify the structures contained within, including the cochlea, arcuate eminence, and contents of the internal auditory canal.

Highlights

1. To decompress the labyrinthine segment of the facial nerve or remove facial nerve lesions.
2. To remove small intracanalicular acoustic tumors in an attempt to preserve residual hearing.
3. To repair large defects of the tegmen and dura that have resulted in cerebrospinal fluid leaks.
4. To section the superior and inferior vestibular nerves and retain hearing.

Procedure

When practicing this approach in the laboratory, placement of the bone within the bone cup is important. Imagine a patient lying supine with the head turned to one side; the surgeon sits at the head of the patient and looks down on the middle cranial fossa floor through the craniotomy opening (described earlier). Hence, the bone needs to be placed in the bone cup so that the surgeon looks directly down upon the floor of the middle fossa (Fig. 5–39*A*). If the dura is still intact, it should be stripped from the exposed floor. As the dura is being elevated, the middle meningeal artery will be found anteriorly as it exits from the foramen spinosum. This represents the anterior limit of an adequate exposure. After all the dura has been removed, the floor should be studied. Laterally, where the floor rises to the pars squamosa, the tegmen overlies the aerated mastoid and the epitympanum. The eustachian tube (covered by thin bone) is located anterior to the epitympanum. Posteriorly, the floor of the middle fossa drops into the posterior fossa. Along this ridge runs the superior petrosal sinus within the reflected dura. Approximately 1 cm medial to the middle meningeal artery lies the greater superficial petrosal nerve, which runs in a posterior to anterior direction as it leaves the geniculate ganglion. This nerve is an important landmark; it can be followed back to find the geniculate ganglion and the facial nerve. In approximately 5% of cases the geniculate ganglion will not be covered by bone. Another important landmark is the arcuate eminence of the superior semicircular canal; usually an obvious feature, it may occasionally be indistinct. It is medial to the aerated bone of the mastoid and epitympanum, and appears as a rounded prominence. It must be remembered that every temporal bone will have its own unique middle fossa topography; no consistent landmark

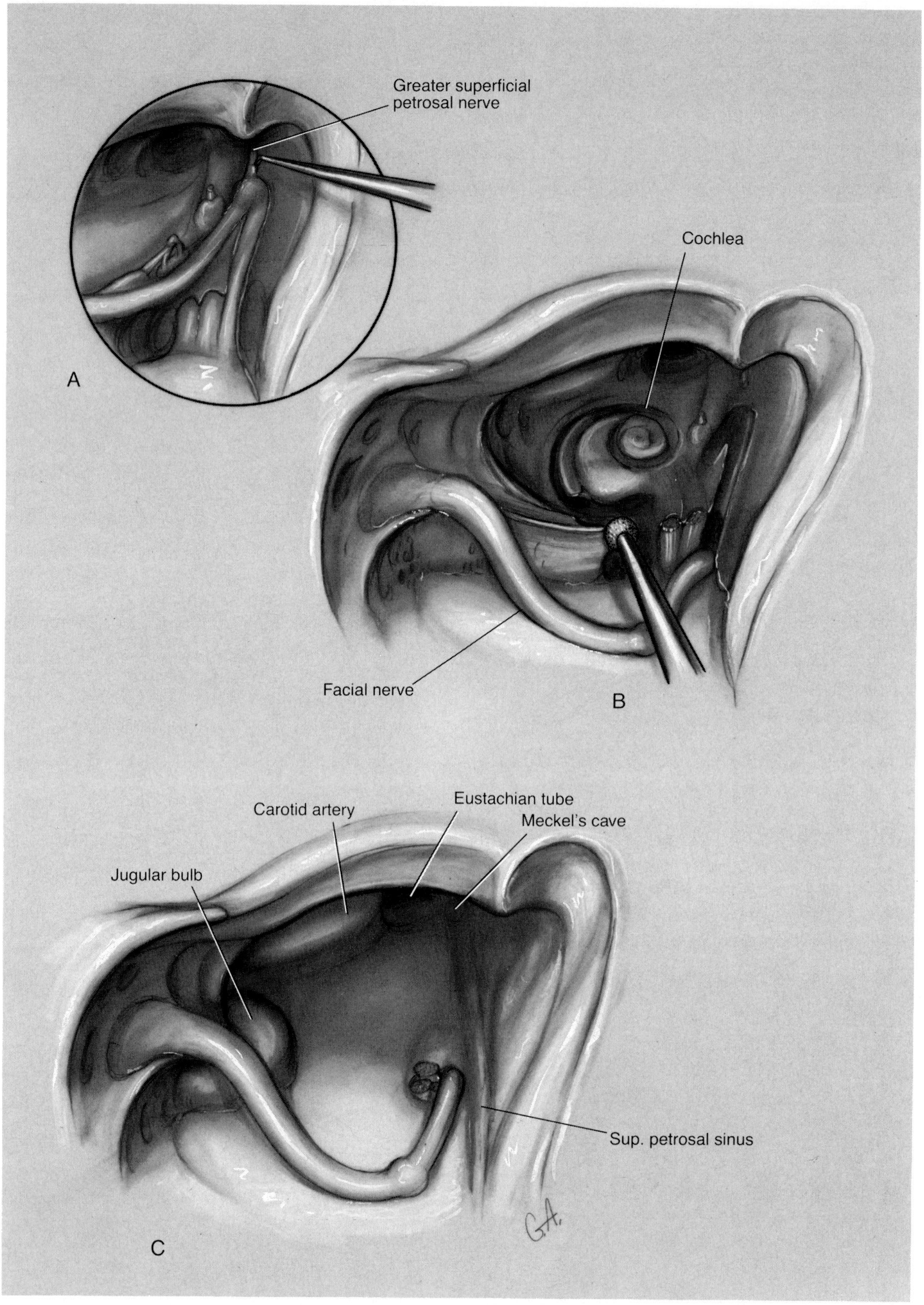
Greater superficial
petrosal nerve
A
Cochlea
Facial nerve
B
Carotid artery
Eustachian tube
Meckel's cave
Jugular bulb
Sup. petrosal sinus
C

FIGURE 5–38.

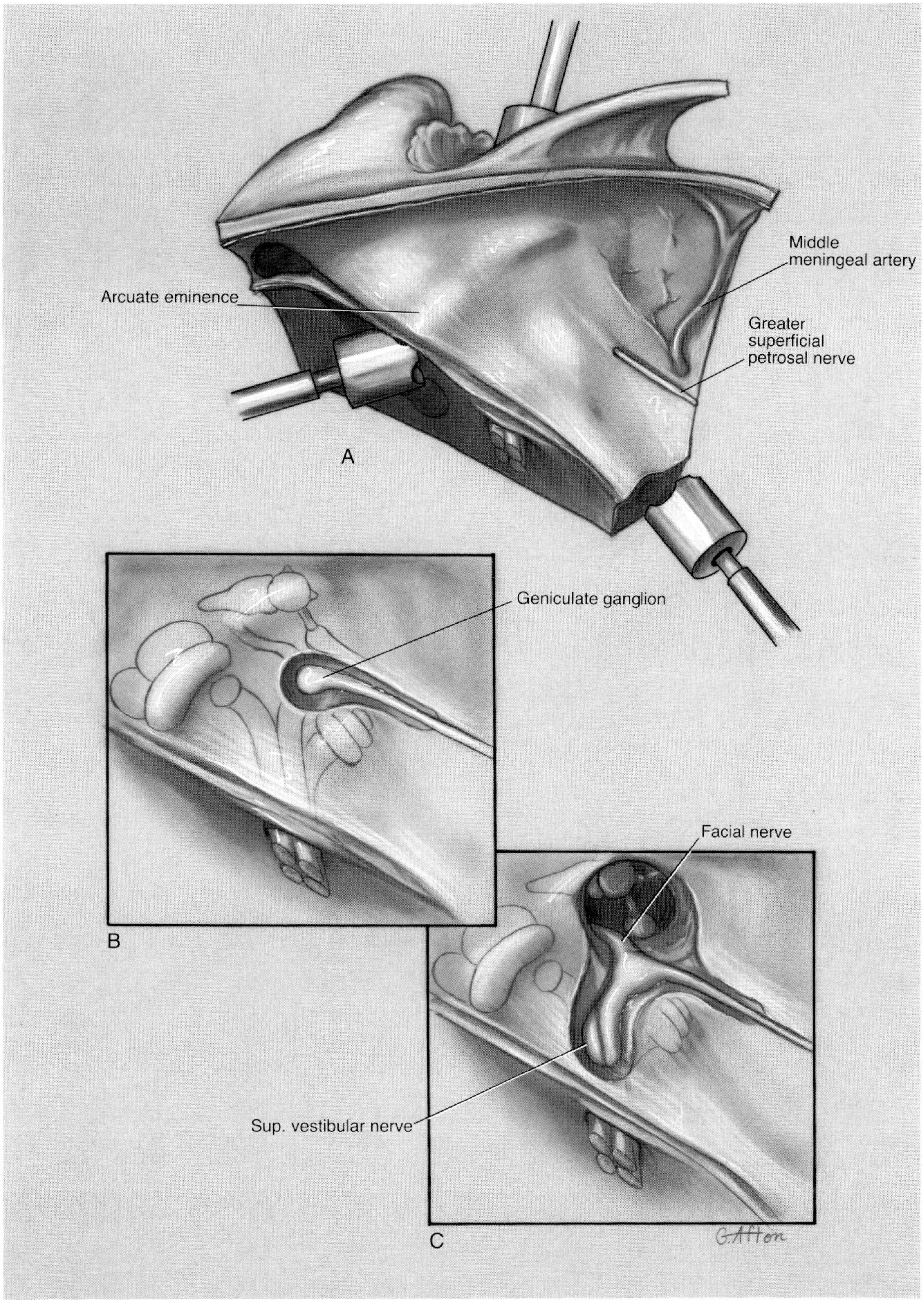
Middle
meningeal artery
Arcuate eminence
Greater
superficial
petrosal nerve
A
Geniculate ganglion
Facial nerve
B
Sup. vestibular nerve
C
G.Afton

FIGURE 5–39.

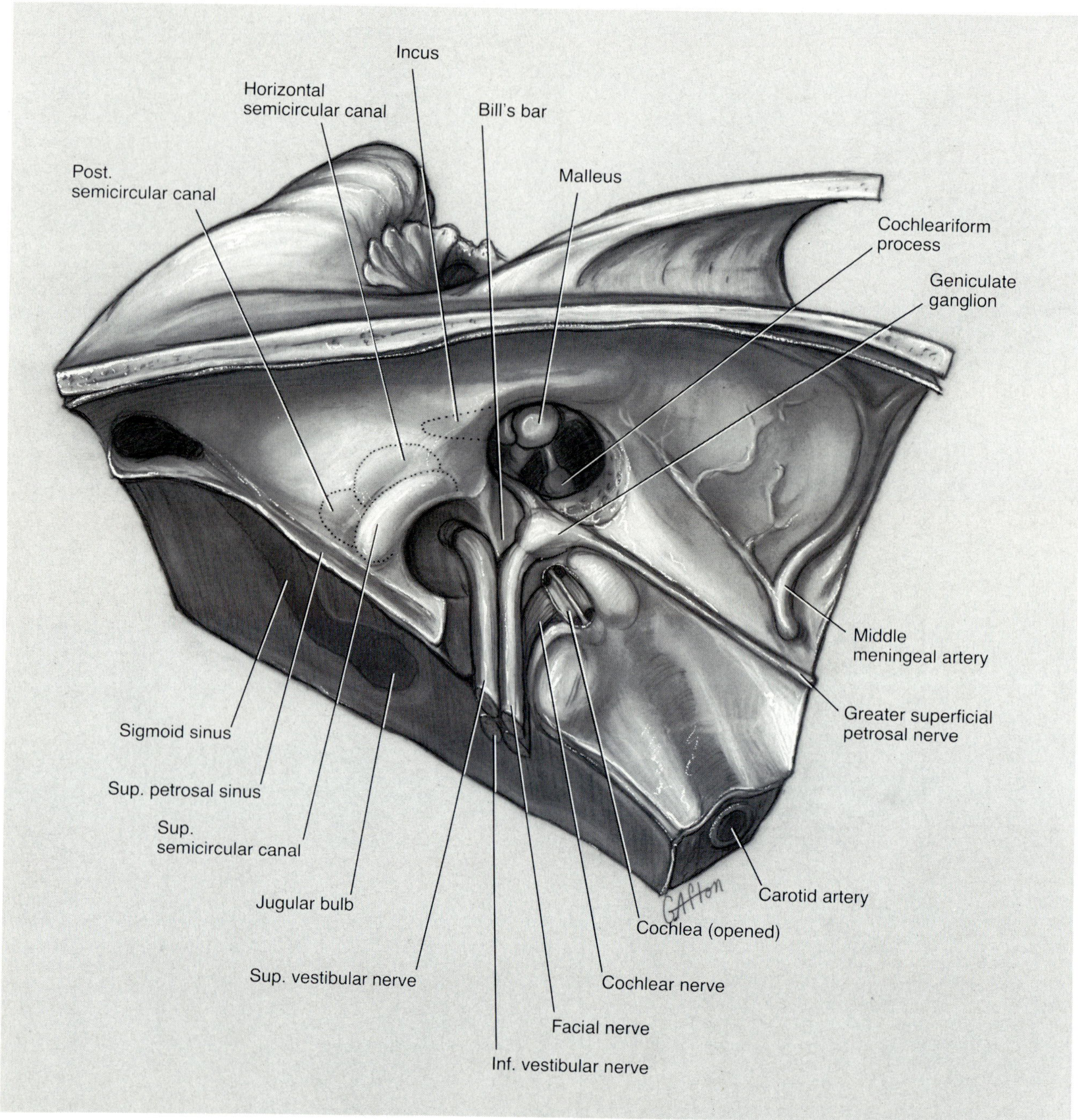

Incus
Horizontal semicircular canal
Bill's bar
Post. semicircular canal
Malleus
Cochleariform process
Geniculate ganglion
Middle meningeal artery
Greater superficial petrosal nerve
Sigmoid sinus
Sup. petrosal sinus
Sup. semicircular canal
Jugular bulb
Carotid artery
Cochlea (opened)
Sup. vestibular nerve
Cochlear nerve
Facial nerve
Inf. vestibular nerve

FIGURE 5–40.

can be relied upon. Familiarity with the middle fossa is accomplished only with repeated inspection and dissection. The major landmarks of the middle fossa have now been identified, including the middle meningeal artery, the greater superficial petrosal nerve with its facial hiatus, and the arcuate eminence.

Dissection begins with positive identification of the facial nerve. The greater superficial petrosal nerve is followed back to the facial hiatus, where it enters and joins the geniculate ganglion. With a large diamond bur and suction irrigation to avoid heat generation and bone dust accumulation, the thin bone overlying the geniculate ganglion is removed (Fig. 5–39*B*). Here the facial nerve turns slightly posterior and inferior as it runs into its tympanic course. The epitympanum may be opened to expose the head of the malleus, tensor tympani, and cochleariform process. The cochleariform process is the limit to which the facial nerve can be adequately decompressed by this approach. Following this, the labyrinthine segment of the facial nerve is exposed; this is a very short segment running from the geniculate ganglion to the lateral end of the internal auditory canal. Care must be taken not to enter the ampulla of the semicircular canal, which lies only a few millimeters posterior, or the cochlea, only a few millimeters anterior. This segment of the facial nerve courses almost parallel to the plane of the semicircular canal. A diamond bur is needed to work in this limited space. Bone is removed medially following the course of the facial nerve, which runs in a posterior and inferior (deeper) direction. When the posterior fossa is reached (medially), the exposure can be widened because the semicircular canal courses posteriorly and the dissection at this point is medial to the cochlea. As the edge of the posterior fossa is reached, remember that the superior petrosal sinus lies in this dural reflection. At this point obtain wide exposure of the internal auditory canal. By carefully removing the final eggshell thinness of bone, the contents of the canal may be identified. The facial nerve occupies the anterosuperior compartment, with the superior vestibular nerve immediately behind in the posterosuperior aspect (Fig. 5–39*C*). At the lateral end of the canal is Bill's bar, the ridge of bone separating these two nerves. Here the superior vestibular nerve runs to the ampulla of the semicircular canal. Immediately below the facial nerve lies the cochlear nerve, and the inferior vestibular nerve lies beneath the superior vestibular nerve. These represent the anteroinferior and posteroinferior compartments respectively.

For the sake of completeness, the following structures should be found and followed in their courses. This will help to further the understanding of temporal bone anatomy in a three-dimensional view (Fig. 5–40). Slightly lateral to the greater superior petrosal, the eustachian tube runs medially from the middle ear cavity to the nasopharynx. Upon dissection of the eustachian tube, the carotid artery may be found on the inferomedial floor of the tube; it courses horizontally from the middle ear to the cavernous sinus. The semicircular canal and cochlea should be entered and followed to gain a clear understanding of their positions within the temporal bone.

SECTION III

General Principles and Approaches

CHAPTER 6

Operating Room Principles and General Concepts

Evaluation

All patients should have a complete history obtained and be given a physical examination. Although proper surgical indications and adequate laboratory studies are essential, their discussion is beyond the scope of this chapter. A complete assessment of the patient's general conditions, as well as of the otologic problem itself, is to be made. It should be remembered that the ear is not an isolated organ; it interrelates anatomically and functionally with other organs and systems—for example, the nasopharynx and nasal cavity—that must be evaluated in detail. The local conditions of the ear, including the skin of the pinna, the ear canal, middle ear mucosa, and so forth, must be improved as much as possible before surgery.

An otologic evaluation includes a number of basic tests in addition to the history and physical examination. A recent complete audiogram that includes pure tones and speech discrimination is essential. Equally important is confirmation of the results by the surgeon, utilizing tuning forks.

Radiologic studies include conventional mastoid x-rays supported by tomograms, computed tomographic scans, magnetic resonance, and other imaging modalities, depending on specific needs such as in cases of retrocochlear lesions, complications of otitis media, and congenital atresia. Specific indications of such studies will not be discussed here except to mention that conventional x-rays remain valuable and essential in many cases, providing information on mastoid aeration, the position of the sigmoid sinus, and other details. X-rays must be available in the operating room. A number of additional tests are used, such as BAER (brainstem auditory evoked responses), electrocochleography, promontory stimulation, and others, the indications for which are outside the scope of this atlas. The essential concept in this section is that the patient must be evaluated from a general as well as a local standpoint, and that tests serve the purpose of screening, ruling out, or confirming specific questions in the mind of the surgeon. They are not a "routine blanket ordered according to trends," nor are they intended to replace common sense and clinical acuity.

Patient Consent

As important as informed consent is from a legal standpoint, it is much more important in that it provides the patient with information. It is essential that the patient (or his or her parents) be aware of the rationale for and purpose of the surgical procedure. Is the aim reconstruction of the ossicular chain? Is it eradication of disease? What are the chances of success and the risks involved?

A well-informed patient is the best guarantee of success. Information on the postoperative course and care is also essential and should be provided by the surgeon. Commercially printed instructions are very helpful; however, they do not approach the usefulness of instructions printed by the surgeon.

Anesthesia

Most otologic procedures can be performed under local anesthesia, with or without sedation. The decision will depend on the specific case and the surgeon's judgment and common sense. It should be remembered that a general anesthetic usually carries a small risk, at times comparable with that of local procedures under sedation. If a local anesthetic is to be used, it is important to know the innervation of the area to be anesthetized. (See the chapters on anatomy and general surgical approaches.) Different agents are utilized; the authors usually use lidocaine (Xylocaine) 1% with 1:100,000 epinephrine in both local and general anesthesia cases, since epinephrine exerts a vasoconstrictive effect essential for microscopic surgery. The maximum safe dose of lidocaine is 3 mg/kg without epinephrine and 7 mg/kg with epinephrine. In cases of myringotomies and tubes, iontophoretic anesthesia is a useful method in the office. It is based on a battery-operated unit (iontophoretic applicator) that generates a constant direct current, allowing ion transfer of a local anesthetic (placed in the ear canal) into the ear canal and tympanic membranes. Because it does not require an injection it is very well accepted by some patients.

Antibiotics

The use of antibiotics is a controversial subject that will not be dwelled upon here. The authors use them prophylactically when there is a risk that infection will extend into the inner ear or intracranially, compromise the survival of a graft or reconstructive procedure, or spread locally—for example, to the auricular cartilage. When antibiotics are used, it is immediately before, during, and after the operation. In chronically draining ears the authors tend to start antibiotic therapy several days prior to the procedure. Use of antibiotics does not mean that strict aseptic techniques are disregarded; they are used only when there are additional risks in spite of a flawless technique that includes asepsis, meticulous hemostasis, and gentleness with tissues.

Equipment and Procedures

The operating table must be comfortable but hard enough to allow for resuscitation procedures if needed. It should be easily adjustable so that it can be raised or lowered or the patient placed in a Trendelenburg or reverse Trendelenburg position (Figs. 6–1, 6–2). The headpiece should be separable in order to change the position of the patient's head independently from the rest of the table (Fig. 6–3).

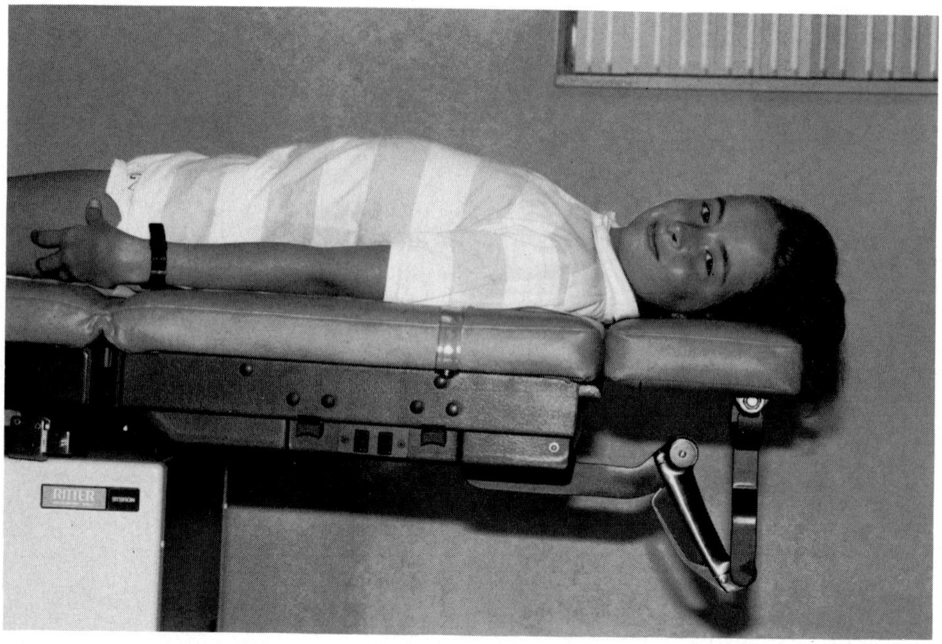

FIGURES 6–1, 6–2.
One of the brands of operating tables with easy adjustments for different positions.

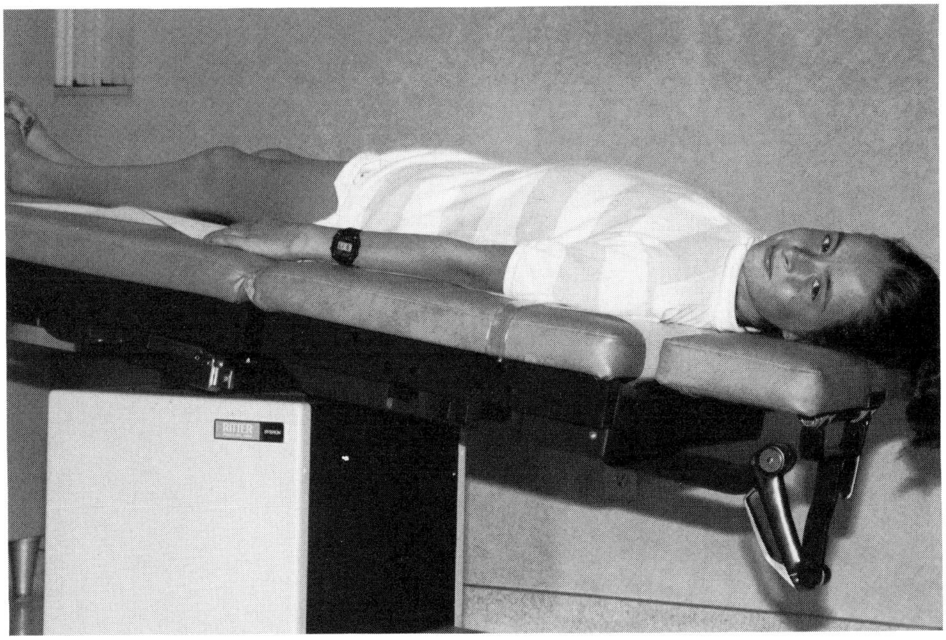

FIGURE 6–2.

At times a simple "donut" will suffice; in general, however, a Juers head holder is more useful, allowing adjustments in angulation of the head as needed (Figs. 6–4, 6–5). The patient's head should be taped to the head holder (which in turn is taped to the head of the table) and moved with the holder as a unit (Fig. 6–6). The patient lies supine with the head turned and lowered in order to bring the external auditory canal, which has a bony orientation that is downward and forward, into a nearly vertical position.

Preparation of the Skin

The skin is prepared after shaving the hair. Shaving of the hair is done with a dry razor blade at the time of surgery, avoiding any lacerations of the skin. Enough hair is shaved to provide a clean operative field. For a postauricular approach the authors shave an area of approximately 2.5 cm. If a large flap is to be raised (for example, for a postauricular cochlear implant) more hair is shaved. For an endaural ap-

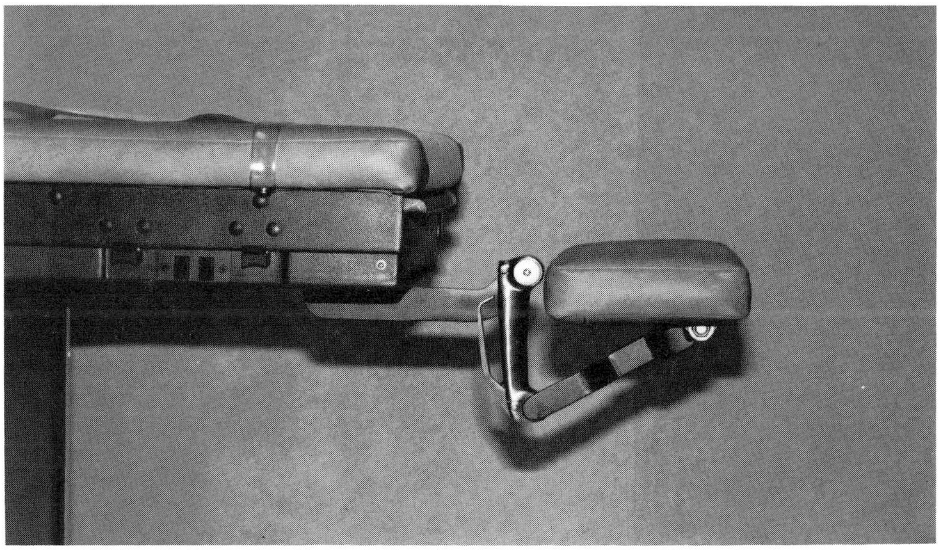

FIGURE 6–3.
A headpiece that can be separated from the table is useful.

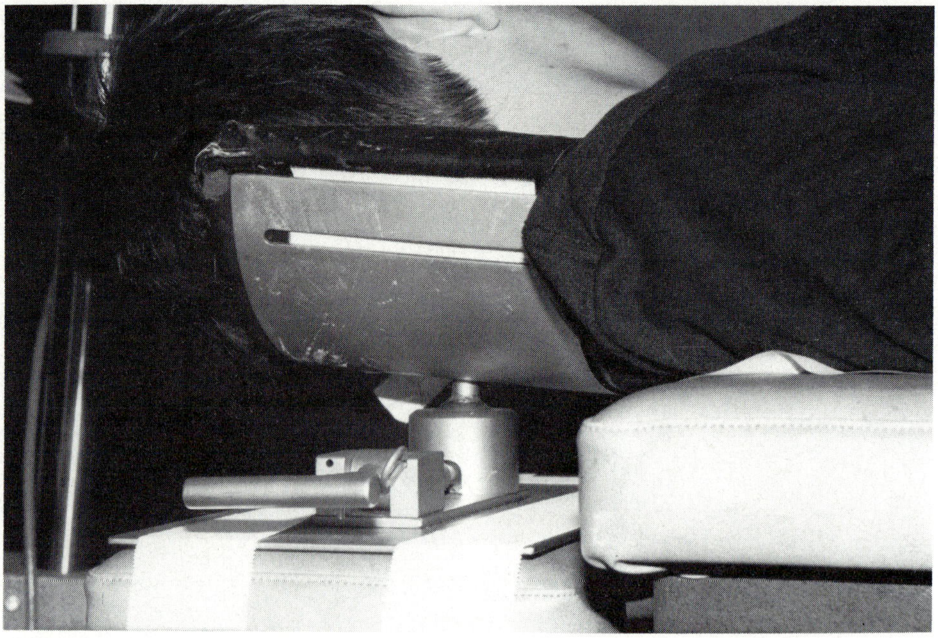

FIGURES 6–4, 6–5.
A Juers head holder allows for maneuverability.

proach 0.5 cm of hair superiorly along the superior helix will suffice. A germicidal soap and solution such as povidone-iodine (Betadine) or hexachlorophene (pHisoHex) is used. Whichever agent is selected, the scrub should be for ten minutes and the solution wiped dry before sterile drapes are applied. The ear canal is cleansed with a solution such as hydrogen peroxide or irrigated with saline, or both.

The operative field is isolated with sterile drapes, avoiding excessive bulk that would compromise mobility. The "hanging drapes" are clamped together in order to allow the surgeon's legs to fit comfortably under the head of the table without interference.

Foreign Body Reaction

Particles contained in gloves (powder), a prosthesis, or surgical instruments can cause inflamma-

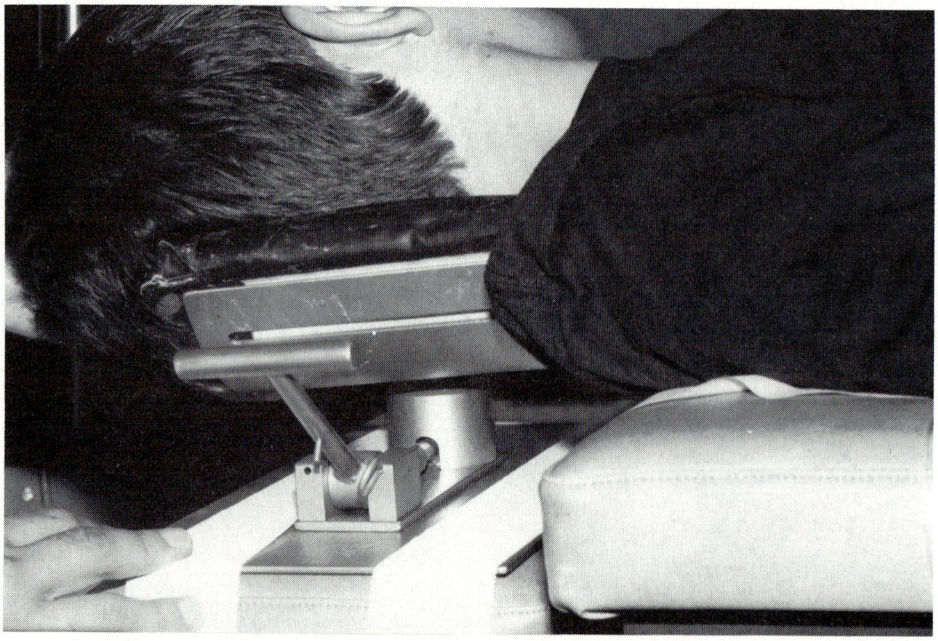

FIGURE 6–5.

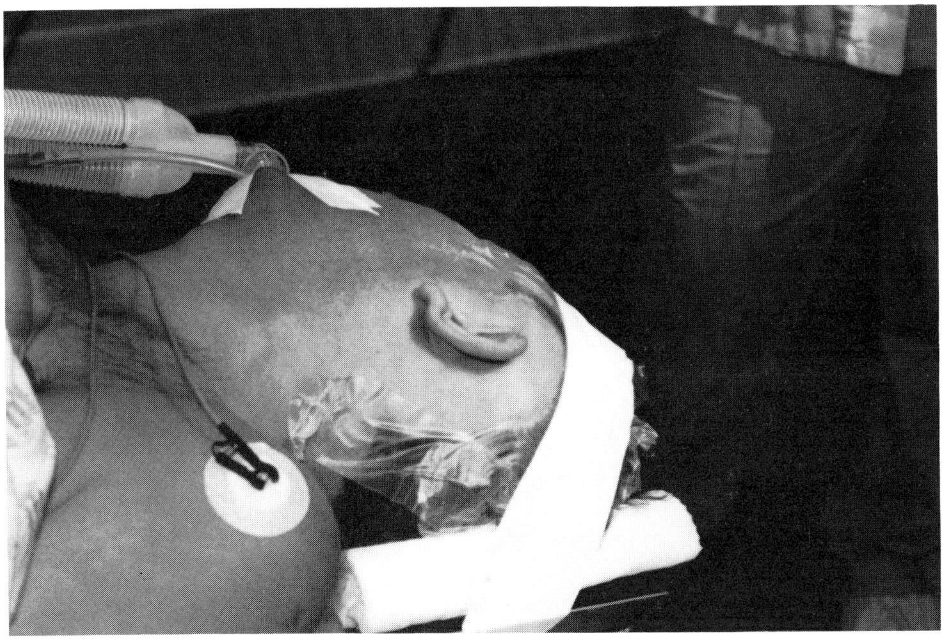

FIGURE 6–6.
The patient's head is taped to the head holder.

tory reactions that are potentially harmful. It is a good habit to keep a sterile solution and a moist towel to rinse and clean the surgical gloves before initiating surgery. The scrub nurse should have on his or her table a container with saline in order to clean the instruments and prosthesis prior to use. Instruments should be rinsed meticulously after the use of sterilizing chemicals, since these can be very damaging to tissues.

Positioning of the Surgical Team

The *surgeon* must be in a comfortable and stable position, with both feet on the floor, and with the back supported by a chair that can be moved easily (by the surgeon) while retaining its position. The patient must be placed so that the surgeon is not bent or forced into uncomfortable positions. This is usually achieved by positioning the head of the operating table virtually over the surgeon's lap, with the surgeon capable of "comfortably writing on a desk" while looking through the microscope.

The *surgical team* is of the utmost importance. A successful surgical procedure represents the combined efforts of a team of surgeons, anesthesiologists, and scrub and circulating nurses. No matter how skilled the surgeon, his or her work is not possible without a safely and adequately anesthetized or sedated patient; no matter how skilled the anesthesiologist, adequate anesthesia will not be possible if the surgeon does not inform him or her of the moment of injection of epinephrine, mobilization of the head of the patient, elevation of the operative table, or other procedures. The same rules apply in principle for the circulating and scrub nurses. The precept of this chapter is that in surgery, teamwork yields better results than "wonder man" or "wonder woman" alone.

The authors' positioning of the team and instruments in the operating room is shown in Figure 6–7. The scrub nurse is at the right of the surgeon and the assistant is at the left. Other surgeons prefer different setups. The best position is one that provides the most comfort and efficiency to a particular team.

Instruments

The *operating microscope* obviously must be binocular with a focal length of at least 20 cm. The authors prefer to use the 25-cm length; it provides a range of magnification from 6× to 40×, with 6×, 10×, and 16× the most commonly used. Along with good light (either bulb or fiberoptic), it requires good handling ability. Both the surgeon and the scrub nurse must be familiar with the different knobs that provide maneuverability. The authors prefer to use an angled eyepiece that provides an angle of 45 degrees and allows a more comfortable head position for the surgeon (Fig. 6–8).

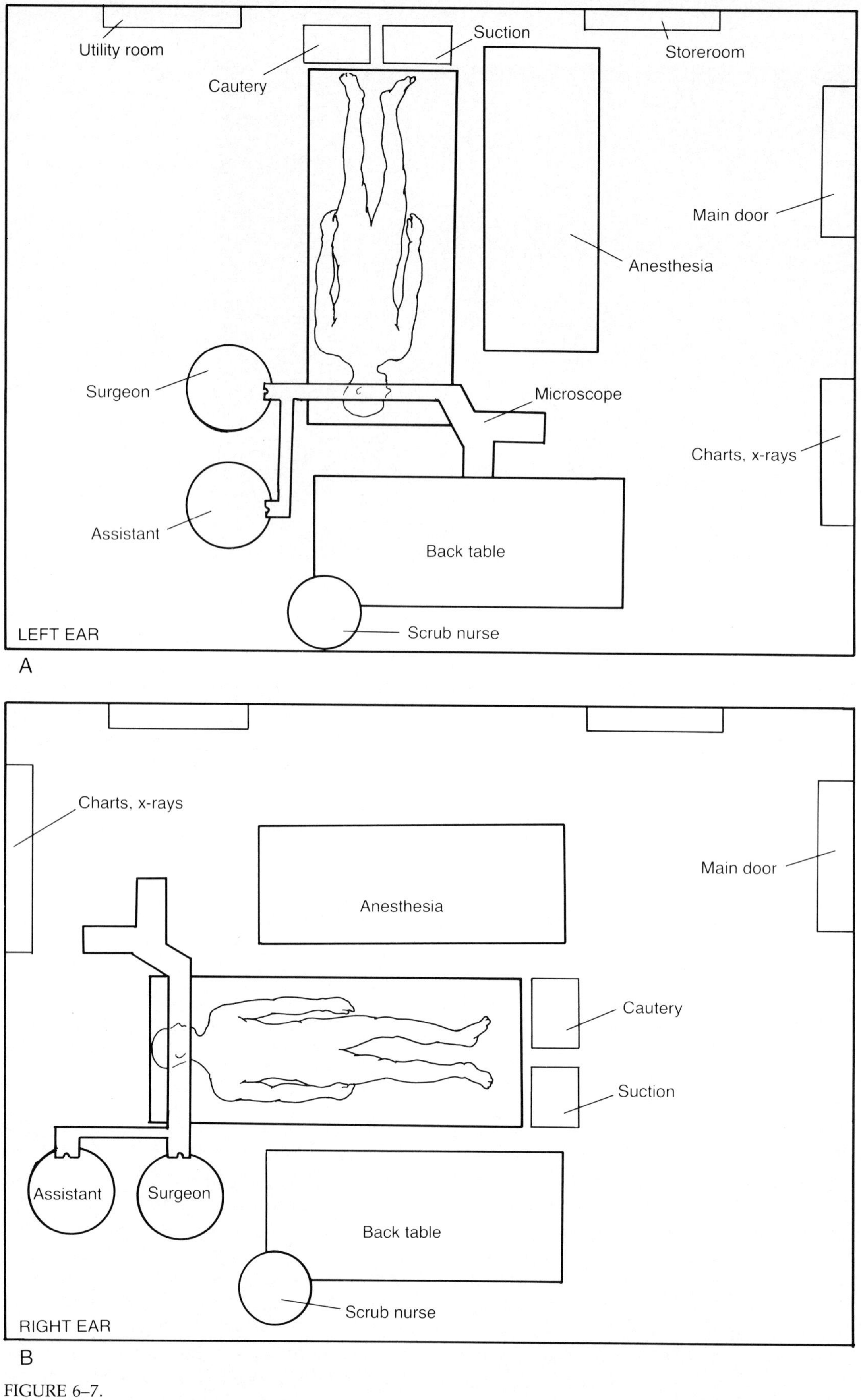

FIGURE 6–7.
Diagram of the authors' positioning of the surgical team and instruments in the operating room.

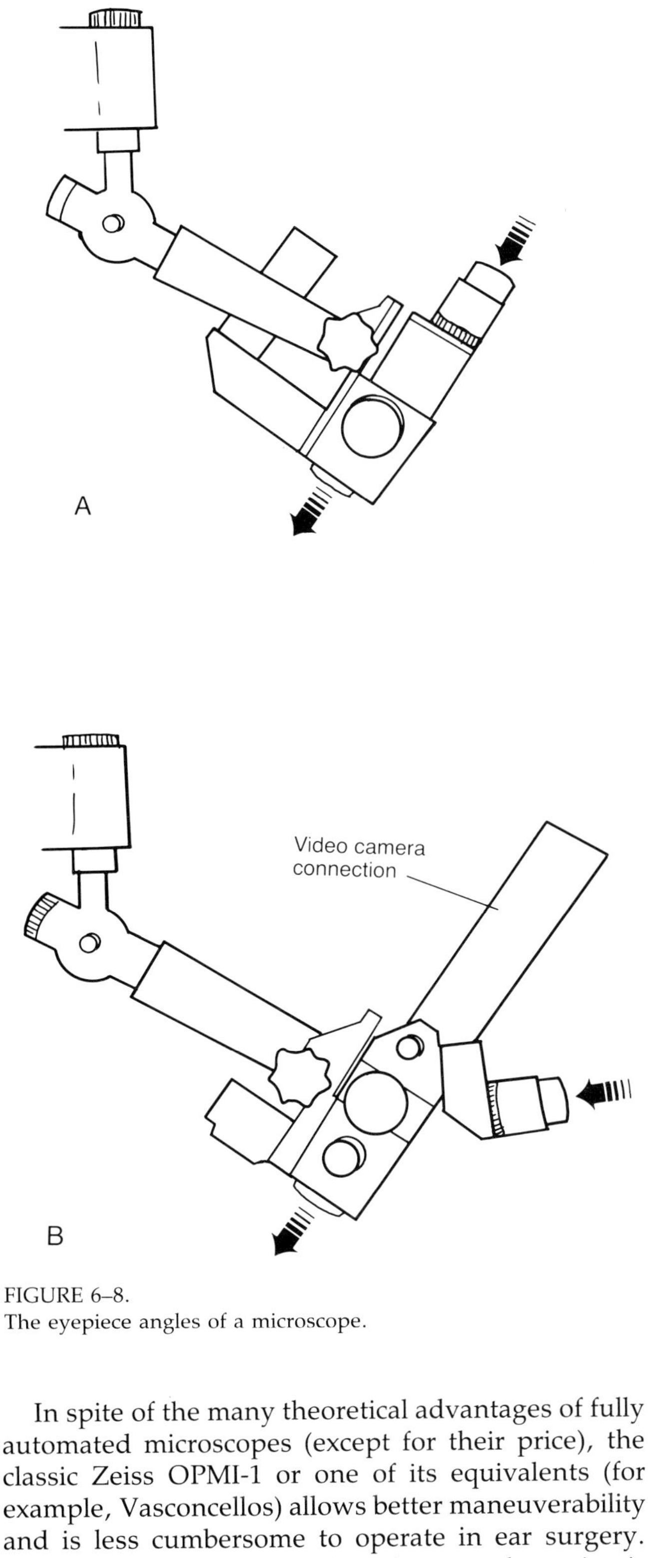

FIGURE 6–8.
The eyepiece angles of a microscope.

In spite of the many theoretical advantages of fully automated microscopes (except for their price), the classic Zeiss OPMI-1 or one of its equivalents (for example, Vasconcellos) allows better maneuverability and is less cumbersome to operate in ear surgery. Again, this is a matter of preference; the point is made because it is not unusual for the "starting surgeon in practice" to be talked into buying a fully automated, "state of the art" piece of equipment.

The position of the microscope is essential. The arms should be at a 90-degree angle, which permits a full range of motion (Figs. 6–9, 6–10). In the case of the OPMI-1 the "longer leg" of the pedestal should point toward the patient's shoulder on the operated side. The side viewer (teaching lens) is placed at the left side; if possible a video camera is attached. This allows the operating team to be aware of the procedure, anticipate the use of instruments, and even maintain a permanent record of the operation. A suitable sterile drape of either cloth or disposable plastic must be used (Fig. 6–11). For insertion of PE tubes, rubber handles for focusing and magnification are useful. If they are not available, a sterile towel will suffice.

A variety of *drills* are commercially available. A high-speed drill should suffice, provided that it is a durable instrument capable of withstanding continuous use. At least two drills should be available in the operating room. The drill handles should be light and easy to manipulate; the instrument should have several speeds, including reverse and forward. Control by a foot pedal is preferable since handle-controlled drills tend to have more vibration. The reverse speed is useful for saucerizing small bleeding points in the mastoid and bony ear canal. It is also important that both the surgeon and scrub nurse should be able to assemble and operate the drill. Different metal burs, usually made out of tungsten or steel, are available. Rounded burs work best for otology; they can be of six or eight teeth. In general, burs with more teeth accumulate more debris and are less effective; however, a bur full of debris is useful in areas requiring gentle work, and is similar in this regard to a diamond bur (a metal bur coated with diamond powder). Burs must be sharp; dulling leads to overheating. The authors favor burs with regular shafts over those with special hooks, which in practice limit the surgeon to particular brands; the more universal the drill, the better. Sizes of burs vary according to need (discussed in specific chapters).

The "suction irrigation" feature is commonly used today. Drills with continuous irrigation (variable flow) are available, and are useful in avoiding drilling over "dry bone," which promotes overheating and necrosis. The authors prefer to use intermittent irrigation with a bulb syringe to provide moisture as needed, thus avoiding the visual distortion that occurs with "underwater drilling." Again, the purpose is to avoid heating and necrosis of bone; that is best achieved in a manner that is efficient for the surgeon.

Good *suction* is essential. The tubing should be flexible, soft but not collapsible, and not too rigid, so that it is easy to handle. A No. 5 suction tip is used for cleansing the ear canal, a No. 20 for raising flaps and for middle ear work, and a No. 24 for work in the oval window. The authors prefer fenestrated

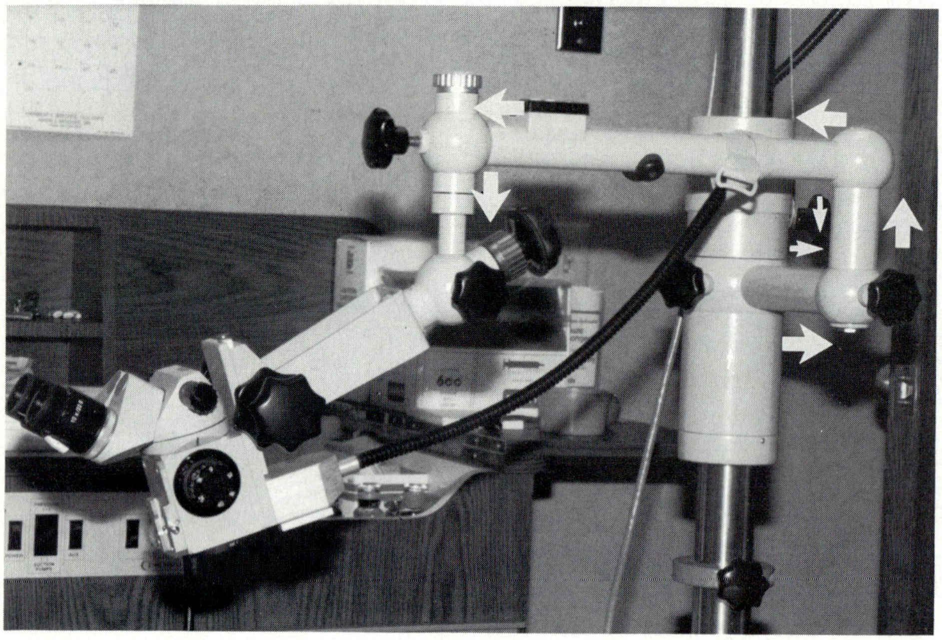

FIGURES 6–9, 6–10.
The positions of the arms of the microscope at 90-degree angles.

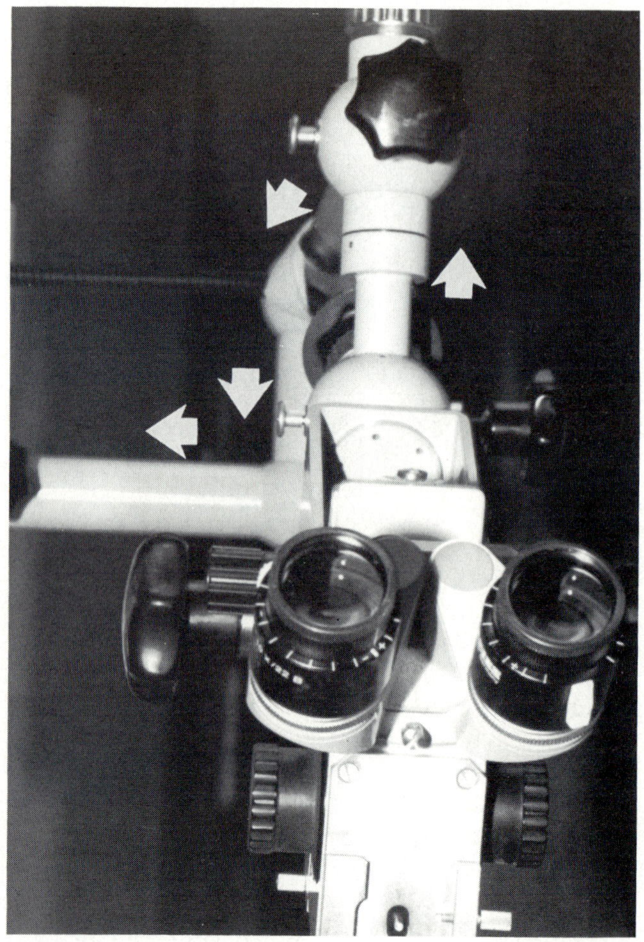

FIGURE 6–10.

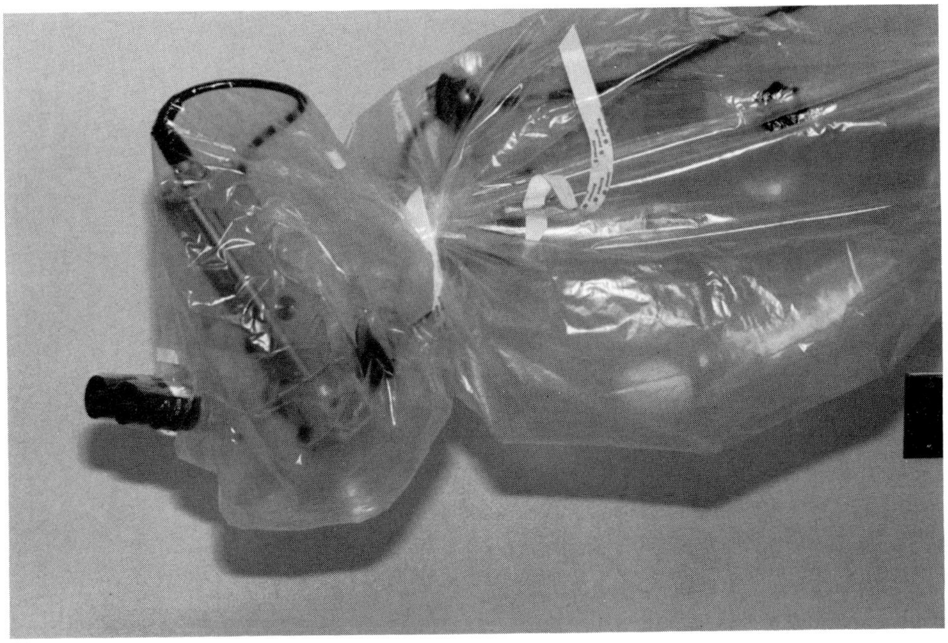

FIGURE 6–11.
A disposable sterile plastic drape has been used with this microscope, which has a video camera attached.

handles, which allow control of the degree of suction; some surgeons prefer to control the degree of suction with a foot control. For drilling, larger suction tips are used (No. 7 to No. 9 French). A syringe for forced irrigation, as well as a wire to clean the suction tip, should be available. Small sponges or cotton balls should be used at the suction tip when working over grafts or prostheses that can be loosened or dislodged by the suction. (Cotton must not be left in the ear since it is a guarantee of infection.) The authors' usual instrument setup is shown in Figures 6–12 and 6–13.

Standard cautery units will not be described; suffice it to mention that the authors routinely use a monopolar unit, but for cases of acoustic neuroma or in which work is to be done near the facial nerve a bipolar unit should be available. Both the suction and cautery units should be adequately positioned and clipped to the drapes, with sufficient length to allow easy handling but short enough to prevent contamination if the units are dropped (Fig. 6–14).

A variety of instrument sets are commercially available. Since the purpose of this atlas is descriptive and not promotional, the authors' specific preferences are not listed; they will be sent upon request. It is important to acquire quality instruments, particularly for work inside the ear. Apparent savings from buying cheaper but poorly made instruments can be illusory. Instruments are designed for specific purposes and should be purchased with them in mind. Instruments bearing the endorsement of a particular surgeon provide a sense of security and should be considered for acquisition; however, they represent the preference of that surgeon and may not necessarily meet your needs.

Operating room cards describing the instruments and materials required for different surgical procedures should be available. They make the nurses' jobs easier and more effective. Ear instruments preferably are placed in a rack and numbered in the order in which they are used—for example, No. 1 straight canal knife, No. 2 curved canal knife, No. 3 duckbill elevator, and so on. If the scrub and circulating nurses rotate or the operating room "committee" believes that nurses can be "jacks of all trades," it is useful to print the names of the instruments (beside their numbers) and to place on the table a plasticized, "sterilizable" card listing the names and positions of instruments and materials. In addition, cards describing the position of the team in the operating room should be taped to the wall in a clearly visible place.

Record of Operation

As important as describing what was done is describing what was found, preferably with a draw-

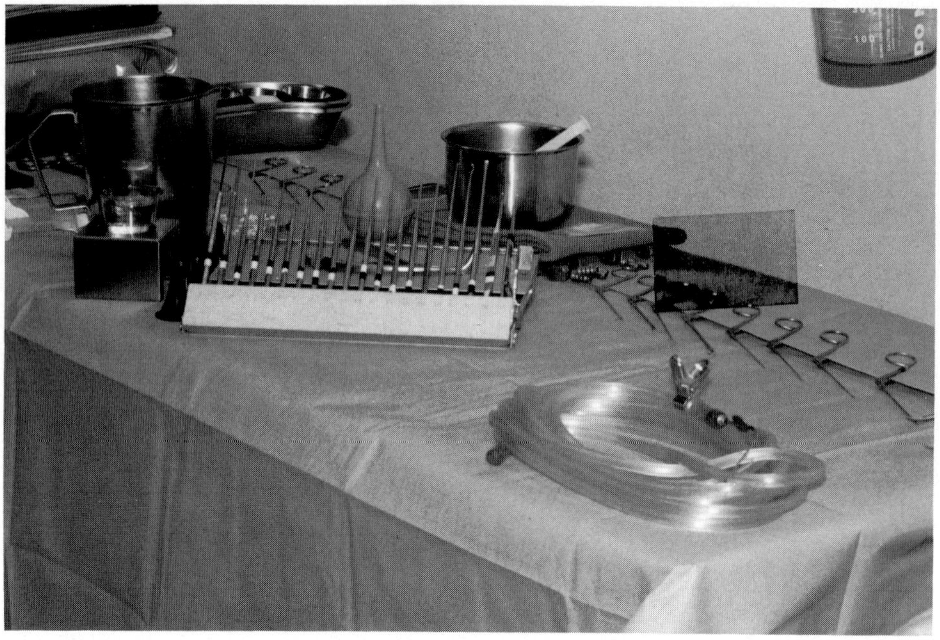

FIGURES 6–12, 6–13.
The authors' usual instrument setup. The suction tubing is included in order to give an idea of the size and type used.

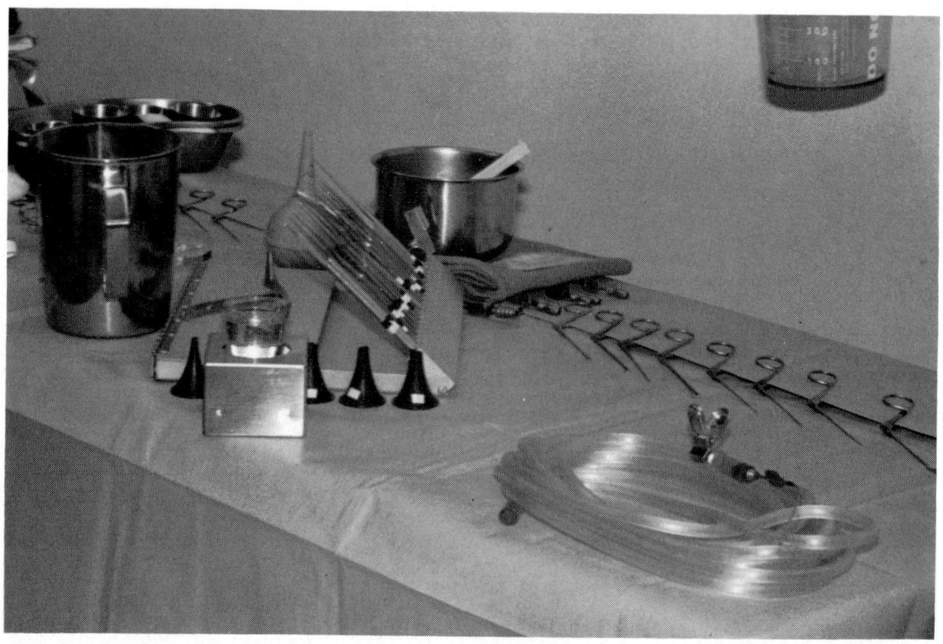

FIGURE 6–13.

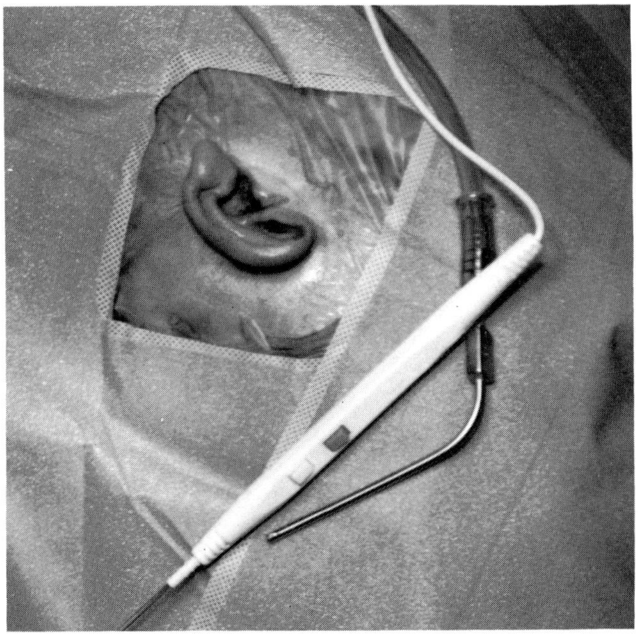

FIGURE 6–14.
Suction tip and cautery "hanging" in the operating field. They are not left in this position during surgery; this figure simply shows that if clipped correctly, the suction tip and cautery will not become contaminated if they fall.

ing. Problem areas should be noted; such records are useful in evaluating prospective causes and factors in both failures and successful results. A stamped or printed drawing or diagram in the operative description is useful. Packing techniques are described in specific sections and will not be discussed here. Illustrations of how to apply an oval eye pad (Figs. 6–15 to 6–17) and a mastoid dressing (Figs. 6–18 to 6–30) are included, as well as two photographs showing the application of ointment with a rubber-tipped syringe (Figs. 6–31, 6–32).

Surgical Time

It is important to develop surgical techniques and habits that allow a systematic and efficient use of time, but completeness and thoroughness are equally essential. In measuring success, results have more weight than speed. Would you prefer to be operated on by a surgeon who is rushing to "finish the schedule" or by one who is more concerned about finishing only when his or her purposes of helping you have been surgically achieved?

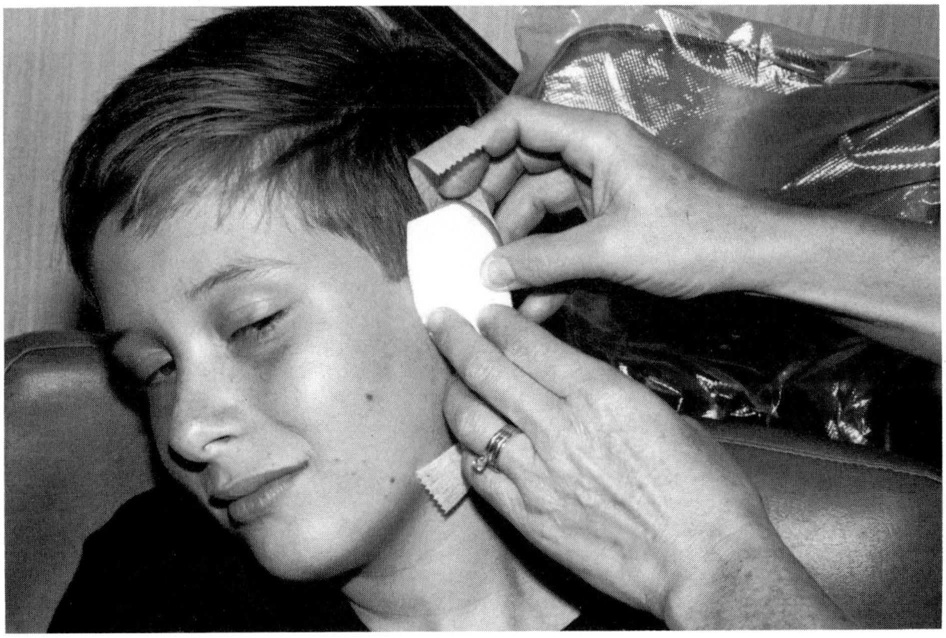

FIGURES 6–15 to 6–17.
Placement of an oval eye pad.

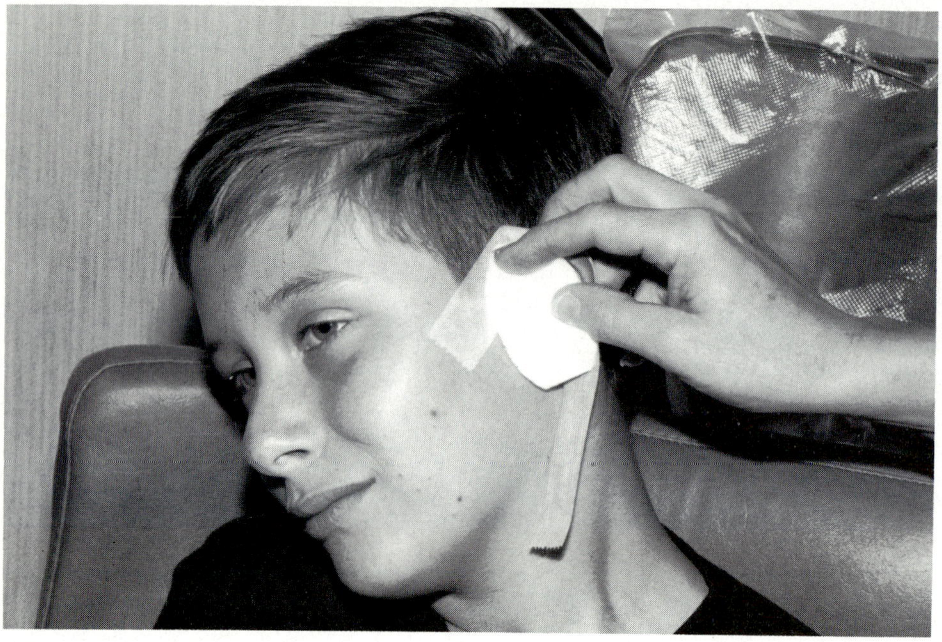

FIGURE 6–16.

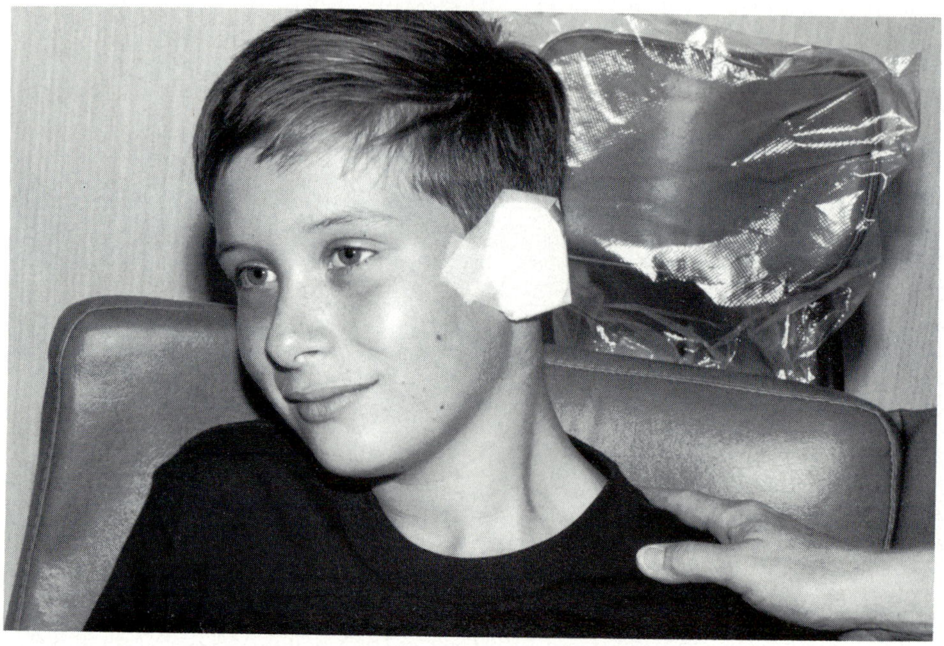

FIGURE 6–17.

FIGURES 6–18 to 6–30.
Placement of a mastoid dressing (self-explanatory). Essential point: Wrap around the ear in a figure of eight while providing some tension with the roller gauze. Figure 6–30 shows where to cut the gauze for removal of the dressing.

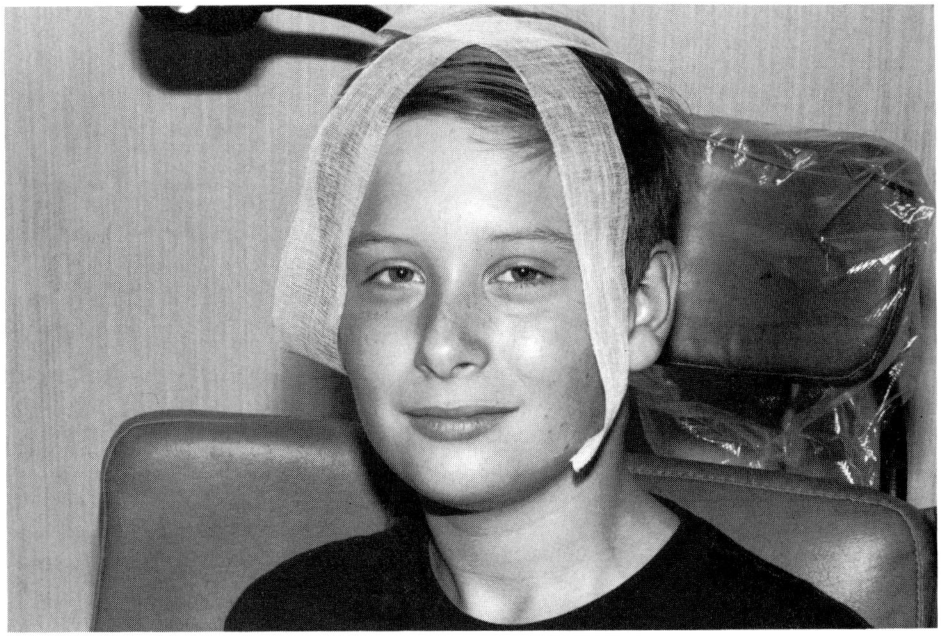

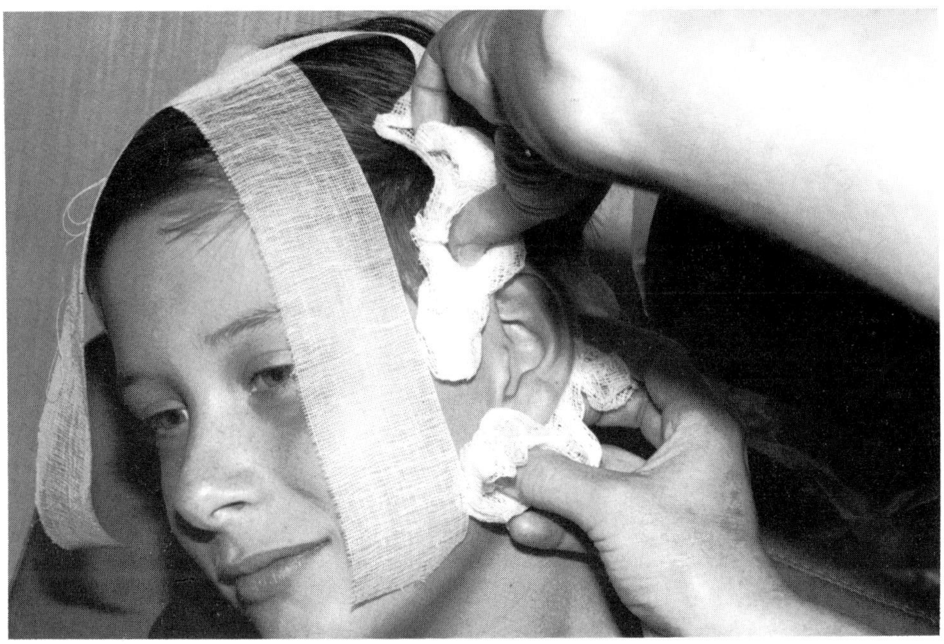

FIGURE 6–19.

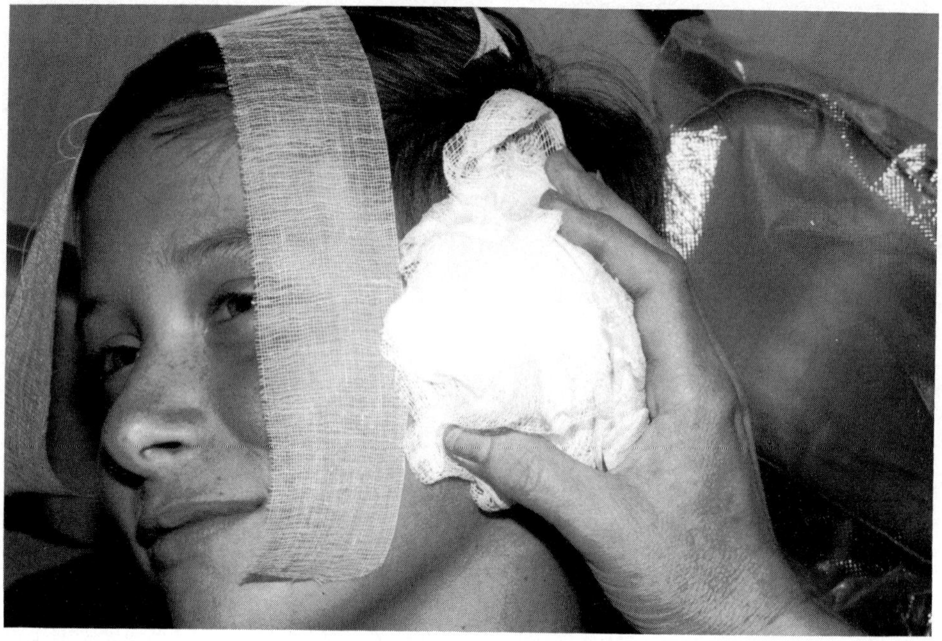

FIGURE 6–20.

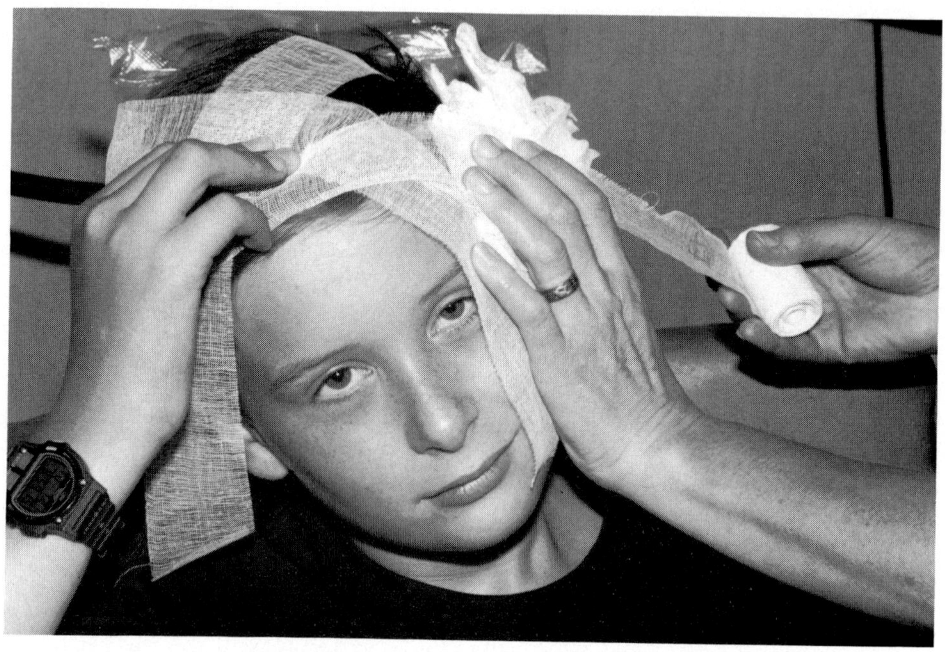

FIGURE 6–21.

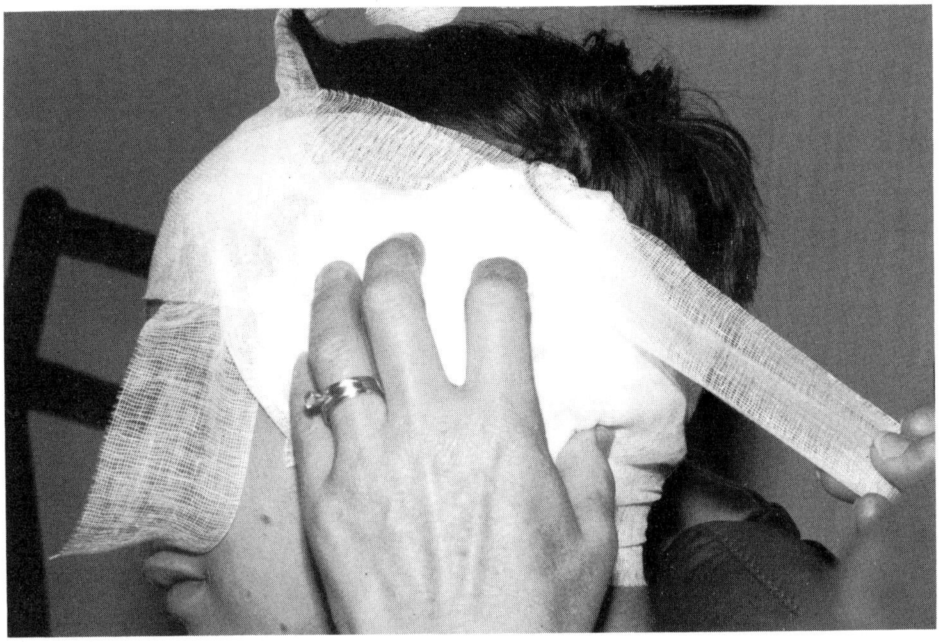

FIGURE 6–22.

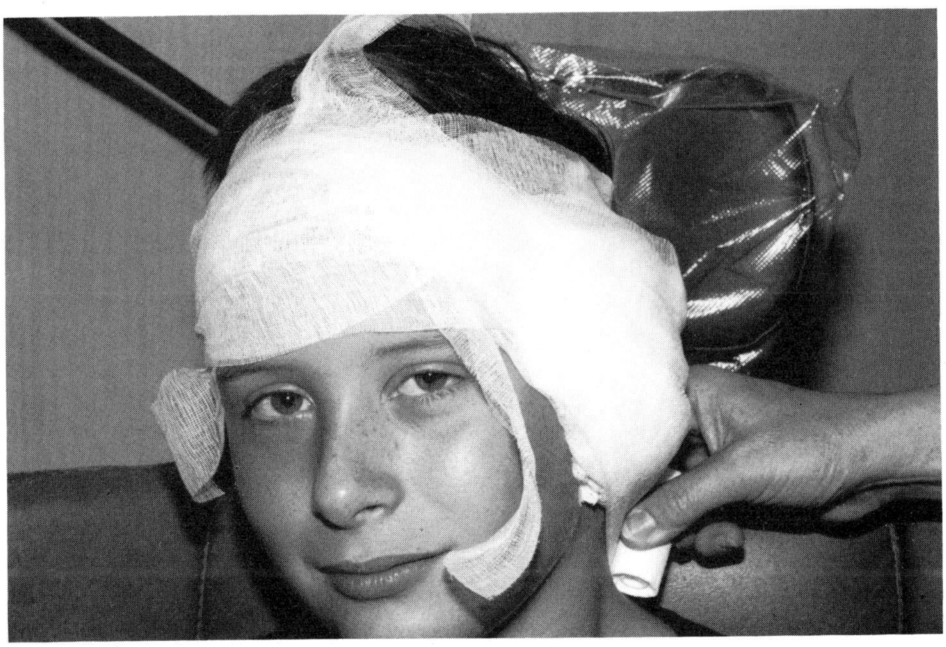

FIGURE 6–23.

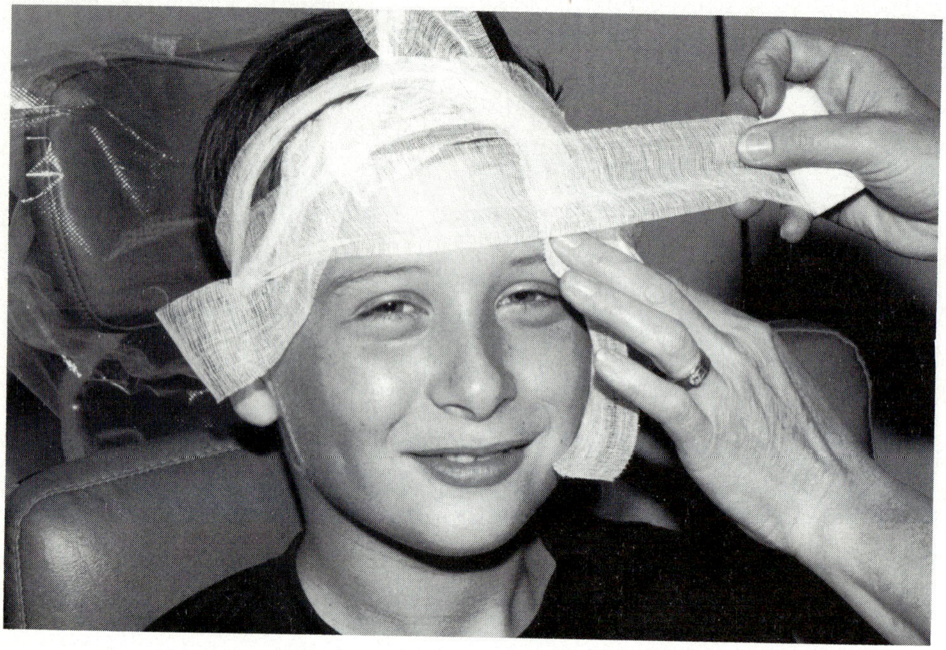

FIGURE 6–24.

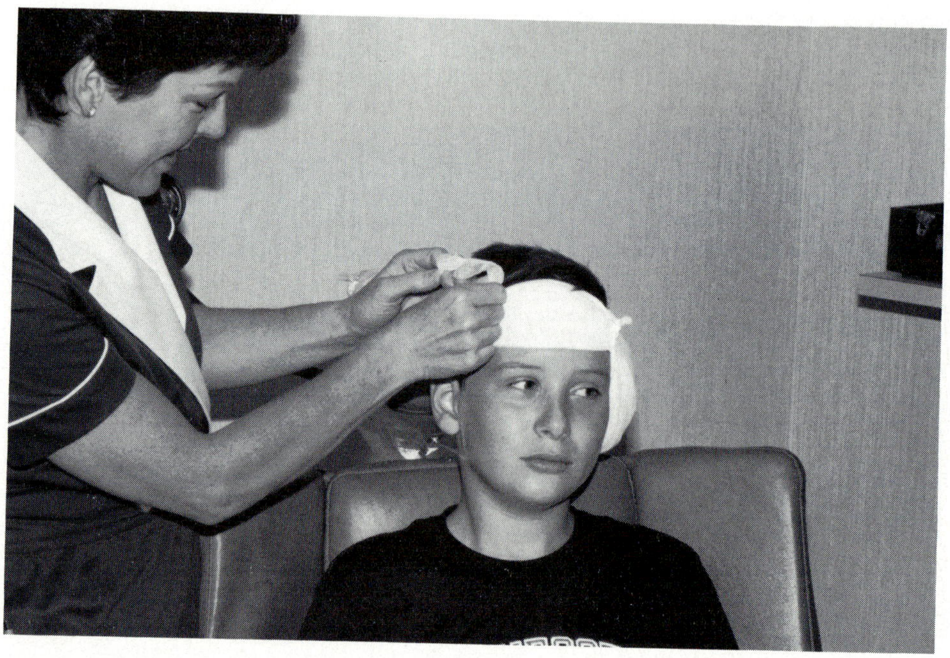

FIGURE 6–25.

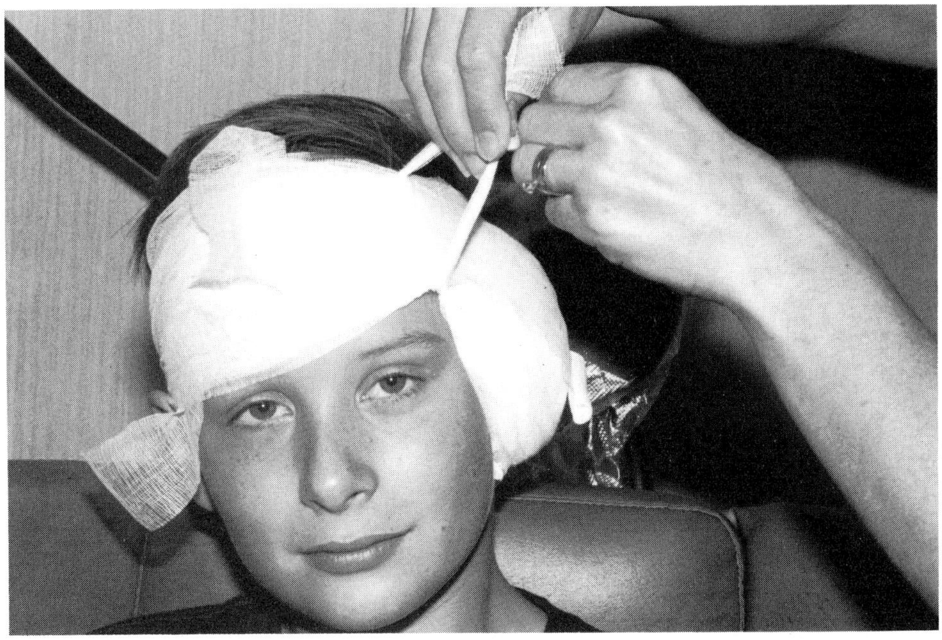

FIGURE 6–26.

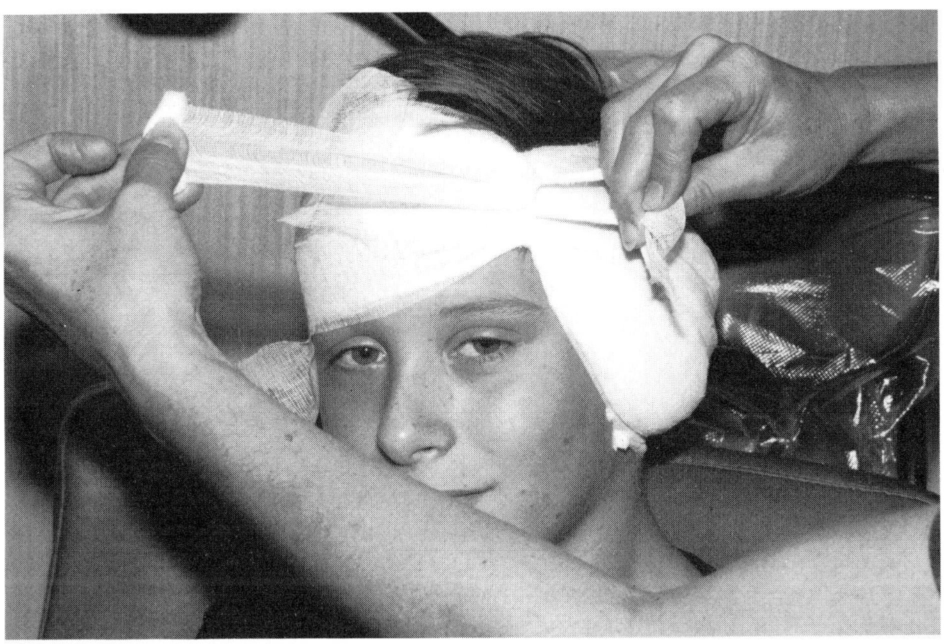

FIGURE 6–27.

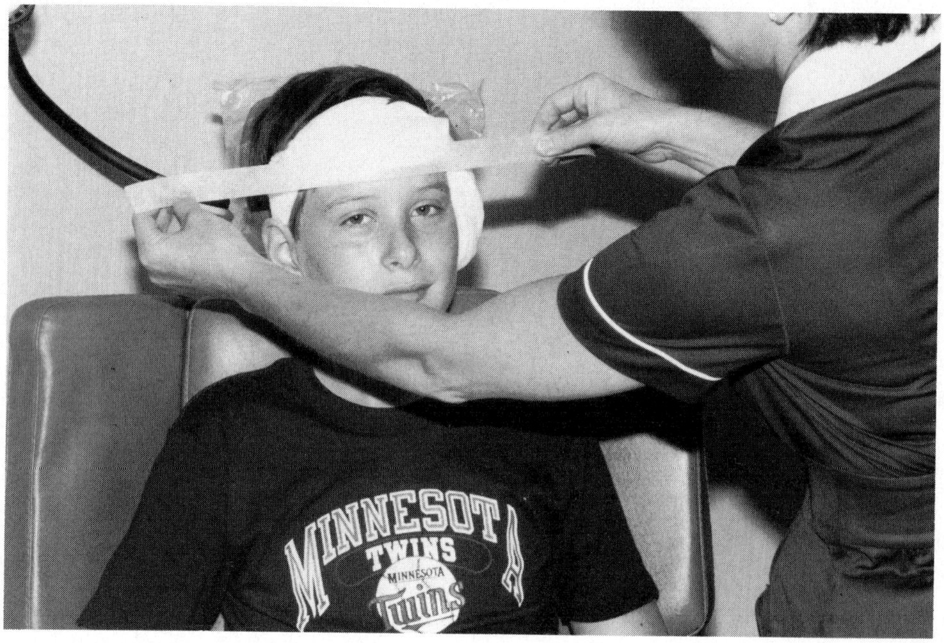

FIGURE 6–28.

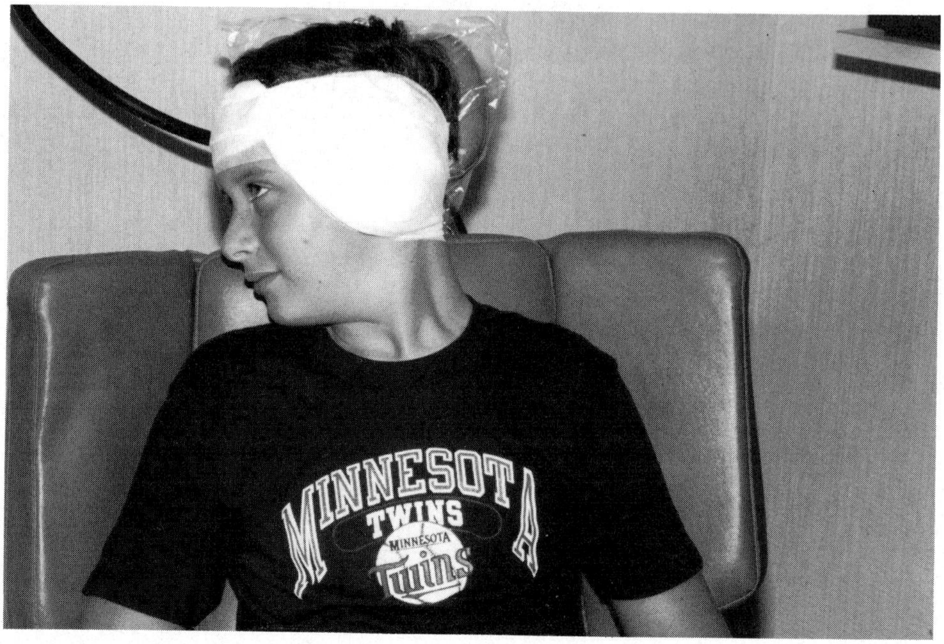

FIGURE 6–29.

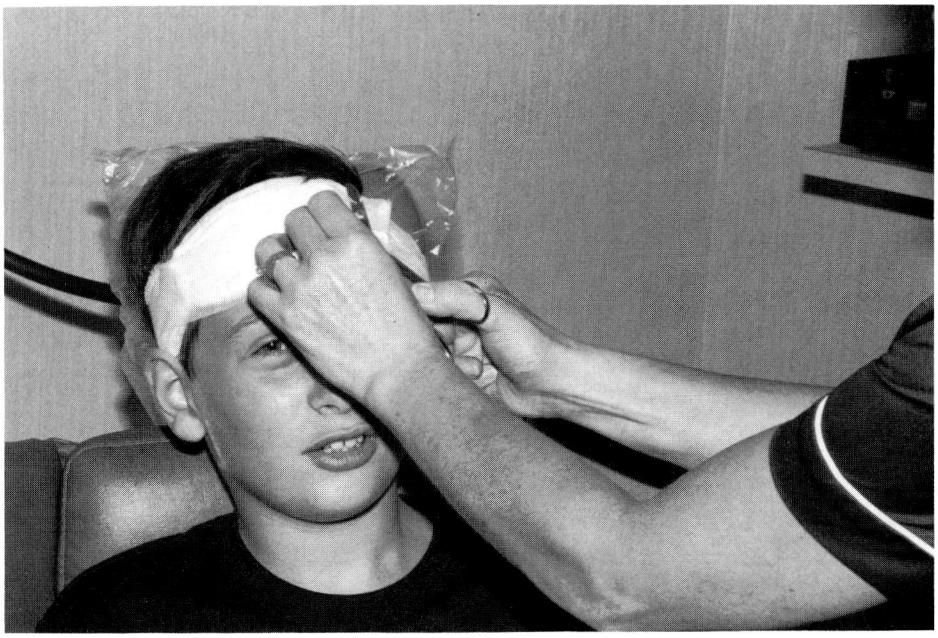

FIGURE 6–30.

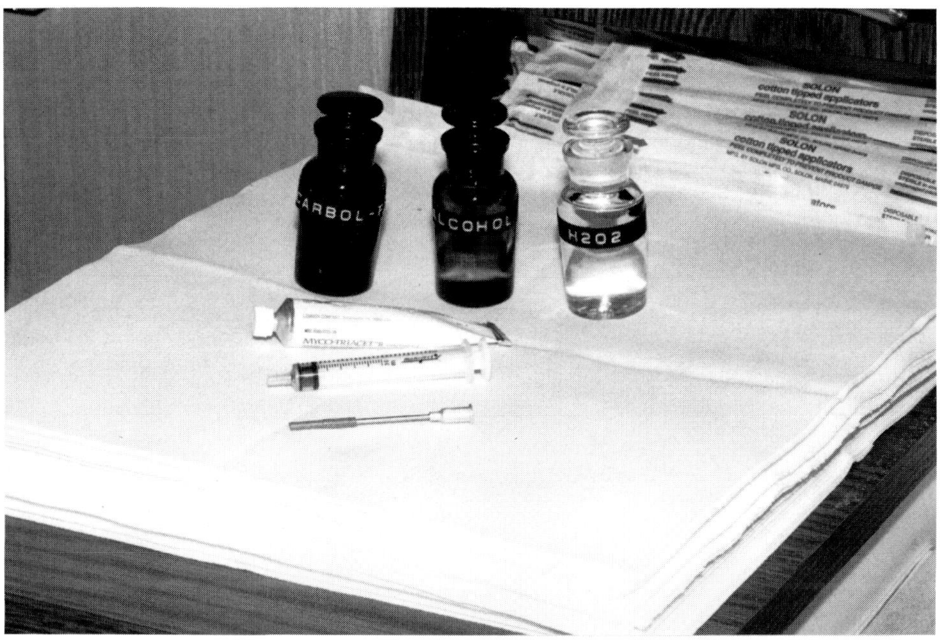

FIGURES 6–31, 6–32.
Along with the usual solutions, the application of ointment with a rubber-tipped syringe is useful in postoperative care.

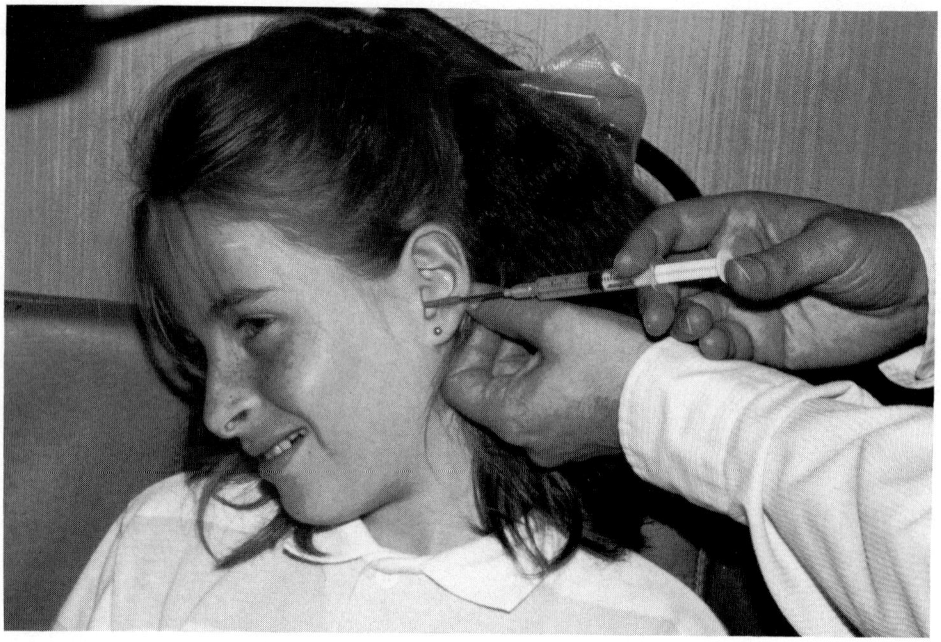

FIGURE 6–32.

CHAPTER 7

Surgical Approaches to the External Ear Canal and Middle Ear

This chapter describes basic general principles underlying the possible alternative approaches to the external ear canal and middle ear. It is obvious that the approach selected will depend upon the type of procedure planned, the needs of exposure, and the surgeon's preference or ability. Specific approaches are described in the chapters in Section IV; however, since these basic principles apply partly or totally in those approaches, they are described separately here in order to avoid repetition.

Three alternative approaches are available to gain access to the external ear canal and middle ear: the transcanal, the endaural, and the postauricular (Fig. 7–1). In all three approaches, all surgical steps are equally important and should be done methodically and carefully, from preparing the patient, draping, and positioning, to applying the last piece of tape to the dressing. Meticulous care should be observed. The procedure is not finished when the flaps are repositioned; it is finished when the ear is healed. All steps, including postoperative care, are essential for proper healing.

Transcanal Approach

Highlights

1. Adequate visualization.
2. Completion of incisions (all the way through).
3. Elevation of an intact flap.
4. Entrance into the middle ear beneath the annulus.
5. Meticulous anatomic repositioning of the flap.
6. Careful packing.

Pitfalls

1. Operating in a small space without visualization.
2. Tearing the flap or tympanic membrane.
3. Suctioning the flap.
4. Making superficial incisions.
5. Entering the middle ear above the annulus.
6. Selecting an inadequate approach.

Inspection and Cleansing

Once the patient has been adequately positioned and the ear has been sterilely prepared and draped, the canal and tympanic membrane are inspected with an ear speculum. An oval, anteriorly beveled, nonreflecting speculum of the largest possible size is used. Too small a speculum provides inadequate vision and is too loose; too large a speculum causes folds in the ear canal that obstruct vision and macerate the skin. The correct size allows satisfactory vision and sufficient tightness to allow bimanual exploration.

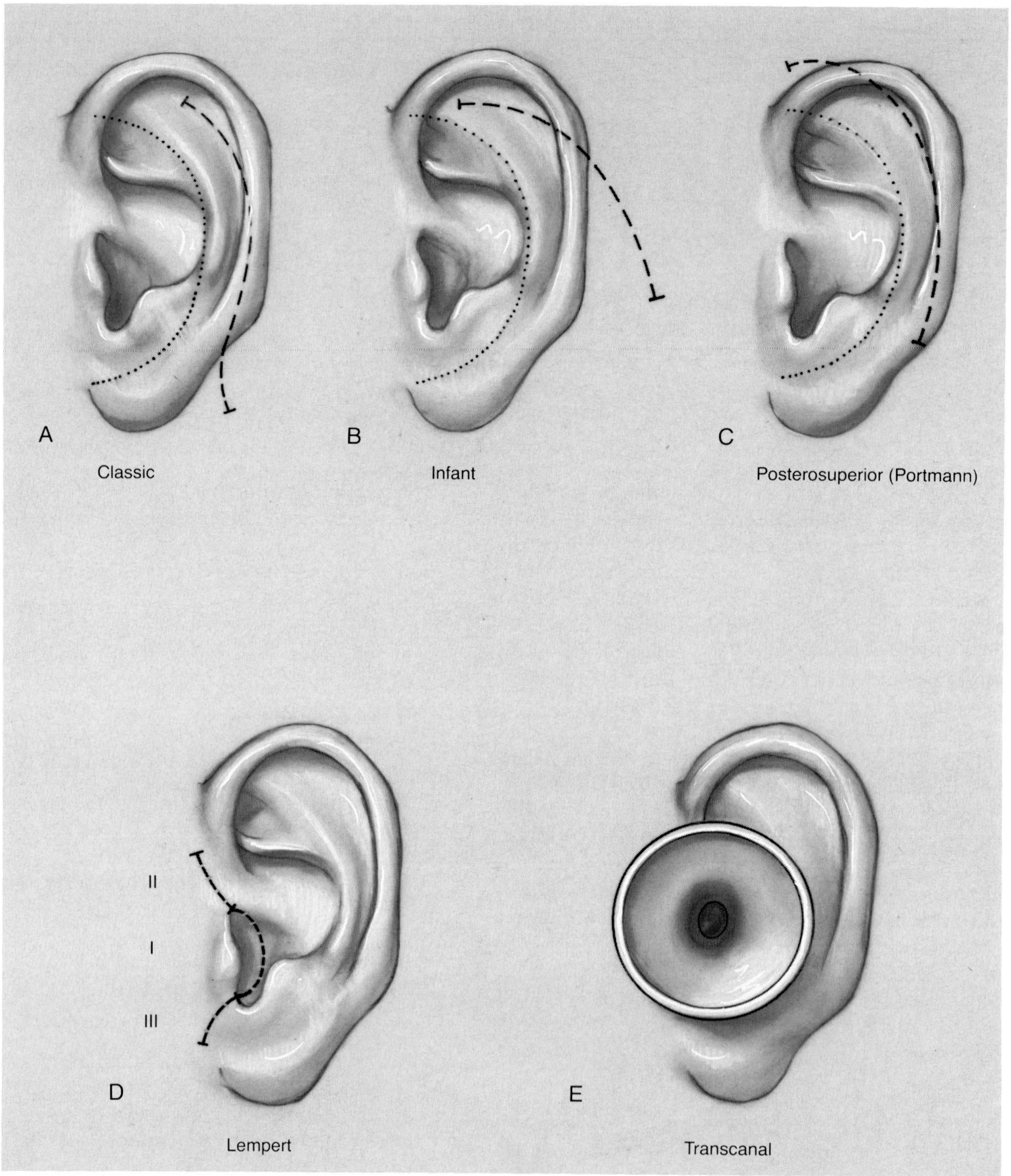
A
Classic
B
Infant
C
Posterosuperior (Portmann)
II
I
III
D
Lempert
E
Transcanal

FIGURE 7–1.

The narrowest portion of the external ear canal is medial to the junction of the bony and cartilaginous canal; it is at this point that placement of the speculum is critical. The canal is carefully cleansed with ring curets, suction (No. 5), or both. The skin and tympanic membrane are carefully visualized, and the size of the canal is appreciated. This visualization is very important, since the surgeon should first think in terms of anatomy. Whatever needs to be done in the middle ear is done best with adequate exposure. Again, positioning of the patient and the surgeon plus adequate angulation of the arm of the microscope are essential. It is a good idea to gently irrigate the canal (with either saline or alcohol).

Injection of Local Anesthetic

Injection of the anesthetic is a skill to be mastered by all means. It is a crucial step that decides if the procedure will be done in a clean, dry field or in a field obstructed by blood and offering inadequate vision. A local anesthetic with vasoconstrictor is used, usually lidocaine 2% with 1:100,000 epinephrine. Alternative anesthetic agents (owing to allergies, desire for a longer-lasting effect, or other reasons) or different concentrations of epinephrine are acceptable, but maximum doses must be kept in mind in order to avoid toxicity or cardiovascular effects, or both. A syringe affording ease of injection (for example, Carpule) is preferred. A 27- or 30-gauge needle is used. A nasal speculum is used for initial injections into the four quadrants of the cartilaginous canal (Fig. 7–2*A*). The bevel of the needle is placed parallel to the surface of the underlying cartilage (or bone), and injection is done very slowly in order to avoid blebs. (If a small bleb is formed, it can be punctured with a needle.) With slow injection under direct vision infiltration and blanching of the skin can be clearly noted; thus the necessary amount of anesthetic can be easily decided. With the aid of an ear speculum, additional injections are done, if needed, into the bony canal under direct vision until blanching of the skin is observed. The skin of the osseous canal is thinner than that of the cartilaginous portion; it is usually simpler and safer to inject into the cartilaginous portion, allowing the injected solution to "dissect its way toward the annulus." On occasion, under local anesthesia a facial paralysis becomes evident at this point. This denotes a dehiscent facial nerve, which should completely recover.

Incisions

With the speculum tightly in the canal and the surgeon working with two hands, the incisions are made. A Paparella No. 1 straight canal knife or sickle knife is used for the first incision at 12 o'clock in a direction straight toward the surgeon (Fig. 7–2*B*). A second incision is made at 6 o'clock, curving toward the vertical incision; this curved incision can be made with a curved canal knife. The length of the flap (distally from the annulus to the horizontal incision) may vary, as well as the location of the vertical incision. In a routine stapedectomy a 6-mm flap should suffice, whereas in a more extensive exploration with a small atticotomy, or if extensive bony canal is to be removed, an 8-mm flap might be necessary. If the canal is wide, a large flap extending even to the cartilaginous canal can be used, since folding it anteriorly will not obscure vision or result in a tight space with no room to work. The length of the flap is then determined by means of exposure and size of the canal.

If attic disease or fixation of the head of the malleus is suspected, a wider flap is elevated, and the vertical incision is made at the 1 or 3 o'clock position in order to provide a flap of sufficient size to cover the defect easily. If more extensive surgery is anticipated, an endaural incision is used. When making the incision, the underlying bone should be "felt" with an instrument, even to the point of producing a sound, to make certain that the skin is completely sectioned. The junction of the skin with the annulus, at 12 or 3 o'clock, is usually thicker and richer in connective tissue. Complete sectioning of this area is very important; a Bellucci scissors is very helpful for this purpose. No attempt to lift flaps or gain entrance into the middle ear should be made until the incisions are completed and the skin flaps are free.

Elevation of Flaps

With the skin edges free, the surgeon takes his or her finger off the hole of the suction tube and holds the speculum and suction in the left hand (for a right-handed surgeon) (Fig. 7–2C). This helpful technique is not difficult to master, and with an adequately sized speculum obviates the need for a speculum holder. The latter is a useful instrument, the most widely used design being the classic Shea

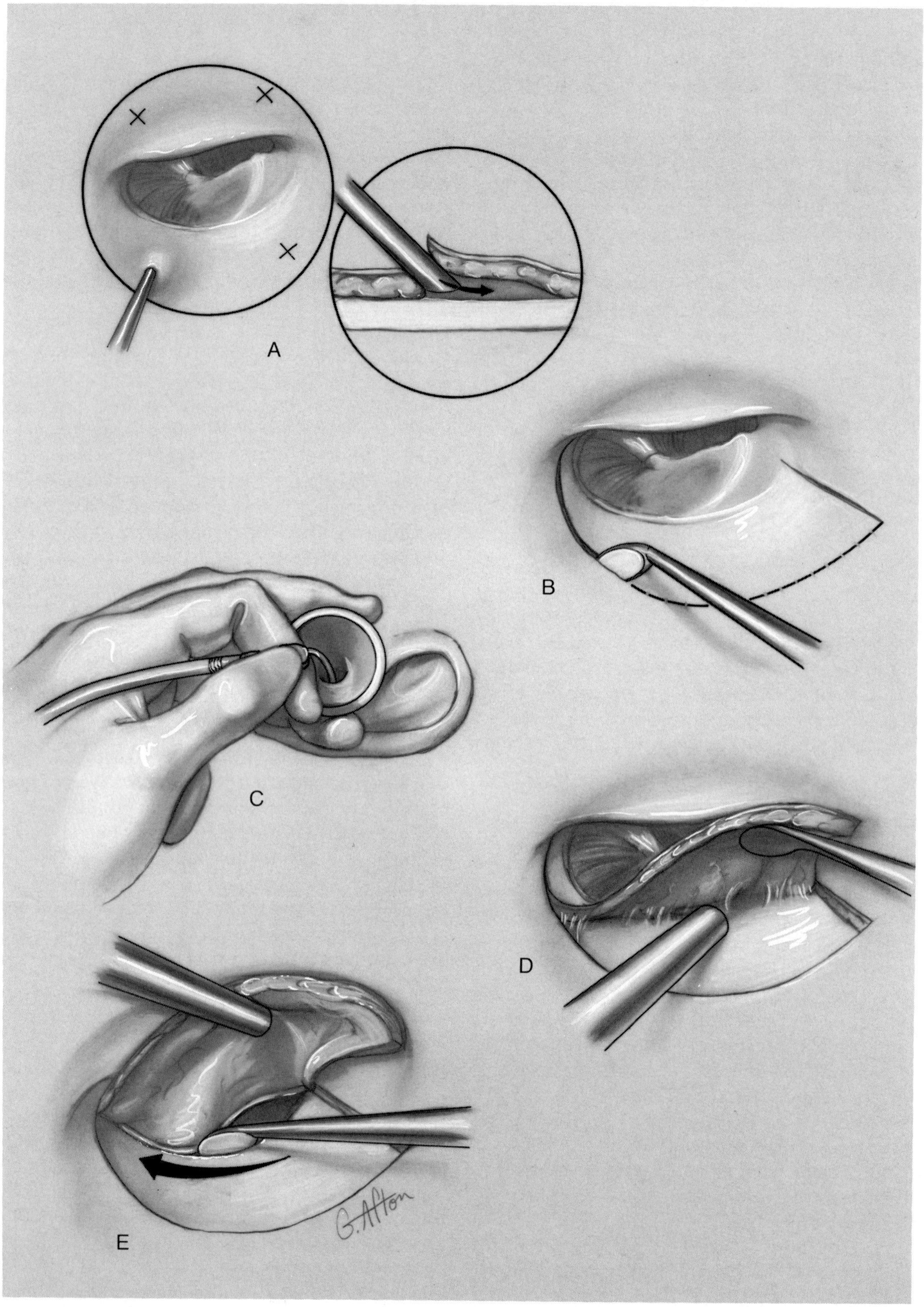

FIGURE 7–2.

speculum holder; other designs are modifications incorporating surgeons' various preferences.

With the use of a flat elevator, preferably a duckbill or large curved canal knife, the skin is gently separated from the underlying bone (Fig. 7–2*D*). Special care must be observed when a prominent tympanomastoid suture is present; simply lifting the skin will cause tears in the flap. A smaller sharp instrument (for example, a No. 1 straight knife or sickle knife) is helpful in releasing connective tissue attachments. Separation must be slow and careful in order to preserve the flap intact. The suction tip (finger off the hole) is used behind (posterior to) the elevator. The skin is elevated evenly, avoiding tunneling, and the flap is elevated until it reaches the annulus. At this point, greater magnification may be used (for example, 16 ×) in the microscope. All bleeding must be controlled, and entrance to the middle ear should be "dry." A No. 20 suction tip is preferred for the middle ear. Small sources of bleeding can be stopped using "Adrenalin tape." Occasionally cautery is needed; however, it is preferable to avoid any edema or necrosis, such as that caused by cauterization, in these thin flaps.

The middle ear is entered *beneath* the annulus with a duckbill or curved canal knife (Fig. 7–2*E*). If there is adequate visualization, the site of entrance is not crucial; in general, however, it is preferable to enter inferiorly toward the round window rather than toward the ossicles. Once the annulus is separated, a drumhead elevator is introduced and the annulus is gently lifted by a sweeping motion from 6 to 12 o'clock through the whole extent of the exposed annulus. The chorda tympani should be gently and carefully moved out of the field of vision; if this would stretch it, the best course is simply to cut it with a Bellucci scissors (Fig. 7–3*A*, *B*). In cases in which adhesions or thickened mucoperiosteum obscure visualization of the middle ear structure, it is imperative to enter the middle ear cautiously and systematically. Avoiding damage, particularly to ossicles (or their remnants) or an exposed facial nerve, is crucial. The cavity is entered inferiorly, where the round window niche area is found; from there the surgeon works toward the ossicles. If they are still obscured, or if the anatomy is (or seems) distorted, a small atticotomy is done. The head of the malleus and body of the incus (which usually are present even if extensive ossicular erosion has occurred) are identified, and the dissection is started from this point. (Beware of the tensor tympani area, where the facial nerve might be dehiscent.) The chorda tympani can also serve as a guide to follow. Whatever the choice, thickened tissue should not be removed blindly.

Exposure of the Middle Ear

The middle ear is visualized and the mucosa as well as the different anatomic structures are identified before any planned procedure is begun (Fig. 7–3*C*). Methodical evaluation of the cavity is good practice. This includes evaluation of ossicular mobility, which is done by mobilizing the long process of the malleus with a drumhead elevator or joint knife (Fig. 7–3*D*), followed by palpation of the incus and stapes (Fig. 7–3*E*). Testing the mobility of the stapes includes the footplate, not the head alone. If more complete exposure of the oval window is needed, the posterior canal wall should be curetted. The tip of the curet should always be in view. A sharp curet that is as large as possible should be utilized. An angled curet is used to remove the bone of the posterior canal, including the area of the scutum. In general, it is better to curet from 12 to 6 o'clock in order to avoid accidental dislocation of ossicles. The curet should not be used in a perpendicular fashion. Special time should be dedicated to completely removing bone fragments, which if left in the middle ear stimulate localized tissue reaction and make the cavity prone to infection. Again, for good visualization it is important to position the patient appropriately, with the surgeon and microscope in the correct position as well.

Closure

Upon completion of middle ear work (procedures are described in specific chapters), the flaps are repositioned. At the same time, they are carefully cleansed, freed of debris with thin suction tips, a joint knife, or both, and examined for tears. The tympanic membrane also is examined for small punctures or lacerations; if any are present, their edges are closely approximated, and small pieces of Gelfoam are used to cover them. The paramount consideration, requiring great care, is anatomic position. The fact that flaps shrink initially must be taken into account.

Revisions

Ideally, previous reports should be available. Revisions should be approached as a "box of surprises" from beginning to end. The main points to keep in

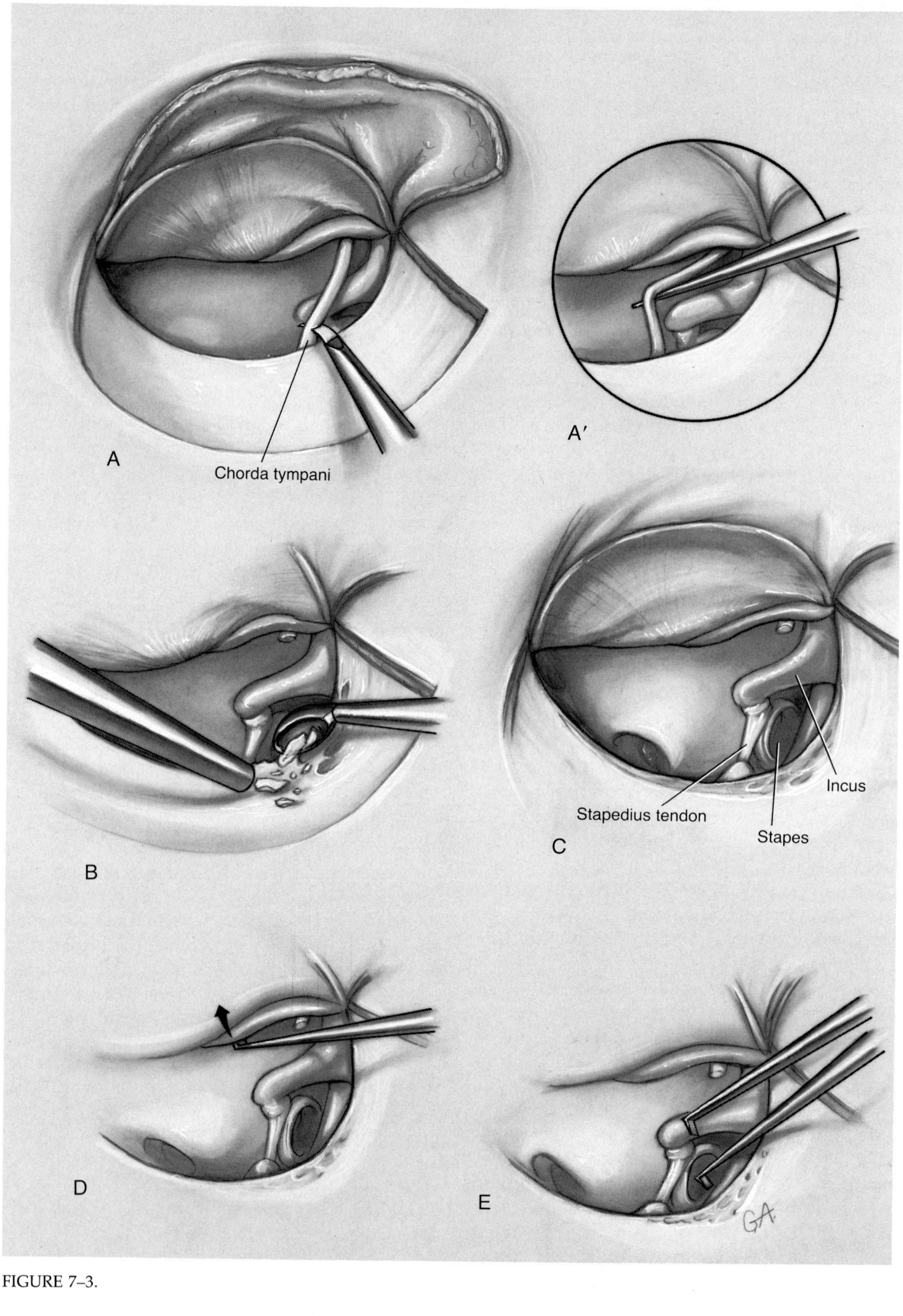

FIGURE 7–3.

mind are that flaps are quite thin and tear easily, and that bony defects of the ear canal are to be expected. Careful incisions and elevation are used. Adhesions are common and should be sectioned carefully and sharply in order to avoid tears. Repositioning of the flaps should be carefully done and anatomically adequate; adequate packing is of the utmost importance as well.

Packing

Alternatives to packing exist, depending upon the particular case and the surgeon's preference. They are all satisfactory and will work if done correctly. Different materials can be utilized; if used properly, most of them suffice. Excessive pressure must be avoided. Antibiotic or steroid ointments or solutions, or both, are useful in preventing localized inflammation and infection. Only the most common packing techniques will be mentioned.

1. A basket is fashioned from surgical rayon or Owen's silk strips moistened with antibiotic or steroid ointment. Cotton soaked in antibiotic solution fills the space, and the silk is used as a rosebud packing. A 1/2-in gauze pack with antibiotic ointment is placed in the lateral third of the canal (Fig. 7–4*A*–*C*). This type of packing provides adequate pressure to keep the flaps flat, but not enough to damage them. It should be removed at intervals of one week for the gauze and two weeks for the rosebud; if left for a longer period granulation tissue invades the silk, making it difficult if not impossible to remove it by simply pulling.

2. The canal is filled with Gelfoam soaked in antibiotic solution. It is placed initially in layers, with Gelfoam strips covering all areas of incision. The lateral aspect of the canal can be filled with ointment, or a piece of sterile cotton can be placed (Fig. 7–4*D*). The disadvantage of this method is that it takes a long time for the Gelfoam to come out spontaneously; thus removal must be done very carefully in order to avoid flap disruption. Gelfoam promotes granulation. This type of packing may require the use of otic drops or ointments.

3. The canal is filled with an antibiotic ointment as the sole packing, and a piece of cotton is placed in the meatus (Fig. 7–4*E*). This method of packing requires perfect approximation of intact flaps.

4. The incisions are completely covered with compressed, dry Gelfoam in strips, and a flat, round piece of Gelfoam is placed over the tympanic membrane. Ointment is then inserted into the canal through a syringe with an 18-gauge needle (Fig. 7–4*F*). Gelfoam provides some stimulation for granulation, favors healing, and discourages maceration of the skin flaps.

Canalplasty in Exploratory Tympanotomy

If the canal is small or "tight" owing to thick skin or anterior bony overhang that prevents satisfactory visualization despite adequate approach and positioning, a canalplasty becomes a very useful procedure (Fig. 7–5).

Highlights

1. Before performing a canalplasty:
   A. Ensure that the approach is the best one.
   B. Ensure that the positioning of the patient and surgeon is adequate.
2. Use curets as needed.
3. Protect the anterior window shade flap.
4. Drill the anterior wall carefully.
5. Carefully remove all debris.

Pitfalls

1. Drilling the skin flaps.
2. Exposing the temporomandibular joint capsule anteriorly.
3. Inadequately removing bone dust and debris, which leads to inflammation and infection.

Procedure

An anesthetic and vasoconstrictors are injected into the anterior wall. The purpose is to expose the bony canal and safely remove as much bone as needed for adequate exposure. This can be accomplished with an "anterior window shade" with a horizontal component and two vertical limbs; the vertical limbs preferably should not involve the vascular strip. The horizontal incision can be made medially or laterally—that is, immediately above the annulus or at the bony cartilaginous junction. In the medial horizontal incision, the skin is gently elevated laterally as a flap with a duckbill elevator or curved

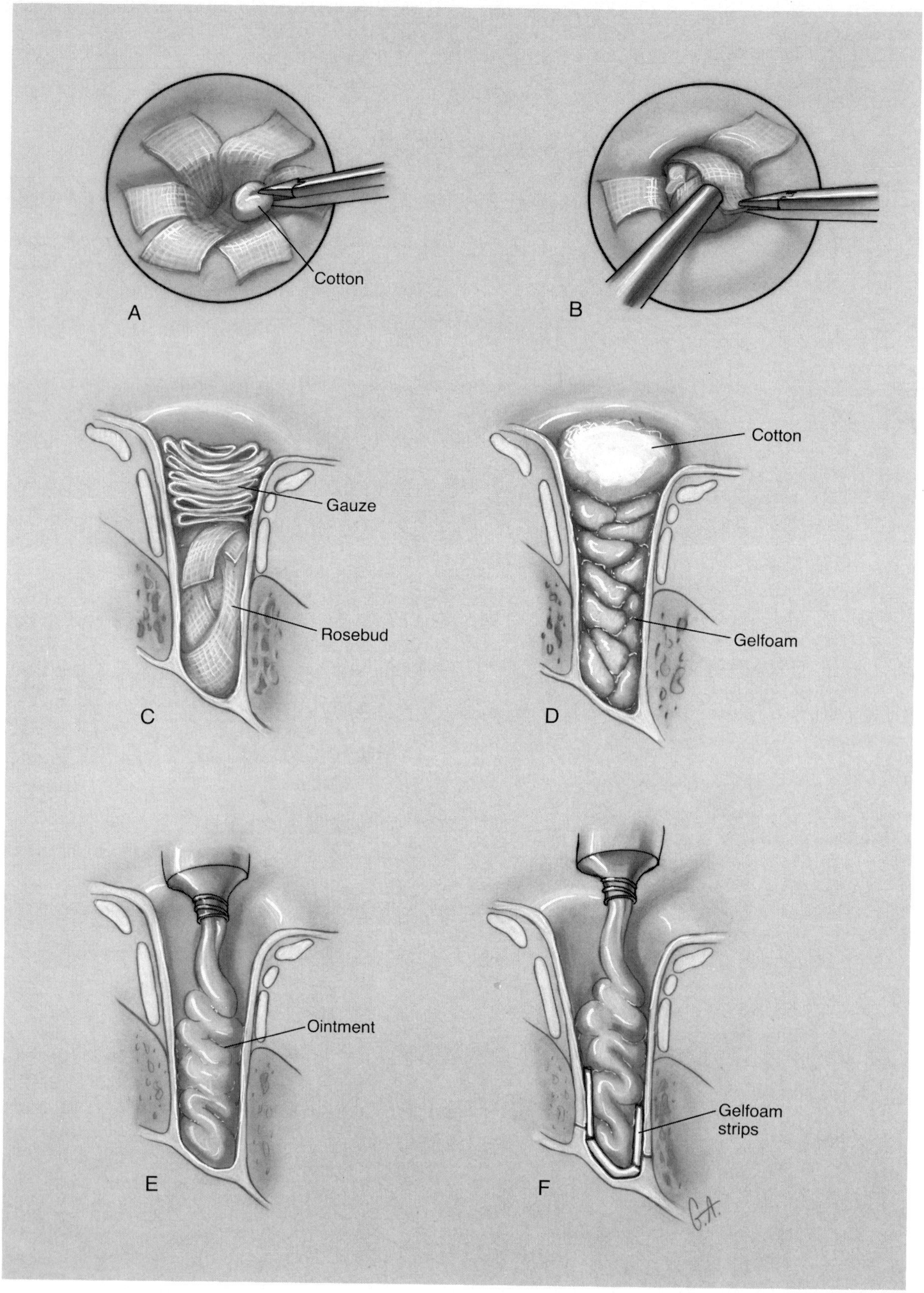
Cotton
A
B
Gauze
Rosebud
C
Cotton
Gelfoam
D
Ointment
E
Gelfoam
strips
F

FIGURE 7–4.

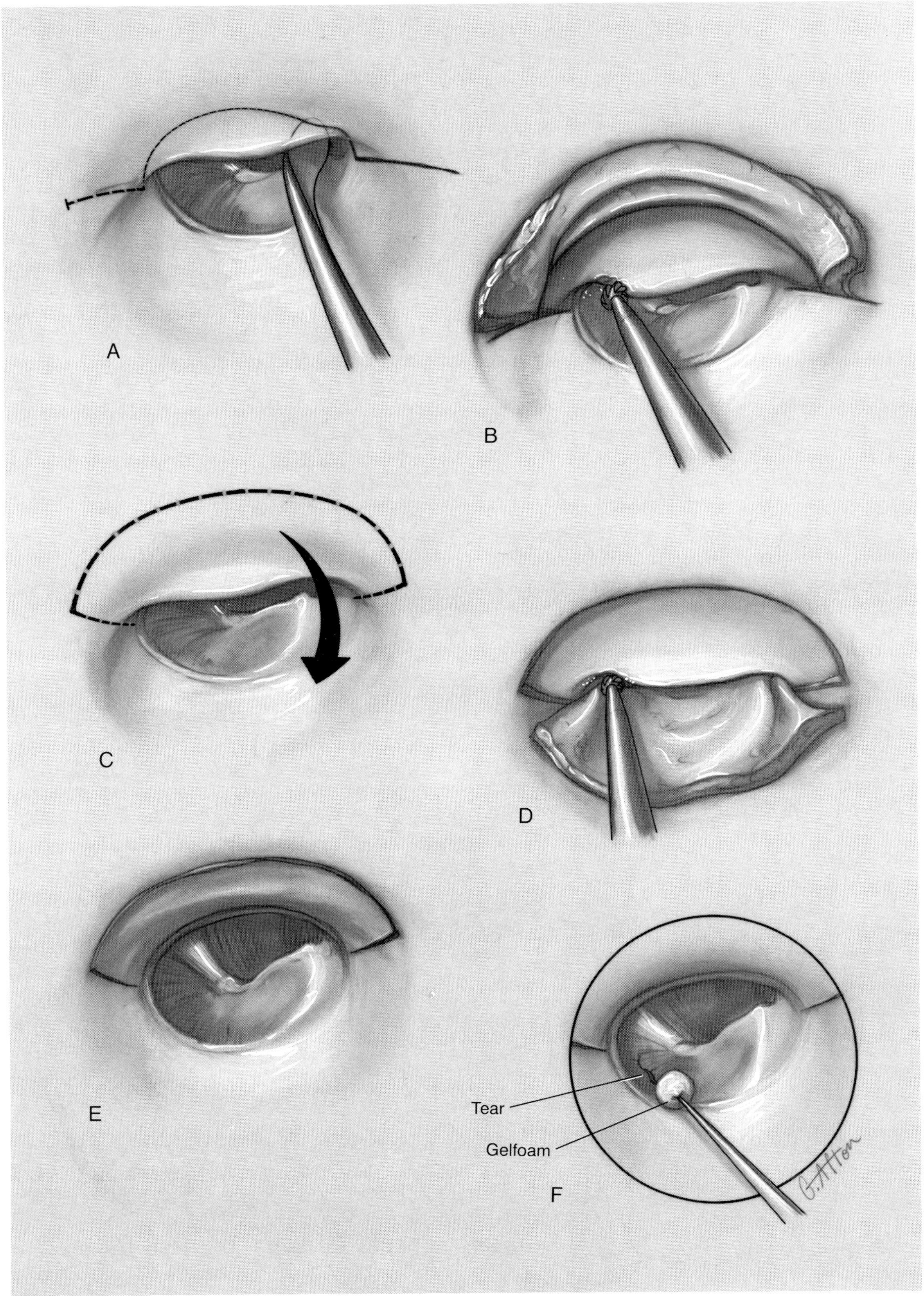

FIGURE 7–5.

canal knife, and gently rolled anteriorly (Fig. 7–5*A*, *B*,). This skin is very thin and tears easily; thus lifting must be done carefully. In the lateral horizontal incision, a flap is developed inferiorly until it reaches the annulus (Fig. 7–5*C*, *D*). Before drilling, the surgeon must ensure that the flaps are safely flattened in order to avoid drilling them. It is a good idea to cover them with a strip of Owen's silk for added protection; if the flaps are touched by the drill bit, the silk will be trapped. A drill bit large enough to be safe but small enough to leave room for drilling should be used; it can be supplemented with curets as needed. Proper use of curets should be learned; they are safe and very effective.

Enough bone should be removed to permit visualization of the anterior annulus. Care must be taken to avoid entering the temporomandibular joint anteriorly. If the temporomandibular joint is entered despite these precautions, a small defect may be created that is extracapsular; if this is the case, no particular coverage is needed except for the flap. In obtaining satisfactory visualization of the entire annulus, it should be remembered that adequate positioning of the patient's head, and of the surgeon, will avoid unnecessary drilling. Exposure of posterior mastoid cells is not a major problem; they should be adequately covered with the skin flap. Once the entire bone work has been done, time should be allotted for complete removal of bone fragments in order to prevent local tissue reaction and possible infection. The flaps are completely elevated posteriorly; the anterior flap ("window shade") is anatomically repositioned and all bleeding vessels are controlled (Fig. 7–5*E*). Then, and only then, can the middle ear be entered.

Endaural Approach

Highlights

1. Same as with the transcanal approach.
2. Control bleeding before entering the middle ear.
3. Position the two-prong retractors properly and carefully.

Pitfalls

1. Same as with the transcanal approach.
2. Exposing or damaging the helix with a Lempert II incision.
3. Inadequately packing and positioning the flaps, resulting in adhesions or stenosis.

The endaural approach can be used for an exploratory tympanotomy, a tympanoplasty, and a mastoidectomy, and is particularly useful and safe for revision surgery. It is useful, as well, for "tight" canals and canals with thick skin. This approach utilizes different sizes of incisions according to need, varying from a minimal to a large Lempert II incision (described below). It is insufficient for large mastoid cavities and does not provide a good view of the anterior annulus unless a canalplasty is done.

Position, inspection, and cleansing are done as in transcanal procedures. Injection of local anesthetic with vasoconstrictors is similar as well, except that additional injections are made between the tragus and helix (at the incisura) and immediately anterior to the helix (Fig. 7–6*A*). The endaural approach avoids the use of an ear speculum and provides a direct view of the middle ear.

Incisions

For purposes of exposure, it is best to use a curved nasal speculum. Incisions are made with a scalpel. The first incision (Lempert I) is made semicircumferentially between 6 and 12 o'clock on the posterior wall at the bony cartilaginous junction (Fig. 7–6*B*). This incision must extend down to the bone. The second incision (Lempert II) runs between the tragus and helix and incisura; care must be taken not to expose or cut the helix. The extension of this incision depends upon the degree of exposure needed, varying from a few millimeters (for an exploratory tympanotomy) to a full 3/4 cm (for a mastoidectomy). This incision is made in the ear. Caution must be exercised not to deepen it immediately after going through the subcutaneous tissue, since branches of the superficial temporal artery and vein are present in this area; too deep a cut also may section the temporal fascia, which might be needed for grafting purposes. It is important to completely section the connective tissue and to expose the bony canal at the level of the incisura, allowing more space. Small bleeding vessels are cauterized. The remaining posterior canal skin (cartilaginous portion) is preserved and gently elevated with a small periosteal elevator, leaving the whole posterior bony canal clearly exposed (Fig. 7–6C). On occasion, a small free skin graft can be taken safely from this area. Two two-prong retractors are used for exposure. It is useful to position them at right angles to each other, one

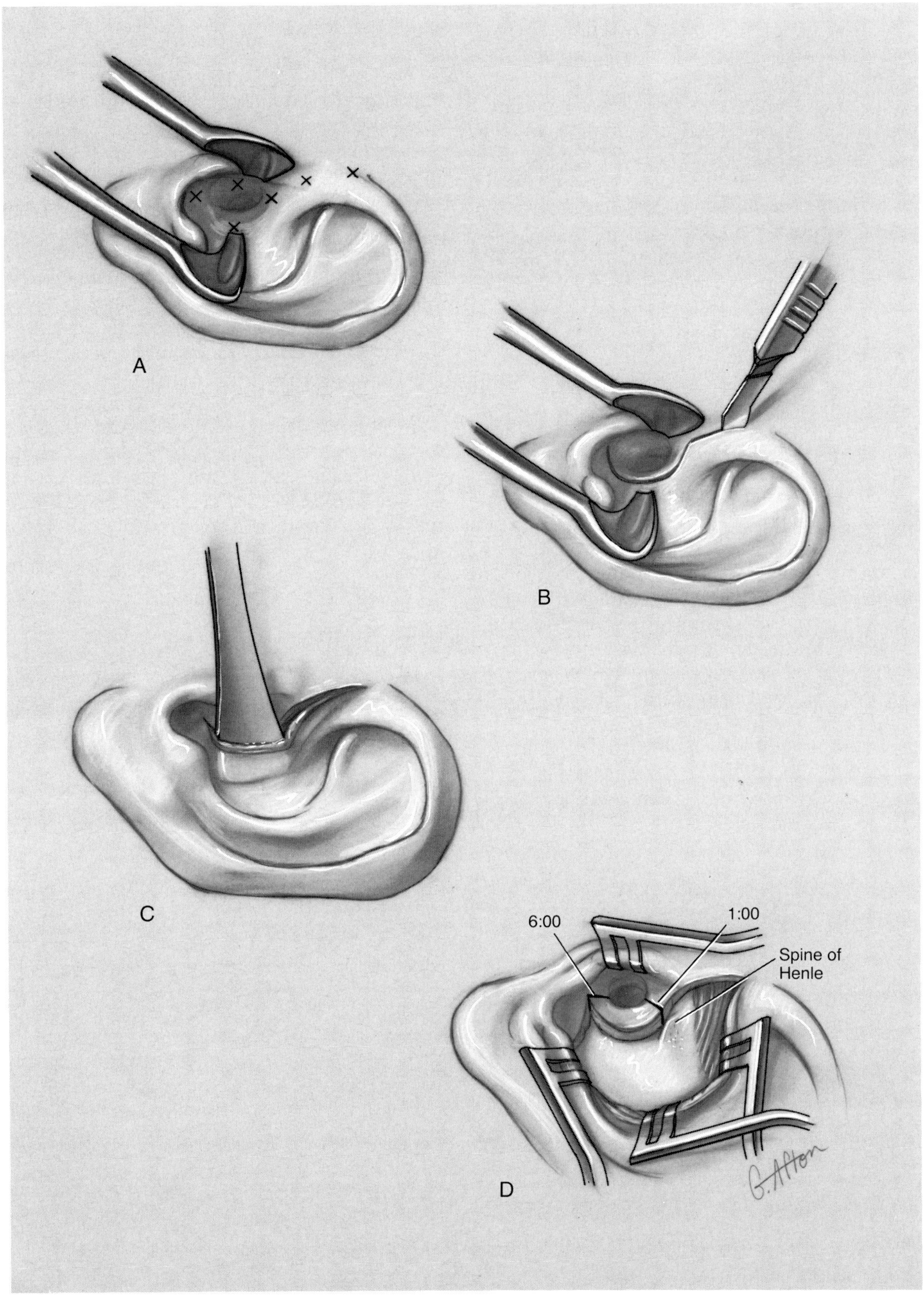

FIGURE 7–6.

pointing cephalad (superiorly) and the other caudad (posteriorly); this provides better exposure and stability and is less inconvenient for the surgeon. Temporal fascia is harvested at this point (discussed in Chapter 12) and all bleeding vessels are controlled. With the scalpel, incisions can be made at 6 and 1 or 2 o'clock (Fig. 7–6*D*). These incisions allow for easier development of the flap; however, the flap can be elevated without the incisions. The flap is elevated in the same manner as in a transcanal incision. The same principles and technique also apply for a canalplasty.

Closure

The flap is repositioned anatomically; particular attention is paid to repositioning the skin, which must cover the cartilaginous canal. Subcutaneous tissues are approximated with interrupted absorbable sutures (for example, 3-0 chromic catgut). Approximation does not need to be very tight at the incisura. Skin is approximated with absorbable 4-0 silk or nylon sutures. The first skin suture should be at the incisura; as in other ear incisions, there is remarkably good healing in this area. Packing is done as in transcanal procedures for the bony canal; however, it is best to use 1/2-in gauze impregnated with antibiotic or steroid ointment in the lateral third (cartilaginous canal), followed by a mastoid dressing. The gauze and the skin sutures are removed one week after the procedure. At this time the authors usually fill the space with antibiotic ointment for one additional week.

Postauricular Approach

Highlights

1. Same as for transcanal and endaural approaches.
2. The postauricular incision should be made plane by plane.
3. The canal should be reached in the "avascular" plane.
4. Cleansing of all debris should be done carefully.

Pitfalls

1. Tearing of the canal with the three-prong retractors.
2. Inadequately cleansing debris, leading to wound infection.

The postauricular approach can be used for an exploratory tympanotomy, a tympanoplasty, and a mastoidectomy. It provides a good view of the anterior rim of the annulus, unless there is a prominent bony overhang or a "tight" canal; however, it is useful for dealing with these two problems as well.

Position, inspection, and cleansing are done in transcanal and endaural procedures; however, patient preparation and shaving of hair is different (see Chapter 6). Injection of a local anesthetic is similar to the transcanal procedure, as far as the canal is concerned; however, a postauricular injection is necessary in the whole area where the incision is to be made, as well as in the posterior aspect of the canal from behind. It is useful to lift the auricle, pull it forward, and inject posteriorly, while feeling the tip of the needle and the flow of anesthetic and vasoconstrictors with the index finger placed in the meatus of the canal; this maneuver ensures adequate injection.

Incisions

The classic incision is made 3/4 cm behind the posterior sulcus, with the inferior end deviating posteriorly. In children, the incision is high and posterior with the inferior limb far posterior, since the facial nerve can be very superficial in its exit at the stylomastoid foramen (because of lack of development of the mastoid tip). For cosmetic purposes the incision can be made in the crease itself, but the cosmetic advantage is relative; this location lends itself to minor healing problems, small epidermal cysts, and so on. An additional incision that can be made is the posterosuperior (Portmann), which is a compromise between the posterior incision and the anterosuperior (Hermann) incision. (In spite of its good exposure, the latter is not used because it may lead to necrosis of the helix.) The posterosuperior incision provides excellent exposure.

Procedure

The incision is made with a scalpel and deepened perpendicularly through subcutaneous tissues without advancing too far. The purpose is to reach the musculo-aponeurotic or "avascular" plane. Cautery can be used for bleeding vessels. If the planes are developed carefully, large branches of the posterior auricular artery usually will not be sectioned; if this does occur, it is best to tie them with a nonabsorbable suture. Many surgeons use cutting cautery in the skin, which is effective in terms of surgical time and dryness of the field. However, this must be weighed against the disadvantage of skin healing secondary to a cutting cautery burn.

If the right plane is reached, the auricle is pulled anteriorly (forward) and the cartilaginous canal is identified, as well as the spine of Henle. (At this point the temporal fascia can be harvested; this is discussed in Chapter 12.) Once this is done, the connective tissue plane behind the cartilaginous canal can be developed sharply and safely. All bleeding vessels, if there are any, should be controlled. Elevating the plane toward the zygomatic root gains room to mobilize the auricle forward (anteriorly) easily (Fig. 7–7*A*). A circumferential incision is made at the bony cartilaginous junction posteriorly, as in the endaural procedure. (We are discussing exploratory approaches alone; other types of flaps for other purposes—for example, Körner's—will be dealt with later.) A piece of twill tape passed gently through the incision ensures that the skin of the meatus posteriorly is not torn when using a retractor, and at the same time serves to keep this flap out of the field of vision (Fig. 7–7*B*). With the use of a three-prong Wullstein retractor, the auricle (pinna) is gently pulled anteriorly with the posterior cartilaginous canal, protected by the twill tape (Fig. 7–7*C*). Care must be taken not to tear this skin and cartilage. If a Wullstein retractor is not large enough, a modified Schuknecht three-prong retractor is used. (This is usually necessary in a mastoidectomy but uncommon in exploratory procedures.)

From this point on, the same procedure is followed as in endaural or transcanal incisions. Closure is preceded by careful removal of debris. The packing of the bony canal is similar to that in other approaches; the lateral aspect of the canal (cartilaginous) is packed as in the endaural approach. Postauricular closure is done with interrupted absorbable sutures for subcutaneous tissues (for example, 3-0 chromic catgut). This layer should be approximated carefully; otherwise, the pinna may lack adequate subcutaneous support and show a tendency to project anteriorly. Skin is approximated with interrupted, nonabsorbable silk or nylon. Some surgeons close the skin with 4-0 catgut sutures; although this method may be adequate, the authors do not use it. A mastoid dressing is applied. Removal of sutures and packing is done as in the endaural approach.

Simple Mastoidectomy as a Surgical Approach

A simple mastoidectomy is described here as a general surgical approach for different procedures; it is discussed as a specific procedure in Chapter 5. Mastoid procedures for chronic otitis are described separately in Chapter 10.

Aim

Exenteration (removal) of all mastoid air cells while maintaining the integrity of the posterior canal.

Highlights

1. Skin incision is performed with the scalpel perpendicular to the skin.
2. Incision should be deepened in layers.
3. Careful elevation of intact periosteum should be done.
4. Retractors must be adequately positioned.
5. Complete exposure of landmarks is important.
6. Carefully close in layers.

Pitfalls

1. Tearing of the skin of the posterior ear canal.
2. Inadequate exposure.
3. Injuring a high sigmoid sinus.
4. Injuring the facial nerve by going:
   A. Deep to the horizontal semicircular canal.
   B. Too far anterior in the digastric ridge.
5. Dislocating the incus by drilling blindly into the antrum area.
6. Exposing the dura mater.
7. Drilling the semicircular canals.

Positioning, patient preparation and draping, and injection have already been discussed. As described in previous chapters, a classic postauricular incision will be used, starting at the level of the linea temporalis and following the contour of the external meatus to turn posteroinferiorly at the level of the mastoid tip.

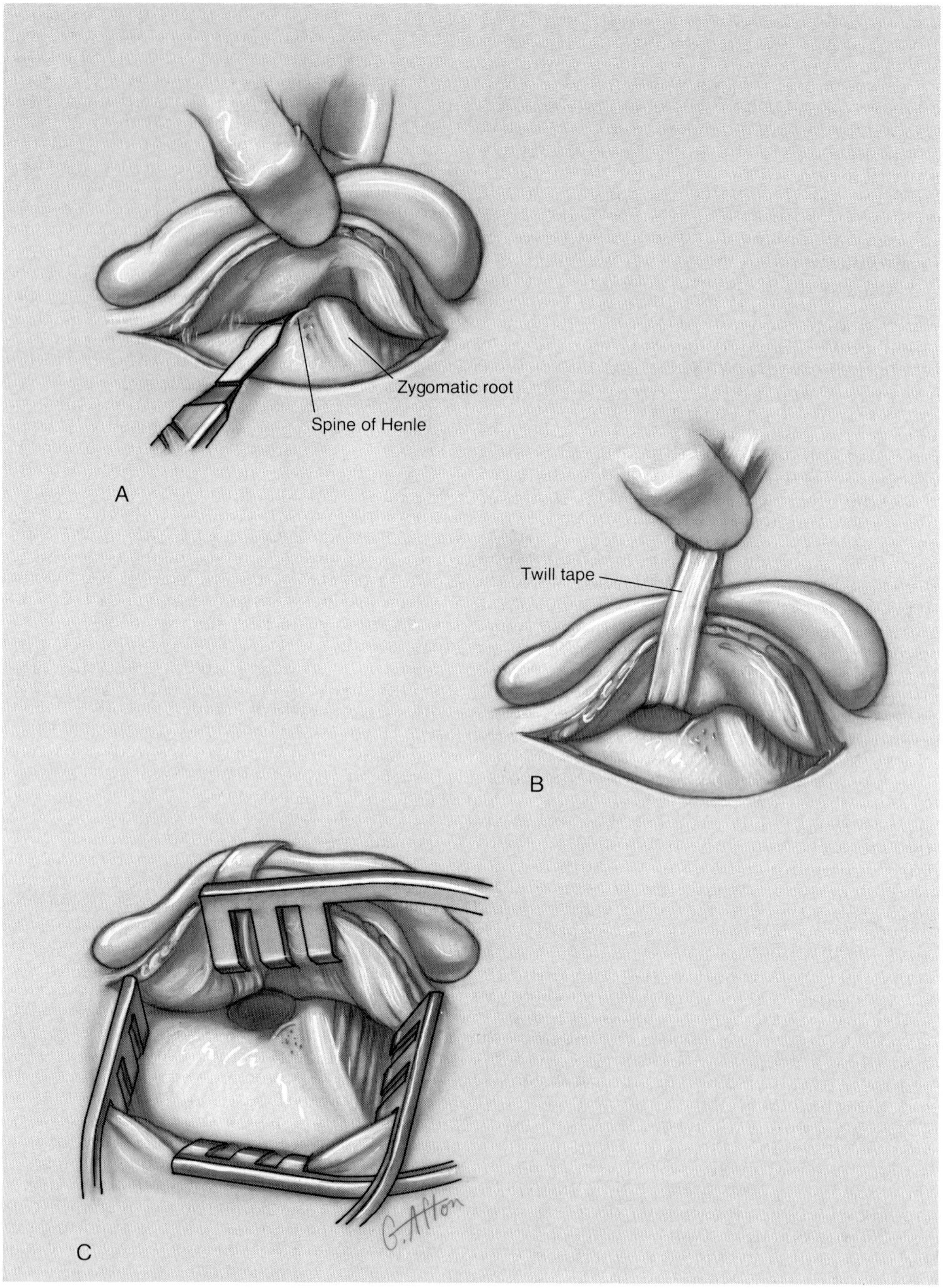

FIGURE 7–7.

Incision and Exposure

Before initiating postauricular work, it is a good idea to place a piece of sterile cotton in the canal in order to avoid accumulation of debris and bone dust.

The incision is made in layers with a scalpel held perpendicularly to the skin. Subcutaneous vessels are cauterized. A plane between the musculo-aponeurotic layer and connective tissue is reached by sharp dissection, and developed. It is possible in this plane to avoid damaging branches of the posterior auricular artery; if damage does occur, it is better to ligate than to cauterize them.

The periosteum is identified and sectioned, following the contour of the external ear canal. Vertical incisions at 45-degree angles are made at 6 and 12 o'clock (toward the linea temporalis and toward the mastoid tip) (Fig. 7–8*A*). The intact periosteum is elevated carefully, using periosteal elevators. This is important for closure, since re-establishing the periosteum in position will avoid a marked postauricular depression. As soon as the periosteum is elevated, the landmarks become apparent. It is useful to expose the root of the zygoma; this provides better mobility when positioning the retractors. Two three-prong retractors are positioned at right angles to one another (Fig. 7–8C).

Specific surgical steps are described in Chapter 5 (pages 45–47). The discussion here will focus on closure and treatment of intraoperative complications.

Closure

Careful washing and thorough removal of all debris and bone dust are of the utmost importance in order to prevent postoperative inflammation and infection. The retractors are removed, and the periosteal flap is repositioned and secured to the posterior canal by nonabsorbable sutures. If the flap is intact and the approximation is adequate, marked postauricular depression will be avoided. Subcutaneous tissues are approximated with layers of interrupted absorbable sutures (for example, 3-0 or 2-0 chromic catgut), and skin with interrupted nonabsorbable sutures (for example, 4-0 silk or nylon), making sure that the skin and subcutaneous sutures do not overlap. A mastoid dressing is then applied.

Intraoperative Complications or Problems

1. Facial nerve trauma.
2. Exposure of the dura mater.
3. Drilling of the semicircular canals.
4. Damage to the sigmoid sinus.
5. Dislocation of the incus.

Facial Nerve Trauma. Inadvertent exposure of the facial nerve sheath does not necessarily imply injury to the nerve and requires no treatment. However, if the nerve itself is injured in its course through the fallopian canal, it should be opened for several millimeters to ensure continuity. *The nerve sheath should not be opened* unless discontinuity of nerve fibers is suspected. Opening of the sheath might allow ingrowth of fibrous tissue, which can compromise nerve regeneration. If discontinuity of fibers exists, they should be apposed cleanly to each other. If the injury is severe and includes maceration, the nerve should be sharply and cleanly incised and an end-to-end anastomosis performed (see Chapter 18). If the traumatized segment is too broad, nerve grafting should be done. Exposed nerve fibers should be covered in order to avoid ingrowth of fibrous tissue. *They should not be covered with fascia,* since fascia provides such ingrowth; materials that discourage fibrous tissue ingrowth (for example, thin sheets of gold foil) should be used.

Facial paralysis that is evident immediately postoperatively may be caused by intraoperative injury, the effect of local anesthesia, or pressure from packing on a dehiscent nerve. Paralysis from such sources necessitates immediate re-exploration unless the surgeon is certain there is no facial nerve damage, in which case packing and pressure should be released. Steroids can be argued against, but in this case the authors believe their use may be beneficial. Delayed facial paralysis (developing after the patient has recovered without paralysis) requires loosening of the packing and should be treated as Bell's palsy.

Exposure of the Dura Mater. Exposure of the dura mater during mastoidectomy can happen at the tegmen (middle cranial fossa dura) and at the posterior cranial fossa dura. Without penetration or rupture of the dura itself, it is of no significance except as a reflection of poor technique. If the dura is torn a cerebrospinal fluid leak will result, with subsequent potential for infection. Small leaks in the middle cranial fossa often cease spontaneously because of the abundant arachnoid that is present. A small piece

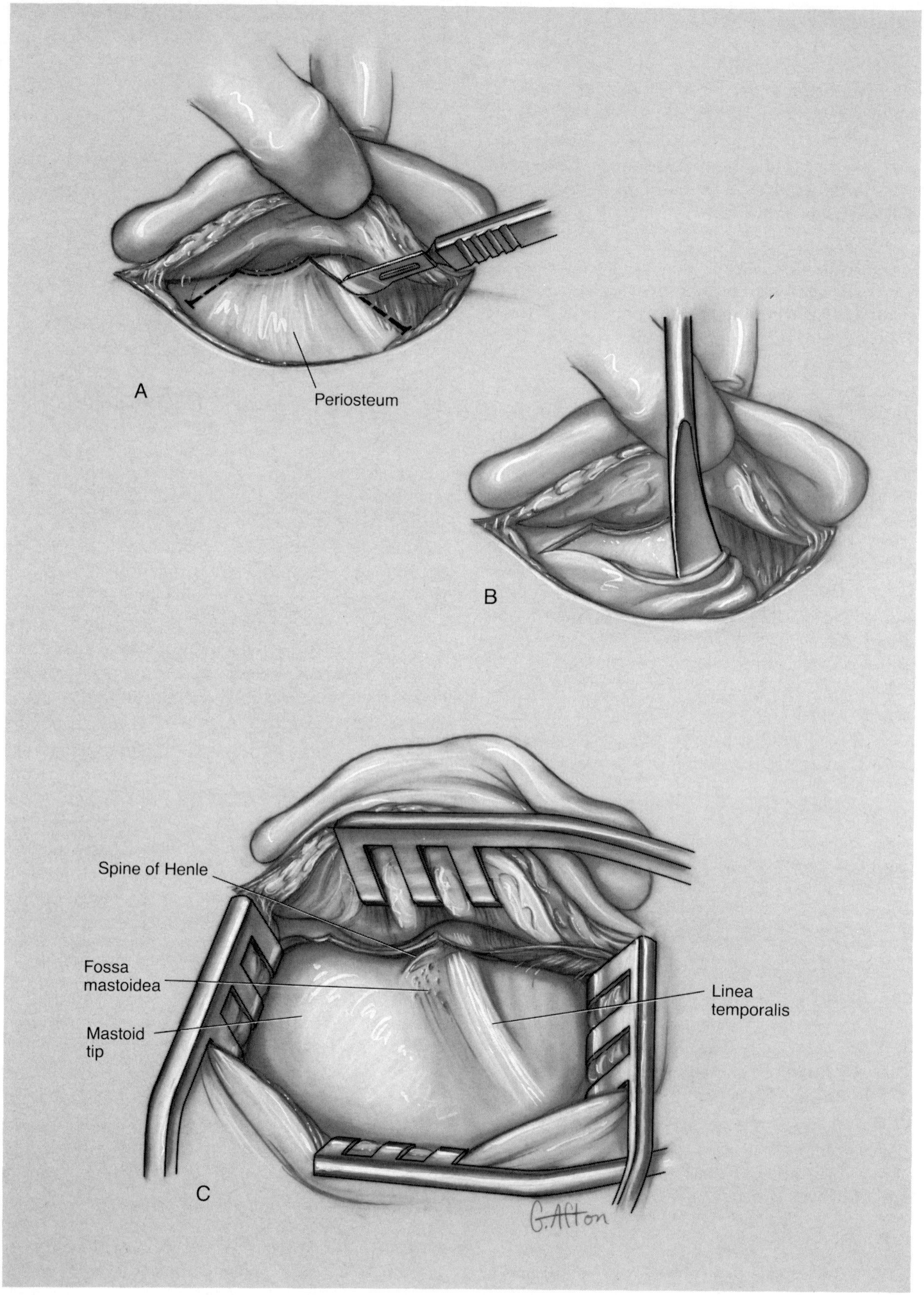
A
Periosteum
B
Spine of Henle
Fossa
mastoidea
Mastoid
tip
Linea
temporalis
C
G. Afton

FIGURE 7–8.

of fascia can be used for coverage, after it is ascertained that the surrounding dura is intact. (Remove a few millimeters in each direction.) The fascia can be tucked in place. Larger defects can be closed by using cartilage or bone lateral to the fascia, or both. Intraoperative and postoperative antibiotics are used as in all other complications involving areas or structures beyond the confines of the mastoid or middle ear cavity. Antibiotics that cross the blood-brain barrier should be used; this is an important but frequently overlooked point.

Posterior cranial fossa dura has less arachnoid, and leaks there are occasionally quite profuse. As soon as the leak occurs, a large piece of Gelfoam or twill tape is placed over the defect and finger pressure is applied. This is followed by tissue grafting with temporal muscle medially and fascia laterally. The cavity is then covered with large pieces of Gelfoam, and, if necessary, filled under pressure. If the flow continues, an indwelling lumbar catheter may be placed in order to diminish the cerebrospinal fluid pressure for several days.

Drilling of the Semicircular Canals. Damage occurs most commonly at the dome of the lateral (horizontal) semicircular canal and occasionally at the posterior semicircular canal when exposing Trautmann's triangle. If the damage is recognized before injury to the membranous labyrinth occurs, sealing the fistula with Gelfoam or tissue graft may prevent serious sequelae. Damage to the membranous labyrinth results in an irreversible disturbance in hearing and balance, except on rare occasions in which previous involvement of the labyrinth has allowed its compartmentalization.

Damage to the Sigmoid Sinus. The best way to deal with this problem, as with all other complications, is to avoid it. This can be achieved by having a good set of preoperative mastoid films that provide information on the location of the sigmoid sinus (for example, "high-lateral," "low-medial," "anterior," etc.), and by developing the mastoidectomy step by step. Ear surgery is not for "racing surgeons."

Laceration of the sigmoid sinus results in profuse hemorrhage. A similar problem can occur with a dehiscent jugular bulb in the hypotympanum. Bleeding can often be stopped by immediate, firm, application of large pieces of Gelfoam and twill tape and by finger pressure, followed by application of oxidized cellulose (oxycel). This in turn is covered by pieces of Gelfoam and fascia if needed. At the end of the procedure, extradural hematoma should be ruled out.

Dislocation of the Incus. This complication entails exploratory tympanotomy and repositioning of the incus in its normal anatomic position (see Chapter 11).

Posterior Tympanotomy (Facial Recess) as a Surgical Approach

The posterior tympanotomy (facial recess) procedure is included here as a general surgical approach for different purposes; aim, highlights, pitfalls, and procedure are described in Chapter 5. Specific indications are discussed in pertinent preceding chapters.

Closure is exactly the same as in a simple mastoidectomy. Management of complications also is identical except for those inherent in this specific approach.

Intraoperative Complications or Problems Inherent in This Approach

1. Damage to the tympanic membrane.
2. Perforation of the bony external ear canal.

Damage to the tympanic membrane implies a transcanal exploration. The borders of a small tear are cleansed and approximated anatomically and covered with Gelfoam. A larger defect necessitates a graft (to be discussed in Chapter 12).

Small perforations of the posterior wall of the bony external ear canal are not significant and need no repair except for adequate coverage with skin flap. Major defects may require posterior wall reconstruction.

Mastoidotomy as a Surgical Approach

Aim

Visualizing the antrum and establishing (or reestablishing) communication between the mastoid and middle ear cavities.

The highlights, pitfalls, technique, and complications of a mastoidotomy are essentially those of a cortical mastoidectomy (see Chapter 5), but the amount of bone removed is much less. This procedure is performed using a postauricular or endaural approach. Drilling is done in the fossa mastoidea toward the antrum. Whether the purpose is to remove tissue blockage, improve aeration to the middle ear, or introduce an electrode into the middle ear, the opening should be large enough to allow visualization of the antrum.

Meatoplasty

Meatoplasty is discussed in this chapter as a general concept owing to its practical and often crucial importance in otologic procedures. The meatus consists of skin, subcutaneous tissue, cartilage, and underlying bone. It is essential to consider all of these structures in a meatoplasty; adequate treatment of the soft tissues combined with insufficient attention to the underlying cartilage or bony meatus, or both, might result in an inadequate meatoplasty. Meatoplasty is essential for obtaining a good surgical result in tympanomastoid surgery and in tympanoplasty (when indicated and usually associated with canalplasty).

Large canals do not need a meatoplasty. The procedure is used for small canal entrances (openings), whether congenital or acquired (by disease or by surgery). A normal-sized meatus allows for proper aeration and self-cleansing of the canal, and adequate sound conduction. The procedures described here (exemplified for practical purposes in open- and closed-cavity tympano-mastoidectomy) apply in principle to other surgical cases as well.

With the understanding that a postauricular and an endaural approach can be used interchangeably, a postauricular approach is described in the meatoplasty for an open-cavity tympano-mastoidectomy, and an endaural approach for a closed-cavity tympano-mastoidectomy. The development of a Körner's flap will be described in the former, as well.

Aim

To provide a well-epithelialized meatus that is wide enough to aerate the ear canal and allow proper sound conduction and self-cleansing.

Highlights

1. Maintain continuity and integrity of the skin flap.
2. Effect meticulous hemostasis.
3. Thin the skin flap.
4. Excise conchal cartilage (the cornerstone of meatoplasty).
5. Drill underlying bone (if necessary).
6. Use sutures to keep the meatus open.
7. Cover all open areas.
8. Postoperative care must be adequate and frequent.

Pitfalls and Complications

1. Leaving skin flap with a thin base.
2. Tearing of skin flap.
3. Excessive bleeding.
4. Leaving open areas with granulation tissue formation.
5. Displacing a flap.
6. Perichondritis.
7. Meatal stenosis.

Meatoplasty in Open-cavity Tympano-mastoidectomy

Since a meatoplasty can cause some bleeding, it can be deferred until the middle ear and mastoid work is completed, grafts are placed, and the distal third of the canal is packed. Meticulous hemostasis should be exercised. In an open-cavity mastoidectomy, a Körner's flap is quite useful in providing skin coverage for the newly created mastoid cavity. The flap is developed by making vertical incisions in the skin of the external auditory canal at 6 and 12 o'clock with a straight canal knife. They are connected by a horizontal incision made with a curved canal knife at 5 mm from the tympanic annulus (Fig. 7–9*A*). The vertical incisions are then extended to the conchal bowl (Fig. 7–9*B*). It is important to keep the base of the flap wide at the conchal bowl level. The subcutaneous tissue of the flap is generally quite thick. It can be thinned carefully with a sharp scissors or scalpel, avoiding damage to the overlying skin (Fig. 7–9*C*).

An opening is considered adequate when the surgeon's index finger can be introduced easily into the meatus. For practical purposes, a meatus cannot be made "too wide"; there is always a tendency toward reduction in size (narrowing). In order to keep the meatus open and provide better apposition of tissues for healing, two permanent sutures can be placed, bringing together the subcutaneous layer with the posterior margin of the postauricular incision (Fig. 7–9*D*). It is important to prevent postop-

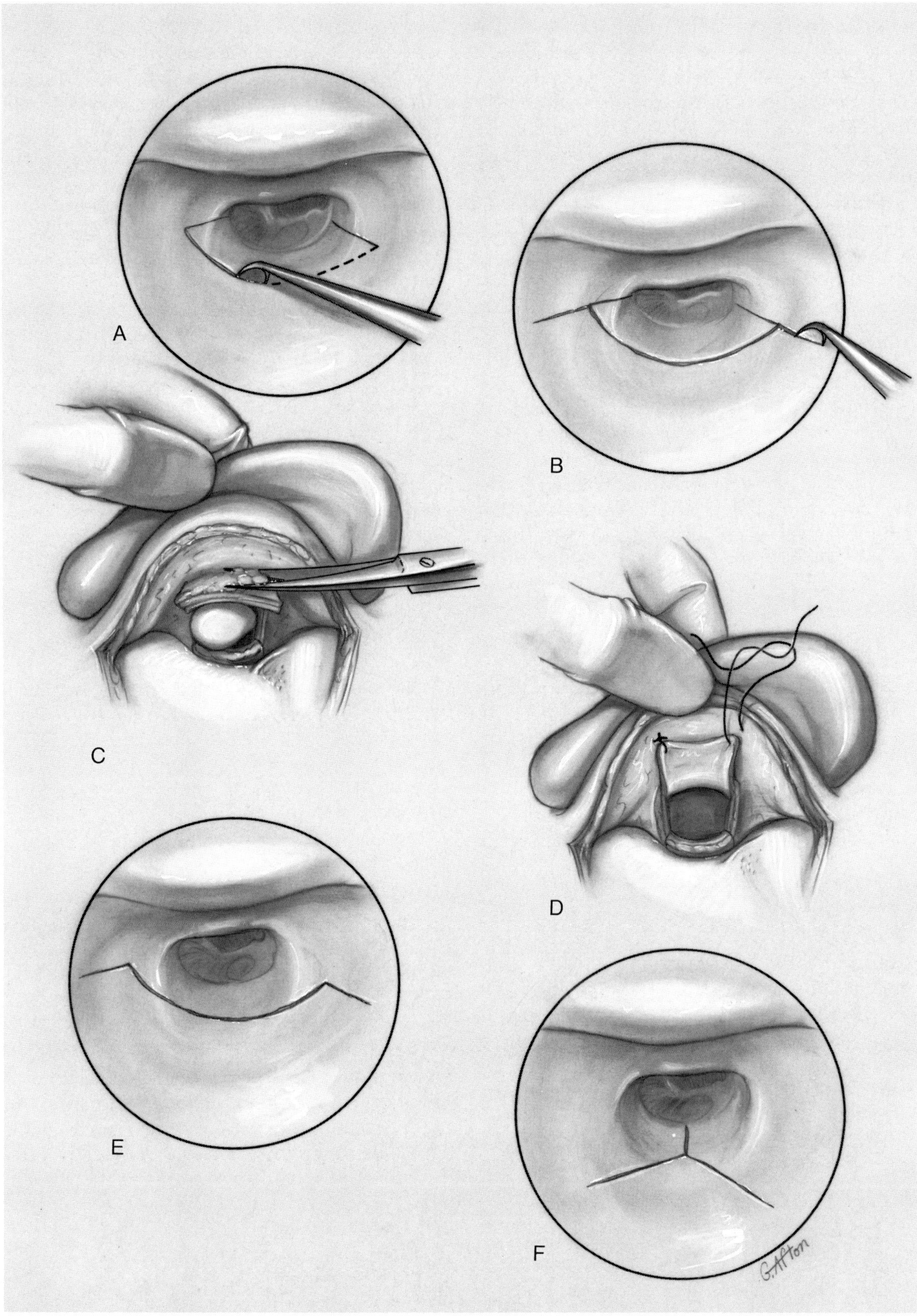

FIGURE 7–9.

erative stenosis by controlling formation of granulation tissue. Clean edges of the flap and good skin coverage of the mastoid bowl are of paramount importance. A Thiersch graft can be performed during the primary procedure for these purposes, or after three weeks if open areas with granulation tissue are present; this should be necessary only occasionally. (See the discussion of the Thiersch graft in this chapter.) A steroid-saturated, *firm* pack is applied and left in place for two weeks; upon its removal, all granulations (if any) are curetted and/or cauterized, and a steroid-antibiotic ointment is applied. Frequent and meticulous postoperative care is basic to successful healing in meatoplasty and in mastoid cavities in general.

An additional point: If a Körner's flap is not used in a postauricular approach, a horizontal incision can be made in the bony cartilaginous junction with two vertical incisions at 6 and 12 o'clock, creating a rectangular flap (Fig. 7–9*E*). With this flap, the basic principles described above apply equally. Other types of flaps can be used according to need, such as a vertical incision, an inverted T, or an inverted Y (Fig. 7–9*F*). Regardless of the flap used, the important point is to provide adequate skin coverage for the newly created surface area. It is crucial to remember that the meatus also comprises cartilage and bone; that the flap is an important part, but only a part, of the meatoplasty. Despite a flap that is beautifully designed "on paper," an inadequate meatoplasty may result because of lack of attention to the underlying subcutaneous tissues, cartilage, or bony meatus.

Meatoplasty in Closed-cavity Tympano-mastoidectomy

An endaural Lempert I incision is made at a level approximately 7 mm below the mastoid cortex level. A Lempert II incision is made that is large enough to admit the surgeon's forefinger freely. The bony canal, especially the posterior bony canal, is enlarged; conchal cartilage is then removed by carefully everting the conchal skin and using a sharp scissors or scalpel (Fig. 7–10). Packing, suturing, and postoperative care are identical to those for an open-cavity mastoidectomy.

Management of Pitfalls and Complications

A torn skin flap or a flap with poor vascularity due to a thin base may not survive; however, a thin flap may, behaving for all practical purposes as a skin graft. Lack of flap survival necessitates surgical debridement and a Thiersch graft. Excessive bleeding may lead to infection or appearance of granulation tissue, or both; if bleeding occurs underneath the flap, the flap may become medially displaced. An "organized clot" often leads to fibrosis, calling for careful elevation of the flap, meticulous hemostasis, debridement, and tight packing. Fibrosis also can occur when using a tight packing, but there will be no secondary problems, provided that the packing is removed at the proper time (no longer than two weeks afterward). Management of open areas with granulation tissue has already been described. On occasion, especially when an infected mastoid has been dealt with, a perichondritis might occur, characterized by edema, induration, and pain over the entire pinna. In early stages, the possibility of allergy to the antibiotic ointment or solution must be considered. These signs (misnamed "cellulitis") require change of antibiotic solution, systemic antibiotics, daily (at least twice) soaks with Burow's solution or any astringent solution, and application of packing saturated with antibiotic steroid solution. If the symptoms progress (which they rarely do), debridement, drainage, and placement of drains may be needed. Cultures should be obtained, if possible.

If general principles, including adequate follow-up, are not observed, meatal stenosis requiring a revision may occur. The meatal skin is carefully elevated, the underlying bone (which usually displays new bone formation, bony spicules, ridges, and so on) widely drilled or curetted, and a large meatus developed. Remember that for practical purposes a meatus cannot be made too large, only too small.

Thiersch Graft

Granulation tissue may develop in the mastoid cavity after canal-wall-down mastoidectomy. Drainage may persist from granulation tissue until the entire mastoid cavity is epithelialized. A Thiersch graft is a thin skin graft that helps to epithelialize and eliminate drainage from the mastoid cavity.

Aim

Placing a thin skin graft in the mastoid cavity in order to achieve complete epithelialization.

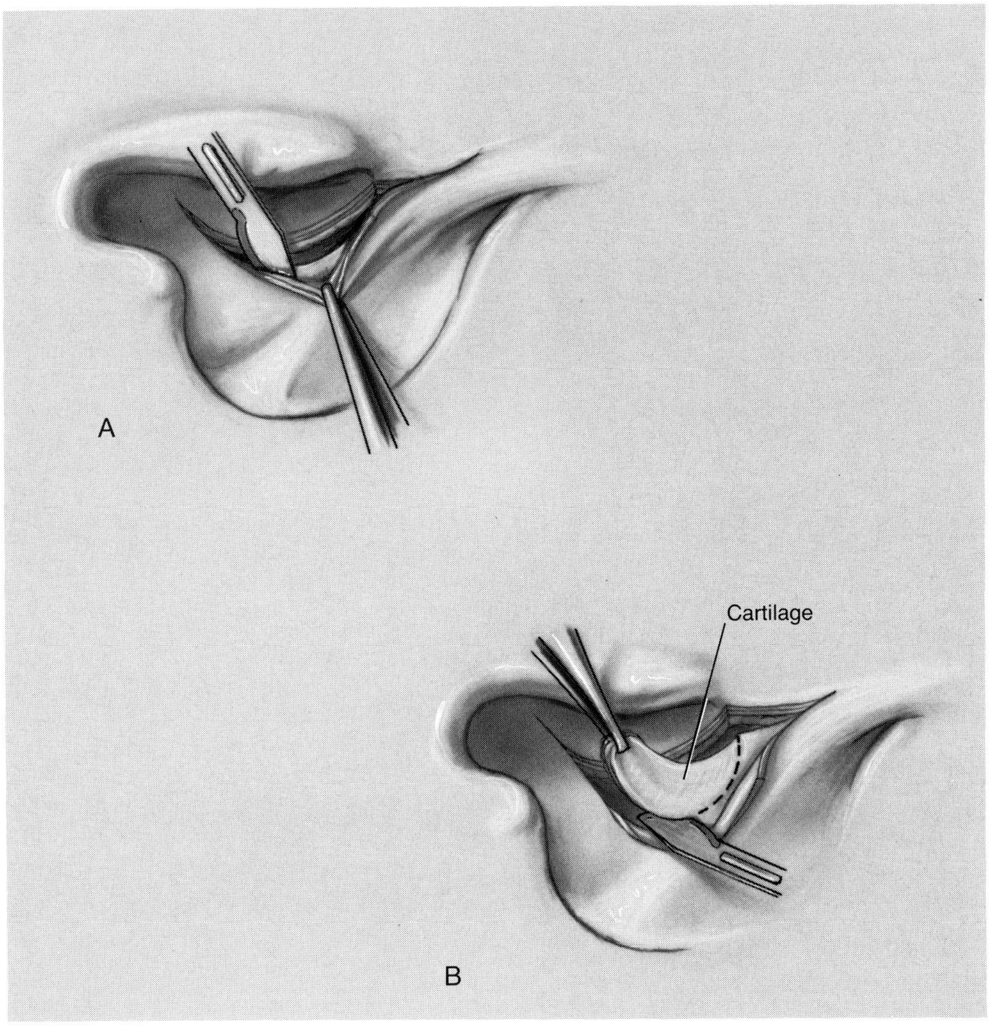

FIGURE 7–10.

Highlights

1. Remove infected granulation tissue.
2. Harvest thin skin from the upper medial arm.
3. Cut the skin into proper sizes on Owen's silk.
4. Cover the entire non-epithelialized mastoid cavity surface with the skin graft.

Pitfalls

1. Inadequately removing infected granulation tissue.
2. Harvesting too-thick skin.

Operative Procedure

The procedure usually is carried out under local anesthesia. Local injection of 1% lidocaine with 1:100,000 epinephrine, combined with topical application of 4% cocaine solution soaked in 1/2-in gauze strip, provides adequate anesthesia.

Debridement of Granulation Tissue from Mastoid Cavity

The mastoid cavity is irrigated with warm saline to remove any debris or mucopus. Using cupped forceps, ring curets, and suction tips, all infected granulation tissue and necrotic tissue is removed;

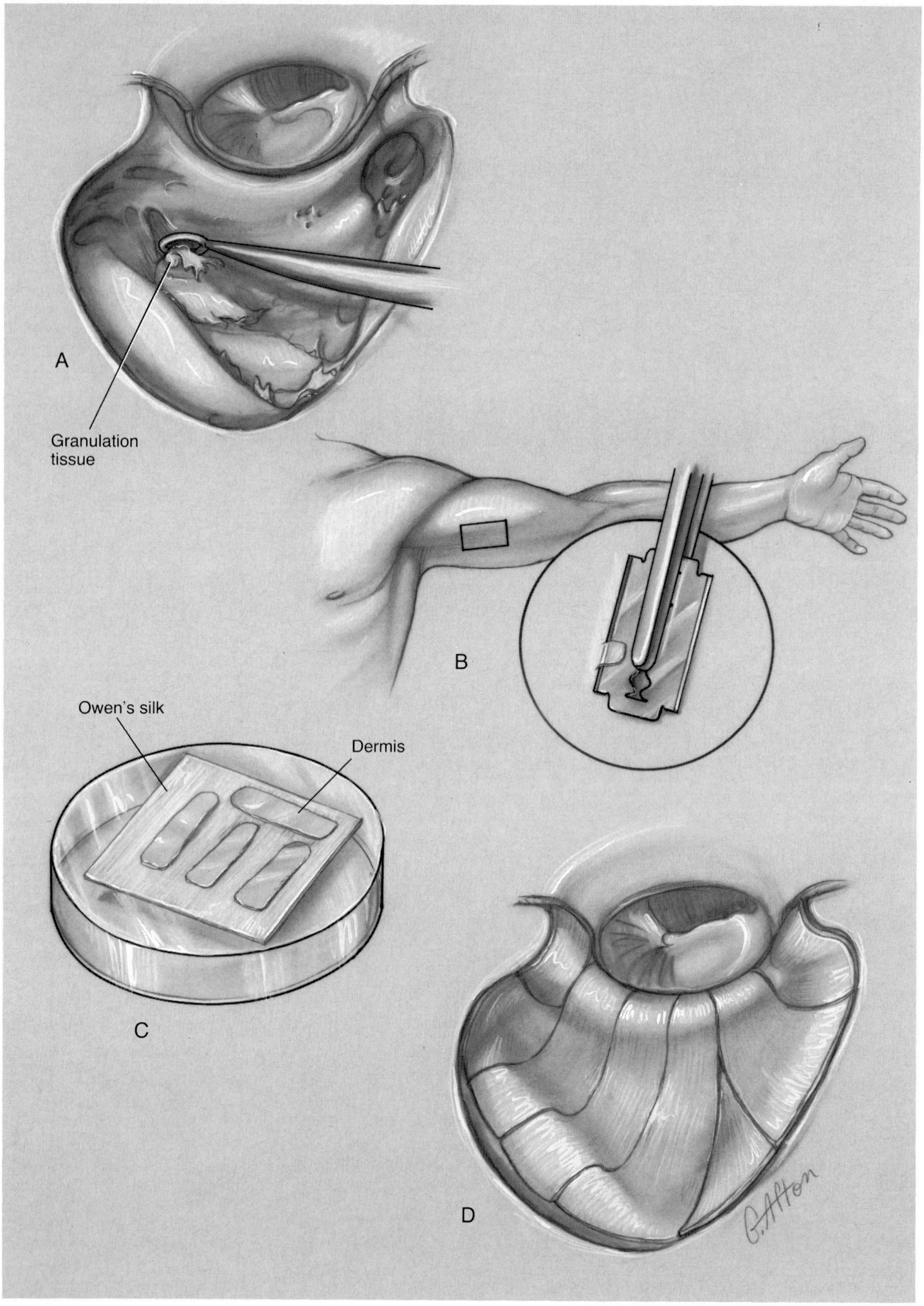

FIGURE 7–11.

any thin, clean, raw tissue over the bone is left intact (Fig. 7–11*A*). Hemostasis is obtained with 1:1000 topical epinephrine (Adrenalin) soaked in 1/2-in gauze strip.

Harvesting Thin Skin

After the mastoid cavity is cleaned out and while hemostasis is being attained, thin skin is harvested from the medial upper arm. Local anesthesia is obtained with 1% lidocaine with 1:100,000 epinephrine injection. The authors use a razor blade held in a clamp to harvest very thin strips of skin (Fig. 7–11*B*). In order to obtain a thin skin graft, the razor blade is pressed down only by the weight of the instrument and a slicing motion is used. The area of the upper arm where the skin is harvested is made tight by pulling the lateral part of the arm with the surgeon's free hand. A thin coat of mineral oil over the skin helps to harvest thin pieces of skin. The area of the mastoid cavity requiring a skin graft determines the amount of skin to be harvested; the donor site is then dressed with scarlet red or Xeroform gauze dressing. The thin pieces of harvested skin are laid on a piece of Owen's silk impregnated with gentamicin sulfate (Garamycin) ointment, and placed on an upside-down Petri dish (Fig. 7–11*C*). Extreme care should be taken to lay the skin on the Owen's silk with the shiny dermis side up. The skin and Owen's silk are then cut into the proper size (usually about 0.5 cm) with a sharp scissors.

Skin Graft of Mastoid Cavity

The gauze strips soaked in topical epinephrine solution are removed from the mastoid cavity. The pieces of skin and Owen's silk are placed over the raw tissue in the mastoid cavity with the dermis side down (toward the bone) and the Owen's silk up (Fig. 7–11*D*). The entire nonepithelialized surface of the mastoid cavity is covered carefully; slight overlap of coverage is acceptable. An eye patch dressing is then applied over the ear.

Postoperative Care

The pieces of Owen's silk are removed in two weeks. If the skin has taken well, drainage is ended and only routine care of the mastoid cavity is required.

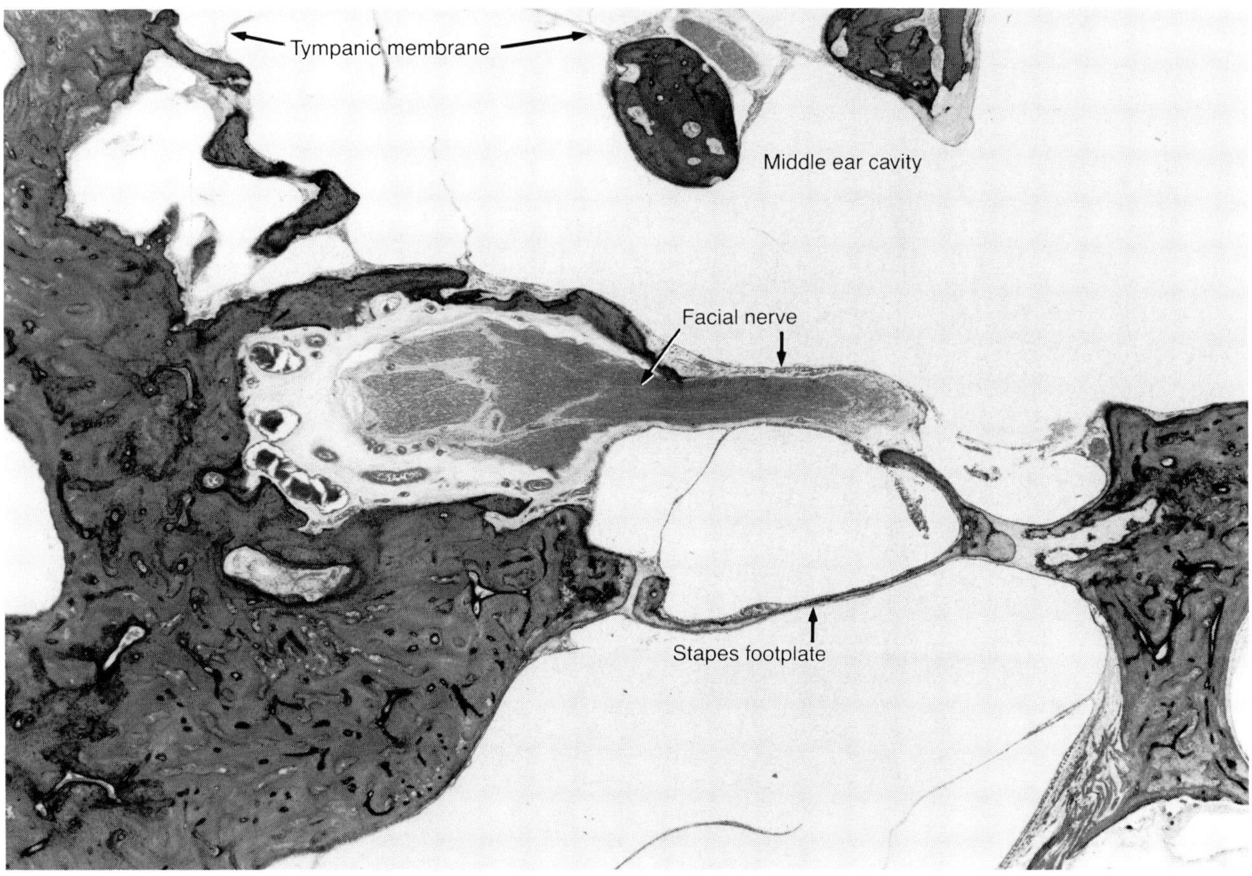

FIGURE 7–12.

Pertinent Histopathology

FIGURE 7–12

This section at the level of the footplate shows a dehiscent and bulging facial nerve over the stapes crura (the most common area of dehiscence). This photomicrograph serves as a reminder of the importance of thorough visualization before any drastic procedures are performed. The facial nerve can be dehiscent in other areas as well, such as adjacent to the tensor tympani, in the facial recess, and in the medial wall of the anterior epitympanic recess. A dehiscent nerve can result in facial paresis or paralysis in cases of acute otitis media, and represents a potential complication in otologic surgical procedures.

FIGURE 7–13

This section shows a focus of otosclerosis, but more importantly a dehiscent carotid artery (*parallel arrows*). Although this is uncommon, there is a risk in working vigorously and blindly in the eustachian tube area since complications could be disastrous.

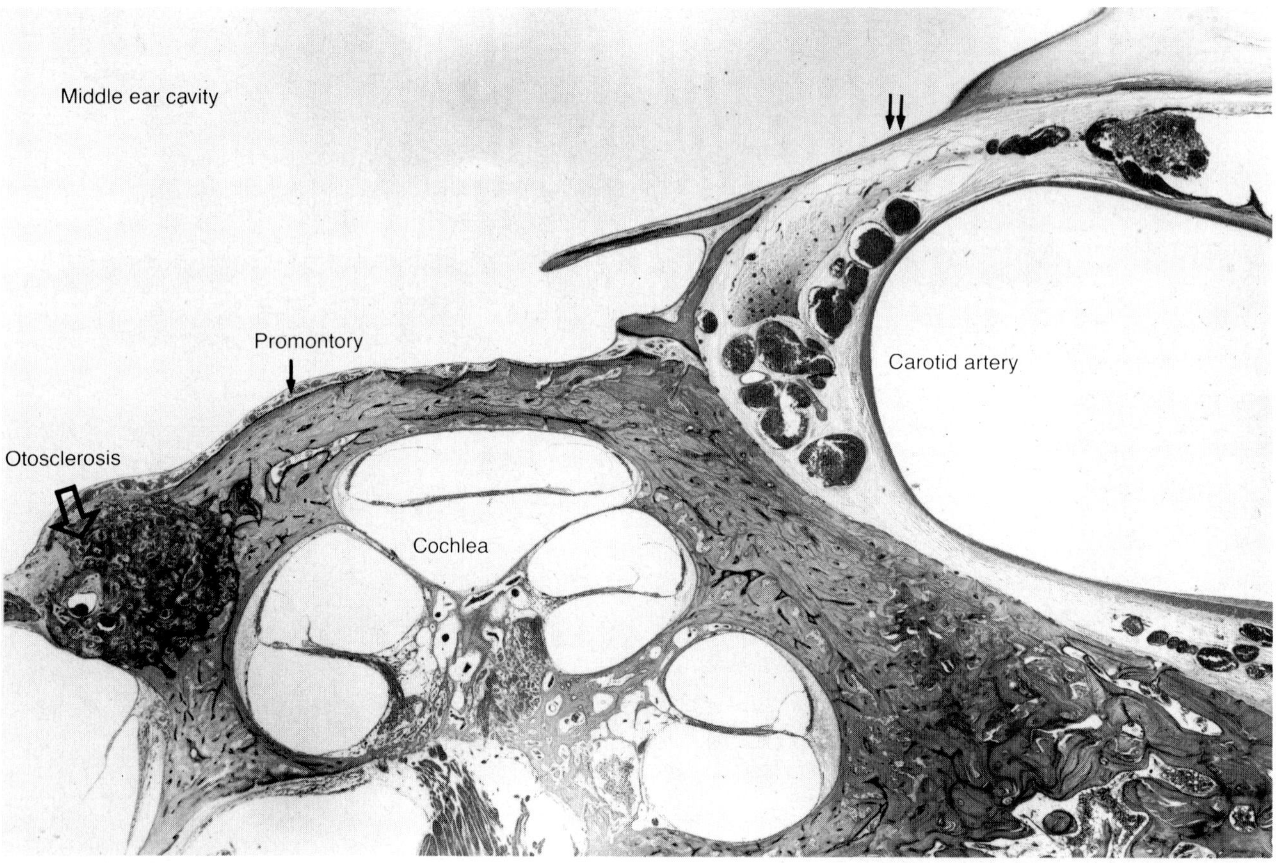

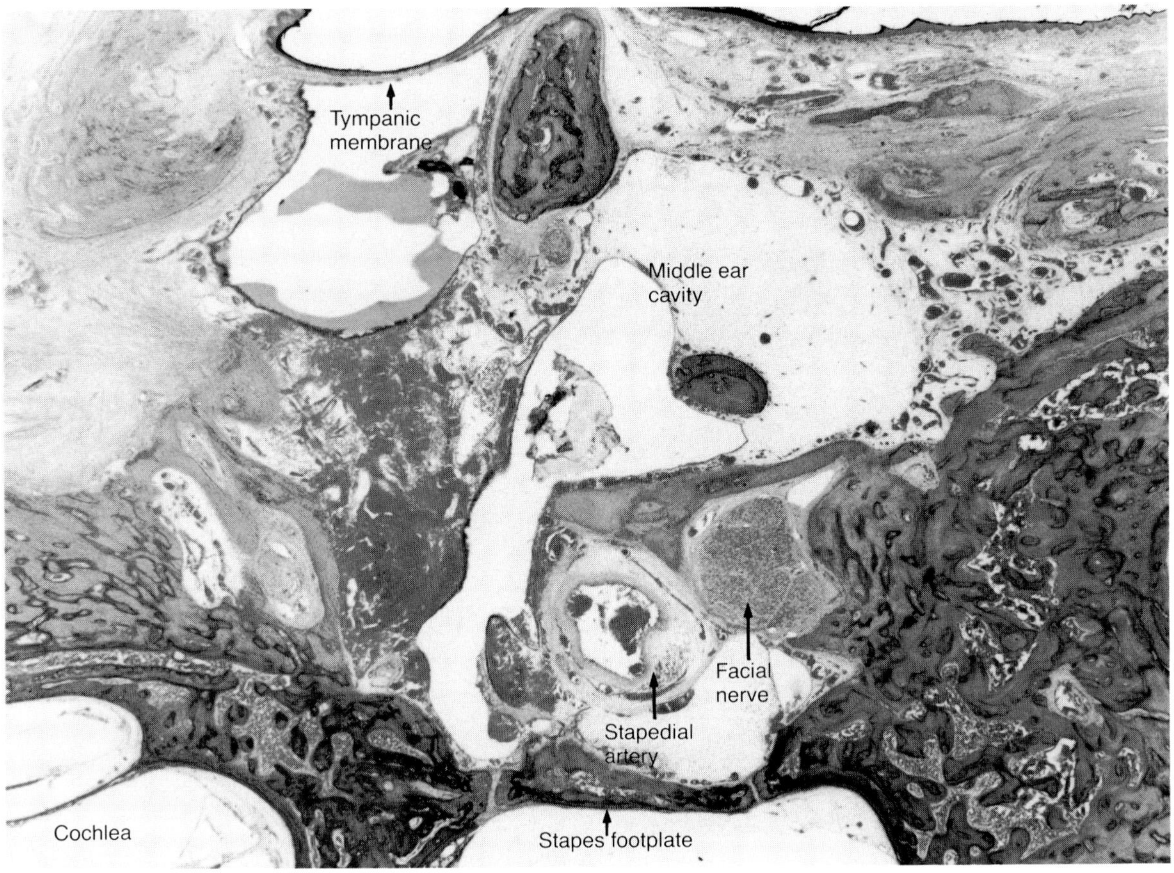

FIGURE 7–14

This section shows the presence of a persistent stapedial artery immediately medial to the footplate in a middle ear with thickened mucosa and a dehiscent facial nerve. This persistence (representing persistence of the embryonal hyoid artery) is rare and should not be confused with a normal small arterial branch that crosses the footplate. Adequate visualization and careful dissection are crucial when exploring an ear with chronic disease.

SECTION IV

Specific Surgical Approaches

CHAPTER 8

External Ear Canal Procedures

Canalplasty

A canalplasty is a procedure that normalizes the external auditory canal by removing abnormal bony growth such as exostosis, removing and replacing intractably infected skin of the canal, or enlarging and straightening a severely stenotic and tortuous canal. Meatoplasty may be done at the same time.

Aim

To restore the normal width and contour of the external auditory canal and, sometimes, to replace diseased with healthy skin.

Surgical Steps

1. Endaural or postauricular incision.
2. Elevation of canal skin flap.
3. Widening of the bony canal.
4. Placing back the canal skin flaps or skin graft.
5. Packing and closure.

Pitfalls

1. Exposing the temporomandibular joint capsule anteriorly.
2. Opening into the mastoid air cells.
3. Damaging the tympanic membrane, ossicles, or skin flaps.

Operative Procedure

The procedure usually is carried out under general anesthesia but can also be done under local anesthesia. In either case, local injection of 1% lidocaine with 1:100,000 epinephrine is made into the four quadrants of the external auditory canal. Either an endaural or postauricular approach can be used.

Exostosis

Large exostoses can cause retention of cerumen, recurrent inflammation of the canal skin, and even conductive hearing loss. An endaural approach usually is adequate. A posterior skin flap is developed from the bony cartilaginous junction to the annulus of the tympanic membrane (Fig. 8–1*A*). The skin over the exostosis is elevated and preserved. When the exostoses are too large to permit a canal incision, a separate incision is made on the top of the exostoses paralleling the annulus of the tympanic membrane. Two skin flaps are developed over each exostosis, one laterally and the other medially based.

When the posterior bony canal with exostosis is exposed, the exostosis is drilled out with a cutting bur and diamond bur under continuous irrigation (Fig. 8–1*B*). As the base of the exostosis is removed, the entire tympanic membrane can be visualized and

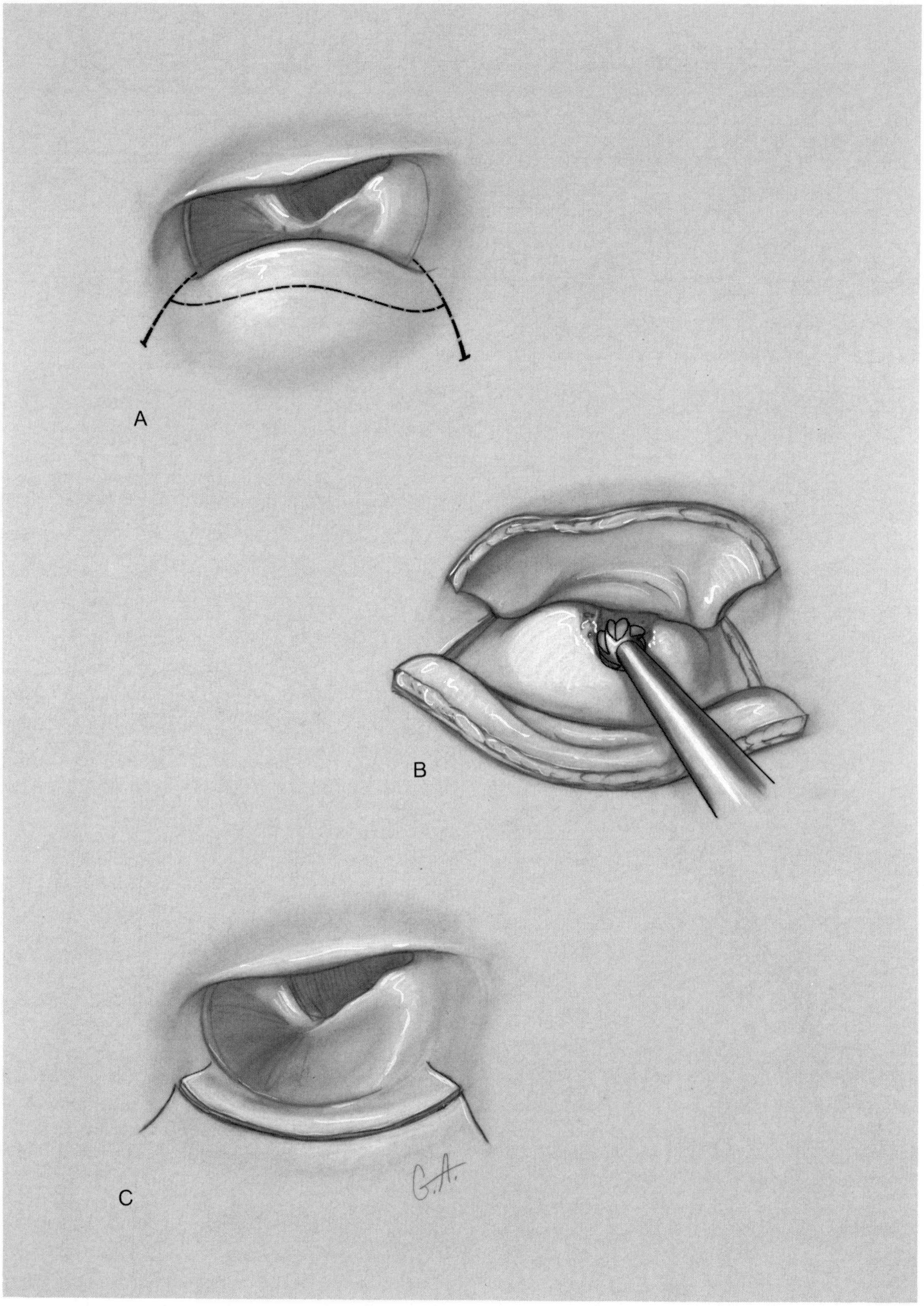

FIGURE 8–1.

the canal skin flap becomes better defined. The annulus of the tympanic membrane is left intact, and the middle ear is not entered. The remaining bony canal wall is smoothed down until the canal has a normal, even contour.

Any other exostoses in the canal are removed in a similar manner. This is usually easier because the canal is less crowded and the tympanic membrane is readily visible. For an exostosis in the anterior canal, a laterally based anterior "window-shade" flap can be developed starting from an area just lateral to the anterior half of the tympanic ring. When drilling the anterior wall of the canal, care must be exercised not to enter the temporomandibular joint.

After all the exostoses are removed and the rest of the canal wall is smoothed down, the skin flaps are laid back (Fig. 8–1C). The external auditory canal is packed with Gelfoam saturated in antibiotic solution and "wrung out"; Owen's silk strips and pieces of cotton packing (rosebud packing) also can be used. The lateral part of the canal and the meatus are packed with 1/2-in gauze strips saturated with antibiotic ointment.

The incision is closed in layers and a mastoidectomy type of pressure dressing is applied.

Intractable External Otitis

This procedure is indicated when chronic external otitis is persistent despite aggressive medical treatment. Usually the canal is obliterated with swollen, thick canal skin. The operation is usually performed under general anesthesia. Local injection of 1% lidocaine with epinephrine helps hemostasis.

A postauricular incision is made for wide exposure. The cartilaginous canal is sectioned at the level of the mastoid cortex through the postauricular incision (Fig. 8–2*A*). An infected stenotic plug of canal skin is removed using an elevator and curets (Fig. 8–2*B*). The thin epithelial layer over the tympanic membrane is also carefully peeled off; this can be done concurrently with canal skin removal or separately. The utmost care must be taken to avoid perforating the tympanic membrane. If a small tear occurs the edges are approximated; for larger defects a fascia graft might be needed (see Chapter 12). The best treatment is prevention.

The bony canal is enlarged with a cutting bur. The canal is drilled as much as possible until the entire tympanic membrane is visible; care must be exercised not to enter the temporomandibular joint anteriorly and the mastoid air cells posteriorly.

A meatoplasty is performed by removing the infected narrow meatus and conchal cartilage (Fig. 8–2C). The anterior cartilaginous canal skin up to the tragus also can be removed if infected. The meatus should be large enough to admit a forefinger.

After the infected canal skin and the meatus are removed and the bony canal wall is smoothed down, a split-thickness patch of skin of 0.01-in thickness is harvested from the upper medial surface of the arm with a DaSilva dermatome. It is better to err on the side of thinness when harvesting since thinner skin takes better than thicker skin. The harvested skin is laid on a wooden tongue blade and cut into two unequal pieces. The larger piece is laid out on the drumhead and covers from the anterior annulus to the entire posterior half of the canal; the smaller piece covers the rest of the anterior half of the canal (Fig. 8–2*D*).

A double packing method is used. The first packing places strips of Owen's silk and antibiotic-saturated cottons through the postauricular exposure. Gelfoam saturated in antibiotic solution and "wrung out" can be used instead of rosebud packing. After this packing is placed, the excess skin is folded over the pack and the postauricular incision is closed (Fig. 8–2*E*). Under the operating microscope, the folded grafted skin is laid over anteriorly toward the tragus and posteriorly toward the concha. Any excess skin can be trimmed off. The second pack is placed endaurally (Fig. 8–2*F*). All raw bone is covered with skin graft, and a pressure dressing is applied over the ear. The packs are removed after two weeks. Crusting may occur for several weeks and requires meticulous removal and cleansing until definite healing is achieved.

Stenotic Canal

The external auditory canal may narrow owing to the presence of scar tissue without infection. This stenosis can cause conductive hearing loss and secondary ear canal cholesteatoma.

The operative procedure is similar to that for exostosis. The posterior canal skin flap is developed from the bony cartilaginous junction to the annulus, from the 12 to the 6 o'clock position. The bony canal is smoothed off with a drill and the skin flap is laid back. Anteriorly a window-shade flap may be necessary. Packing, dressings, and postoperative care are the same as for exostosis.

Tumors of the External Auditory Canal

The external auditory canal may be involved with benign or malignant tumors. The surgical treatment

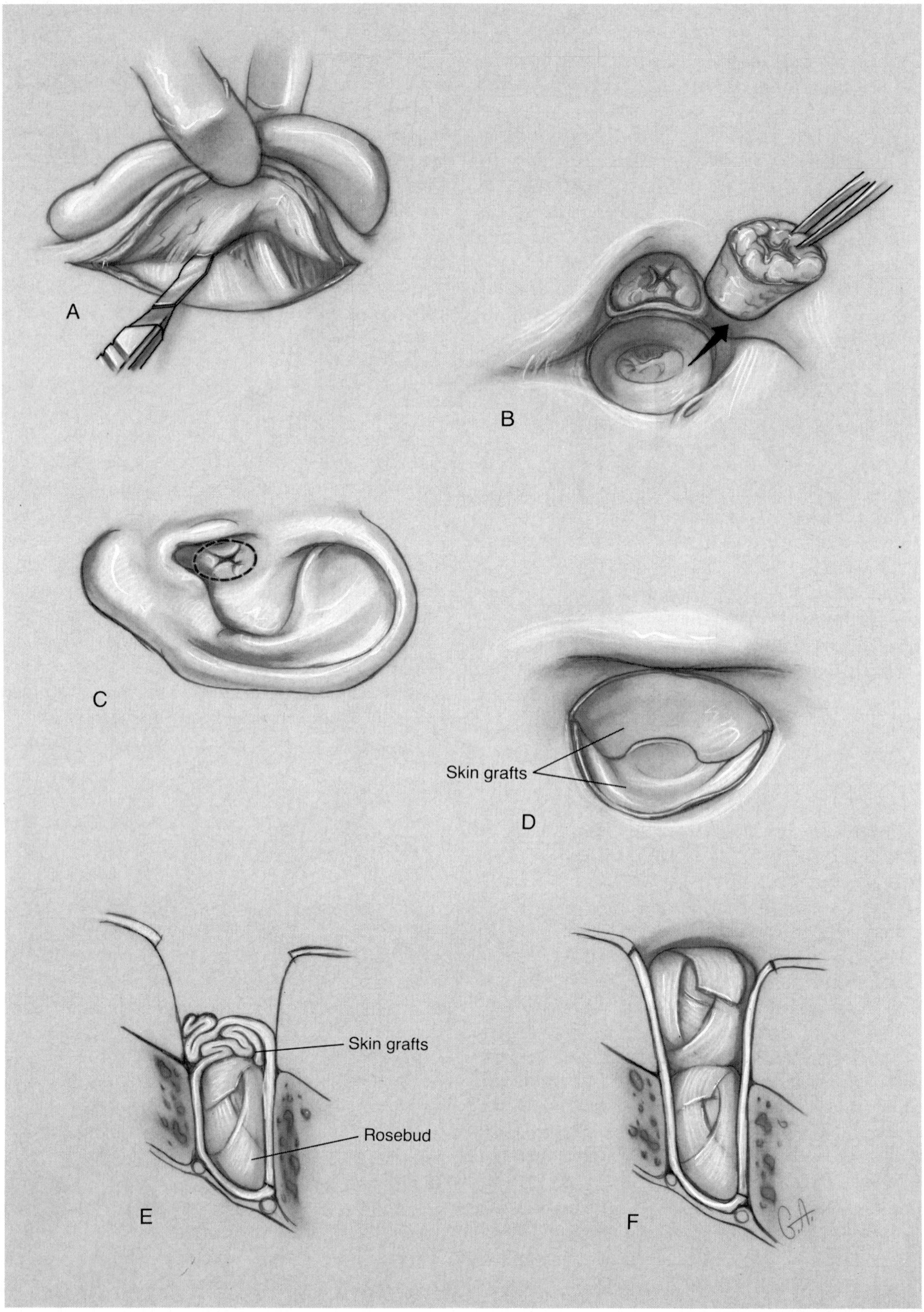

FIGURE 8–2.

of these tumors depends on the type and their location in the canal.

Aim

To achieve complete removal of the tumor and restore a normal external auditory canal whenever possible.

Surgical Steps

1. Biopsy of the tumor.
2. Complete removal of tumor with or without parotidectomy, mastoidectomy, or temporal bone resection.
3. Split-thickness skin graft.
4. Packing and closure.

Pitfalls

1. Inadequately excising a malignant tumor.
2. Delaying the diagnosis.
3. Causing unnecessary damage to the tympanic membrane, ossicles, or temporomandibular joint.
4. Leaking of cerebrospinal fluid after temporal bone resection.

Operative Procedure

Biopsy

The location, size, and extent of a tumor in the external auditory canal should be thoroughly evaluated. If otalgia or bleeding is associated with the tumor, malignancy should be suspected. New imaging techniques such as computed tomography (CT) or magnetic resonance (MR) are helpful in defining the extent of the tumor. Biopsy should follow after a thorough examination under an operating microscope, and can be done under local anesthesia using a cup-biting forceps (Fig. 8–3*A*). If the lesion is small and has not penetrated to the underlying bone, an excisional biopsy that includes removal of surrounding canal skin should be adequate (Fig. 8–3*B*).

Anterior Canal Tumors

If benign, the tumor with surrounding anterior canal wall skin is removed. The excision can be extended up to the tragus and over the tympanic membrane by denuding the epithelial layer of the drumhead (Fig. 8–3*C*). The bony canal is widened with a drill, and a split-thickness skin graft of 0.01-in thickness from the upper medial arm is used to cover the exposed bone and the drumhead (Fig. 8–3*D*).

If the tumor is malignant, lymphatic spread through Santorini's fissures into the preauricular nodes can be assumed. Adequate excision may include a superficial parotidectomy and removal of the anterior canal wall. If a CT scan shows the tumor has extended anteriorly and medially, the excision should include the cartilaginous and bony anterior canal wall, the anterior drumhead, the superficial lobe of the parotid gland, and the condyle of the mandible (Fig. 8–3*E*). The facial nerve is preserved whenever possible; if involved with tumor, it is included in the excision and repaired with a cable graft. The canal defect is covered with a split-thickness skin graft.

Posterior Canal Tumors

Benign tumors involving the cartilaginous posterior canal can be excised with a margin (Fig. 8–3*F*). If the defect is large, a split-thickness skin graft may be used. When a tumor is in the posterior bony canal closer to the tympanic membrane, wide areas of posterior canal skin with the epithelial layer of the drumhead can be removed and a split-thickness skin graft is applied. The posterior canal can be widened with a drill before the skin graft is applied.

When a malignant tumor is small and has not extended to the drumhead, a complete modified radical mastoidectomy is done. If the tumor is close to the drumhead a radical mastoidectomy is done.

If a malignant tumor is extensive and involves the middle ear or mastoid, a subtotal or total temporal bone resection may be necessary.

Subtotal Resection of Temporal Bone

The external auditory canal with surrounding skin and bone is removed, leaving the facial nerve intact. The incision is made anterior and posterior to the auricle, with the inferior extension along the anterior border of the sternocleidomastoid muscle (Fig. 8–4*A*). The auricle is elevated superiorly, leaving a cuff

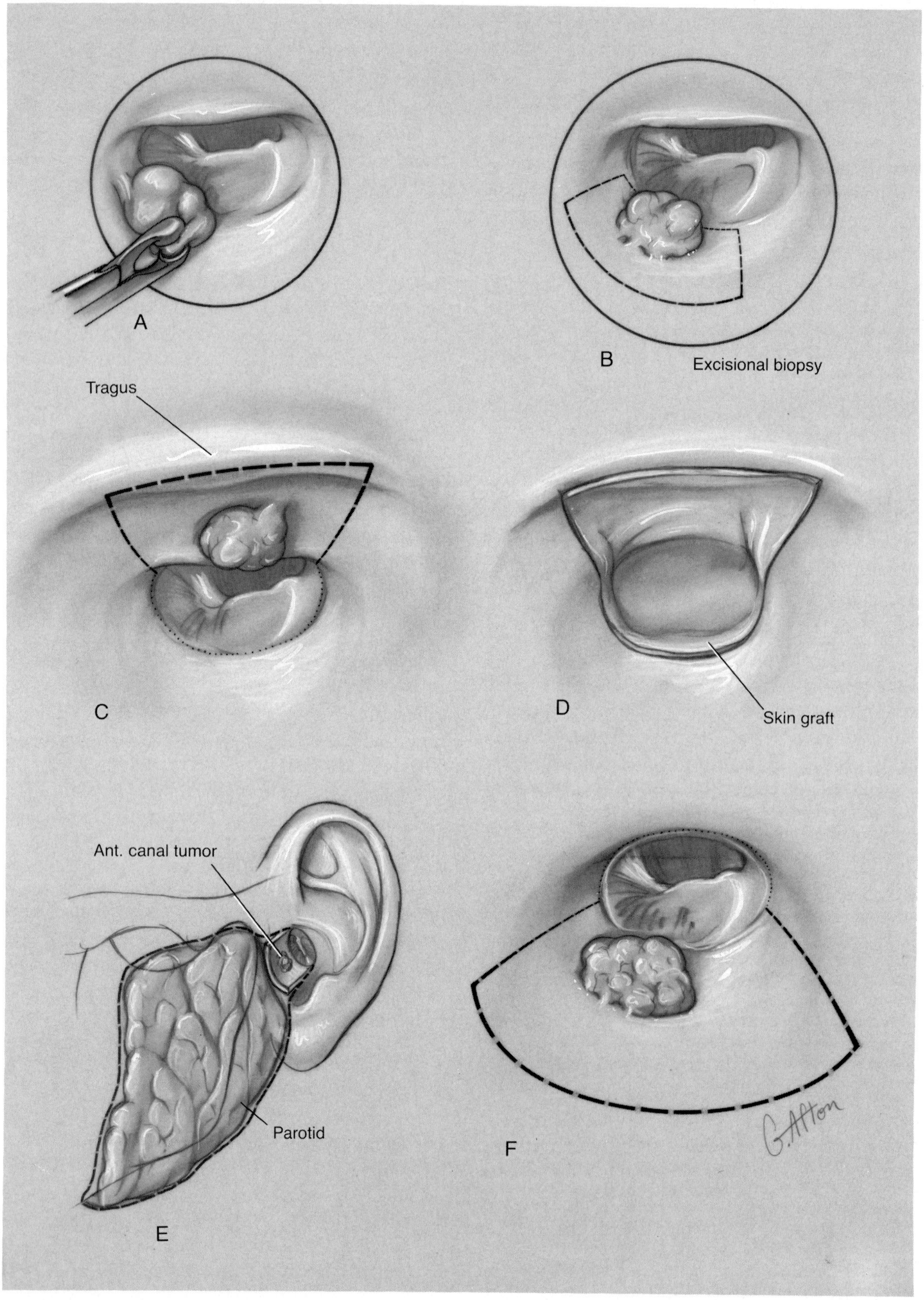
A
B
Excisional biopsy
Tragus
C
D
Skin graft
Ant. canal tumor
Parotid
E
F
G.Alton

FIGURE 8–3.

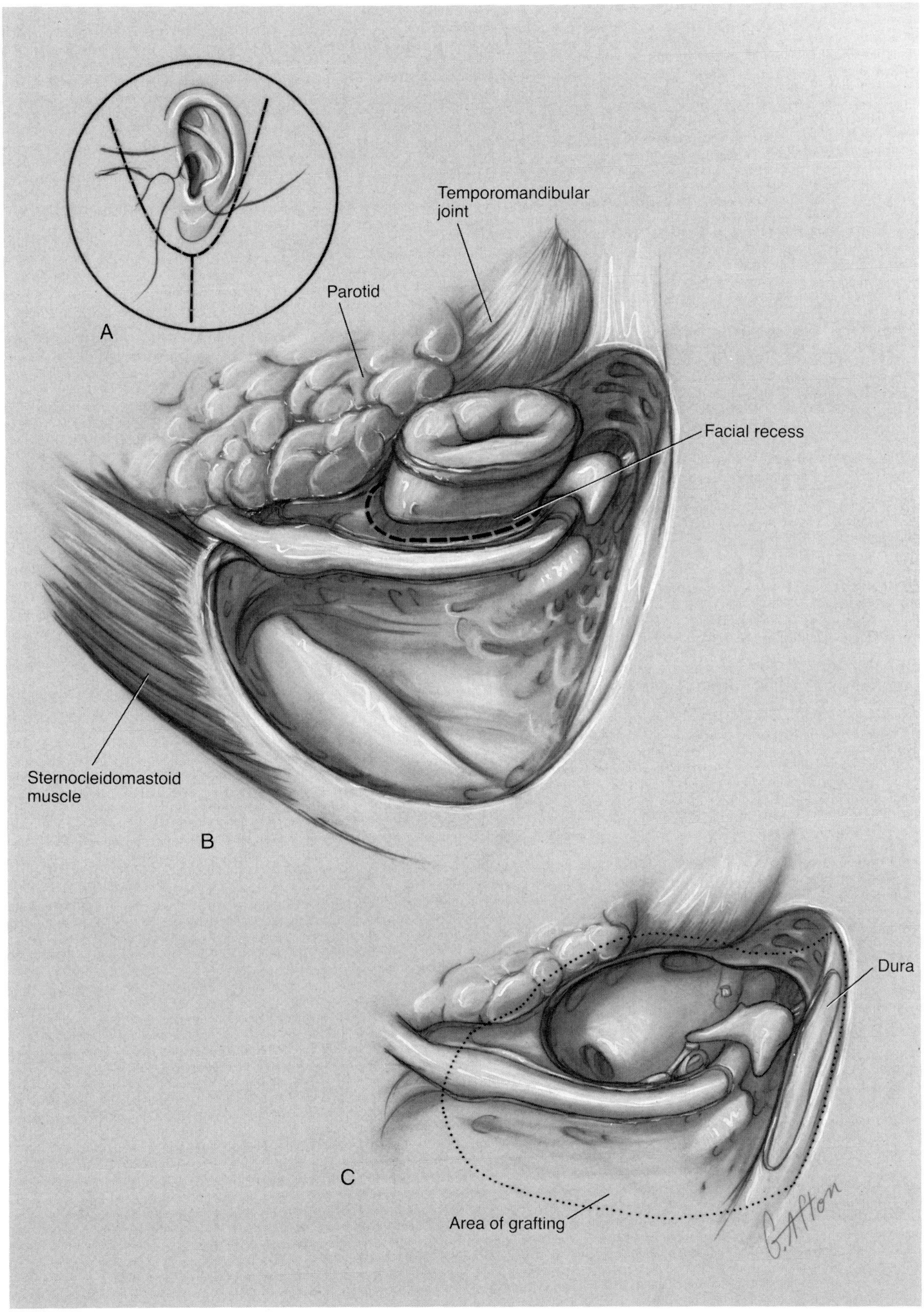
A
Temporomandibular joint
Parotid
Facial recess
Sternocleidomastoid muscle
B
Dura
C
Area of grafting

FIGURE 8–4.

of tissue from the canal and meatus. A wide area of mastoid cortex is exposed, along with the parotid gland and the facial nerve as it exits from the stylomastoid foramen. Using the operating microscope and drill, the entire mastoid portion of the facial nerve is exposed. The bony canal is isolated and separated from surrounding structures. Anterosuperiorly, the bony buttress of the zygomatic process of the temporal bone is drilled down. Anteriorly, the capsule of the temporomandibular joint is separated from the canal wall. The malleus is removed along with the tympanic membrane; the incus may be left intact or removed, depending on the extent of the tumor. Drilling is continued just anterior to the facial nerve, as in the extended facial recess approach. Inferiorly, the dissection is limited by the jugular bulb. The specimen is separated as drilling continues just above the bony annulus (Fig. 8–4*B*). After the specimen is removed, the middle ear space and exposed dura are covered by a large temporal fascial graft (Fig. 8–4*C*). The fascia is held in place by a rosebud or Gelfoam pack and the wound is closed.

Total Temporal Bone Resection

After the incision is made, the auricle is elevated with the superiorly based flap. Wide areas of the zygomatic arch, the squamous portion of the temporal bone, and the mastoid are exposed by elevating the temporal muscle (Fig. 8–5*A*). The lower limb of the incision is made and the parotid gland is exposed. The internal jugular vein is exposed by detaching the sternocleidomastoid muscle from the mastoid tip. The arch of the zygoma is removed and the middle fossa dura is exposed by drilling on the squamous portion of the temporal bone; this opening is enlarged with a rongeur. Elevation of the dura from the temporal bone allows the tumor to be evaluated for possible intracranial extension (Fig. 8–5*B*). The head of the mandible is removed. If the tumor has invaded the anterior canal, a total parotidectomy is done; the facial nerve is resected and the posterior belly of the digastric muscle is severed (Fig. 8–5*C*). The internal carotid artery is exposed with a drill; during this procedure the bony eustachian tube is transected (Fig. 8–5*D*). The bone over the internal carotid artery is removed with the points of the artery's entrance into the foramen lacerum defining the anterior and superior limits of the resection (Fig. 8–6*A*). A mastoidectomy is performed, exposing the sigmoid sinus with a drill (Fig. 8–6*B*). The specimen is removed by fracturing the temporal bone through the otic capsule with a chisel placed just posterior to the internal carotid artery. Hemorrhage is controlled with packing. The boundaries of the resection are the internal carotid artery anteriorly, the middle fossa dura superiorly, the posterior fossa dura and sigmoid sinus posteriorly, and the petrous apex medially (Fig. 8–6*C*). The line of resection as seen from above, passes through the petrous portion of the temporal bone just lateral to the internal auditory canal. If the tumor extends to the dura, the involved portion may have to be resected; if there is evidence of metastasis to the neck, a radical neck dissection may be necessary. The wound is closed after the defect is filled with temporal muscle and a large meatoplasty is done (Fig. 8–6*D*). A split-thickness skin graft over the temporal muscle will shorten the healing time. If the tumor extends to the auricle, the entire auricle and its surrounding skin are excised (Fig. 8–6*E*). The defect is best covered with a myocutaneous flap from the greater pectoral muscle.

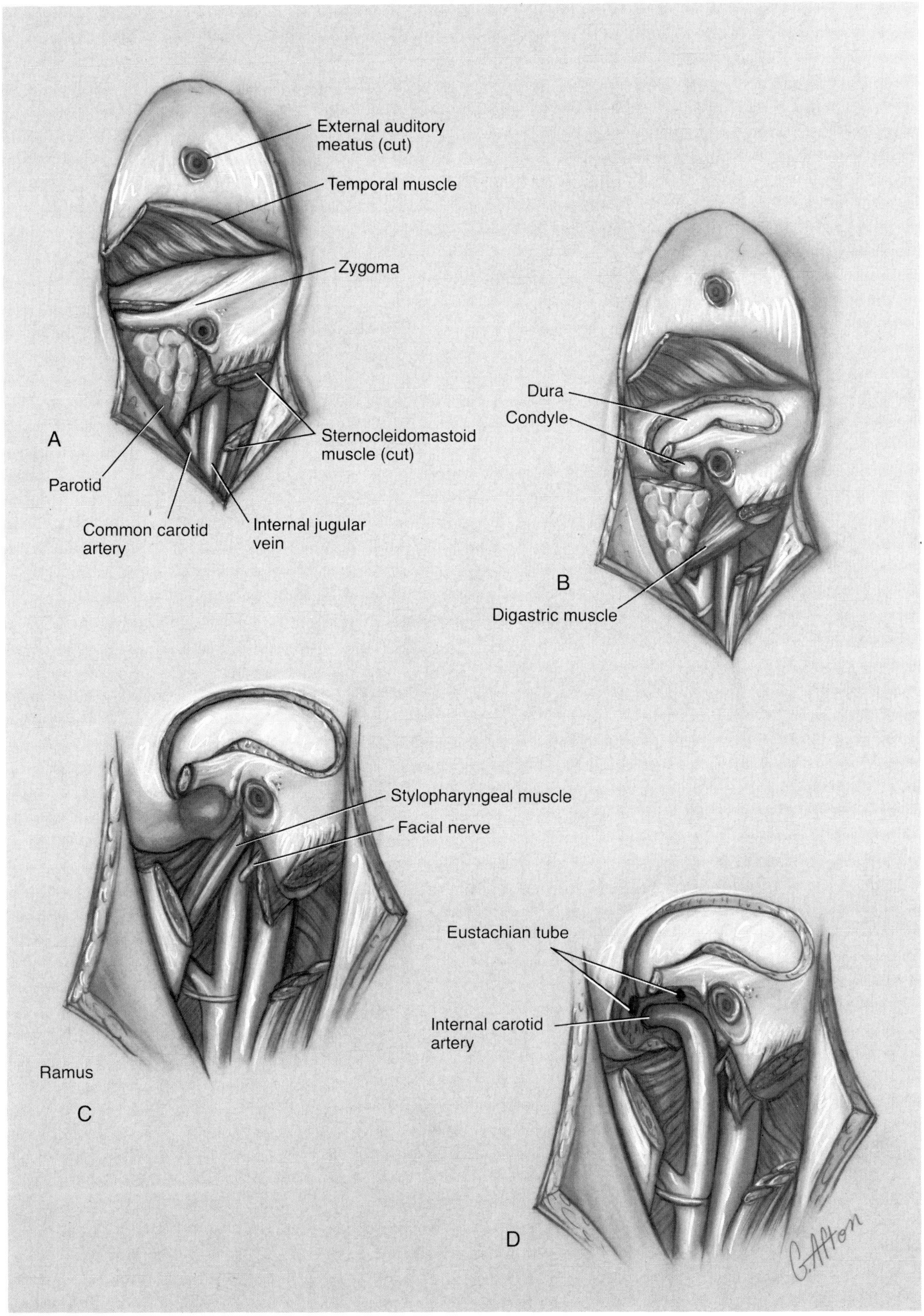

External auditory meatus (cut)
Temporal muscle
Zygoma
A
Sternocleidomastoid muscle (cut)
Parotid
Common carotid artery
Internal jugular vein
Dura
Condyle
B
Digastric muscle
Stylopharyngeal muscle
Facial nerve
Ramus
C
Eustachian tube
Internal carotid artery
D
G.Alton

FIGURE 8–5.

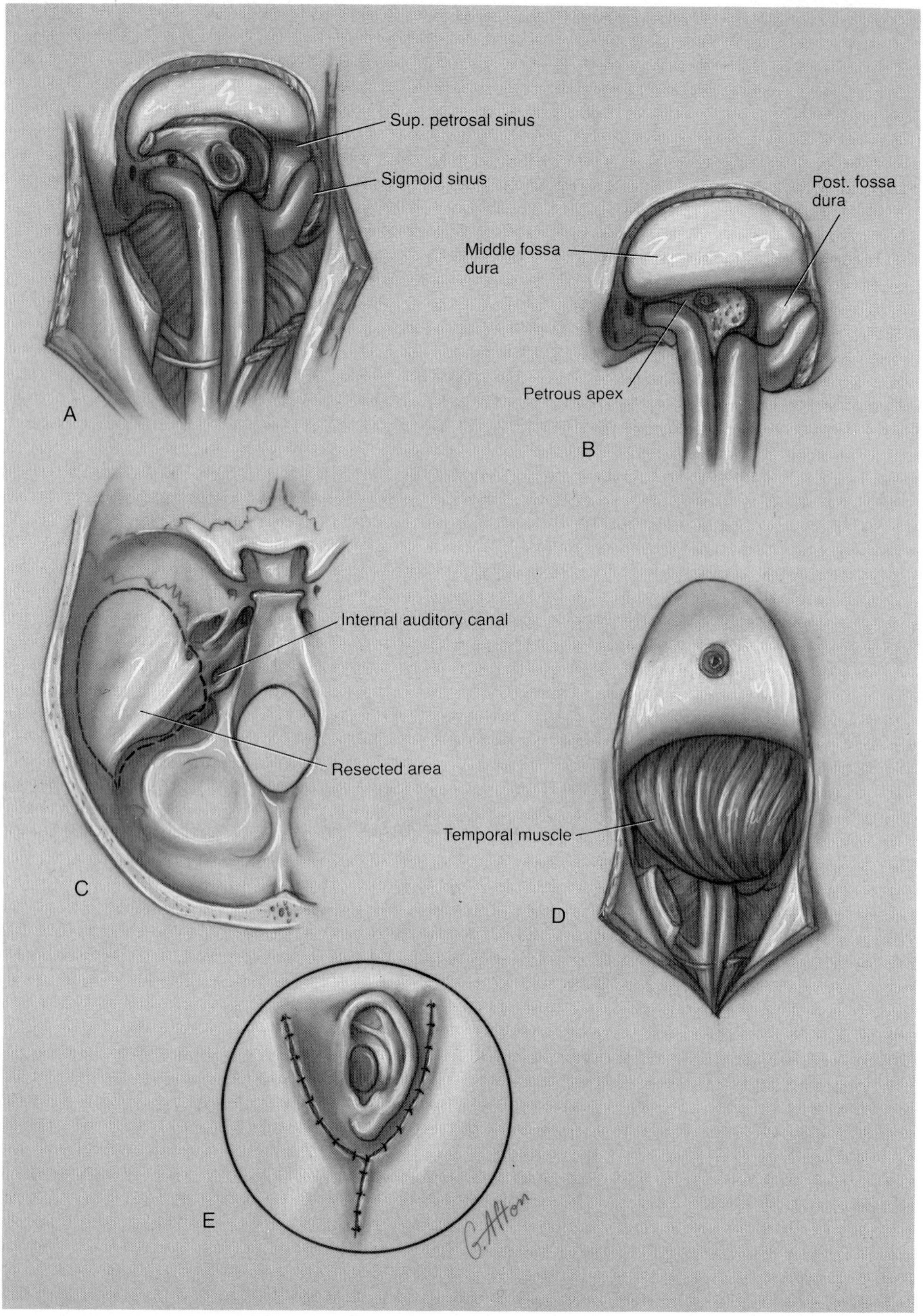
Sup. petrosal sinus
Sigmoid sinus
A
Post. fossa dura
Middle fossa dura
Petrous apex
B
Internal auditory canal
Resected area
C
Temporal muscle
D
E
G. Alton

FIGURE 8–6.

CHAPTER 9

Congenital Atresia

Congenital aural atresia remains one of the most challenging (and rewarding) of all otologic problems. With the eventual incorporation of fully developed bone conduction aids, the indications for surgery may vary; it is essential, however, to have a clear understanding of the main surgical points and concepts. A full discussion of the subject would require a detailed review of embryology types and forms of atresia and their surgical indications and timing. This is outside the scope of this atlas.

The basic requirements for undergoing surgery include:

1. Pneumatization of the mastoid.
2. Adequate cochlear function.
3. A cooperative patient with a supportive family.

Surgical Technique

Aims

1. To achieve a large meatus.
2. To achieve a self-cleansing mastoid cavity that can be easily visualized through the meatus.
3. To avoid post-operative stenosis. A large meatoplasty, skin grafting of the cavity, and close follow-up are important favorable factors.

Highlights

1. The middle ear cavity is approached from the mastoid and not by drilling directly over the atretic canal.
2. In many patients the temporomandibular joint is posterior to the auricular remnant. This requires surgical incisions that allow final positioning of the ear canal anteriorly to the remnant, and of the remnant posteriorly to the temporomandibular joint.

Procedure

The Z-plasty technique shown in Figure 9–2*A* allows repositioning of the auricle posteriorly and of the ear canal anteriorly to the auricular remnant. When the Z-plasty is completed, self-retaining retractors are applied and the mastoid cortex is identified. This is a crucial point. It is essential to have a clear anatomic picture before initiating any drilling. The linea temporalis usually is identifiable; drilling is begun anterior to it. The absence of adequate landmarks can lead the surgeon to explore, and become lost in, the temporomandibular joint space without finding the middle ear cavity. This potentially can result in transection of the facial nerve.

Another important precept is that the atretic canal must not be drilled directly. Pneumatization of the mastoid is required because the essential procedure to be done is an open-cavity mastoidectomy, which allows safe drilling and identification of the facial nerve, lateral semicircular canal, and middle ear "from behind" (Fig. 9–1). Drilling directly into the atretic plate carries a significant risk of damaging these structures. The atretic plate is removed carefully while the mastoid drilling is being done (Fig. 9–2). A tympanic remnant may or may not be present, and the middle ear cavity may be quite small. Extreme care must be taken not to injure the ossicles, which may be wholly or partially present, fused, or absent. Once the ossicles have been identified, their mobility is assessed and reconstruction of the os-

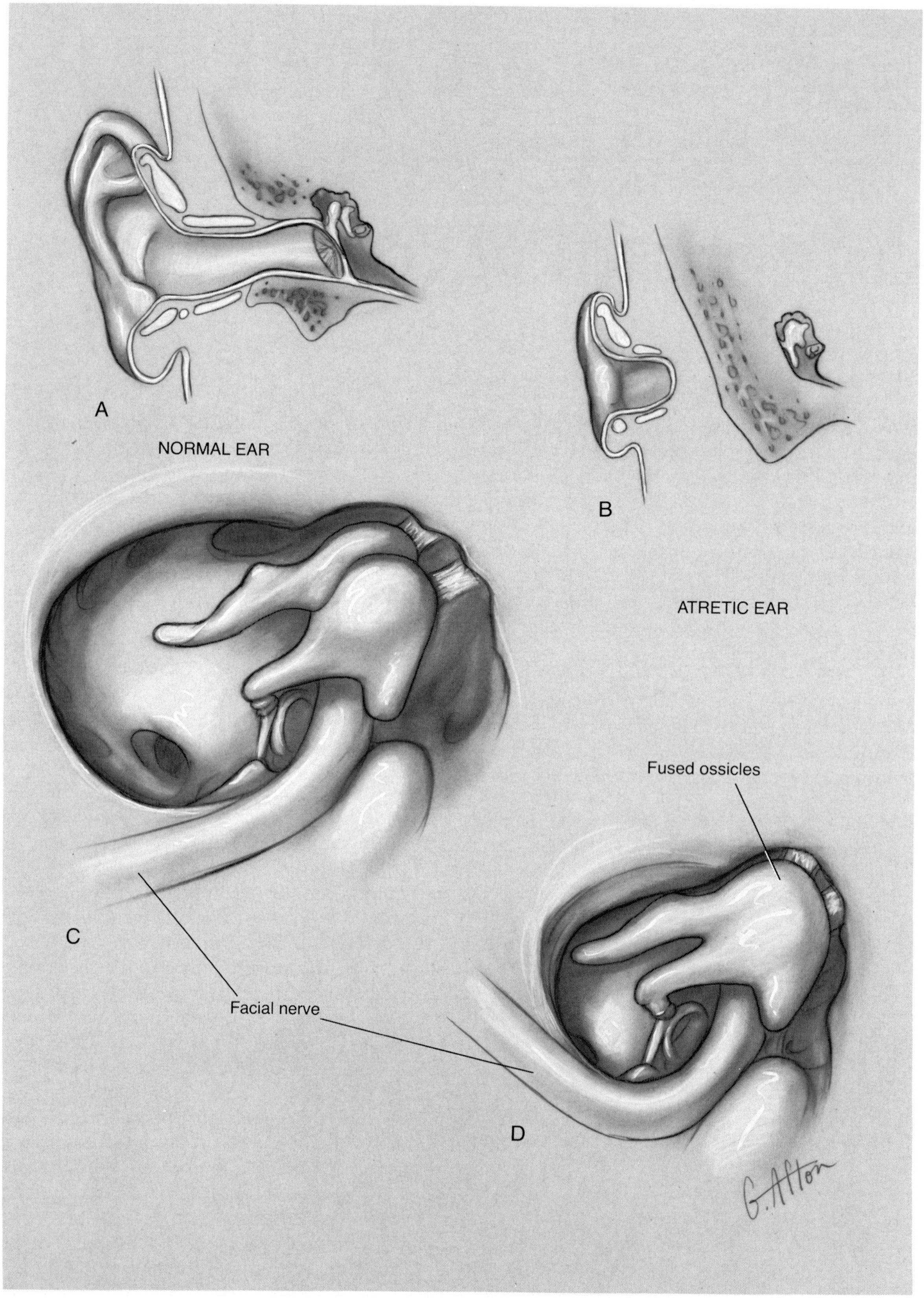
A
NORMAL EAR
B
ATRETIC EAR
C
Fused ossicles
Facial nerve
D
G. Afton

FIGURE 9–1.

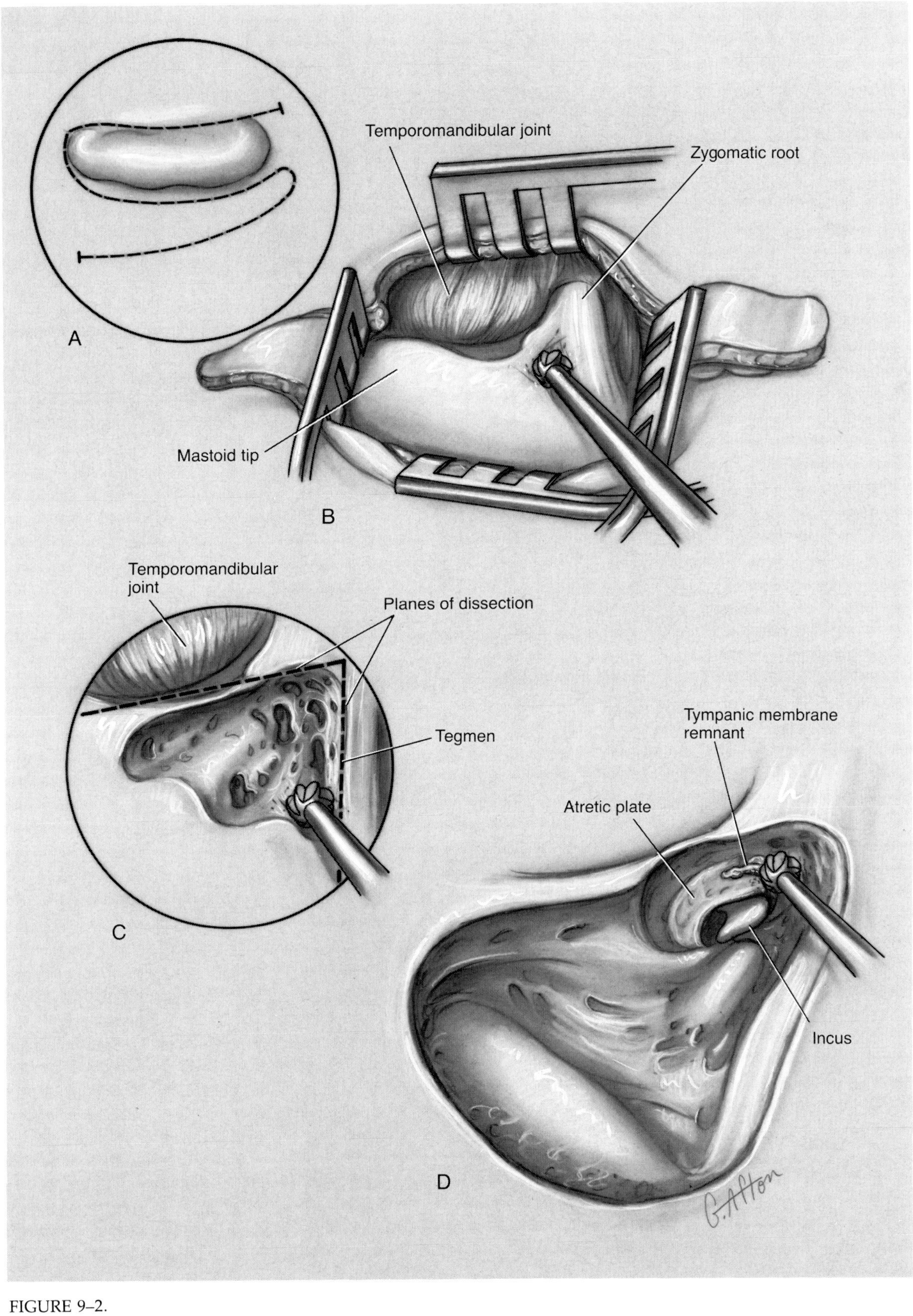
A
Temporomandibular joint
Zygomatic root
Mastoid tip
B
Temporomandibular joint
Planes of dissection
Tegmen
C
Tympanic membrane remnant
Atretic plate
Incus
D
G. Afton

FIGURE 9–2.

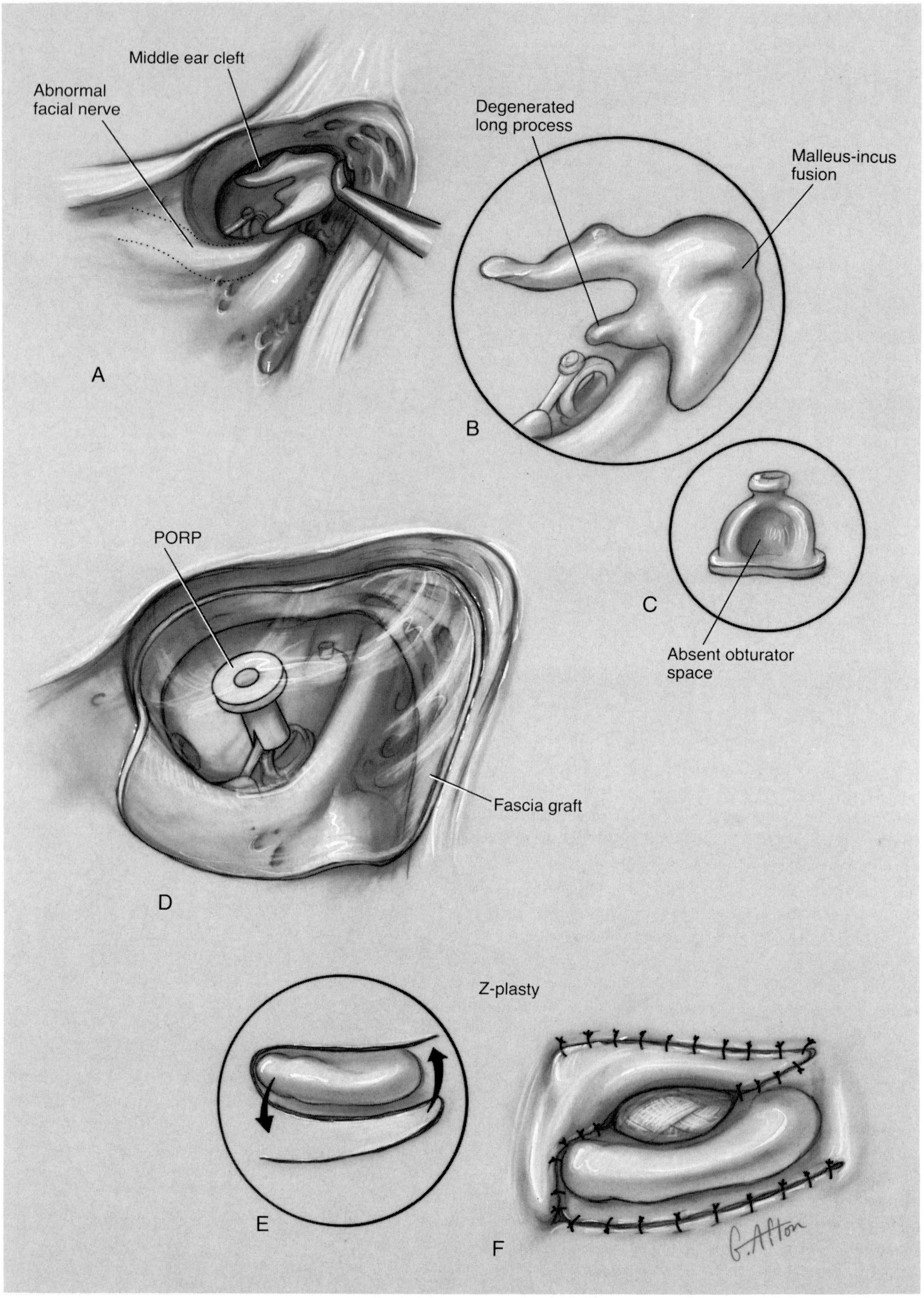
Middle ear cleft
Abnormal facial nerve
A
Degenerated long process
Malleus-incus fusion
B
C
Absent obturator space
PORP
Fascia graft
D
Z-plasty
E
F

FIGURE 9–3.

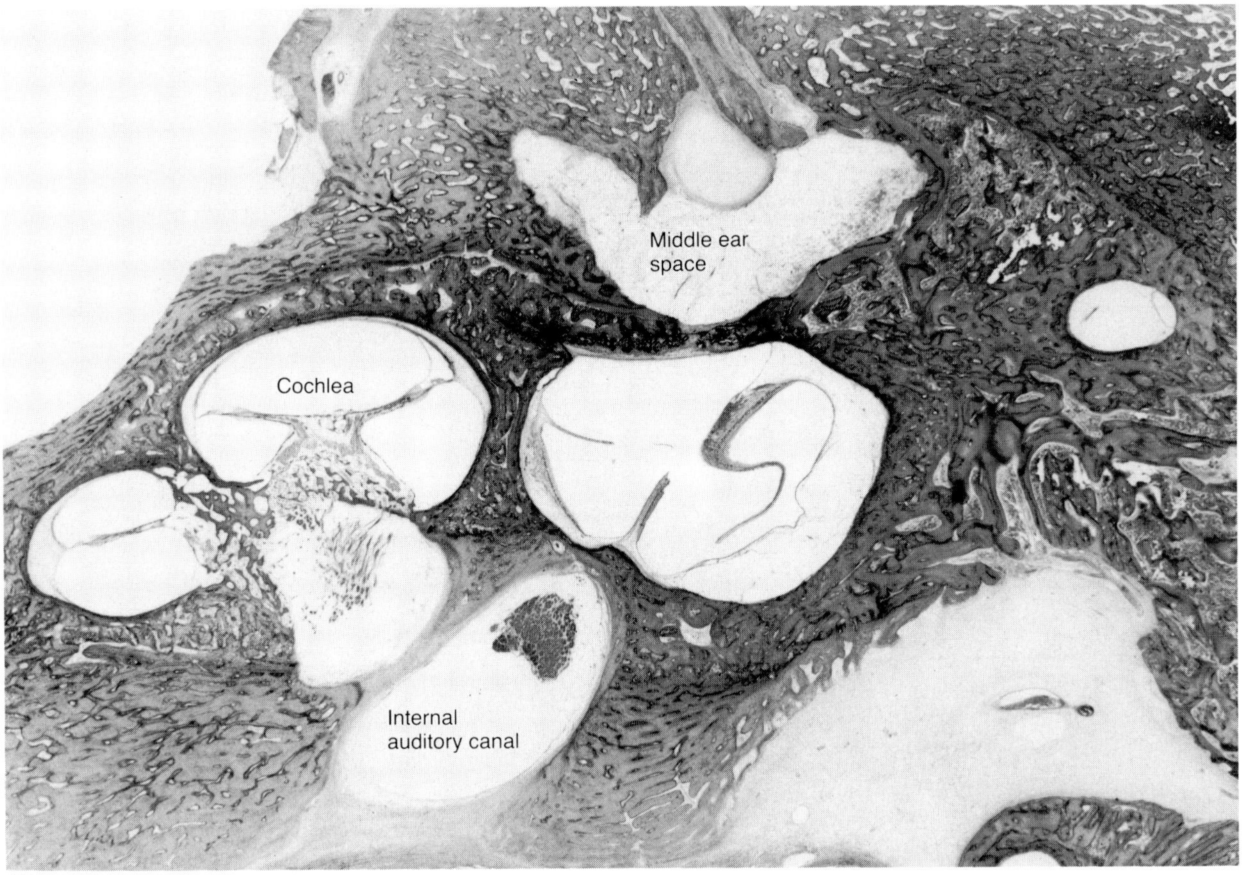

FIGURE 9–4.

sicular chain is planned accordingly (see Chapter 5). The facial nerve not uncommonly is found to have an abnormal angulation in the second genu, making a turn of 60 degrees rather than 120 degrees (Fig. 9–3*A*). This occurs because the nerve has a smaller middle ear cleft to encircle; therefore it makes a sharper angle (60 degrees) and exits inferiorly near the glenoid fossa, in a more lateral position.

Once the mastoidectomy has been performed, the lateral semicircular canal and facial nerve identified, the middle ear cavity enlarged, and an ossiculoplasty done, grafting of the tympanic membrane is performed. Temporal fascia is placed over the reconstructed ossicles; the fascia must not be excessive, in order to avoid adhesions and lack of ossicular mobility (Fig. 9–3*D*). The mastoid cavity itself either is left "raw" for an eventual Thiersch graft or is grafted primarily at the same time. The cavity is packed as described in previous chapters, and the incisions are closed with appropriate sutures (Fig. 9–3*E*, *F*).

Once again it should be mentioned that a large meatus is very important; for practical purposes a meatus can almost never be made too large.

Pertinent Histopathology

FIGURE 9–4

A horizontal section of the temporal bone of an individual with congenital atresia and malformation of the auricle. Mondini's dysplasia also is present. The magnitude of compromise is severe. Absence of the incus, stapes, and oval window can be noted. The facial nerve also is absent; this can be seen only in the internal ear canal (not shown here), since the facial nerve does not course through the temporal bone.

CHAPTER 10

Surgical Procedures in Different Forms of Otitis Media

Clinical experience and laboratory studies indicate that middle ear effusions, far from being innocuous, are slightly delayed reflections of severe underlying histopathologic changes in the mucoperiosteum. They are part of a continuum in which some forms of otitis lead to others, resulting in complications or sequelae. The immediate purpose of the surgical procedures described in this chapter primarily is to halt this process, and to help in the regression of middle ear histopathologic changes. The ultimate goal is to arrest the continuum medically, thus reserving surgery for the restoration of function rather than the mere eradication of active disease.

This chapter begins with a description of a myringotomy and insertion of ventilation tubes. Because this seems on the surface to be the simplest of surgical procedures, it can be, and usually is, treated lightly by surgeons. The procedure is detailed purposely in excess in order to develop a "conscience" in surgeons about the significance and extreme importance of this "little operation," which has changed the course of otologic practice and helped to reduce significantly the number of major otologic procedures for complications or sequelae of otitis media. The chapter concludes with a series of horizontal sections of temporal bones, highlighting the underlying changes in the mucoperiosteum that take place behind an apparently benign "middle ear fluid."

Myringotomy and Tubes

Myringotomy is an incision of the tympanic membrane.

Aim

To substitute for the function of the eustachian tube—that is, to provide ventilation and drainage for the middle ear. By providing aeration to the middle ear space, the intent is to reverse the pathologic changes of the middle ear mucosa and prevent subsequent complications or sequelae. A myringotomy also provides symptomatic improvement, confirms a diagnosis, and allows aspiration of middle ear fluid (which can also be diagnostic) and insertion of ventilation tubes.

Indications

1. Persistent effusion that has failed to respond to adequate nonsurgical therapy.
2. A poorly ventilated middle ear even when fluid

is absent, but the patient is symptomatic or the tympanic membrane is retracted, or both. A good and not uncommon example is that of airline pilots or attendants with eustachian tube dysfunction (or individuals subjected repeatedly to pressure changes), who are otherwise asymptomatic.

3. Recurrent otitis media, even when normal conditions exist between episodes.

4. Acute suppurative otitis media with a bulging or insufficiently perforated tympanic membrane; the patient is markedly symptomatic. (A myringotomy alone is performed.)

5. For diagnostic purposes in infants with fever of unknown origin.

6. To correct conductive hearing losses due to effusions.

7. A retracted tympanic membrane before the stage of atelectasis.

8. With a tympanoplasty in patients with tubal dysfunction.

9. Otitis media with facial paresis or paralysis or other impending complications.

Instruments

1. Set of aural specula.
2. Suction tubes (5- , 20- , and 7-gauge).
3. Myringotomy knife.
4. Baby alligator forceps.
5. Blunt pick (straight or angled).
6. Small ring curet.

Procedure

First, inspect and visualize (this means to purposefully look and screen and *not* to glance casually) the ear canal. Cleanse the cerumen and epithelial debris very carefully; dry, crusty cerumen can be washed and loosened with saline or hydrogen peroxide. Abrupt cleansing can cause bleeding or small hematomas in the ear canal. Insert the proper ear speculum (see Chapter 6) and carefully scrutinize the four quadrants of the tympanic membrane (Fig. 10–1*A*). Look for perforations, retraction, and retraction pockets, and for characteristics of the drum itself, such as myringosclerosis, monomeric areas, atrophic changes, evidence or suggestion of a dehiscent jugular bulb, evidence of a reddish mass in the anterior or anteroinferior areas (dehiscent carotid artery), or myringostapediopexy. Once it becomes a habit, this inspection does not take time and can avoid a number of problems. Look first; do the preparatory work; then—and *only* then—proceed with the operation.

Initially, a magnification of 6× will suffice. In general, the authors tend to use higher power, which provides a better view of sections of the membrane (once the area has been inspected and the site of incision selected).

Incisions

The incision should not be made in the posterosuperior quadrant because of the underlying incudostapedial joint and stapes, nor should it be made too close to the annulus because this favors early extrusion of the tube (unless that is the purpose). An incision should not be made in the presence of acute infection, again because of the risk of early extrusion (unless only drainage is intended).

Epithelial migration can be considered for practical surgical purposes as radiating from the umbo. Migration is slowest in the anterosuperior quadrant, followed by the anteroinferior and posteroinferior. For this reason, the incidence of persistent perforation is higher in the anterosuperior quadrant. Since migration is not the only factor in extrusion of the tubes, the benefits of using this quadrant should be judged on a case-by-case basis. In addition, surgical repair of perforations in this quadrant is not so simple as in other quadrants. The surgeon must decide whether, in a particular case, a larger flange tube (for example, a Paparella No. 2) in the anteroinferior or posteroinferior quadrant would be more beneficial than a No. 1 tube in the anterosuperior quadrant.

In the middle ear space, incisions should not be made in the umbo because of its close proximity to the promontory. The widest space available is the hypotympanum (Fig. 10–1*B*); this must be considered when there is retraction of the tympanic membrane. In such a case, incisions in this area allow better drainage and more space, and carry less risk of middle ear structural damage.

The length of the incision depends partly on the type of tube to be used; in general, it should be the same as the diameter of the inner flange of the tube. Too short an incision can precipitate tears when the tube is placed, especially in a weakened or atrophic membrane (Fig. 10–2*A*). Too long an incision might preclude a tight fit around the tube, allowing it to extrude or even fall into the middle ear cavity (Fig. 10–2*B*). Paparella-type tubes that have a small indentation in the inner flange can be placed through a small incision and rotated with baby alligator forceps or a blunt pick ("screwing motion").

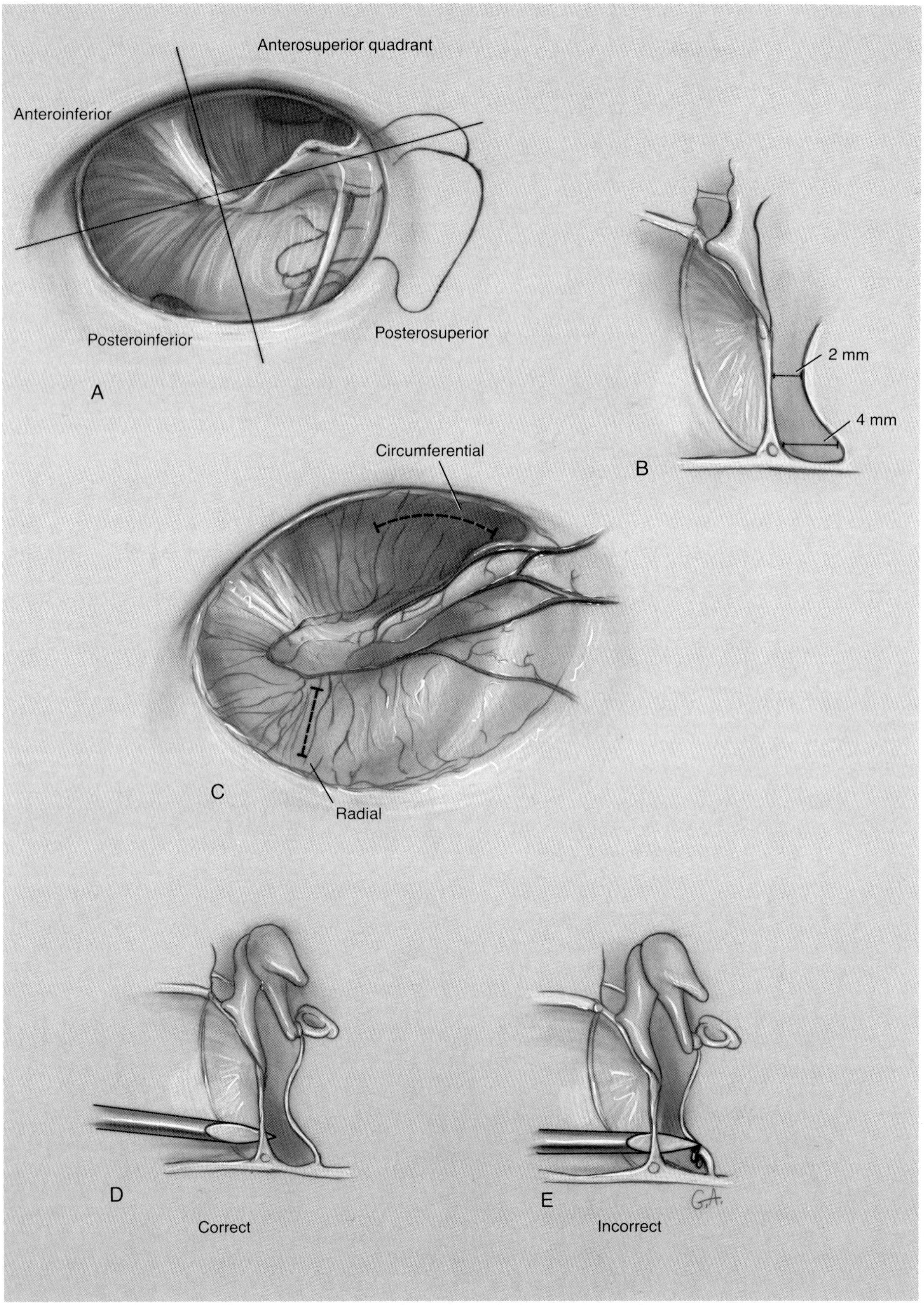
Anterosuperior quadrant
Anteroinferior
Posteroinferior
Posterosuperior
A
2 mm
4 mm
B
Circumferential
C
Radial
D
Correct
E
Incorrect
G.A.

FIGURE 10–1.

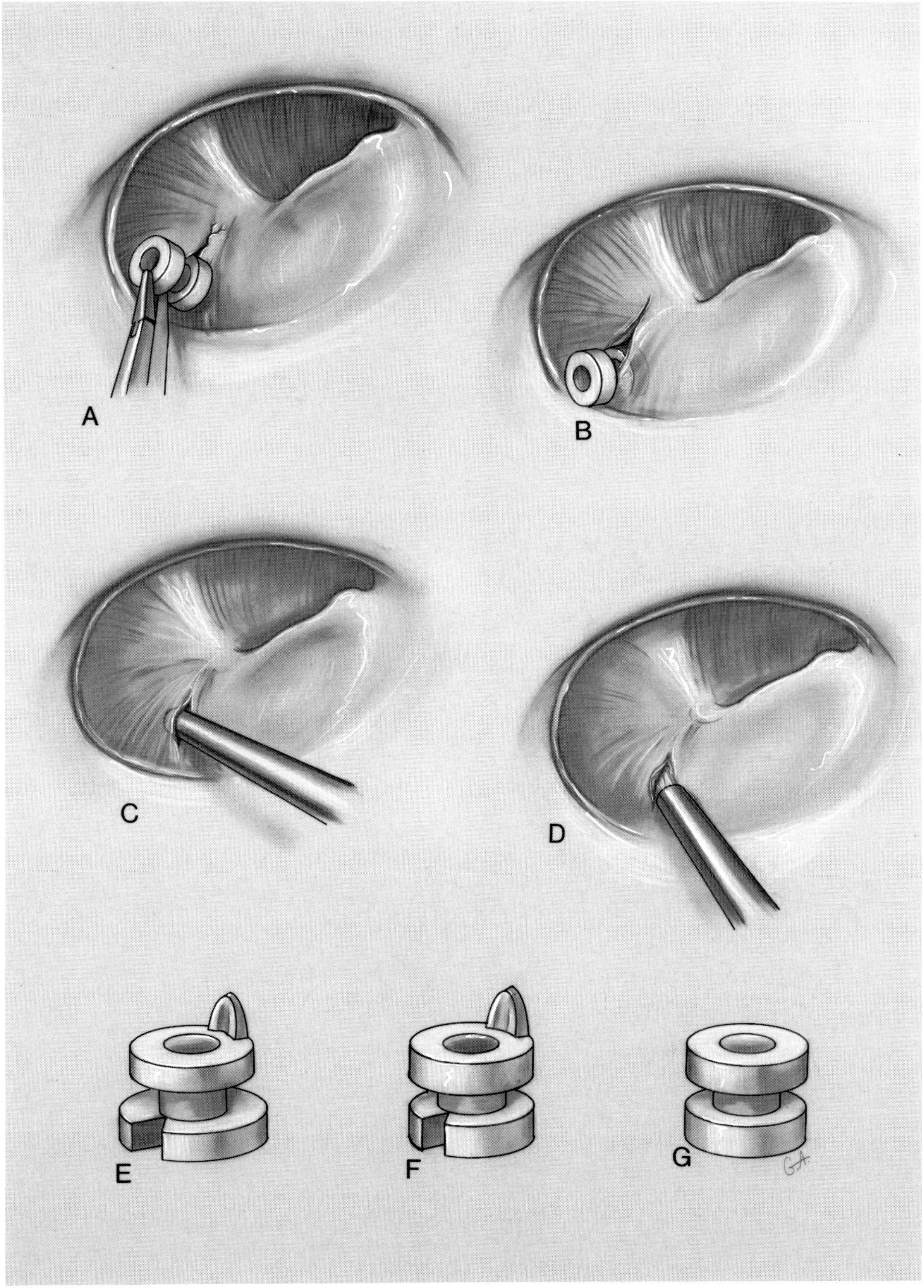

FIGURE 10–2.

A sharp myringotomy knife should be used. Incisions can be made radially or circumferentially (Fig. 10–1*C*). Circumferential incisions tend to accumulate more epithelial debris, leading to earlier extrusion of the tube. In cases of acute purulent otitis a wide circumferential (smile) incision is preferred, since drainage alone is the purpose and prompt closure is desired. In all other circumstances, a radial incision is preferred, since it sections fewer fibers, runs parallel to most of the blood vessels irrigating the membrane, and causes less scarring.

The tip of the knife should be inserted just far enough to section the membrane; deeper incisions might damage the middle ear mucosa (Fig. 10–1*D*, *E*). If there is localized bleeding (thicker membranes sometimes bleed) and blood obscures the incision, hydrogen peroxide or cotton saturated with epinephrine, or both, will control it.

Tubes

Tubes should be placed in a normal area of the membrane. Special care should be taken to avoid atrophic or monomeric areas. Myringosclerotic areas tear easily and tubes do not hold well. In contrast, tubes in normal areas that are surrounded by sclerotic plaques tend to stay in place for long periods.

Before inserting the tube, as much middle ear fluid as possible should be removed. Markedly retracted tympanic membranes tend to have small amounts of this serous fluid. A No. 5 suction tip can be used, placed barely through the incision while trying to avoid enlarging the incision or causing localized bleeding (Fig. 10–2*C*). If the middle ear cavity is to be entered with a suction tip, the smaller No. 20 is preferable. Excessive suctioning can also cause mucosal bleeding. With thick mucoid effusions, a No. 5 suction tip may be insufficient. In some cases a baby alligator forceps, or a No. 7 suction tip placed immediately above (not through) the incision, can be useful (Fig. 10–2*D*). Occasionally a counterincision that allows air to enter the middle ear cavity while the fluid is suctioned is helpful. When fluid is not completely removed by one incision, a small incision in a different quadrant may be more effective in removing loculated fluid than "fishing" in the middle ear cavity with a suction tip. Some authors consider counterincisions undesirable, but in the authors' experience a small incision consistently heals well. It is important to make a clean incision and to approximate the edges carefully. A small piece of Gelfoam saturated with a drop or two of blood can be used to cover the incision. In thick, cloudy mucoid effusions, a No. 2 tube is placed; this tube is also used in infected effusions with facial palsy. Cultures also should be obtained in these cases. It is a good habit to visualize the middle ear mucosa through the incision.

The canal, the tympanic membrane, and even the middle ear cavity can be irrigated with saline, antibiotic-steroid solutions, or hydrogen peroxide as needed. When used in the middle ear cavity, antibiotic solutions should be neutral (not acid); otherwise there may be considerable postoperative pain (or intraoperative pain if local anesthesia is used). Ophthalmic drops are useful. Ototoxic antibiotics should be avoided.

Types of Tubes

There are many kinds of tubes of different shapes, sizes, and materials, ranging from "homemade" polyethylene to Silastic, Teflon, or metal; some examples are shown in Figure 10–2*E–G*. The type of tube is less important than the rationale for using it. In terms of size and shape, three types can be considered: short- , medium- , and long-term. Length of stay depends partially on the type of tube (except for permanent tubes, which are described elsewhere in this chapter). Additional important factors to be considered include the quadrant of insertion, conditions of the membrane, and individual tympanic membrane migration, among others. The authors have seen many so-called long-term tubes lead to eventual perforations requiring tympanoplasty. It has also been observed that shorter tubes with wide lumens tend to plug less and collect less epithelial debris than long-term tubes protruding from the tympanic membrane. In general, however, most well-designed tubes work well if they are properly used.

Cost of the tubes is also a factor. Variations in price sometimes seem illogical. The authors have designed and used 18-karat gold tubes handmade in Chile that are 200% cheaper than the least expensive plastic tube.

Placement of the Tube

With a baby alligator forceps, the tube is grasped gently from its outer border or from a special lip. The incision should be clean and free of blood. The inner flange is laid sideways on the incision (proximal end) (Fig. 10–3*A*). Sometimes it can be "popped" or "screwed" in with a gentle motion (Fig. 10–3*B*). Usually it can be laid over the proximal lip of the incision and then pushed in with a blunt pick, either by pressing it from its superior surface or by gently

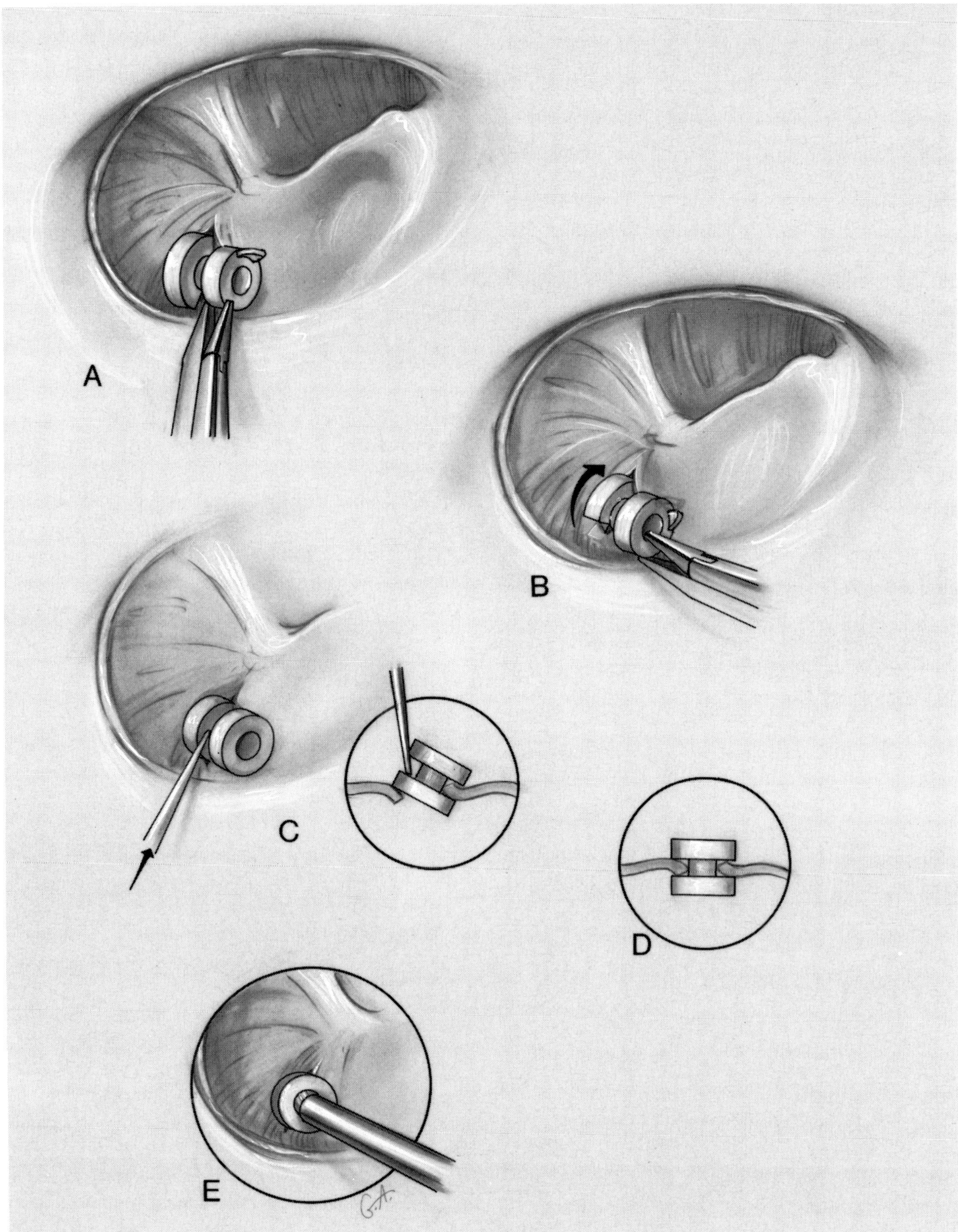

FIGURE 10–3.

twisting it around (Fig. 10–3*C, D*). Once the tube has been inserted, it is a good idea to rotate it to ensure that it is in position.

Once it has been verified that the tube is in place, it is a good idea to place a No. 20 (or smaller if needed) suction tip through the opening of the tube (Fig. 10–3*E*). Any middle ear fluid or blood should be suctioned and a few drops of hydrogen peroxide left in place. Postoperatively, the authors tend to recommend neutral pH drops for two or three days to ensure that patency is maintained. If there is any pain or discomfort with the drops, they are discontinued. If the fluid is cloudy or shows any signs of infection, do not hesitate to keep the patient on antibiotics (and culture the effusion). These apparently small details in technique can make a big difference in ventilation tube insertion.

Complications

Potential

As in most surgical procedures, the best treatment for complications is to prevent them. Excessive desire for speed is a potential surgical enemy, particularly harmful in tube insertion. Many unnecessary problems arise in training programs because this "simple procedure" is left to the most junior and inexperienced surgeons. It takes time to learn how to use an operating microscope properly and to see all that must be seen. Mutual coordination and understanding with the anesthesiologist are essential. The resident should ask for help if his or her orientation and timing are inadequate; the anesthesiologist should understand that the purpose of the procedure is to protect the patient's ears, not the anesthesiologist's hand.

Intraoperative

1. A small ear canal can make it difficult to visualize the whole tympanic membrane. Extreme care should be taken to avoid damaging the skin of the ear canal; bleeding will further obscure vision. A small ear speculum can be gently "screwed" in, and the speculum size gradually increased.

2. For lacerations, bleeding, or hematoma of the ear canal, carefully irrigate with hydrogen peroxide or apply small cotton balls saturated with epinephrine, or both.

3. Facial paralysis due to injection of local anesthetics is a temporary phenomenon of no consequence, but the surgeon must be aware of this annoying possibility.

4. For bleeding from the incision, use hydrogen peroxide or cotton balls saturated with epinephrine, or both.

5. If an incision is too long, approximate the borders carefully; if necessary, place small pieces of Gelfoam saturated with a few drops of blood and select a different site for the incision. Large tears and tears in myringosclerotic areas may require a tympanoplasty.

6. For a too-deep incision causing mucosal bleeding, aspirate fluid and irrigate the middle ear with hydrogen peroxide or a few drops of epinephrine solution, or both. Use postoperative antibiotic-steroid drops.

7. If a tube has fallen into the middle ear cavity, carefully recover it through the available incision or make a new incision if necessary. However, if it is lost in the cavity, it is better to leave it in or (rarely) perform an exploratory tympanotomy than to fish blindly for it.

8. If bleeding occurs because of damage to a jugular bulb occupying the hypotympanum (either in a high location or medial to the tympanic membrane), immediate packing should be done, initially with Gelfoam and then with tight gauze packing. The Gelfoam layer helps to avoid further bleeding when removing the gauze pack. Do not panic, just pack.

9. Damage to the ossicular chain and damage to the facial nerve are uncommonly seen complications that require exploration; they are dealt with in different chapters.

Postoperative

1. Short-term:
   A. Infected ear drainage (purulent otorrhea) immediately after surgery usually means that an infected middle ear effusion or silent otitis media was present. Antibiotics (orally and topically) should be used. The same treatment should suffice for late purulent otorrhea.
   B. Forcing the footplate into the vestibule in cases of previous myringostapediopexy (either spontaneous or postsurgical) has been described. The best treatment here, as for all other complications, is prevention; once it has occurred, exploration is indicated.
   C. Otalgia usually occurs with acid otic drops. Neutral drops or ophthalmologic drops usually suffice. The value of drops should be assessed on a case-by-case basis. On occasion, the dis-

comfort is caused by the drops dripping into the nasopharynx.

2. Long-term:
   A. Epithelial debris or cerumen blocking the tube can be removed with a small hook under the microscope. It is a good idea to use otic drops and sometimes hydrogen peroxide to soften this debris before removal. Occasionally it dissolves by itself and can be gently suctioned.
   B. Treatment of a permanent perforation of the tympanic membrane varies. If the patient is a child with eustachian tube dysfunction and the perforation is clean and small, it may serve the purpose of a tube and should be observed carefully. If the perforation is larger or if the exposure of the mucosa requires further action, a tympanoplasty should be done, and possibly a tube should be placed at another site in the tympanic membrane.
   C. Skin migrating into the middle ear cavity via the tube opening is a rare event that requires middle ear exploration, removal of tympanic membrane edges around the tube, and tympanoplasty. On occasion, a congenital cholesteatoma appears as an apparent complication of tubes. Adequate preoperative radiologic evaluation and thorough middle ear exploration are crucial in such cases.
   D. Extrusion of the tubes may be followed by recurrence of the original problems. In some cases tubes must be reinserted. In other cases, tubes are poorly tolerated or are extruded shortly after insertion; these might require so-called "transmeatal permanent aeration tubes." The indications are relative and should be assessed on a case-by-case basis. Some surgeons utilize "permanent" tubes through the tympanic membrane; these have a high incidence of persistent perforation requiring an eventual tympanoplasty. Transmeatal tubes are preferred, but the indication for their use also is relative. The authors do not use permanent tubes, preferring instead to reinsert a No. 2 tube in such cases. Because of their common use, however, insertion of permanent tubes is described below.

Transmeatal Permanent Aeration Tubes

Instrumentation is similar to that for stapedectomy.

Aim

To place a tube beneath the annulus in the posteroinferior quadrant.

Technique (Portmann)

With a curved canal knife, a horizontal incision is made parallel to the annulus, approximately 10 mm lateral to it in the posteroinferior quadrant (Fig. 10–4*A*). A small flap is elevated and the middle ear cavity is entered *beneath* the annulus (Fig. 10–4*B*). A small bur is used to drill a canal in the posterior bony wall. The tube is placed with the inner flange medial to the annulus (in the middle ear) (Fig. 10–4*C*). The flap is repositioned and held in place with Gelfoam and antibiotic-saturated gauze (Fig. 10–4*D*). After one week the gauze is removed.

Complications

1. Those of pressure-equalizing (PE) tubes.

2. Edema of the skin that obscures the tube. Treatment with topical antibiotics and steroids usually solves the problem, allowing the tube to become visible again.

3. Blockage with debris or cerumen, or both. This complication is more common with permanent tubes than with regular tubes. Measures for removal of the blockage are similar to those for regular tubes; however, removal with hooks, requiring a local or general anesthetic, is more common. (This is equivalent to reinserting a No. 2 tube.)

In addition, a number of patients over time develop complications or sequelae involving the tympanic membrane or middle ear, or both. These include an atrophic or atelectatic tympanic membrane, myringosclerosis, chronic otitis media, cholesterol granuloma, disruption or fixation of the ossicular chain or tensor tympani tendon, and so on. Such complications highlight the need for periodic checkups and close observation in the treatment of otitis media. In unresponsive cases or in those in which underlying middle ear pathology is suspected, there should be no hesitation in proceeding with exploratory tympanotomy; the surgeon should not sit and wait for a localized disaster to occur. Exploratory tympanotomy, tympanoplasty, and ossiculoplasty are described in different chapters in this book. Persistent dysfunction of the eustachian tube may lead to tympanic membrane retraction, thinning, and

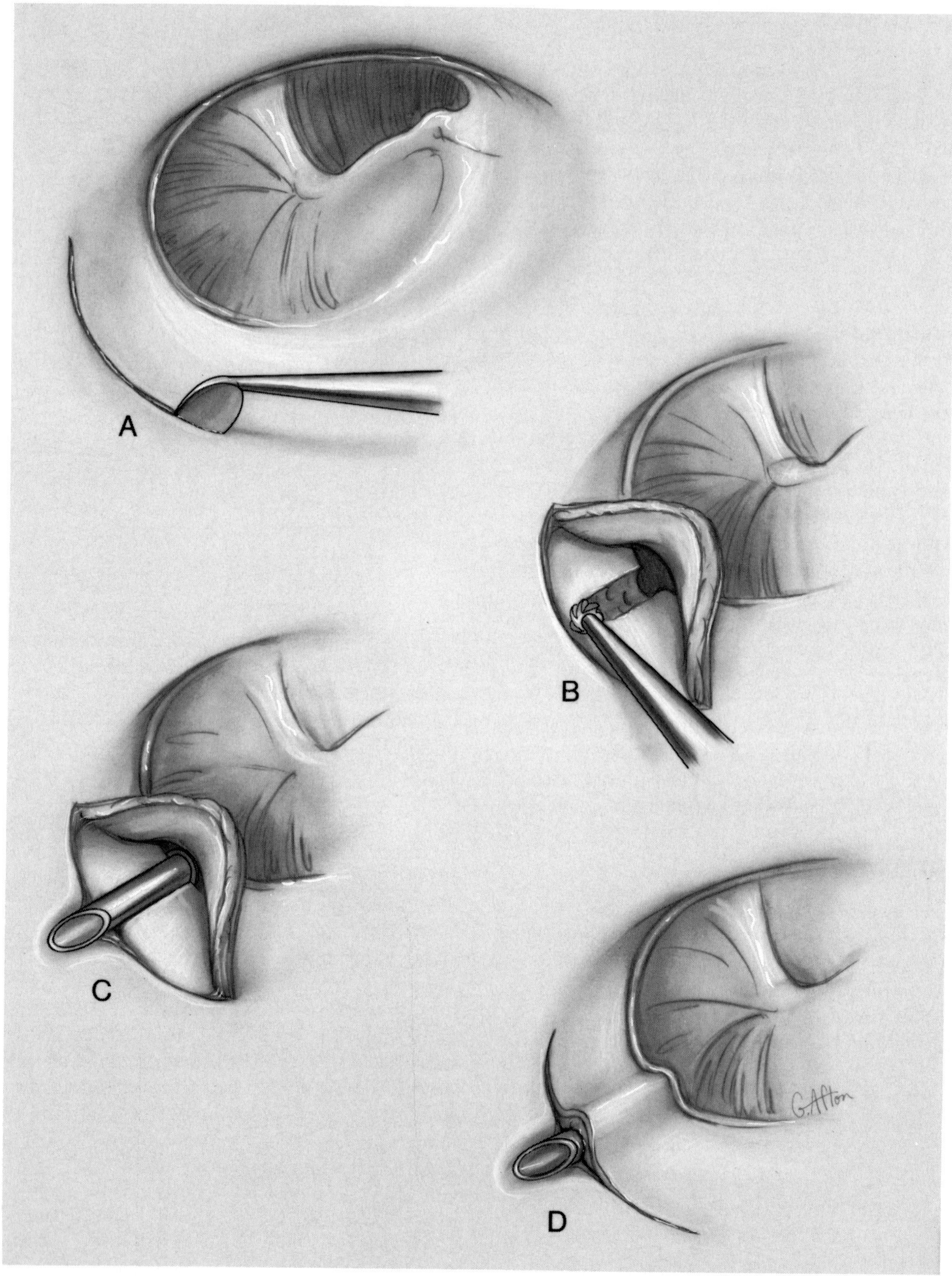

FIGURE 10–4.

formation of adhesions of the membrane to the promontory. A tympanoplasty for an atrophic or atelectatic tympanic membrane (described below) may be required. On occasion, persistent effusions and underlying histopathologic changes may lead to hypocellularity of the mastoid and lack of aeration of the middle ear cavity. Once these are clinically and radiologically documented, surgical procedures to increase aeration—either a mastoidotomy or a cortical ("intact wall") mastoidectomy (described below)—are recommended. Surgery for major complications of otitis media is described elsewhere in this chapter.

Surgery for an atrophic or atelectatic tympanic membrane can be performed using a transcanal, endaural, or postauricular approach. Different methods can be used; two of the most common, cartilage tympanoplasty and tympanoplasty for atelectatic tympanic membrane, will be described. The basic objectives are (1) to reinforce an exceedingly weak tympanic membrane, which is usually collapsed and not uncommonly attached to the medial wall of the middle ear; (2) to inspect the middle ear cavity, repair ossicles, and lyse adhesions (re-establishing function); and (3) to re-establish the middle ear space and prevent further disease.

These measures, in turn, can be combined with aeration procedures such as a cortical mastoidectomy or mastoidotomy. The procedure and approach to follow depend on the judgment, expertise, and preference of the surgeon.

A cartilage tympanoplasty will be described as a transcanal procedure and a tympanoplasty for atelectatic tympanic membrane (adhesive otitis) as an endaural approach, with the understanding that they can be done either way or even by a postauricular approach. Similarly, a cortical mastoidectomy or a mastoidotomy can be done by an endaural or postauricular approach. It is important for the surgeon to realize that different approaches can be used interchangeably or combined as necessary; there are so many forms of presentation in otitis media that a "single surgical approach" can be, at times, a very limiting concept. The two methods described only suggest alternatives. The surgeon should decide what is best for the patient and modify these approaches according to need.

Cartilage Tympanoplasty for Atrophic Tympanic Membrane

Surgical Steps

1. Transcanal incisions.
2. Tympanomeatal flap.
3. Widening of the bony canal.
4. Harvesting tragus (cartilage-perichondrium graft).
5. Elevation of the tympanic membrane.
6. Inspection of the middle ear cavity.
7. Inspection of the antrum and atticotomy-mastoidotomy, if necessary.
8. Placement of Silastic, Gelfilm, graft, and PE tube (optional).
9. Packing and closure.

Highlights

1. Create a large tympanomeatal flap.
2. Carefully harvest and prepare a cartilage-perichondrium graft.
3. Perform a canalplasty.
4. Carefully elevate the thin tympanic membrane.
5. Adequately position the cartilage-perichondrium graft.

Procedure

A large tympanomeatal flap is elevated with vertical incisions at 6 and 1 or 2 o'clock (Fig. 10–5*A*). A large flap is useful since an underlay cartilage-perichondrium graft extending into the posterior canal is to be used. The posterior canal may need to be widened. If necessary, the approach can be turned into a postauricular or endaural approach. If the posterior canal is not wide enough, the canal wall can be widened carefully with a bur (after elevating the flap). If an anterior bony overhang is present, a window shade is developed and the overhang removed (see Chapter 8). A wide and open canal favors visualization, postoperative healing, and even hearing (to a small degree).

A cartilage-perichondrium graft is harvested. This can come from different sources, the most common being the tragus. An incision is made in the dorsal (posterior meatal) side of the tragus, and by gentle, sharp dissection the tragus is isolated and a piece harvested (Fig. 10–5*B*). The tragus has perichondrium on both sides. An incision is made with a scalpel in one of the borders and the perichondrium on one side is elevated (under the microscope) with a duckbill, leaving the perichondrium as a single continuous strip with one side attached to the cartilage (Fig. 10–5C). The cartilage can be left as is or carefully thinned with a scalpel. It can also be compressed *briefly* and *gently*; if compressed firmly or for

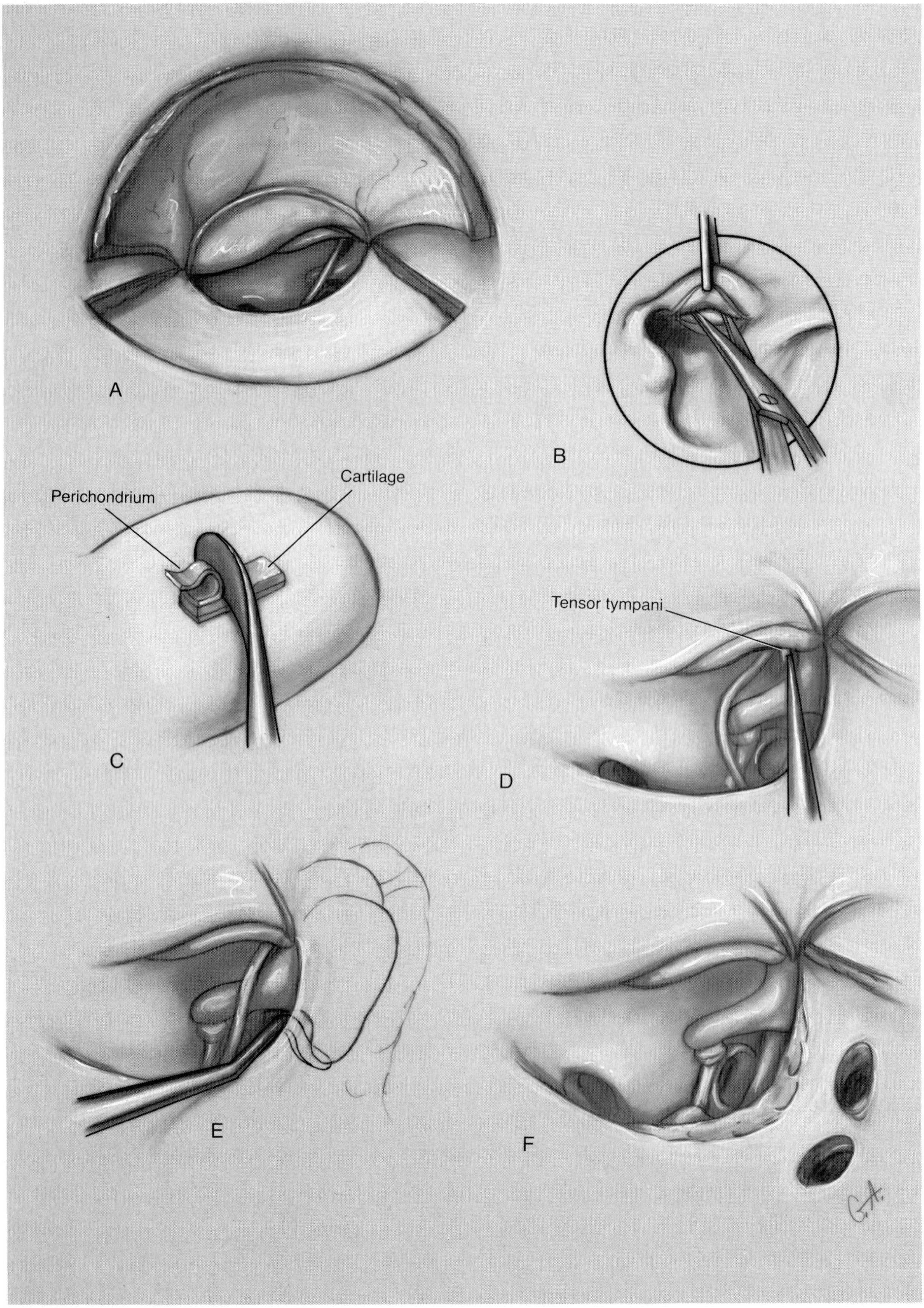

FIGURE 10–5.

too long, the cartilage will separate from the perichondrium. The graft is preserved in saline. The tragal incision is closed with appropriate sutures after meticulous hemostasis with cautery (or ligation); otherwise, a localized hematoma may develop postoperatively.

The tympanic membrane is very carefully elevated while trying to maintain its integrity. If the membrane has sclerotic plaques, they can be gently and meticulously removed with a joint knife or its equivalent. It is not imperative to remove all plaques; excessive removal can cause tears in the membrane. (To make matters worse, the membrane is poorly vascularized, so the surgeon must be careful here.)

Any adhesions are carefully sectioned. A No. 20 or 24 suction tip with the finger "off the hole" is used. The ossicular chain is inspected and, if necessary, reconstructed (see Chapter 12).

If the tympanic membrane is retracted or the tensor tympani is fixed, or both, the tendon is sectioned (Fig. 10–5*D*). The main aim of this procedure is to mobilize the malleus and widen the mesotympanic space. (This does not produce increased aeration.)

At this point, the attic and antrum are inspected (Fig. 10–5*E*). Palpation with a Whirlybird can give a good idea of the adequacy of communication between the middle ear and the mastoid antrum. If there is any question, further inspection is made. It is not uncommon to find a so-called "aditus block" that obstructs communication and significantly impairs aeration despite the presence of an adequately sized mastoid cell system. An atticotomy is done, the extent of which depends on the degree of visualization needed. The attic is gently curetted down with stapes curets in a superior to inferior direction (away from the ossicles), which helps to avoid ossicular disruption. The attic is then inspected, adhesions are sectioned and removed, and the ossicles are freed of excessive adhesions and connective tissue. If there is any question of insufficient passage, the mastoid should be inspected. Some authors create "observation windows" by drilling openings in the posterior superior bony canal (over the antrum) (Fig. 10–5*F*). Others advocate the use of mirrors. While these methods are acceptable and work well, the authors prefer a complete inspection that at the same time provides a solution. This is achieved by a mastoidotomy (see Chapter 7), which provides direct visualization, ease of cleansing, and removal of any blocks; increases aeration; and permits irrigation of the mastoid and middle ear (Fig. 10–6*A*). An antibiotic-steroid solution should flow freely between these two cavities. On occasion, a small strip of thin Silastic can be placed between the antrum and middle ear to ensure patency. If a wider communication is needed, a mastoidectomy and a facial recess opening could be helpful, but usually this is not the case in the types of problems discussed here. If the mastoid is found to be involved with disease, a mastoidectomy is done.

Once the ossicles are reconstructed, communication of the middle ear and mastoid is ensured, and aeration is felt to be adequate, a thin Silastic sheeting is placed that extends from the eustachian tube to the tympanic sinus and round window niche (Fig. 10–6*B*). The cartilage-perichondrium graft is laid over a piece of Gelfilm, which is placed over the long process of the incus under the tympanic membrane (Fig. 10–6*C*). The perichondrium that is not attached to cartilage is placed over the posterior canal wall (Fig. 10–6*D*). This type of graft also is very useful in covering atticotomy defects, and in areas where retraction pockets tend to occur or recur. It is an easy and very effective resource for ear surgery.

A slightly thicker anterior tympanic membrane remnant usually is present, through which a No. 1 ventilation tube can be inserted (Fig. 10–6*E*). The authors prefer to do this since it helps to ensure postoperative aeration and healing of the middle ear. The flap is then repositioned covering the graft, and the ear canal is packed. If endaural or postauricular incisions were used, they are closed in layers and a dressing is applied.

Tympanoplasty for Atelectatic Tympanic Membrane (Adhesive Otitis)

Surgical Steps

1. Endaural incisions (Lempert I and II).
2. Harvesting of temporal fascia.
3. Tympanomeatal flap.
4. Widening of the bony canal.
5. Elevation of the tympanic membrane.
6. Repair of ossicles.
7. Inspection of the antrum.
8. Placement of Silastic, Gelfilm, underlay fascia, and pharyngoesophageal tube.
9. Packing and closure.

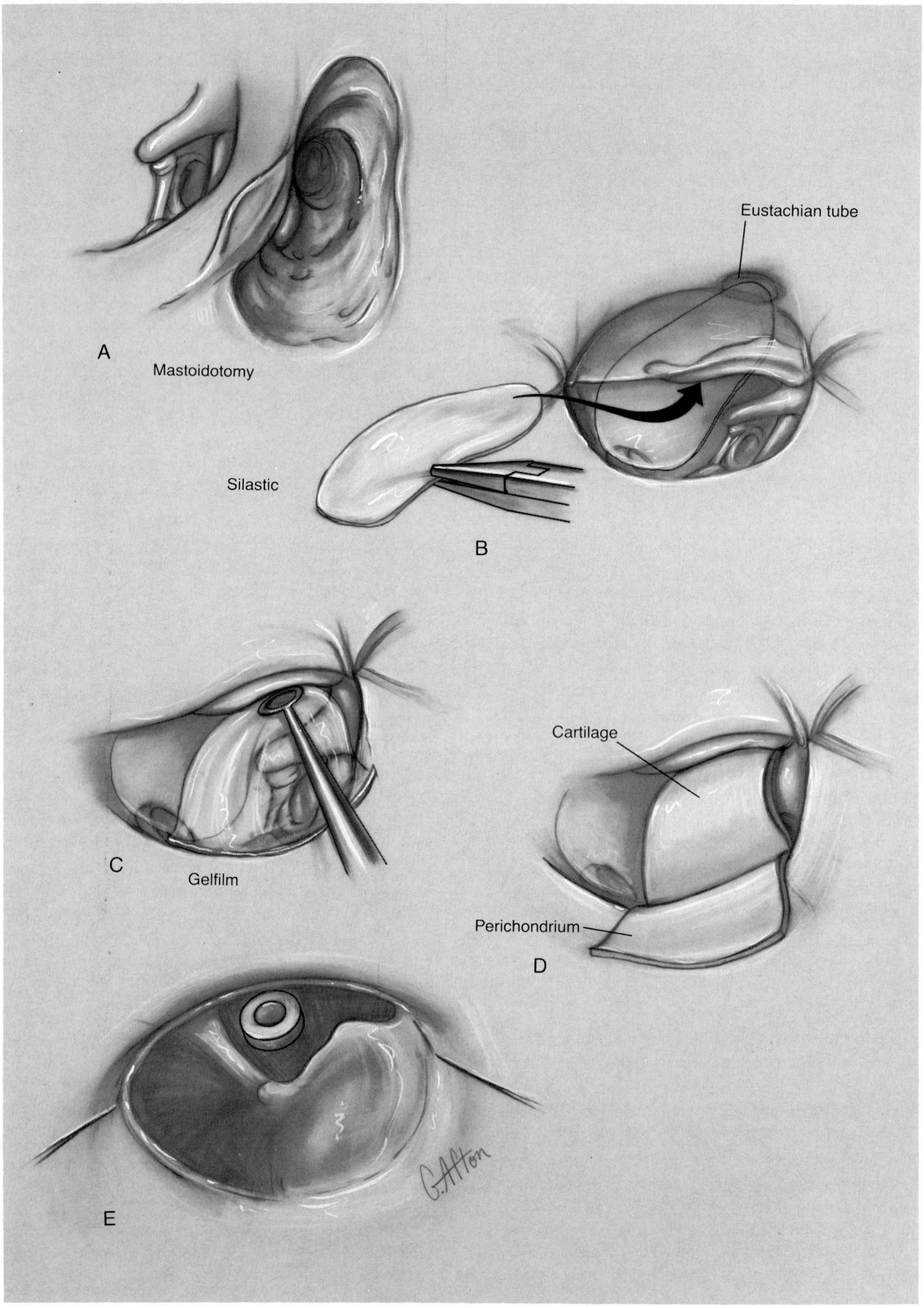
Eustachian tube
A
Mastoidotomy
Silastic
B
Cartilage
C
Gelfilm
Perichondrium
D
E
G. Afton

FIGURE 10–6.

Highlights

1. Create a large tympanomeatal flap.
2. Perform a canalplasty.
3. Carefully elevate the thin tympanic membrane.
4. Section the tensor tympani tendon.

Procedure

Endaural incisions (Lempert I and II) are made. Using two-prong self-retaining retractors, temporal fascia is harvested via the Lempert II incision, placed in Ringer's solution, and pressed for two to three minutes before being used (Fig. 10–7*A*). A tympanomeatal flap is elevated with vertical incisions at 6 and 1 o'clock; a large flap is best since a large underlay fascia will be placed extending into the posterior canal. The posterior canal wall is widened carefully with a bur (Fig. 10–7*B*). If an anterior bony overhang is present, a window shade is developed and the overhang is removed (see Chapter 8). The canal should be wide and open. This is true for all middle ear reconstructive procedures except for some cases of stapedectomy.

The thin tympanic membrane is very carefully elevated; an attempt should be made to maintain its integrity. Meticulous sectioning of adhesions is the key to this elevation. A No. 24 suction tip with the finger "off the hole" is used. The field should be as dry as possible; any bleeding is treated with cotton saturated in epinephrine solution.

The ossicular chain is inspected. Necrosis of the lenticular process often is found; if so, the area is reconstructed. If tympanosclerosis is fixating the ossicles, this also is corrected (see Chapter 12).

Fixation of the tensor tympani tendon, including the cochleariform process, is a common finding and requires a tympanoplasty. The tendon is severed, which mobilizes the malleus and widens the mesotympanic space (Fig. 10–7*C*). If the malleus adheres to the promontory, the adhesions are freed. If necessary, the distal tip of the long process of the malleus is severed after being carefully separated from the overlying tympanic membrane (Fig. 10–7*D*). At this point the attic and antrum should be inspected (as discussed in the previous procedure for an atrophic tympanic membrane).

Once the ossicles have been reconstructed and the tympanic membrane has been elevated, a piece of thin Silastic sheeting is placed extending from the eustachian tube to the tympanic sinus and round window niche (Fig. 10–7*E*). Gelfilm that was kept in Ringer's solution for softening is placed above the ossicles between the eustachian tube and the facial recess (Fig. 10–8*A*), and the fascia is placed beneath the thin tympanic membrane (Fig. 10–8*C*). Usually a slightly thicker anterior tympanic membrane remnant is present through which a No. 1 ventilation tube can be inserted (Fig. 10–8*D*). (Some surgeons thread a small piece of synthetic nonabsorbable suture through the tube and into the canal in order to avoid plugging of the tube with packing and debris. The authors have not observed plugging to be a problem in these cases.) The ventilation tube helps ensure postoperative aeration and healing of the middle ear. The ear canal is packed, the Lempert II incision is closed in two layers, and a mastoid dressing is applied.

Figure 10–9 depicts three alternative methods for improving aeration of the middle ear.

Mastoid and Tympanomastoid Procedures in Otitis Media

If intractable disease develops in the mastoid and middle ear cavity, more extensive surgical procedures are necessary. These may range from a cortical mastoidectomy to a tympanomastoidectomy and even a radical mastoidectomy. The comments below are intended to contribute to the overall concepts of specific procedures; a complete discussion of specific indications for these surgical alternatives is beyond the scope of this atlas.

The basic aims of mastoid surgery for chronic, medically intractable otitis media cannot be emphasized enough. The first is the eradication of disease; the second is functional reconstruction.

Both endaural and postauricular incisions and their corresponding approaches have already been described. It should be mentioned that if a mastoid obliteration procedure is planned, a postauricular incision is made far behind (posterior to) the sulcus preparatory to the use of a muscle flap (described below). Although the authors tend to prefer postauricular approaches for tympanomastoid surgery, the endaural approach provides easy access to the middle ear and mastoid, and is very useful in revision surgery as well. It can be limited in exposure posteriorly in cases of large, well-pneumatized mastoid cavities.

It is useful to describe the alternative approaches in mastoid surgery. The simple mastoidectomy (which derives its name from its original use for simple drainage and *not* from the simplicity of the procedure) was described in Chapter 7; it involves

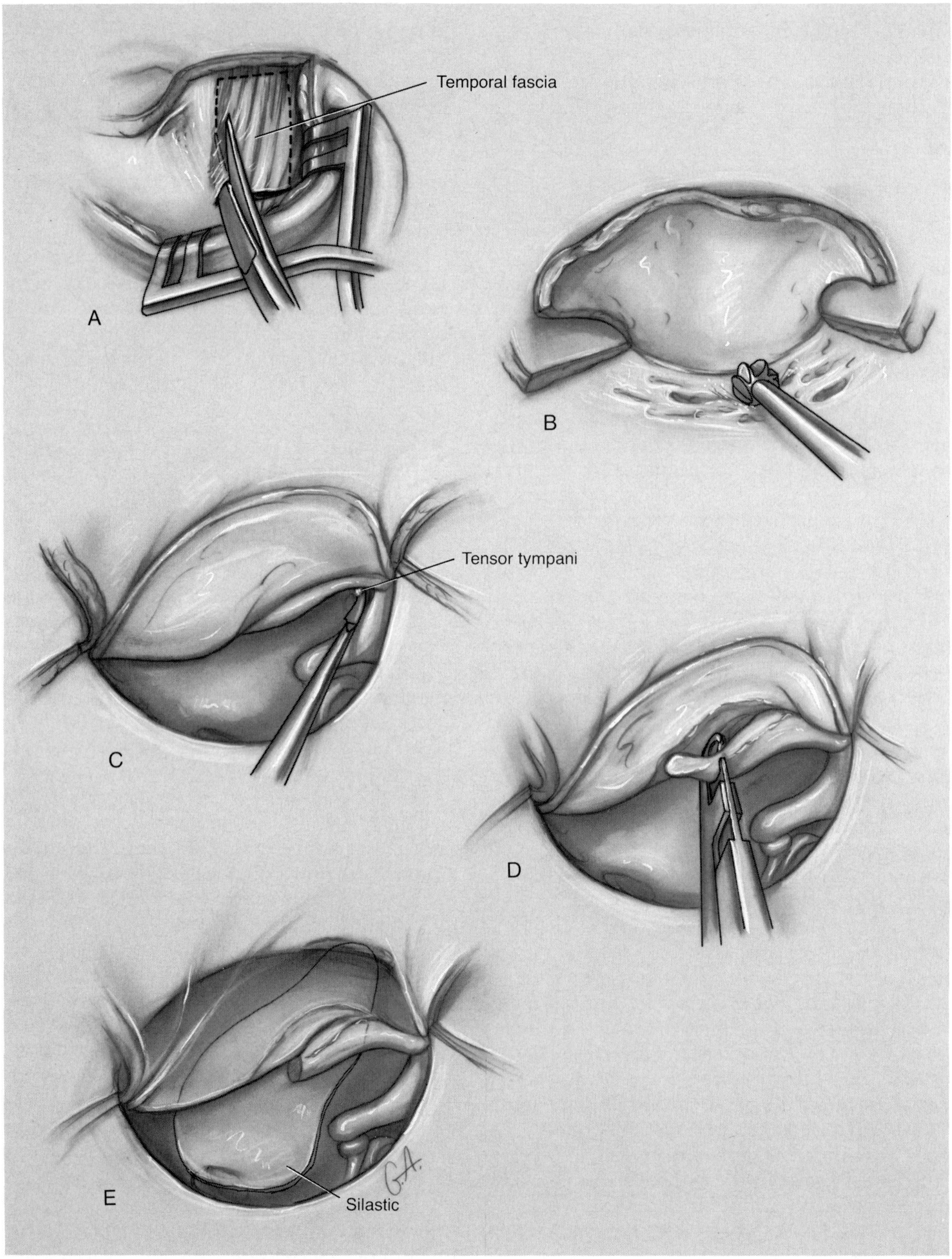

FIGURE 10–7.

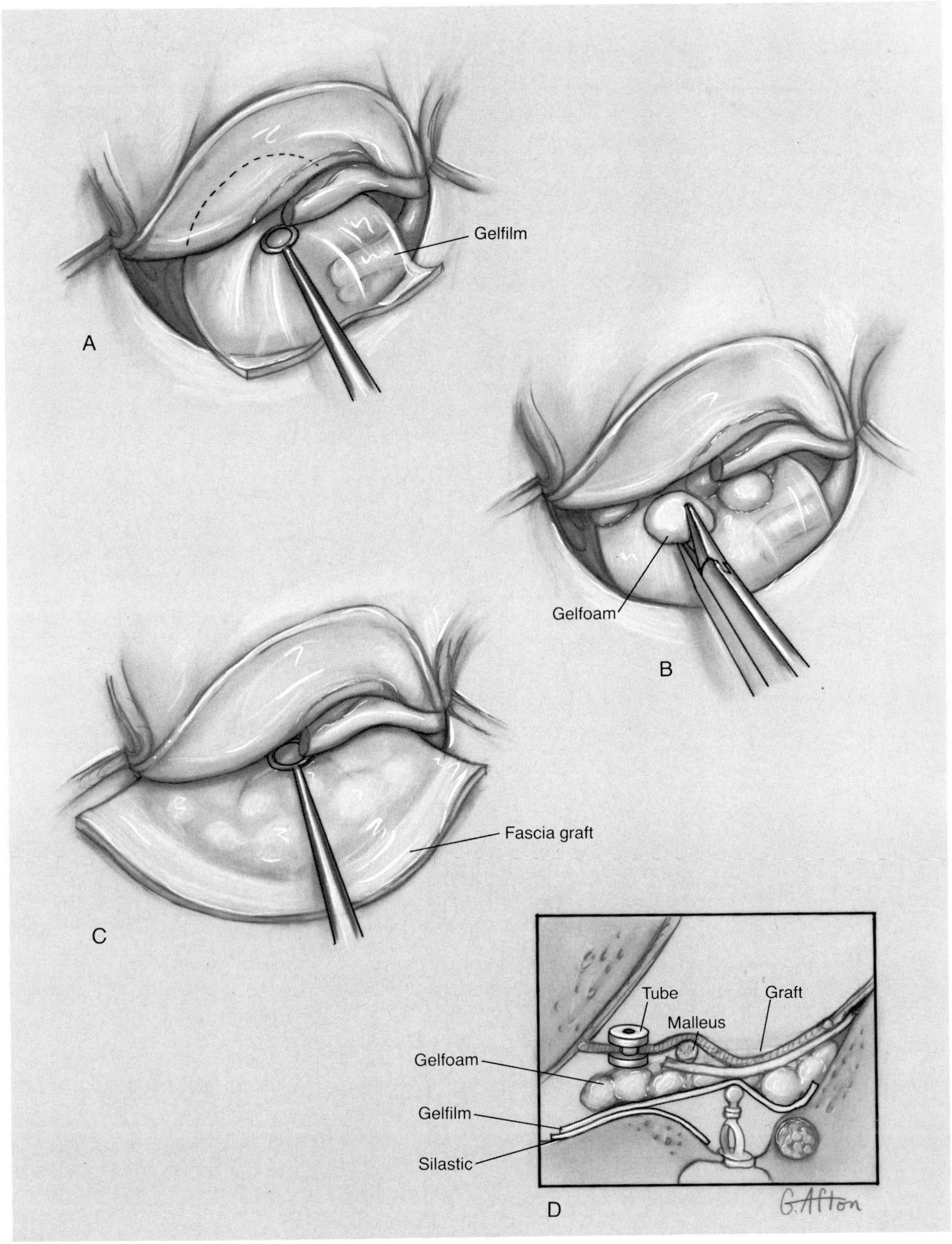
Gelfilm
A
Gelfoam
B
Fascia graft
C
Tube
Graft
Malleus
Gelfoam
Gelfilm
Silastic
D
G. Afton

FIGURE 10–8.

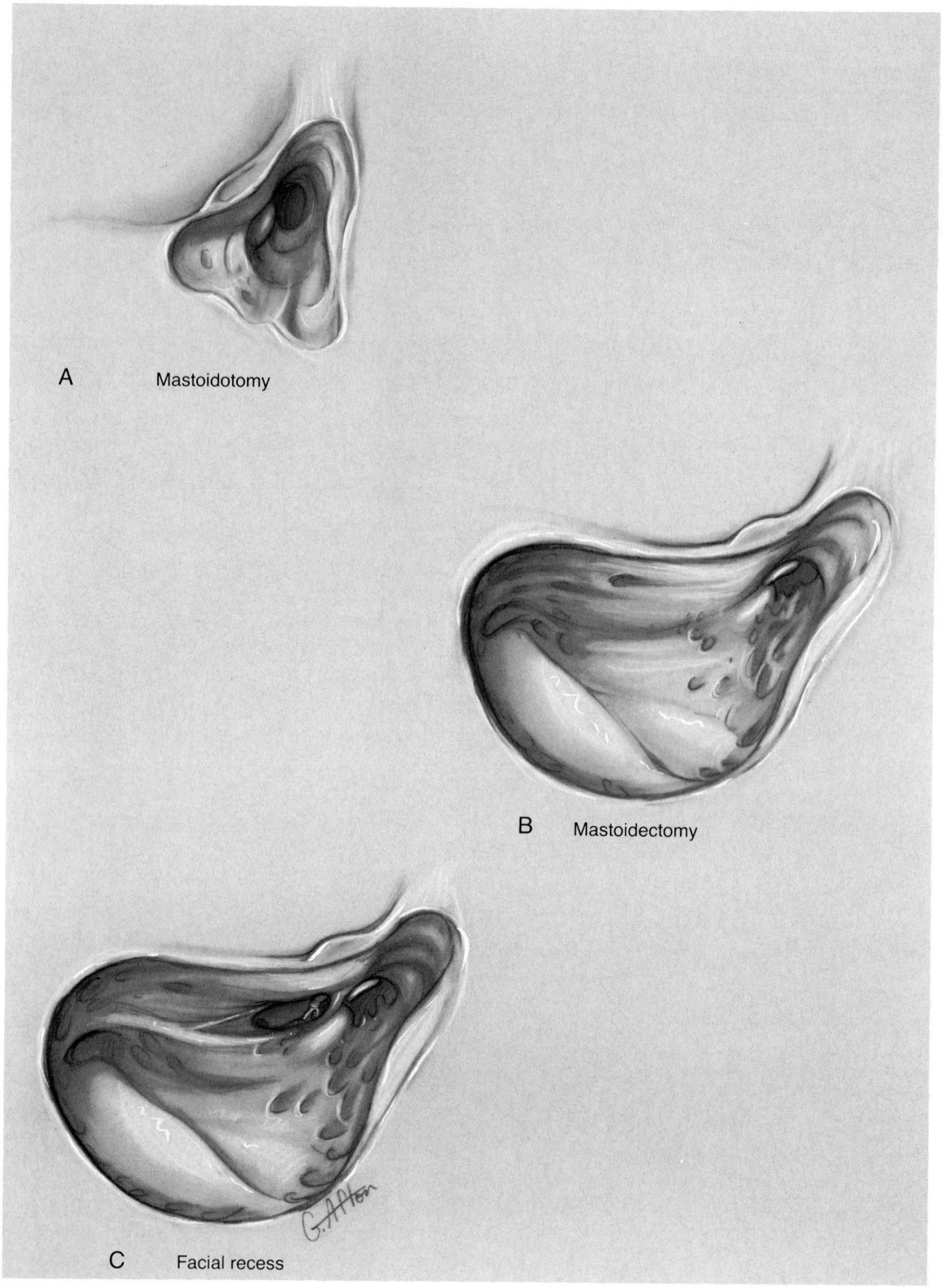

FIGURE 10–9.

opening the mastoid and exenterating all air cells. This approach can be used for purposes of aeration or removal of disease, such as in acute coalescent mastoiditis. It does not involve entering the middle ear, except when combined with a facial recess approach (posterior tympanotomy). The facial recess approach allows exploration of the middle ear and removal of diseased tissue; however, it must be kept in mind that in cases of chronic ear disease this access often is limited and removal of diseased mucosa may be incomplete. Nevertheless, this can be a very useful approach, depending on what the surgeon wants to achieve in a specific case.

Since chronic otitis involves both the middle ear and mastoid, it is often necessary to directly approach both cavities; hence the term tympanomastoidectomy. If the posterior canal wall is left intact and both cavities are entered independently, the procedure is termed "canal wall up," "intact canal wall mastoidectomy," or "closed-cavity tympanomastoidectomy." Intact canal wall procedures are preferable since they prevent an open mastoid cavity. They should be performed if there is a good possibility of eradication of disease (the first aim of mastoidectomy) and if the mastoid is sufficiently pneumatized to allow a safe procedure. A sclerotic mastoid presents a serious risk of complications. In these cases, a tympanomastoid procedure is not recommended unless the otologist is extremely familiar with the approach, its risks, and its limitations. Use of a "canal wall up" or "canal wall down" approach will depend upon each individual case. The primary aim of the procedure is to eradicate disease, not to maintain an intact posterior canal wall. In other words, what should be done is what the patient needs and not what the surgeon would like to do. For practical purposes, this procedure will be described as an endaural approach.

Procedures that involve removal of the posterior canal wall are known as "canal wall down" or "open-cavity" mastoidectomies. They include the Bondy procedure, the intact-bridge tympanomastoidectomy, the modified radical mastoidectomy, and the radical mastoidectomy. The procedure originally described by Bondy is indicated only for an unusual case of primary cholesteatoma, and involves "exteriorizing" the cholesteatoma while preserving the inner matrix or capsule. The posterior bony canal wall is removed, but the middle ear cavity is not entered. The modified radical mastoidectomy involves entrance into the middle ear cavity, allowing tympanoplasty procedures. The intact-bridge tympanomastoidectomy is a contemporary version of the modified radical procedure in which a bridge of bone is left when the posterior canal wall is removed; this allows more effective tympanoplasty (reconstruction) procedures. Finally, the radical mastoidectomy is the same as a modified radical mastoidectomy, with the addition of removal of middle ear mucosa and ossicles (excepting the stapes), and closure (plugging) of the eustachian tube. The mastoid and middle ear become an open (exteriorized) cavity with, obviously, a loss of hearing.

Cortical Mastoidectomy

A cortical mastoidectomy with or without a facial recess approach (posterior tympanotomy) has been described in detail and will not be repeated here. Suffice it to mention that drilling should be done carefully in the presence of diseased tissue, since complications are easily caused. The use of curets to unroof mastoid cells that are full of granulation tissue is a good and safe habit, especially when there are doubts as to the underlying structures. If in doubt, palpate the air cell with a Whirlybird and then curet. Special considerations in mastoid procedures are described elsewhere in this chapter. For an overall view of these cases, it is recommended that the entire chapter be read, not just individual approaches.

Closed-cavity Tympanomastoidectomy

Incisions are made with a scalpel, and exposure is improved by using a curved nasal speculum. The first incision (Lempert I) is made semicircumferentially between 6 and 12 o'clock on the posterior wall at the bony cartilaginous junction. The second incision (Lempert II) runs between the tragus and helix and incisura; the extent of this incision depends upon the degree of exposure of the mastoid needed, but a length of 0.75 cm is not uncommon. Temporal fascia is harvested through this incision for grafting purposes. The remaining posterior canal skin (cartilaginous portion) is preserved and gently elevated with a small periosteal elevator, leaving the whole posterior bony canal clearly exposed. (On occasion, a small free skin graft can be removed safely from this area.) The spine of Henle is identified and the periosteum elevated off the mastoid, exposing its lateral surface (cortex) in its entirety from the temporal line (linea temporalis) superiorly to the mastoid tip inferiorly.

Three-prong self-retaining retractors are used. It is helpful to position them at right angles to one

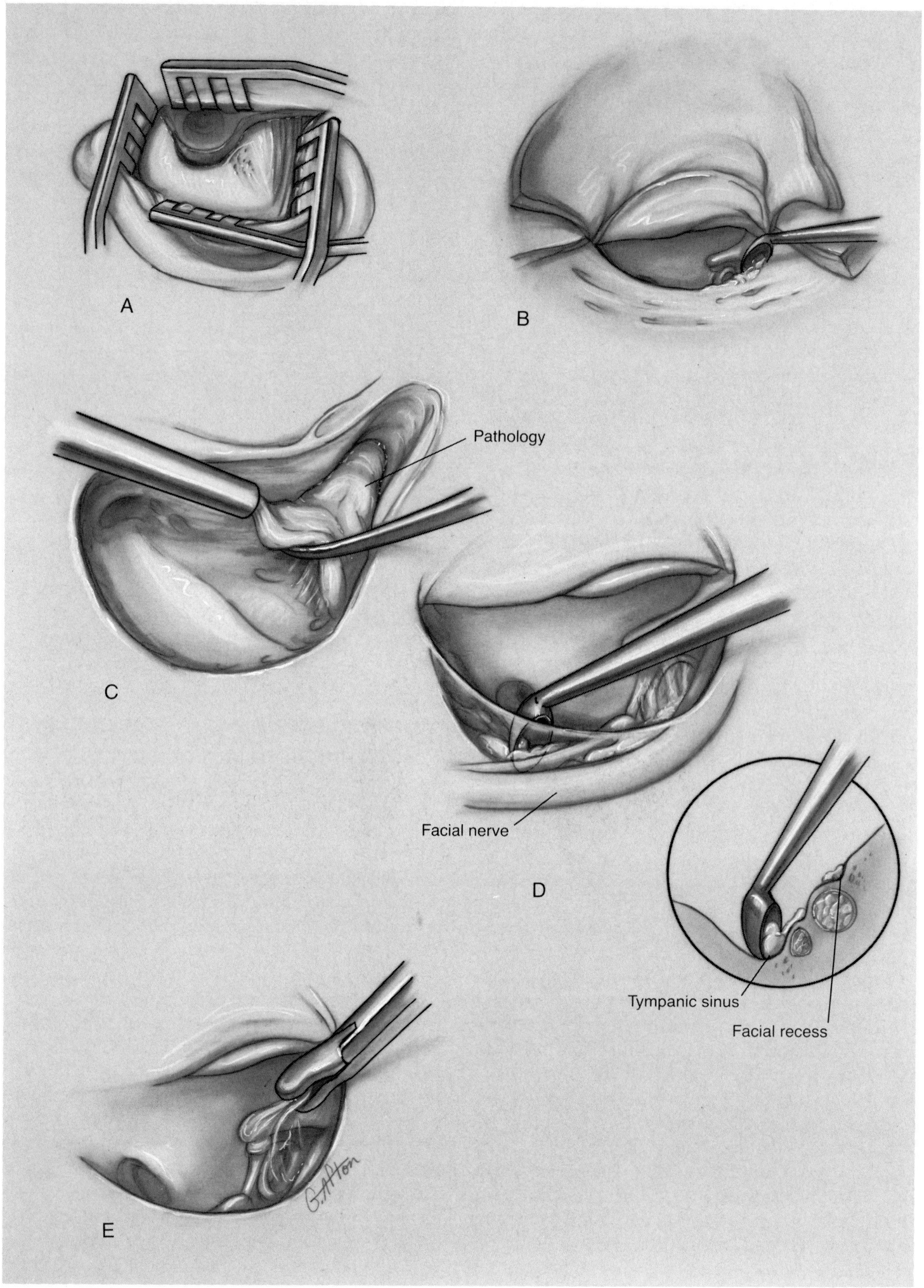
A
B
Pathology
C
Facial nerve
D
Tympanic sinus
Facial recess
E

FIGURE 10–10.

another, with one pointing cephalad (superiorly) and one caudad (posteriorly) (Fig. 10–10*A*). Schuknecht retractors allow wider exposure than Wullstein retractors in these cases. At this point, the mastoid and ear canal are well exposed.

If needed for exposure, a canalplasty (previously described) is done, and the entire fibrous and bony annulus is exposed without entering the temporomandibular joint space.

With the scalpel, incisions can be made at 6 and 1 or 2 o'clock. These incisions allow for easier development of the flap; however, the flap can be elevated without these incisions. After the middle ear cavity is entered (beneath the annulus), the aditus is enlarged so that the incus is readily seen, allowing inspection of the epitympanum through the aditus ad antrum (Fig. 10–10*B*). The technique of a mastoidectomy has been described. Cortical white bone should be obtained in all directions, but saucerization of the outer cortex is not so important as in a complete mastoidectomy since there is no residual open cavity. The same principles described for mastoidectomy as an approach apply here. However, some important points relative to chronic otitis should be mentioned.

1. In cases in which the mastoid is full of inflammatory tissue, the surgeon can easily lose momentarily the sense of depth and location of the antrum. Since the middle ear is clearly exposed, a Whirlybird can be introduced into the antrum via the middle ear side and visualized or palpated to help regain surgical orientation.

2. Inflamed tissue must be removed carefully, in a step-by-step fashion (Fig. 10–10*C*). Do not "pull" large pieces of tissue or drill into "holes."

3. Special attention should be given to identifying the location of the facial nerve at all levels. Its bony canal may be eroded (exposing the nerve) or the nerve may be out of its usual anatomic position, or both.

4. Cleansing of all diseased tissue in the area of the facial recess (suprapyramidal recess) and the tympanic sinus (infrapyramidal recess) should be thorough (Fig. 10–10*D*). The surgeon must be especially careful in cleansing this area; this is a common site for iatrogenic injury to the facial nerve. With this surgical approach, removal of diseased mucosa in this area sometimes is difficult.

5. Ossicles should be carefully cleansed of diseased mucosa (Fig. 10–10*E*). It is crucial to avoid both dislocation of the ossicular chain (or its remnants) and removal or dislocation of the stapes, which would have obviously catastrophic consequences for hearing. If the stapes is accidentally removed, the oval window is sealed with collagen tissue and covered with Gelfoam saturated in antibiotic solution.

6. In surgery for chronic ear disease, the surgeon should give special attention and care to three areas or structures: the facial nerve, the horizontal semicircular canal, and the stapes (Fig. 10–11). These areas require early and clear identification during the procedure and very careful management when involved with disease.

7. It is unwise to remove too much of the attic wall for purposes of exposure; this may result in a potential retraction pocket area. If this occurs, a cartilage-perichondrium graft (described earlier in this chapter) can be placed to cover the defect.

8. Cholesteatomas and granulation tissue have the capacity to erode bone and result in fistula formation. There is no agreement as to the management of these fistulae. In general, when a cholesteatoma erodes the promontory the matrix (capsule) should be left in place, owing to the high frequency of total hearing loss associated with its removal. If a fistula of the (small) horizontal semicircular canal exists with no apparent involvement of the underlying membranous labyrinth, the matrix can be removed. Very many fistulae are identified in surgery for which there were no preoperative symptoms or diagnostic suspicions based on laboratory studies.

9. Once again, the primary aim of these procedures is to eradicate disease. Reconstruction is the second aim and will be described in Chapter 12. Maintaining the posterior canal wall intact is not an aim; it is a preference if conditions allow it to be done safely and properly.

Closure and the technique of meatoplasty have already been described.

Intact-bridge Tympanomastoidectomy (IBM)

This procedure is described here as a postauricular approach. Its aims will be listed and the basic steps only touched upon since they have been described earlier (see Chapter 5). The same principles as for a closed-cavity tympanomastoidectomy for chronic otitis media apply here. As discussed previously, different skin flaps can be used—a Körner's flap or a flap made by an incision in the posterior canal wall skin at the bony cartilaginous junction. This incision can be made when the postauricular flap is lifted, or through the canal before lifting the flap.

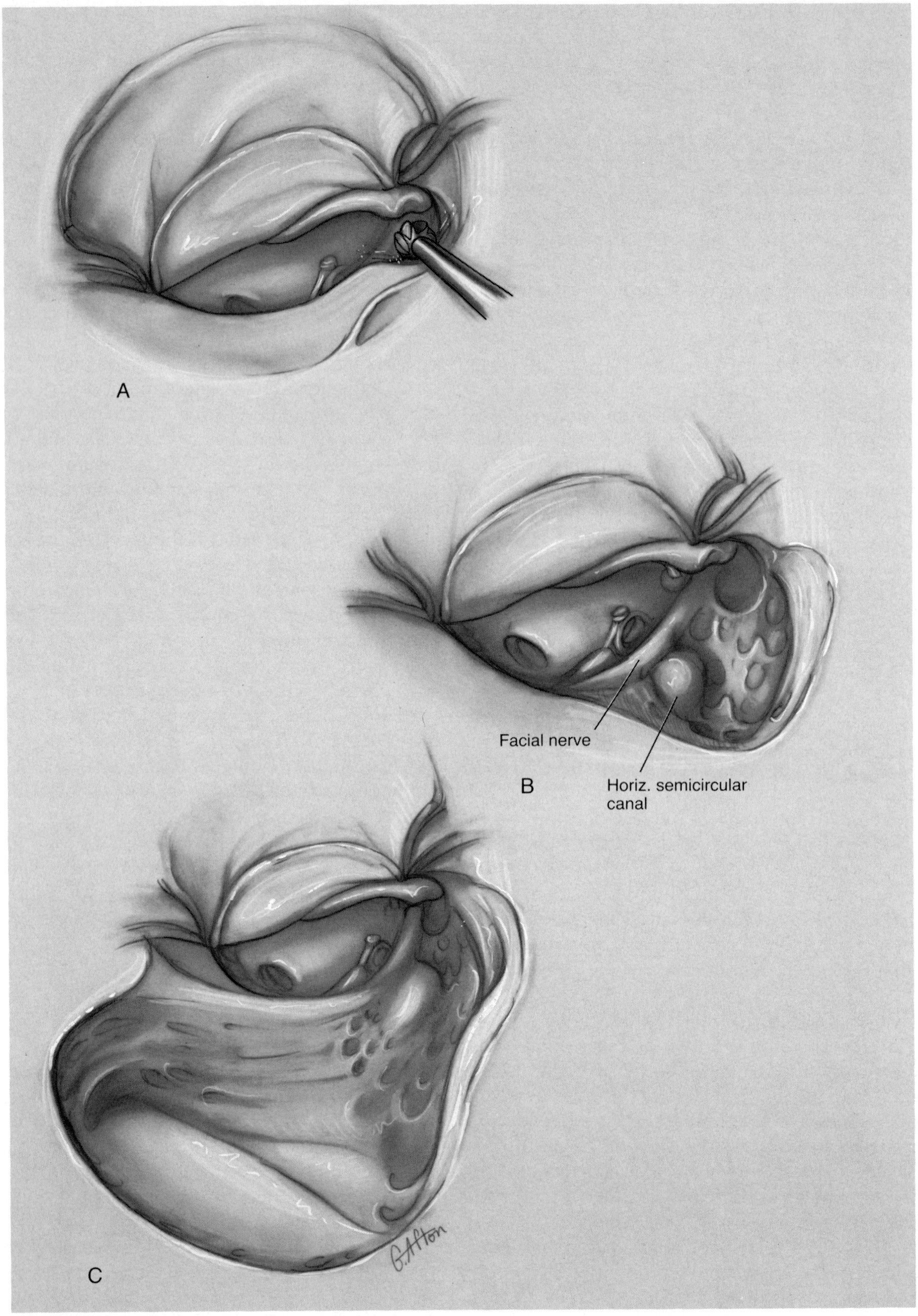

FIGURE 10–11.

Aim

To exteriorize the disease process within the epitympanum, antrum, and mastoid to the meatus. The IBM is a contemporary version of the modified radical mastoidectomy with bridge preservation, allowing a better tympanoplasty repair.

Highlights

1. Enlarge the anterior canal wall without opening the temporomandibular joint, and visualize the entire fibrous and bony annulus.
2. Perform a large meatoplasty; this is crucial for the success of the procedure.

Pitfalls

1. Incompletely removing the posterior meatal wall.
2. Performing a poor meatoplasty.

Surgical Steps

1. Meatoplasty.
2. Canalplasty.
3. Circumferential saucerization of the mastoid.
4. Enlargement of the aditus and sculpturing of the bridge to widen the mesotympanum.
5. Removal of all disease.
6. Preservation, when possible, of the anterior tympanic membrane and manubrium.
7. Use of a ventilation tube.
8. Ossiculoplasty, tympanoplasty.
9. Obliteration of the aditus with periosteum or cartilage.
10. Mastoid obliteration (usually not necessary).
11. Thiersch graft (three to four weeks postoperatively).

Procedure

This procedure involves removal of the posterior meatal wall with preservation of the "bridge."

Exposure of the mastoid cortex with a postauricular approach has already been described. The type of flap to be used is selected and appropriate incisions are made (Fig. 10–12*A*). This is followed by a meatoplasty (see Chapter 7) and a canalplasty, until the entire fibrous and bony annulus is fully visualized without entering the temporomandibular joint space (Fig. 10–12*B–E*). This is the time to trim and "freshen" the edges (if necessary and if possible) of a perforated tympanic membrane.

The mastoid work is now begun; Figure 10–13*A* shows the site of the opening to be made. In these cases, the surgeon usually is dealing with sclerotic small mastoids (large, well-pneumatized mastoids lend themselves better to intact canal wall procedures). Figure 10–13*B, C* shows the removal of diseased tissue from the mastoid and antrum. It is important to saucerize the edges (Fig. 10–13*D*), since this leads to a smaller cavity and frequently makes it unnecessary to obliterate the cavity with muscle (mastoid obliteration procedures are described below). This mastoidectomy implies leaving the "bridge" intact (Fig. 10–13*E*). The bridge is the most medial portion of the posterosuperior meatal wall, and crosses the attic toward the tegmen. It has both anterior and posterior buttresses. The anterior buttress is the superior portion where the posterior bony canal meets the tegmen; the posterior buttress is the inferior portion where the posterior bony canal meets the floor of the external auditory canal, lateral to the facial nerve (Fig. 10–14*A–C*).

Once diseased tissue has been removed, an ossiculoplasty is done; Figure 10–14*D, E* and Figure 10–15 show preparation for and placement of a partial ossicular replacement prosthesis (PORP). A tube is then placed in the tympanic membrane, followed by a graft and the obliteration of the aditus (with either periosteum or cartilage) (Fig. 10–16). The cavity (by now the "open" or "exteriorized" mastoid cavity) is covered by the flap. A Thiersch graft can be placed primarily but is usually done after six to eight weeks, when healthy granulation tissue is covering the mastoid cavity ("bowl"). On occasion, coverage with the flap alone allows adequate epithelialization of the cavity, and skin grafting (Thiersch graft) is not necessary. The aim is to obtain a well-epithelialized, safe, "exteriorized" mastoid cavity.

Modified Radical Mastoidectomy

The same principles observed in an intact bridge mastoidectomy apply here. In this procedure, however, the bridge is removed. Two approaches are possible for the mastoidectomy in the modified radical approach: (1) the "inside-out" or atticotomy-antrotomy, and (2) the "outside-in" or antrotomy-atticotomy (starting from the mastoid side). The latter is the approach that has been described previously for mastoidectomy—that is, drilling is initiated from the mastoid side toward the antrum.

Text continued on page 191

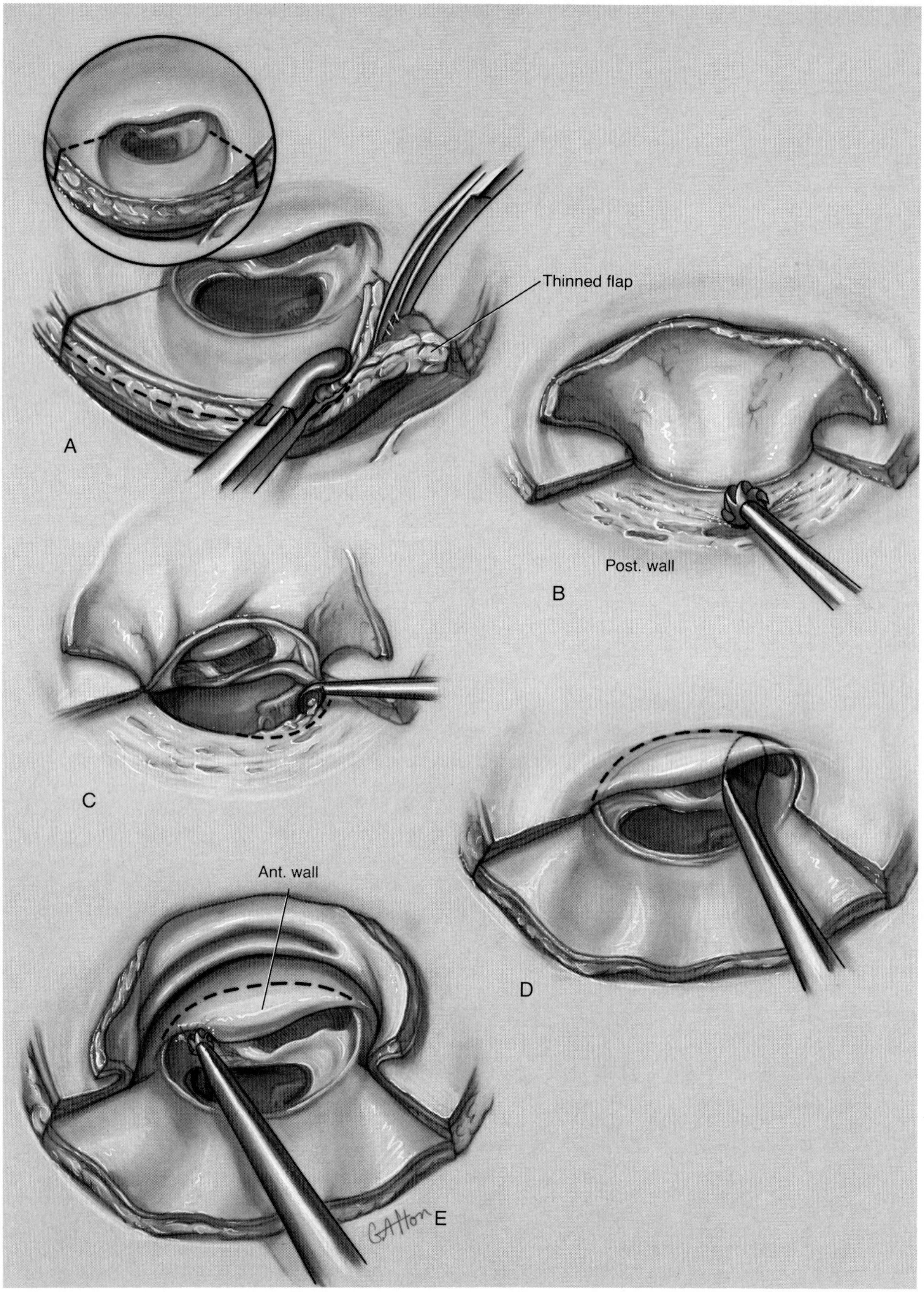

FIGURE 10–12.

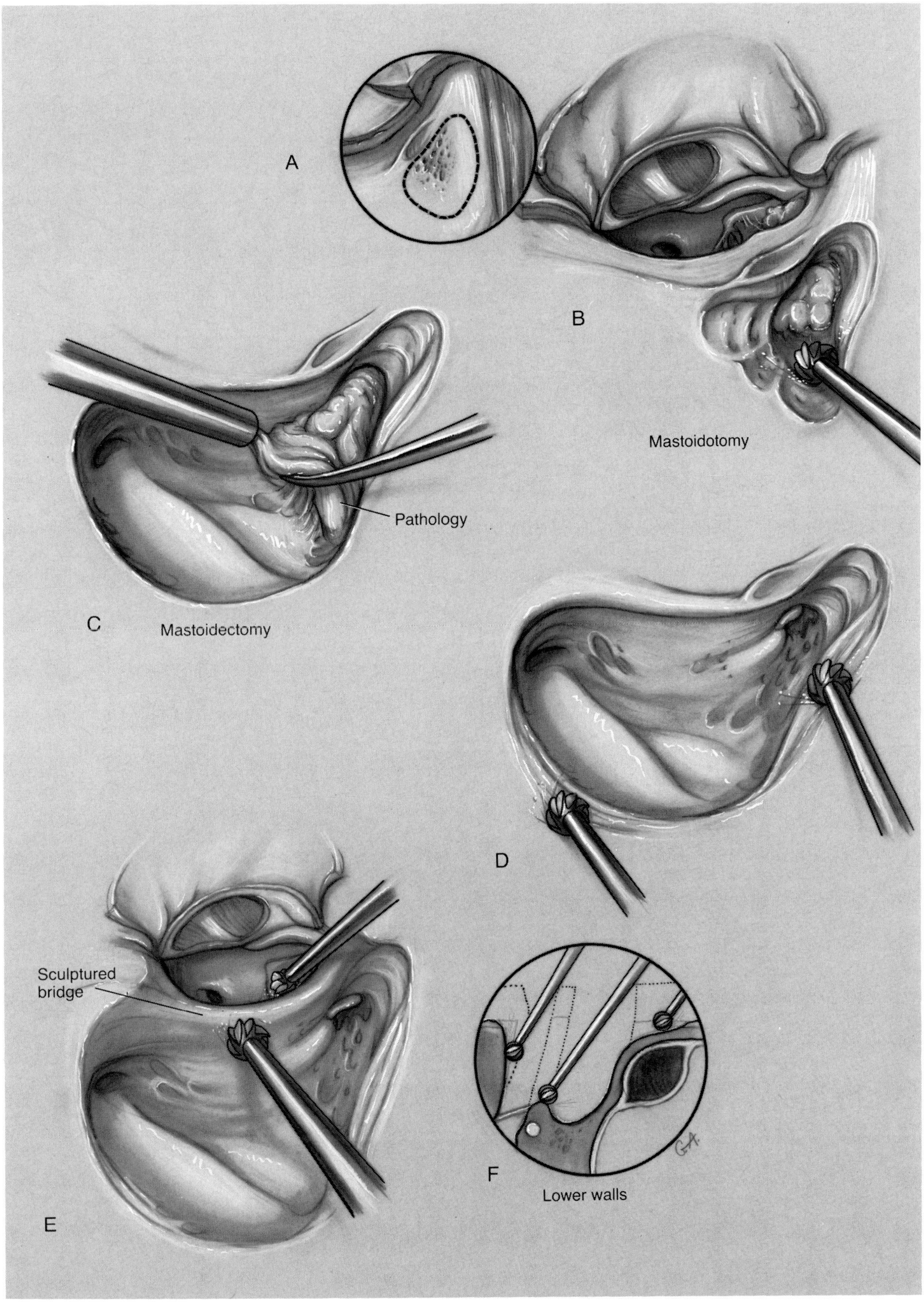
A
B
Mastoidotomy
Pathology
C
Mastoidectomy
D
Sculptured bridge
E
F
Lower walls

FIGURE 10–13.

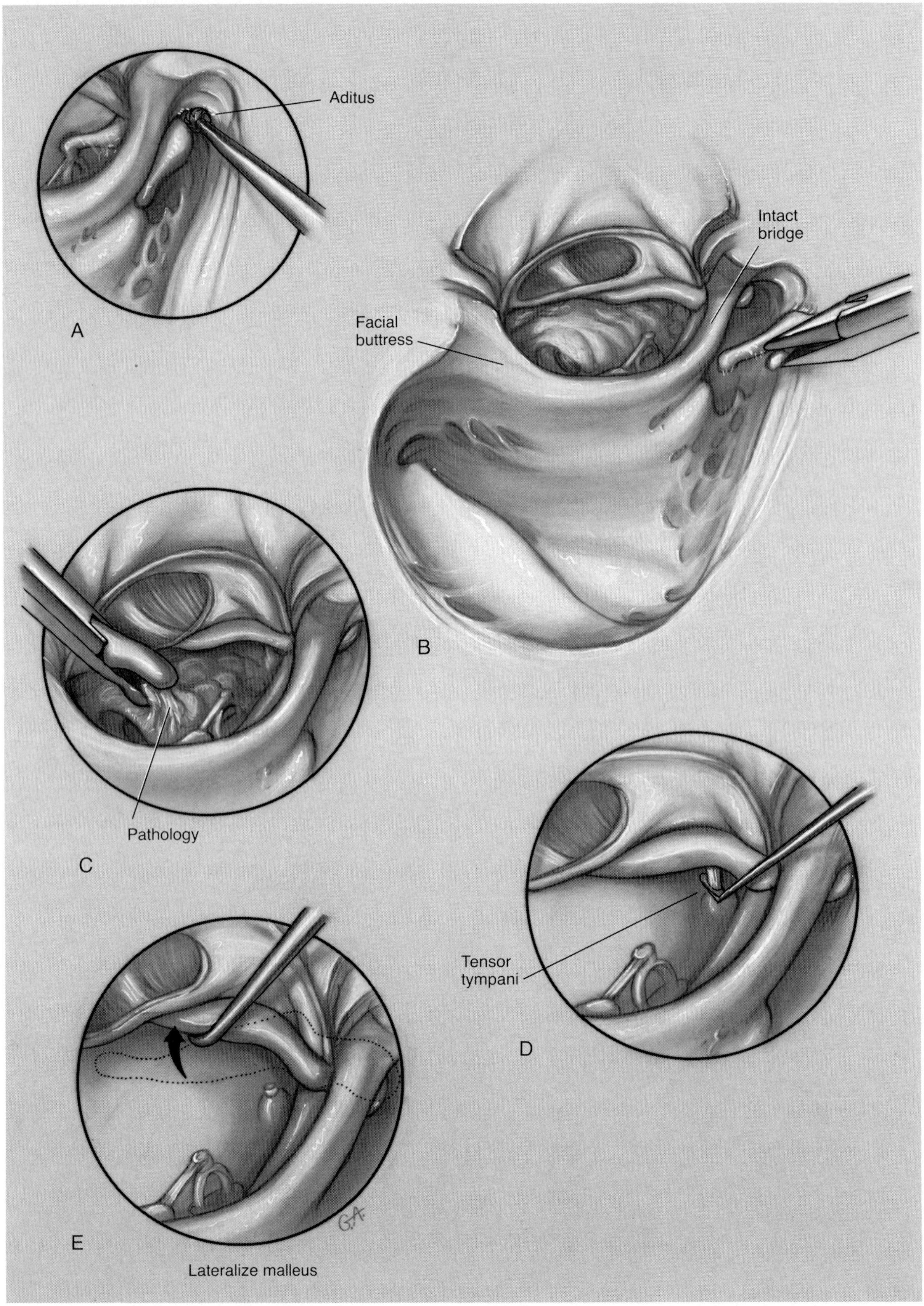
Aditus
A
Intact
bridge
Facial
buttress
B
Pathology
C
Tensor
tympani
D
E
Lateralize malleus

FIGURE 10–14.

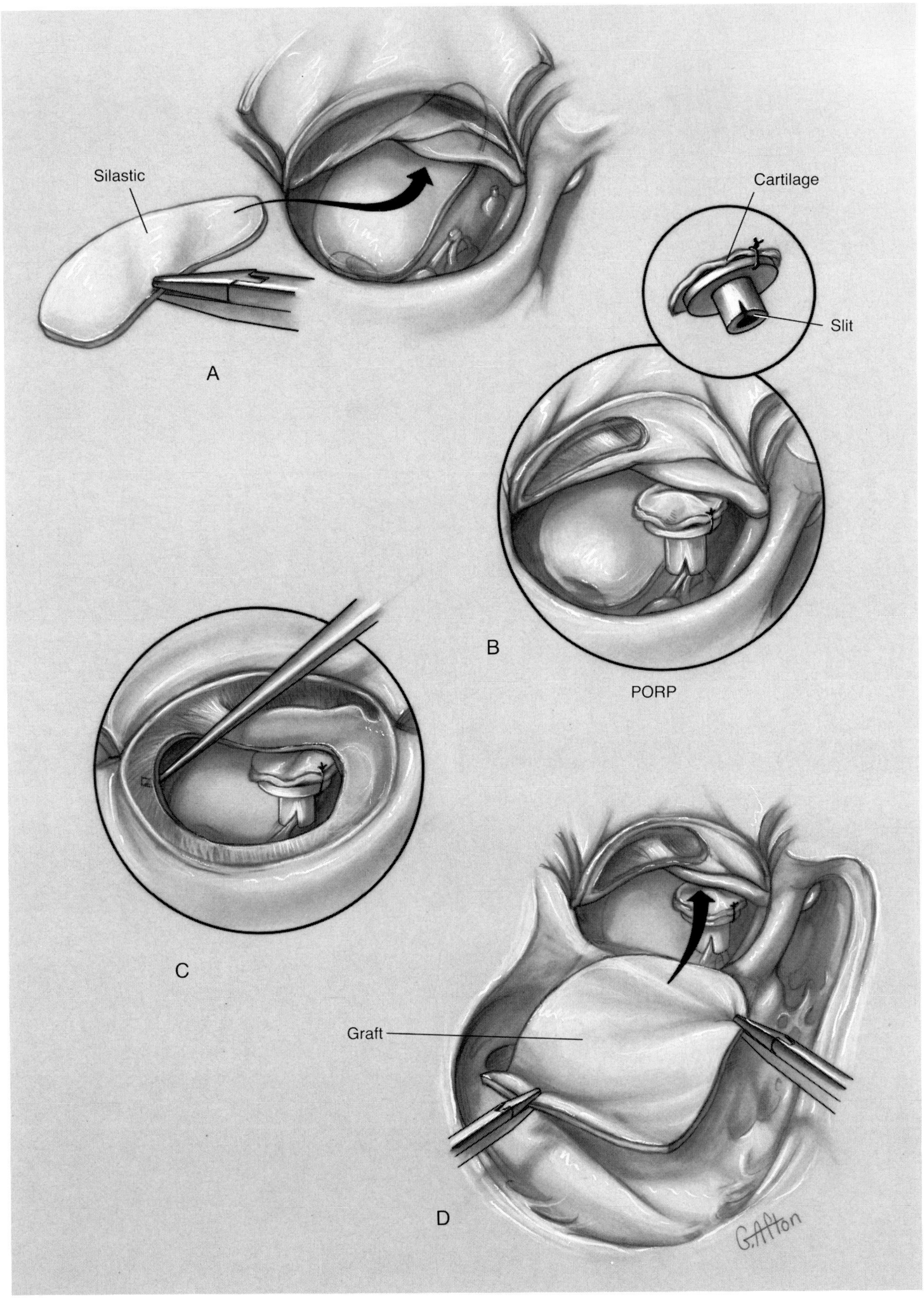

FIGURE 10–15.

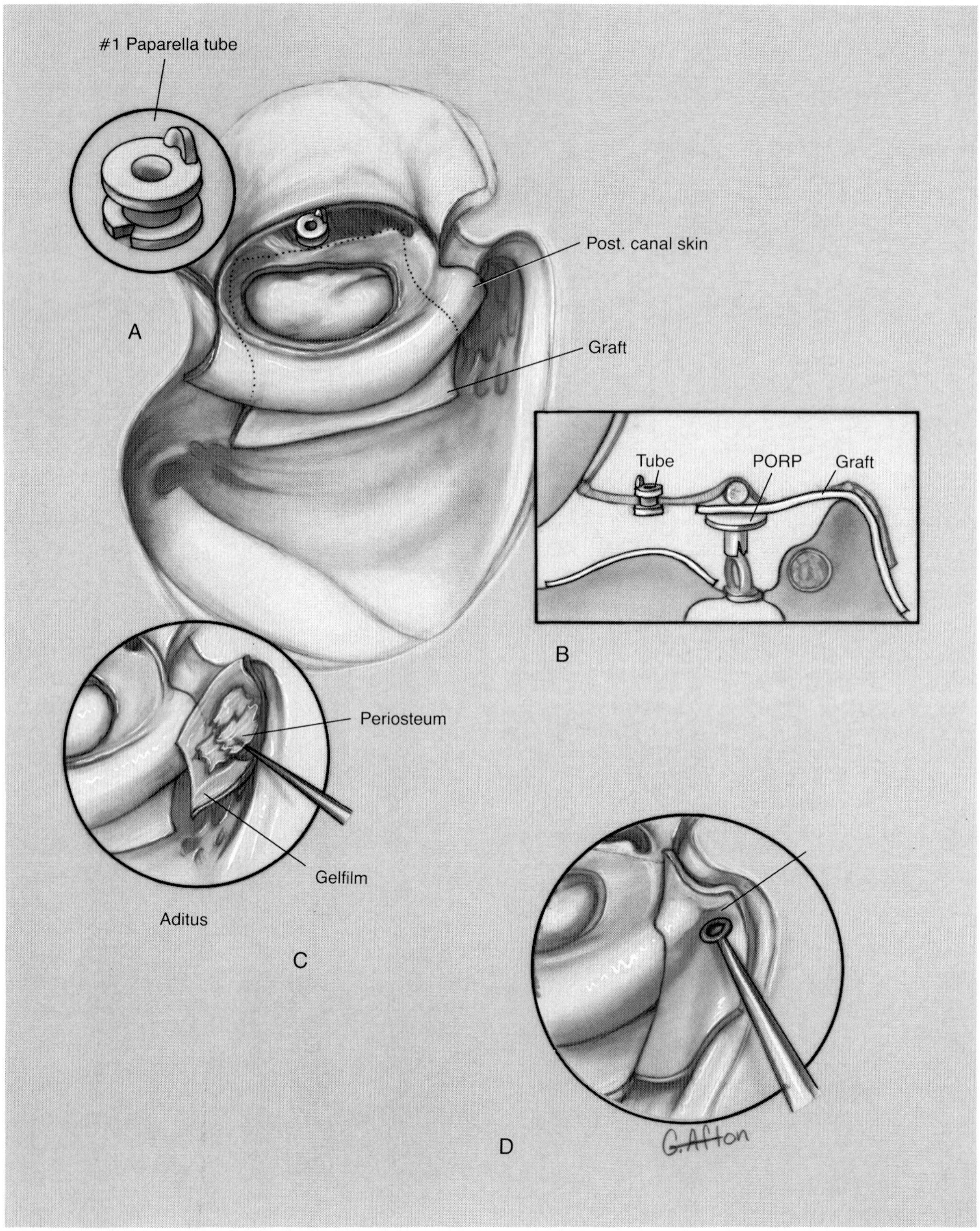

#1 Paparella tube
Post. canal skin
A
Graft
Tube
PORP
Graft
B
Periosteum
Gelfilm
Aditus
C
D
G.Afton

FIGURE 10–16.

In sclerotic mastoids with scarce air cells or cells filled with diseased tissue, a safe outside-in procedure can be extremely difficult. In such cases, the inside-out approach is utilized. In terms of orientation, it is easier to start drilling at the epitympanum, moving in the direction of the antrum. This allows immediate identification of the antrum, the dome of the semicircular canal, and the position of the facial nerve. With these landmarks under direct vision, the mastoidectomy is more easily performed, and the posterior wall is lowered to the level of the facial ridge. As mentioned earlier, this approach involves removal of the bridge. In an intact-bridge mastoidectomy, however, it may be possible to palpate the antrum with a Whirlybird, identify the antral space, and drill an opening immediately superior to the bridge (as in the so-called "observation windows"). This opening is carefully enlarged and an inside-out procedure initiated, thus leaving the bridge intact. Tympanoplasty procedures can be performed in a modified radical mastoidectomy.

Radical Mastoidectomy

This procedure is seldom performed at present. Eradication of disease can be achieved by the procedures described above; these in turn allow reconstruction, thus avoiding the hearing loss inherent in a radical mastoidectomy.

The aim of this procedure is to create an exteriorized cavity that includes the mastoid, antrum, epitympanum, and mesotympanum, leaving a dry, epithelialized cavity continuous with the external meatus. This approach is similar to the modified radical procedure, but also involves removal of the mucosa, the malleus, and the incus while leaving the stapes intact. The eustachian tube opening is obliterated with a bone plug.

The "Exteriorized" Mastoid Cavity

Postoperative care of an open (exteriorized or "canal wall down") cavity is of the utmost importance. Not infrequently, a satisfactory procedure fails owing to lack of adequate postoperative local care. The importance of a meatoplasty has already been stressed. Care of the mastoid cavity is initiated during the procedure itself by obtaining an even, smooth mastoid bowl (cavity) surface, adequate flap coverage, and packing that favors epithelialization. The primary objective is a well-epithelialized, dry mastoid cavity. Epithelialization is achieved by a generous flap (with further epithelialization) or by skin (Thiersch) grafts done during the primary procedure or six to eight weeks after surgery. Once epithelialization is achieved, open cavities tend to accumulate epithelial debris and cerumen and require cleansing every six months to one year. Because a small cavity is desired, adequate saucerization is important. If a large cavity is to be obtained, mastoid obliteration (described below) preferably should be done.

Packing of the cavity varies according to the surgeon's preference and expertise. Gelfoam with antibiotic ointment or solution can be used; other surgeons prefer a rosebud pack fashioned from Owen's silk and cotton saturated with an antibiotic-steroid solution. (Free cotton encourages infection and formation of granulation tissue.) This packing is advantageous when a tympanoplasty is done and a certain degree of pressure is desirable; this is also true for apposition of the skin flap to the wall of the newly formed cavity. The outer one-third (meatal area) usually is packed with gauze saturated with an antibiotic ointment. Owen's silk must be removed a maximum of two weeks after surgery; otherwise it adheres to the walls of the cavity and necessitates a new procedure to remove it (such as curetting or cleansing). The packing used is not so crucial as the rationale for selecting it.

Topical antibiotics, steroids, and prophylactic antibiotics are used routinely, since these procedures are performed in severely infected tissues. External dressings are removed seven days after surgery and inner dressings at 10 to 14 days. Thorough cleansing of the cavity is essential. Removal or cauterization (or both) of any small areas of granulation tissue is crucial. If necessary, local acidification with solutions of boric acid powder should be done; at times, daily cleansing is needed. This meticulous care is essential until epithelialization occurs. If skin grafting is needed (see the discussion of Thiersch grafting in Chapter 7), it is done six to eight weeks after surgery. Skin coverage prevents infection of exposed areas.

Mastoid Obliteration Procedure

When the mastoid cavity is small, an obliteration procedure is not needed. If a mastoid obliteration procedure is necessary, it usually is done in the course of a tympanomastoidectomy. During the mastoidectomy every effort should be made to make the mastoid cavity small. Wide drilling around the mastoid cavity helps to reduce its size.

Aim

To make the mastoid cavity smaller or to minimize problems arising from a large mastoid cavity.

Surgical Steps

1. Postauricular approach.
2. Elevation and insertion of a musculofascial flap.
3. Split-thickness skin graft.
4. Closure and packing.

Pitfalls

1. Incomplete removal of underlying disease.
2. Infection of the flap.
3. Resorption and retraction of the graft.
4. Swelling of the flap, causing disruption of ossicles.

Procedure

Before a postauricular incision is made, the type of muscular flap that will be used to obliterate the mastoid cavity should be decided upon. The flap can be based either superiorly or inferiorly, but in general an inferiorly pedicled flap is more useful (Fig. 10–17*A*). The flap includes muscle, fascia, and periosteum. Before the flap is turned into the mastoid cavity, all disease, especially a cholesteatoma in the cavity, should be removed. The pedicled flap is elevated from the bone, rotated, and inserted into the mastoid cavity; it can then be covered with epithelium previously elevated from the mastoid cavity or the posterior canal.

A Palva's flap is broadly based on the concha. A wide area of the postauricular musculoperiosteum is included in this flap (Fig. 10–17*B*).

A large meatoplasty should be done as part of an obliteration procedure. A large piece of conchal cartilage is removed without tearing or penetrating the conchal skin (Fig. 10–17*C*). A Körner's flap is developed by making longitudinal incisions at 12 and 6 o'clock in the canal extending out to the auricle (Fig. 10–17*D*). The meatus should be large enough to admit the surgeon's forefinger. The Körner's flap is placed between the musculoperiosteal flap and the packing (Fig. 10–17*E*). The postauricular incision is closed and the lateral canal is packed with ½-in gauze strips saturated with antibiotic ointment. The outer packing is removed in one week and the inner packing in two weeks.

Surgery for Complications of Suppurative Otitis Media

Complications of suppurative otitis media are classified into two major categories, intratemporal and extratemporal. Intratemporal bony complications include coalescent mastoiditis, facial nerve paralysis, petrositis, and labyrinthitis. Extratemporal bony complications are divided into intracranial and extracranial. Intracranial complications include extradural, subdural and cerebellar abscesses, meningitis, sigmoid sinus thrombophlebitis, and otitic hydrocephalus; extracranial complications include subperiosteal, postauricular, Bezold's, and zygomatic abscesses. Owing to the use of antibiotics, these complications are relatively rare but still occur. New imaging techniques (CT scan and MRI) have revolutionized the treatment of these complications, especially intracranial complications. Surgical treatments pertinent to otologic surgeons are described below.

Coalescent Mastoiditis

Patients with coalescent mastoiditis are treated with a complete mastoidectomy (see Chapters 5 and 7). Communication should be established between the mastoid and the middle ear cavity. The facial recess may have to be opened. A large myringotomy and insertion of a tympanostomy tube help drainage after surgery.

Facial Nerve Paralysis

Facial nerve paralysis may develop in association with an acute suppurative otitis media, especially in younger (pediatric) patients. A wide myringotomy is done and pus is drained. A large-bore tympanostomy tube may be inserted at the same time to help further

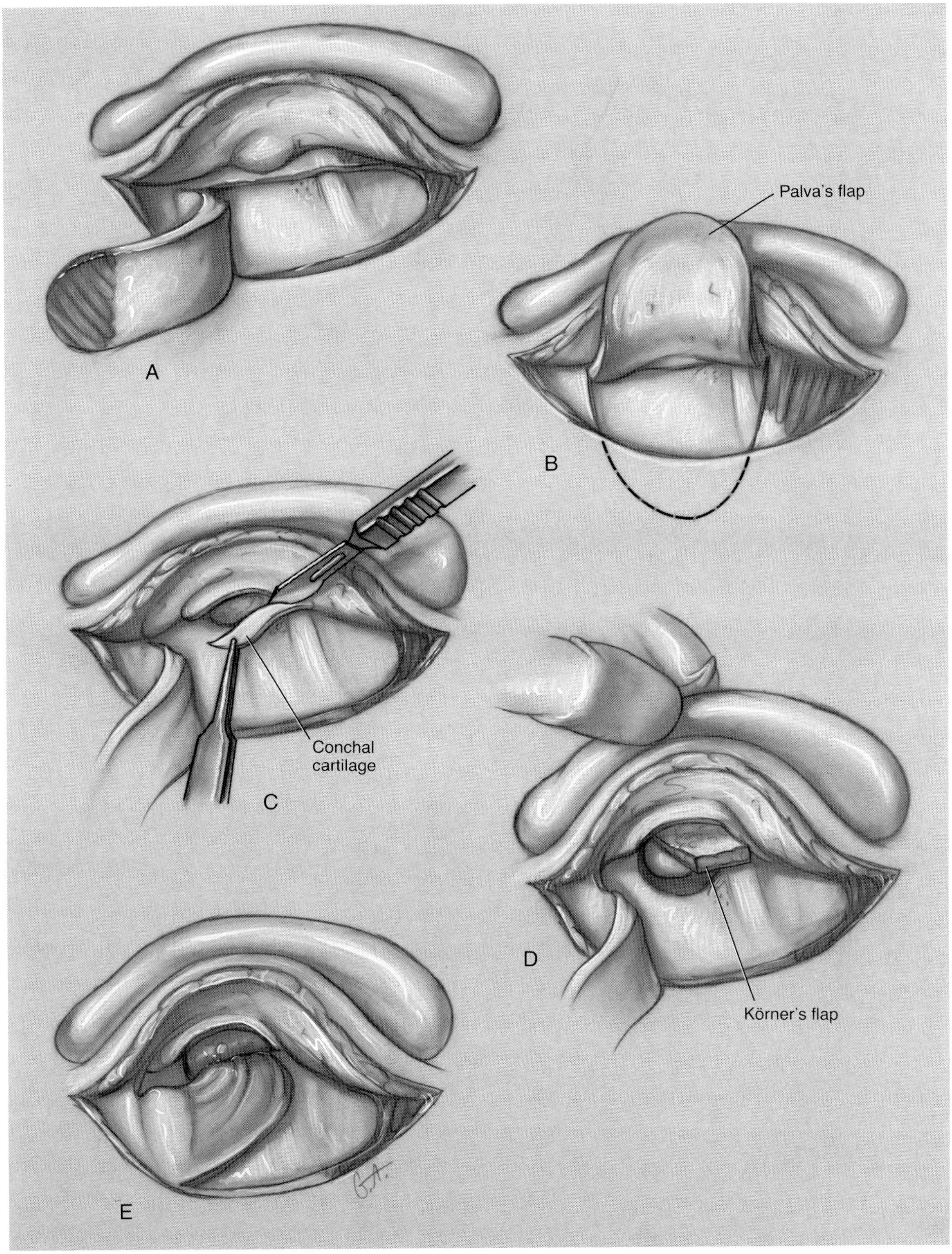

FIGURE 10–17.

drainage. Intensive parenteral antibiotics are given; after several doses, corticosteroids are added. The patient is followed with electrodiagnostic tests. Decompression of the facial nerve rarely is necessary. On the other hand, facial paralysis occurring with chronic otitis media requires prompt exploration and decompression of the nerve.

Petrositis

Petrositis manifests itself clinically with deep pain, palsy of cranial nerve VI, and otorrhea (Gradenigo's syndrome). Pain may be the only complaint. Once the diagnosis is made, the patient with petrositis is treated with intensive antimicrobial therapy and surgery. A complete extended mastoidectomy is done, with special emphasis on location and exenteration of the cell tracks around the semicircular canals; if this is unsuccessful, an apicectomy might be necessary. Surgical approaches to the petrous apex may be made through the subarcuate air cell tract; the sinodural angle; the tract beneath the posterior canal and vertical portion of the facial nerve; the hypotympanic cells; the peritubal cells to the petrous apex between the cochlea and the carotid artery; and the middle fossa (Fig. 10–18).

Labyrinthitis

Patients with labyrinthitis present with sensorineural hearing loss, tinnitus, and vertigo. Initial treatment includes hospitalization, hydration, antimicrobial therapy, antivertiginous medications, and a myringotomy; if there is no improvement, surgical intervention should be considered. A complete mastoidectomy is done. The labyrinth can be drained with a labyrinthectomy approach. In this procedure, the posterior and horizontal semicircular canals are opened. The bony wall between the oval and round windows is removed, along with the lateral end of the internal auditory canal. In addition, the sigmoid sinus and dura of the middle and posterior cranial fossa are exposed to identify and drain any pus in these areas.

Intracranial Abscess

Intracranial abscesses may occur at an extradural or a subdural site, or in the brain itself (Fig. 10–19*A*). An extradural location is the most common.

The extradural (epidural or subperiosteal) abscess may be at the middle or posterior fossa. Surgical steps include a postauricular incision, a complete mastoidectomy, exposure of dura, and drainage of the abscess. The bony plate over the dura is carefully removed with a diamond bur and curet (Fig. 10–19*B*). Granulation tissue over the dura can be carefully peeled off or left alone.

A subdural or brain abscess is managed in cooperation with neurosurgical colleagues. It can be drained to the mastoid cavity.

Meningitis

Meningitis is the most common intracranial complication. The primary mode of treatment is intensive antimicrobial therapy; when surgical intervention is indicated, the procedure is essentially the same as that for an extradural abscess.

Sigmoid Sinus Thrombophlebitis

Suppurative otitis media can cause inflammation around the sigmoid sinus, resulting in a localized phlebitis. Phlebitis promotes formation of a mural thrombus, which may enlarge, occlude the lumen, and become infected. Symptoms of sigmoid sinus thrombophlebitis include spiking fever, chills, headache, increased intracranial pressure, and postauricular edema (Griesinger's sign).

The treatment is appropriate antimicrobial therapy and surgery. Surgical steps include a complete mastoidectomy, exposure of the sigmoid sinus, needle aspiration of the sinus, evacuation of the thrombus, ligation of the internal jugular vein, and packing and closure.

After a complete mastoidectomy is done, the bony plate overlying the sigmoid sinus is thinned with diamond burs and removed proximally and distally with a curet or elevator until normal sinus appears. After the sigmoid sinus is exposed, a needle (with syringe) is inserted into the sinus distally. If blood is aspirated freely, no further procedure is necessary and the wound is closed. If there is evidence of a clot, the sinus is opened and the thrombus is removed until blood flows freely (Fig. 10–19*C*, *D*). Packing impregnated with antibiotics is inserted between the wall of the sinus and the overlying bony plate.

If there is no retrograde bleeding and thrombus is suspected at the bulb or inferior location, the internal jugular vein is ligated in the neck; the incision is made along the anterior border of the sternocleidomastoid muscle (Fig. 10–20*A*). The muscle is retracted

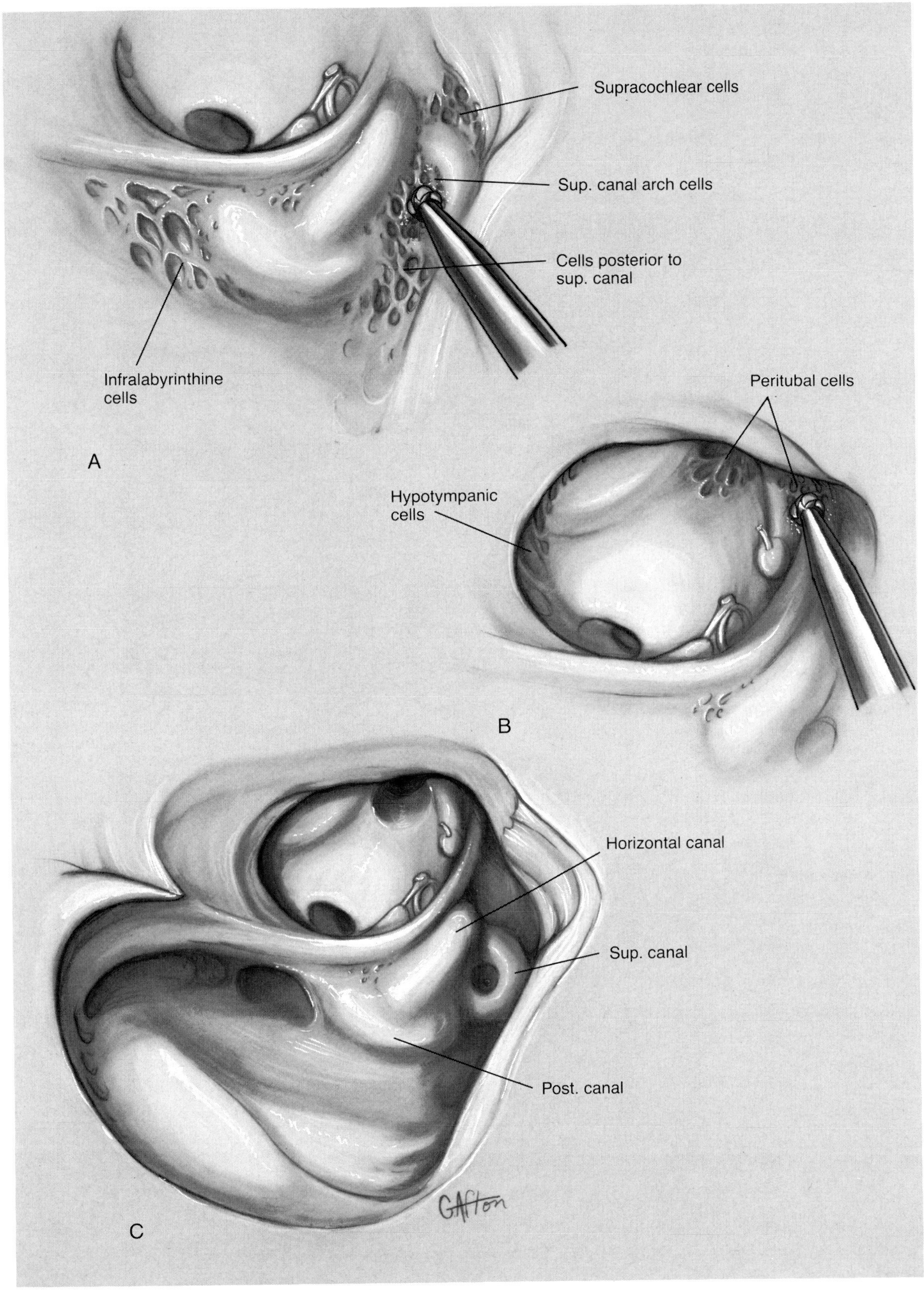
Supracochlear cells
Sup. canal arch cells
Cells posterior to sup. canal
Infralabyrinthine cells
A
Peritubal cells
Hypotympanic cells
B
Horizontal canal
Sup. canal
Post. canal
C

FIGURE 10–18.

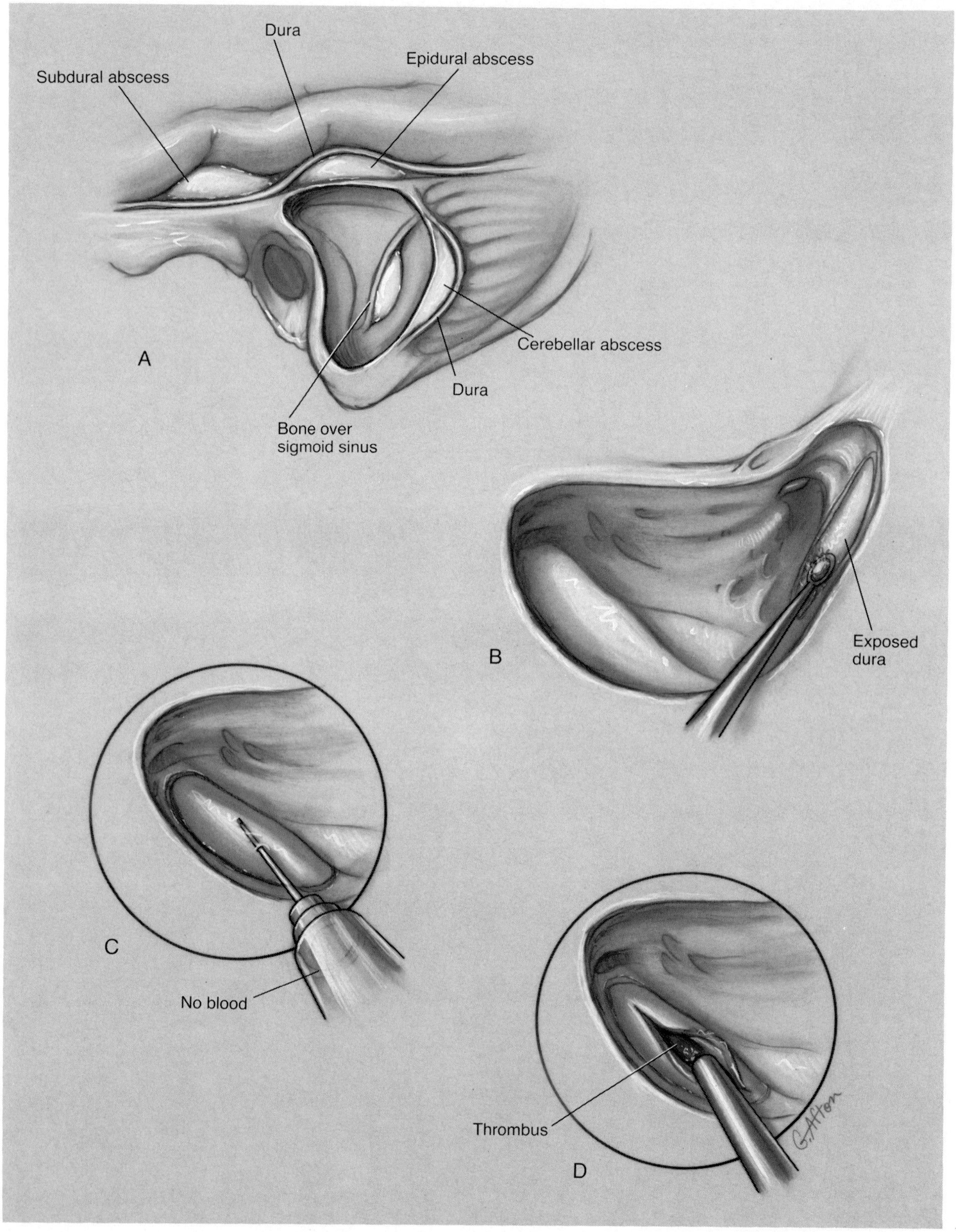
Dura
Epidural abscess
Subdural abscess
A
Cerebellar abscess
Dura
Bone over
sigmoid sinus
Exposed
dura
B
C
No blood
Thrombus
D

FIGURE 10–19.

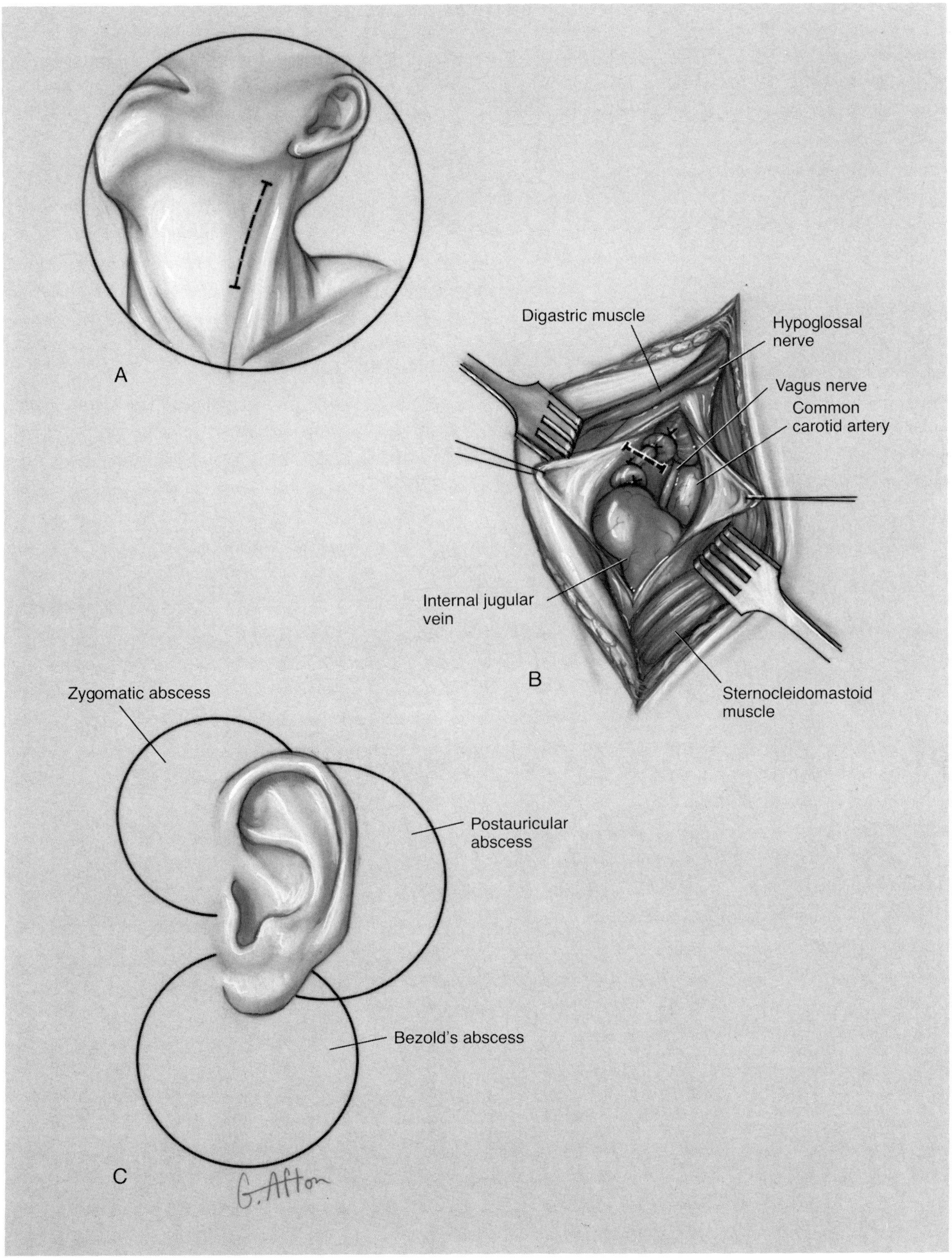
A
Digastric muscle
Hypoglossal nerve
Vagus nerve
Common carotid artery
Internal jugular vein
B
Sternocleidomastoid muscle
Zygomatic abscess
Postauricular abscess
Bezold's abscess
C
G. Afton

FIGURE 10–20.

posteriorly, and the internal jugular vein is identified and doubly ligated (Fig. 10–20*B*). The vagus nerve should be positively identified before the vein is ligated.

The wound is partially closed. Packings on the sinus are removed in 7 to 10 days; this should be done in the operating room owing to the possibility of bleeding.

Periauricular Abscesses

Infection of the middle ear and mastoid can cause abscess formation around the auricle. An abscess may develop posteriorly (postauricular), anteriorly (zygomatic), or inferiorly (Bezold's) (Fig. 10–20*C*). The postauricular abscess is the most common.

Treatment includes antimicrobial therapy and surgery. Surgical treatment consists of incision and drainage of the abscess, a myringotomy, and insertion of a tympanostomy tube with or without a simple mastoidectomy.

Frequently the mastoid returns to normal by the time the abscess is drained. However, a mastoidectomy is helpful in removing any remaining focus of infection or underlying pathology. Any blockage at the aditus ad antrum is removed. A myringotomy and insertion of a tympanostomy tube help further drainage. A Penrose drain may be inserted into the abscess cavity during surgery; it is advanced gradually and removed in two to three days.

Pertinent Histopathology

FIGURE 10–21

This section shows an episode of acute otitis media with perforation of the tympanic membrane. Note that the mucoperiosteum overlying the promontory is thickened.

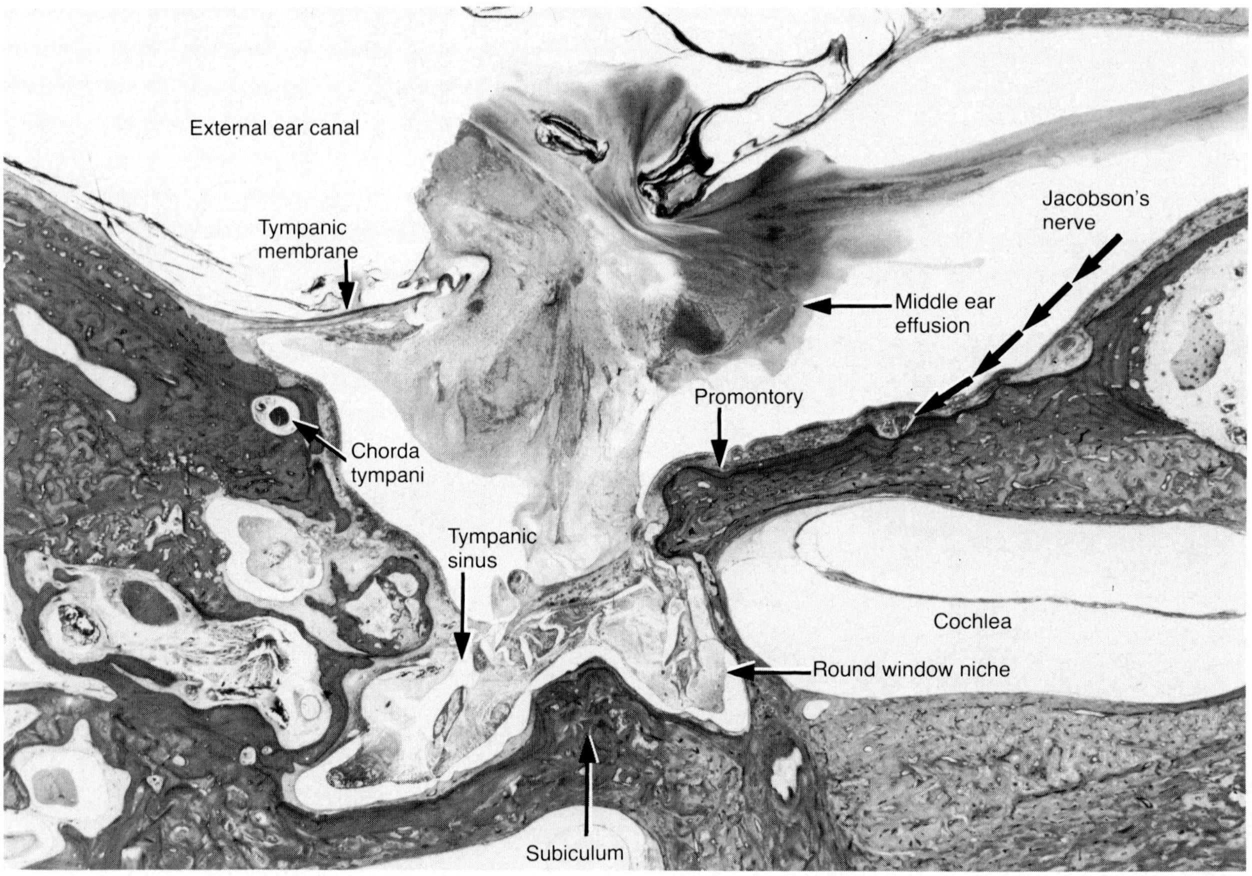

FIGURE 10–21.

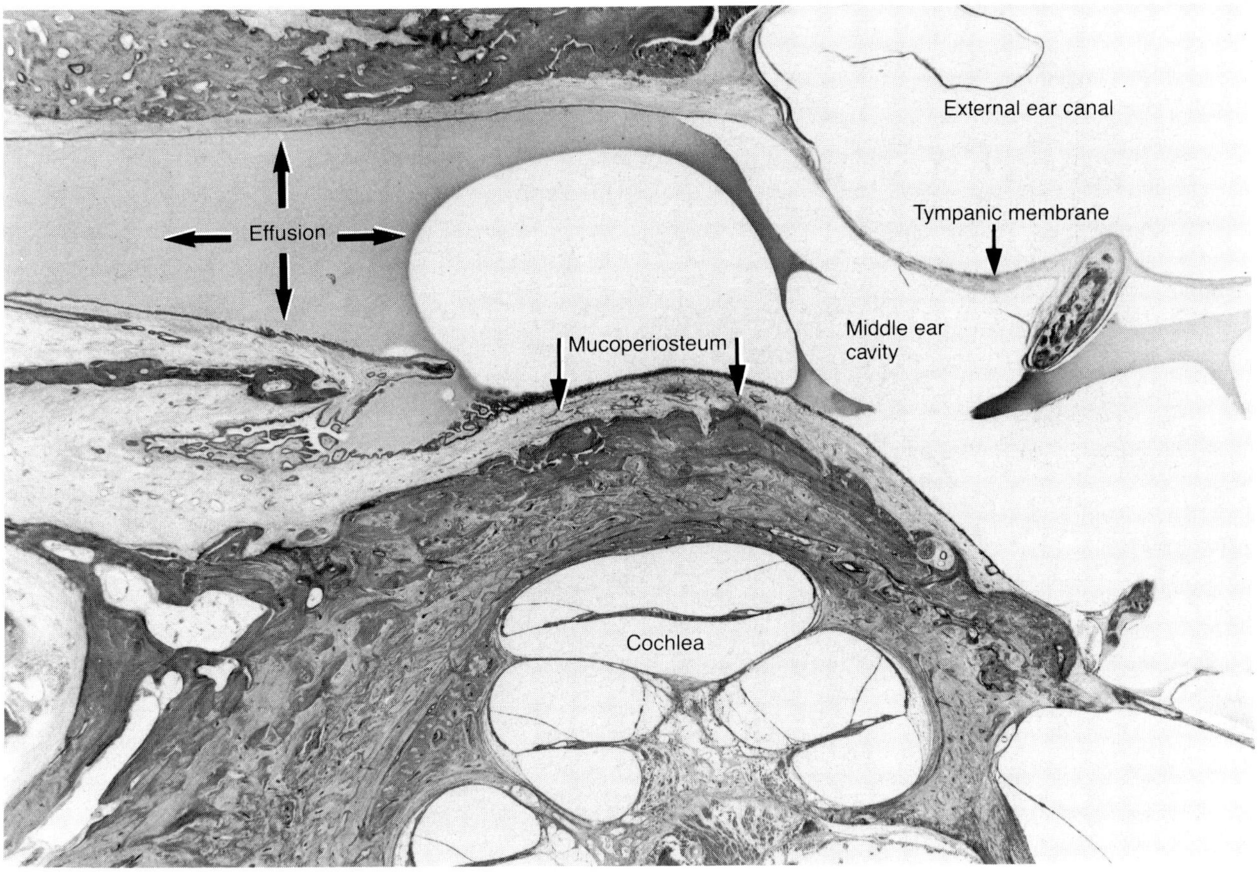

FIGURE 10–22

This section shows a middle ear effusion occupying the middle ear cavity. The mucoperiosteum is thickened. This is a typical image of mucoid otitis.

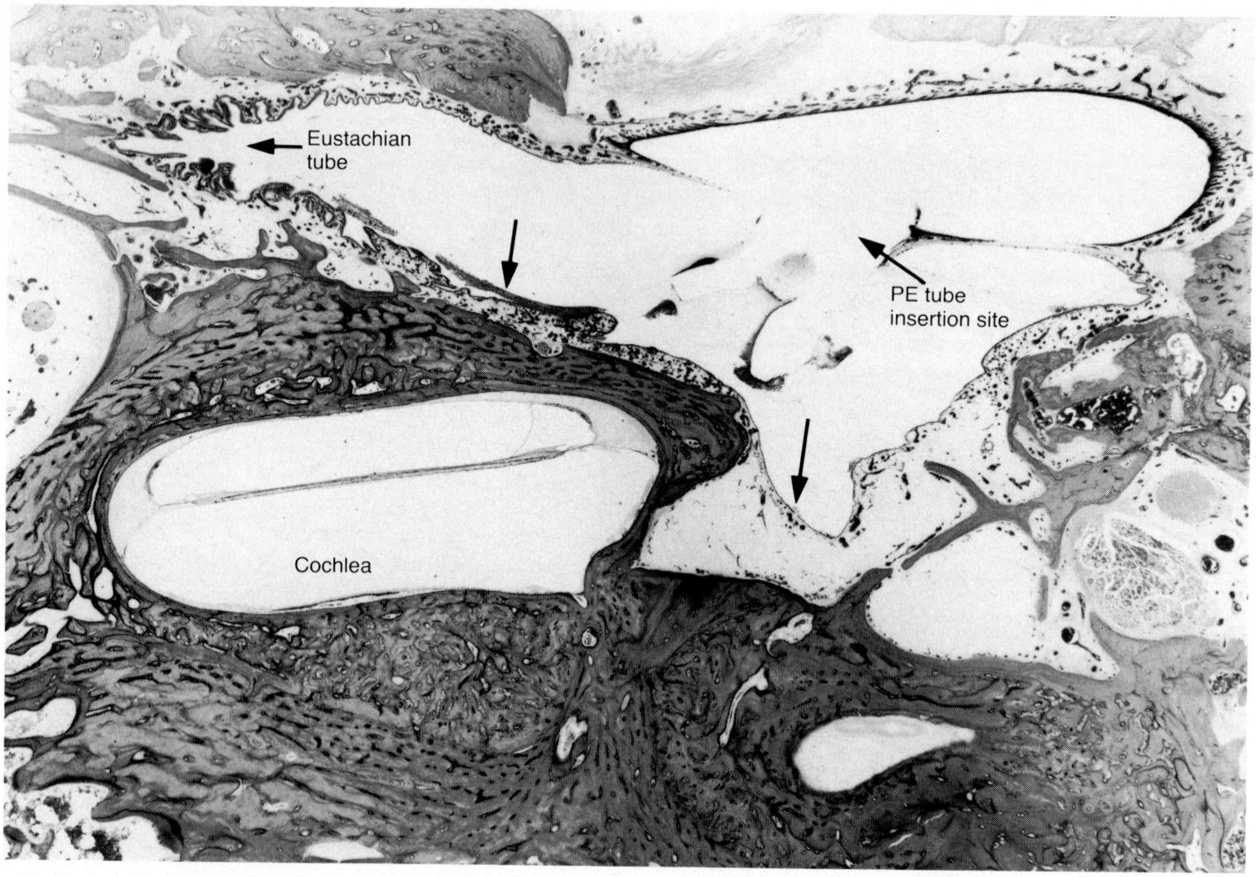

FIGURE 10–23

This 18-month-old baby had a pressure-equalizing (PE) tube inserted; the site of insertion can be identified. There is no middle ear effusion but the mucoperiosteum remains thickened (*arrows*); thus, either the underlying process has not been relieved by insertion of the tube or the process is in a regression phase.

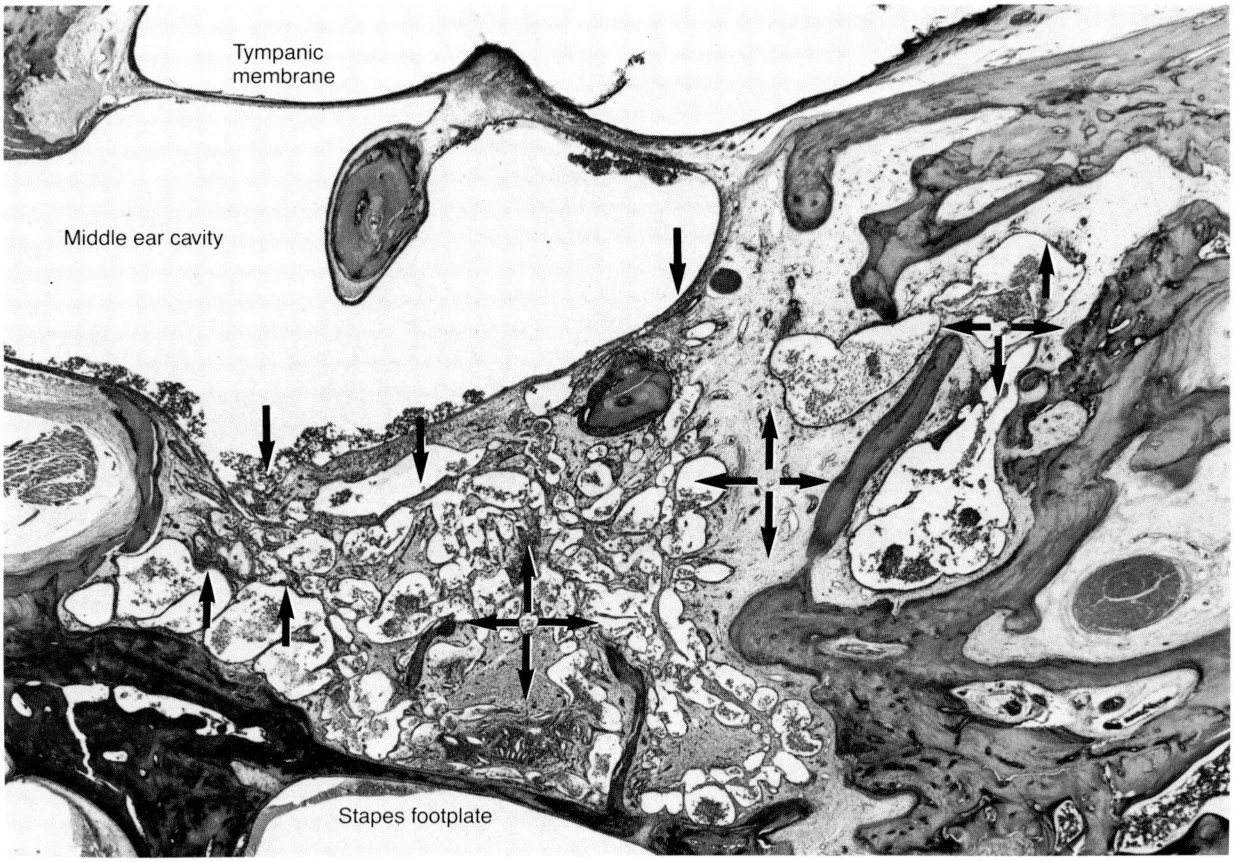

FIGURE 10–24

This horizontal section belongs to the temporal bone of an 18-year-old individual with a history of recurrent episodes of otitis media. He had a mild conductive hearing loss and a slightly retracted tympanic membrane with decreased mobility. The middle ear cavity and mastoid are full of chronic inflammatory tissue (*single arrows*). Would insertion of a PE tube help?

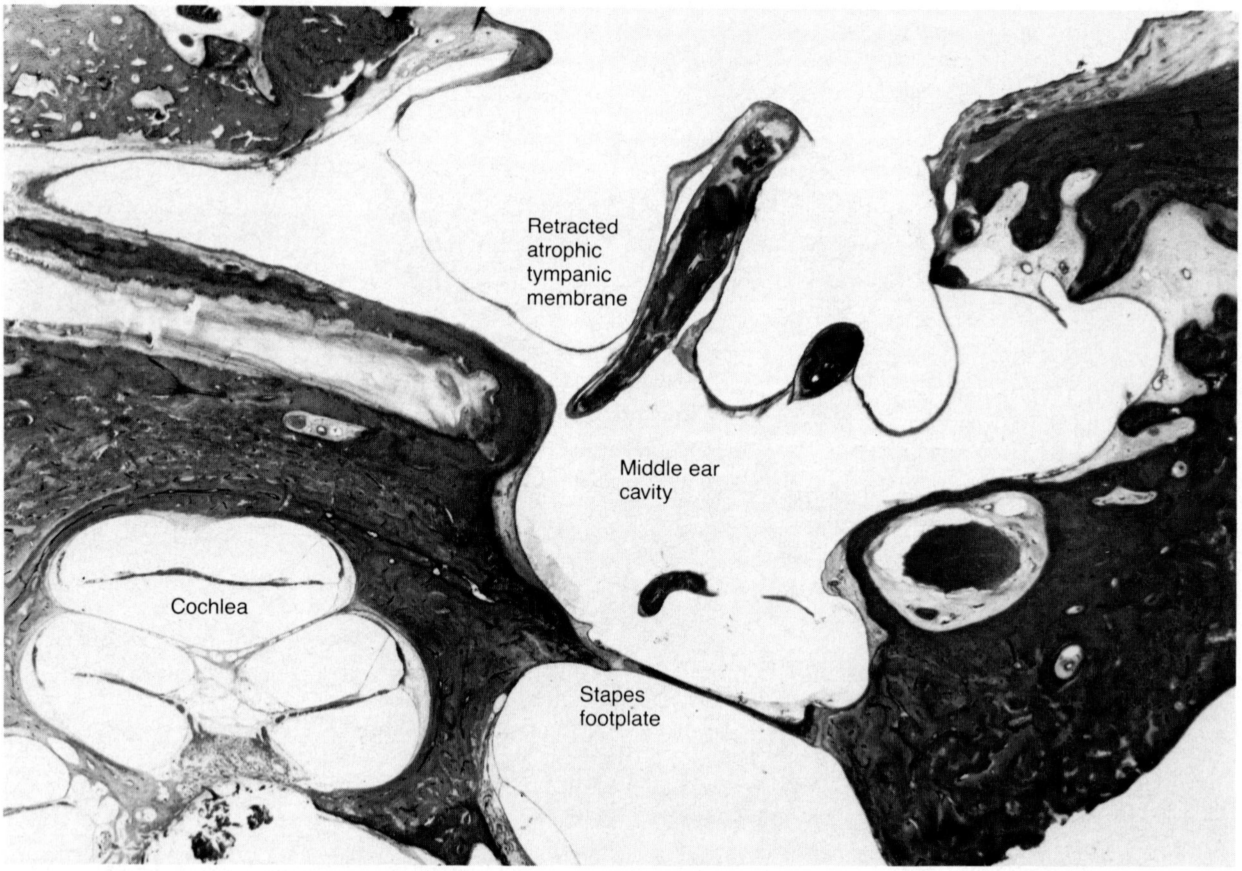

FIGURE 10–25

This section shows a markedly retracted, atrophic tympanic membrane with a so-called "retraction pocket." Note the small middle ear space available. Elevation of this membrane without any tears is obviously a difficult task to perform properly. The thinness of the membrane justifies reinforcement with fascia during surgical repair (even if the membrane is elevated intact).

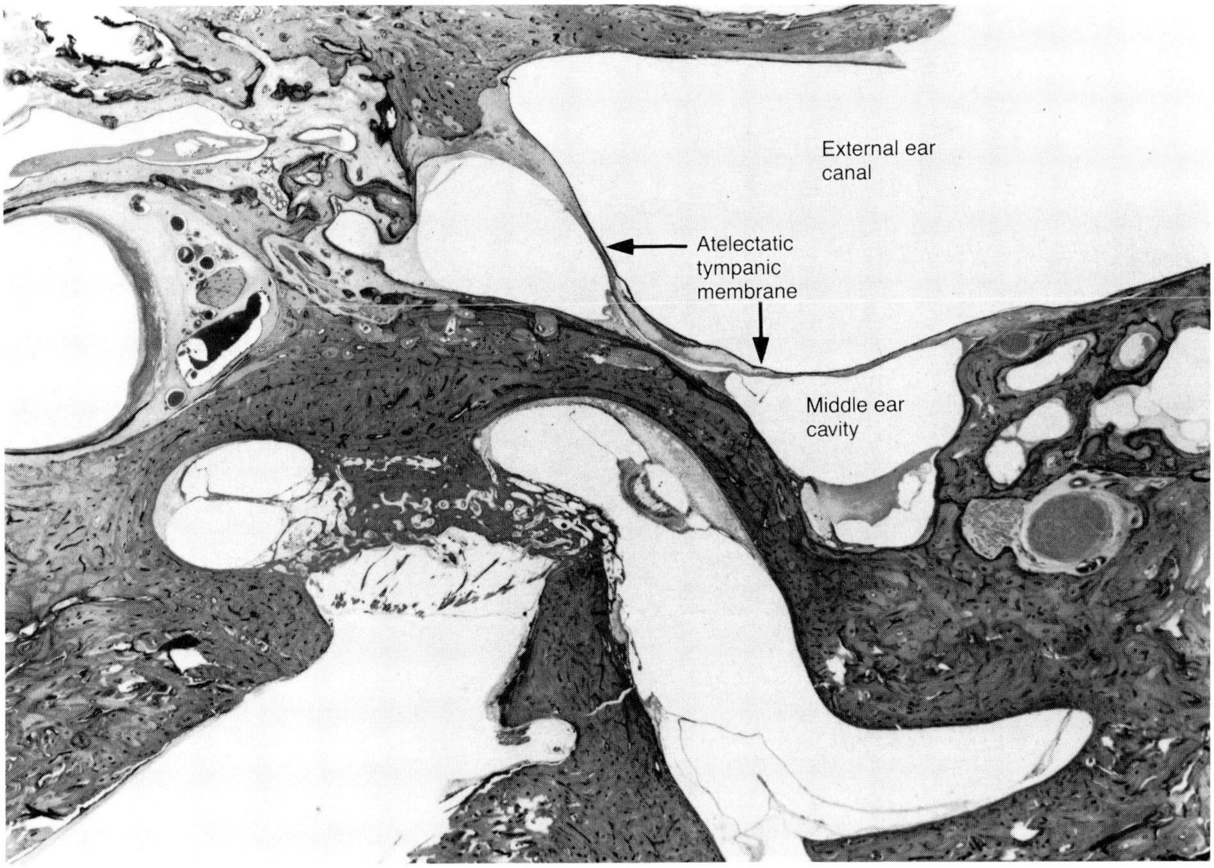

FIGURE 10–26

This section shows an atelectatic tympanic membrane against the promontory. Atelectatic or retracted membranes tend to have small amounts of middle ear effusions. The "adhesiveness" of the tympanic membrane and the common formation of adhesions in otitis media processes justify the use of thin Silastic sheets, which tend to preclude these formations, thus maintaining a middle ear space and the free mobility of the tympanic membrane and ossicles. Sectioning of the tensor tympani (when there is fibrous involvement) also allows a larger middle ear space and better tympanic membrane mobility (not shown in this figure).

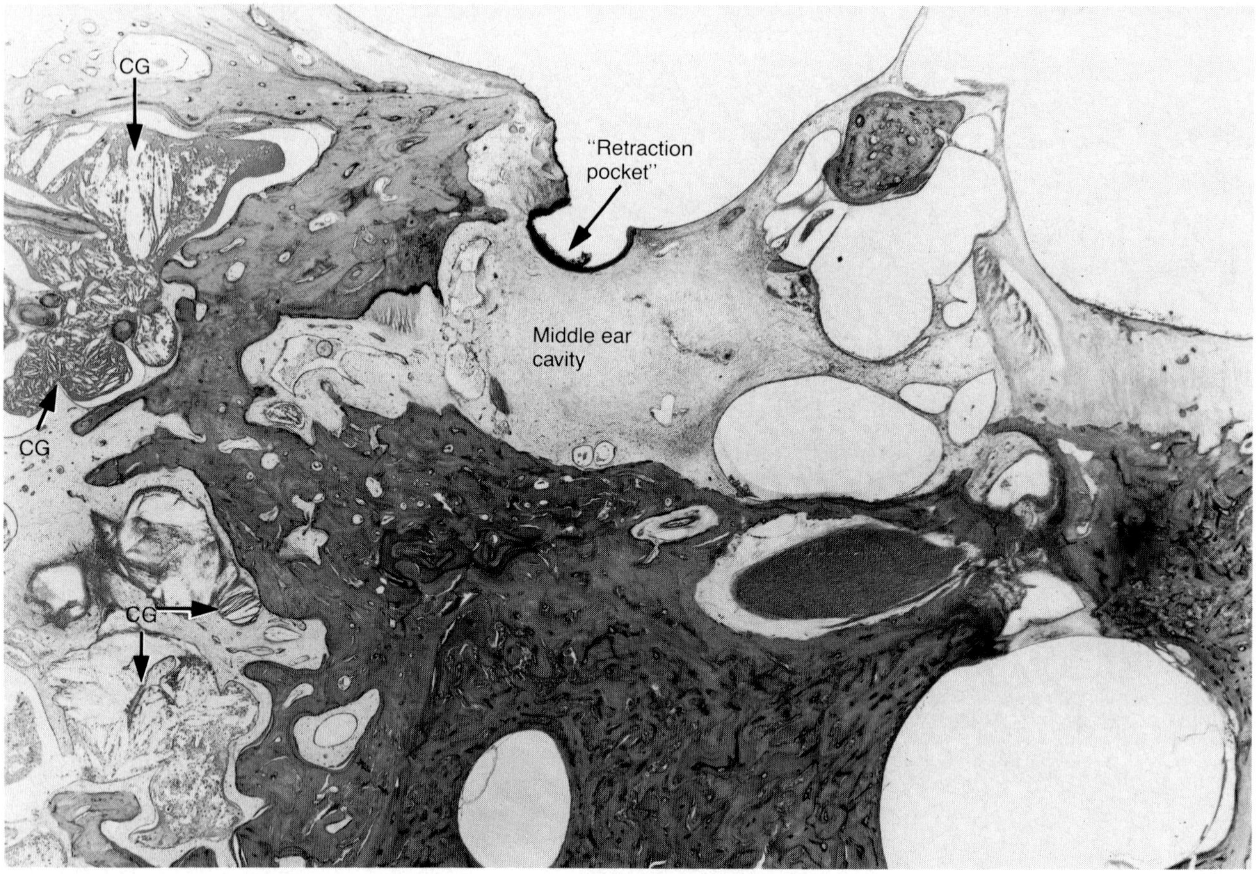

FIGURE 10–27

Beneath the small "retraction pocket" lies a middle ear cavity filled with connective tissue and a diseased mastoid containing a cholesterol granuloma (CG) and other changes. This requires eradication of disease from both the middle ear and mastoid. The gradual systematic approach described in this chapter allows the surgeon to deal with this case properly. Simple insertion of a tube or exploration of the middle ear not only would not suffice but would leave diseased mucoperiosteum with all of its potential complications.

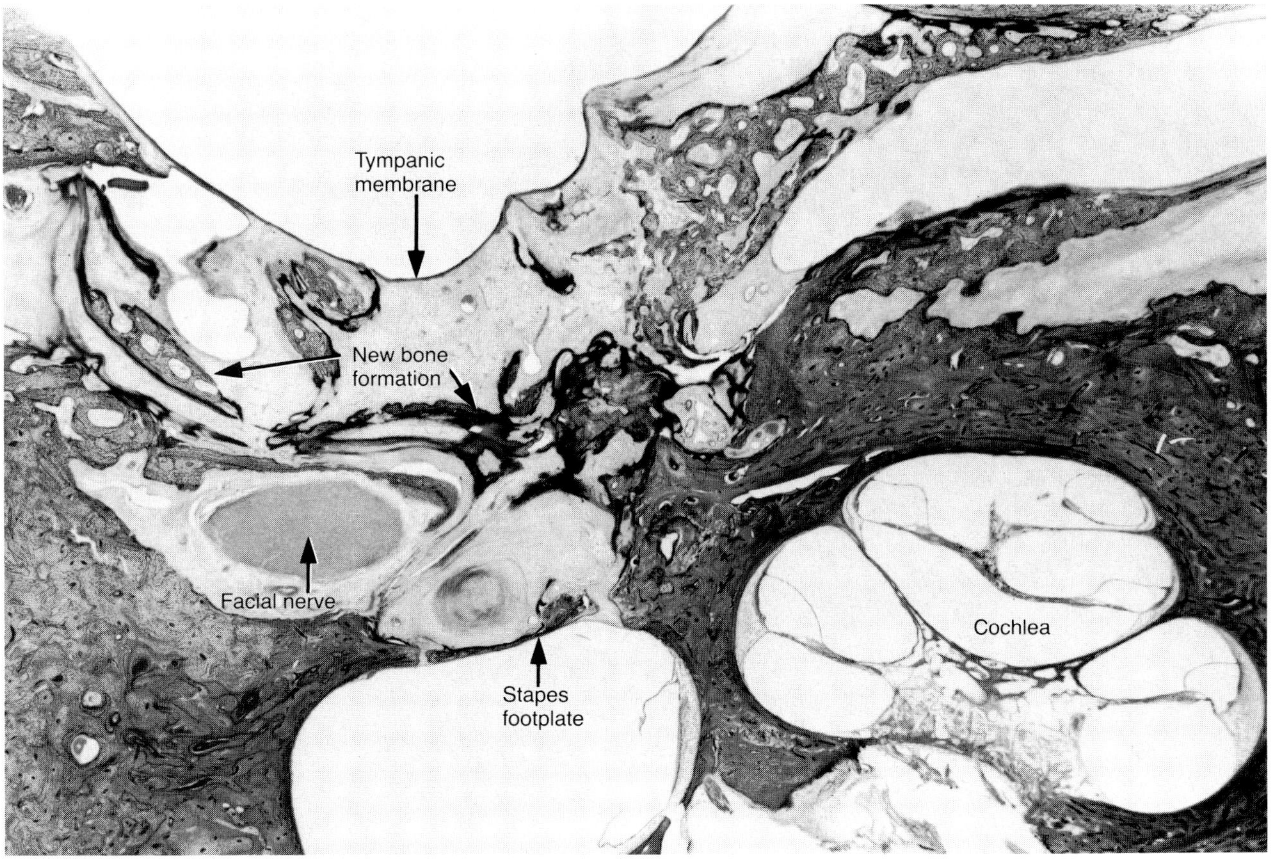

FIGURE 10–28

This section shows another case of otitis media chronic middle ear involvement that requires removal. New bone formation in the cavity makes the surgical task difficult, requiring the utmost care. Incomplete removal of diseased tissue will leave disease behind; too aggressive an approach can expose and compromise the facial nerve, which has a very thin, bony covering laterally and is dehiscent toward the oval window. The stapes footplate is fixed by fibrous tissue. Removing this stapes and replacing it with a prosthesis would turn this case into a surgical tragedy because of the middle ear process involving the vestibule. In chronic otitis, the stapes footplate and the malleus tend to become fixed by fibrous tissue. The long process of the incus and stapes head and crura undergo resorption, resulting in ossicular discontinuity.

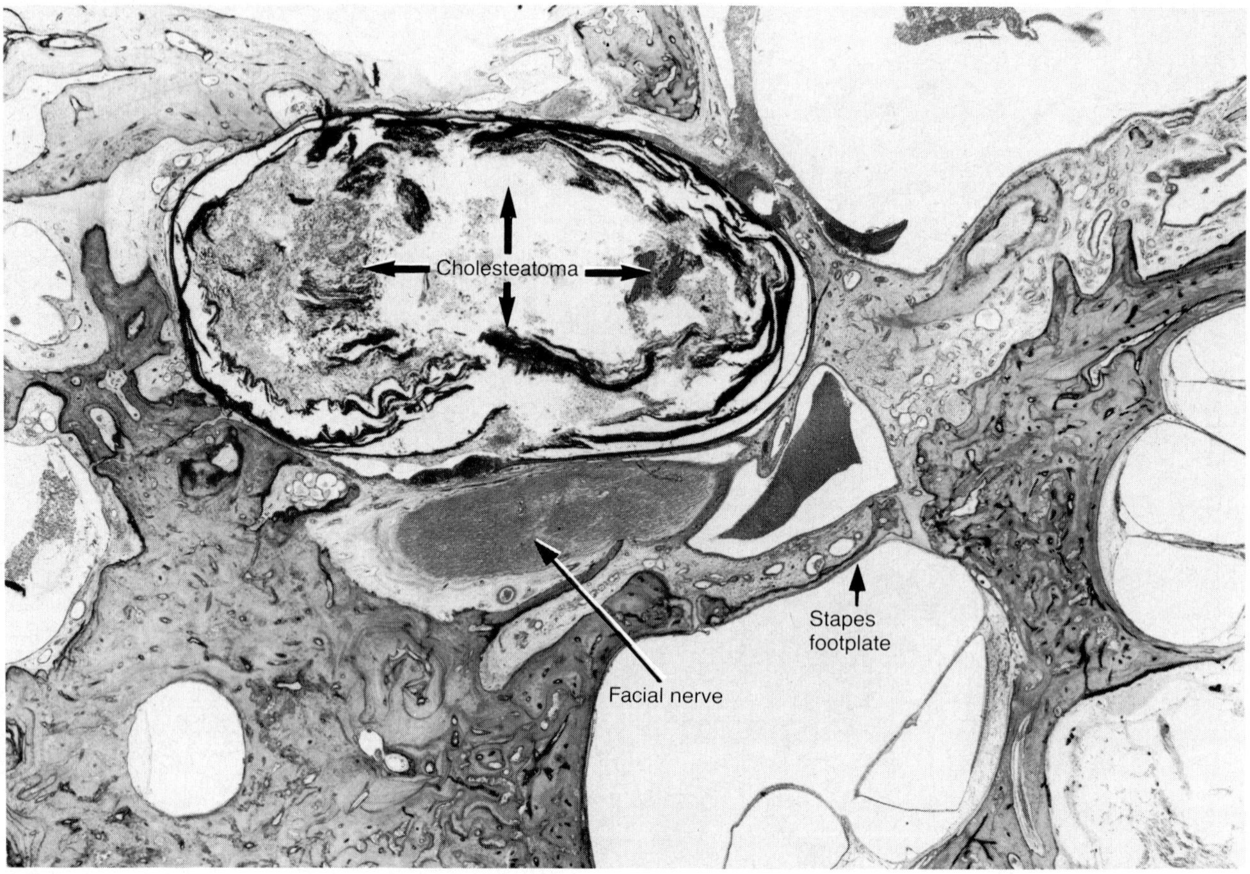

FIGURE 10–29

This section shows a middle ear cavity containing not only thickened mucoperiosteum but also a cholesteatoma eroding into the facial nerve. This lesion, if untreated, will lead to facial paralysis. Careful dissection of the cholesteatoma is important since facial paralysis is a likely complication of such a procedure.

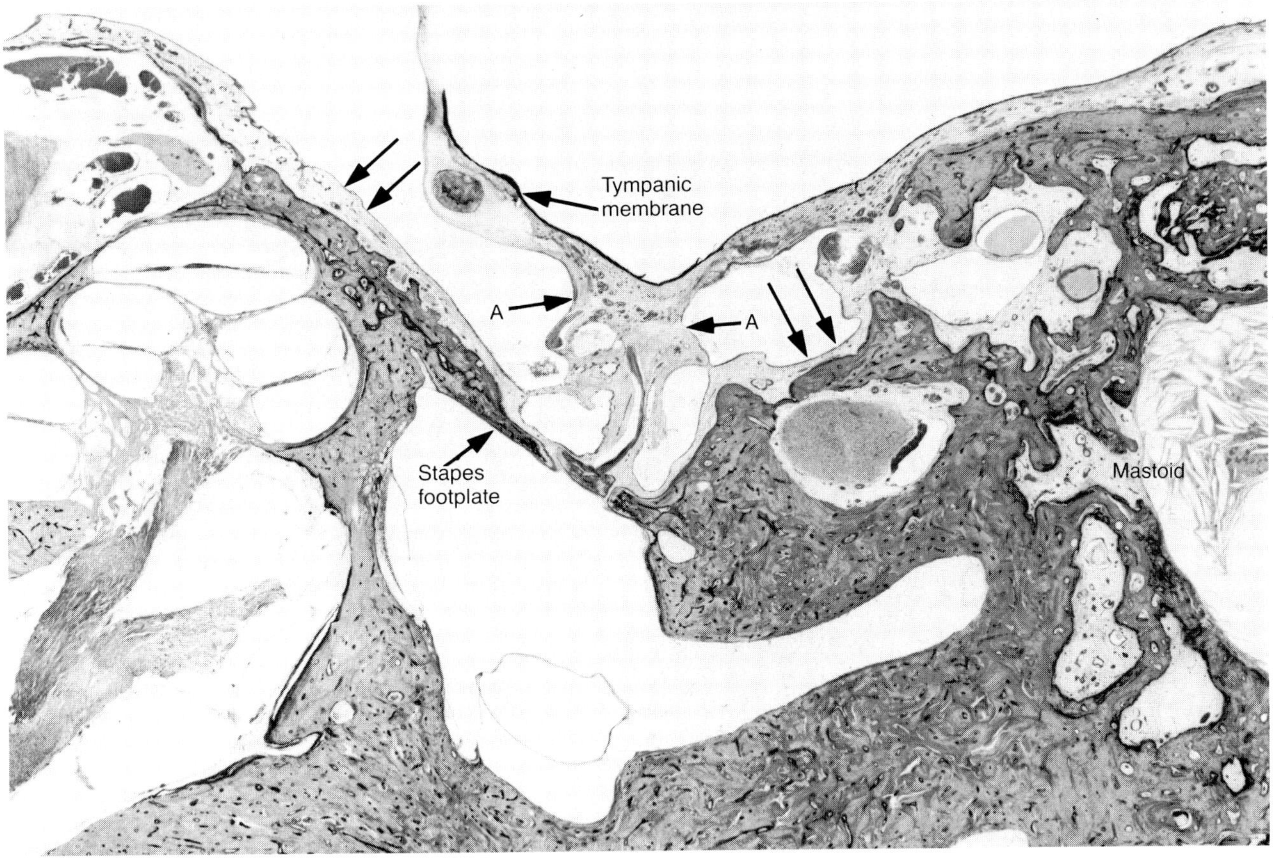

FIGURE 10–30

This section shows a thickened, retracted tympanic membrane with adhesions (A) (spontaneous type III tympanoplasty), a thick middle ear mucoperiosteum (*parallel arrows*), and involvement of the mastoid with a chronic inflammatory process. If the mastoid and antrum are not explored, disease will be inadvertently left behind and the procedure will be inadequate. This case should be approached systematically as described in the text.

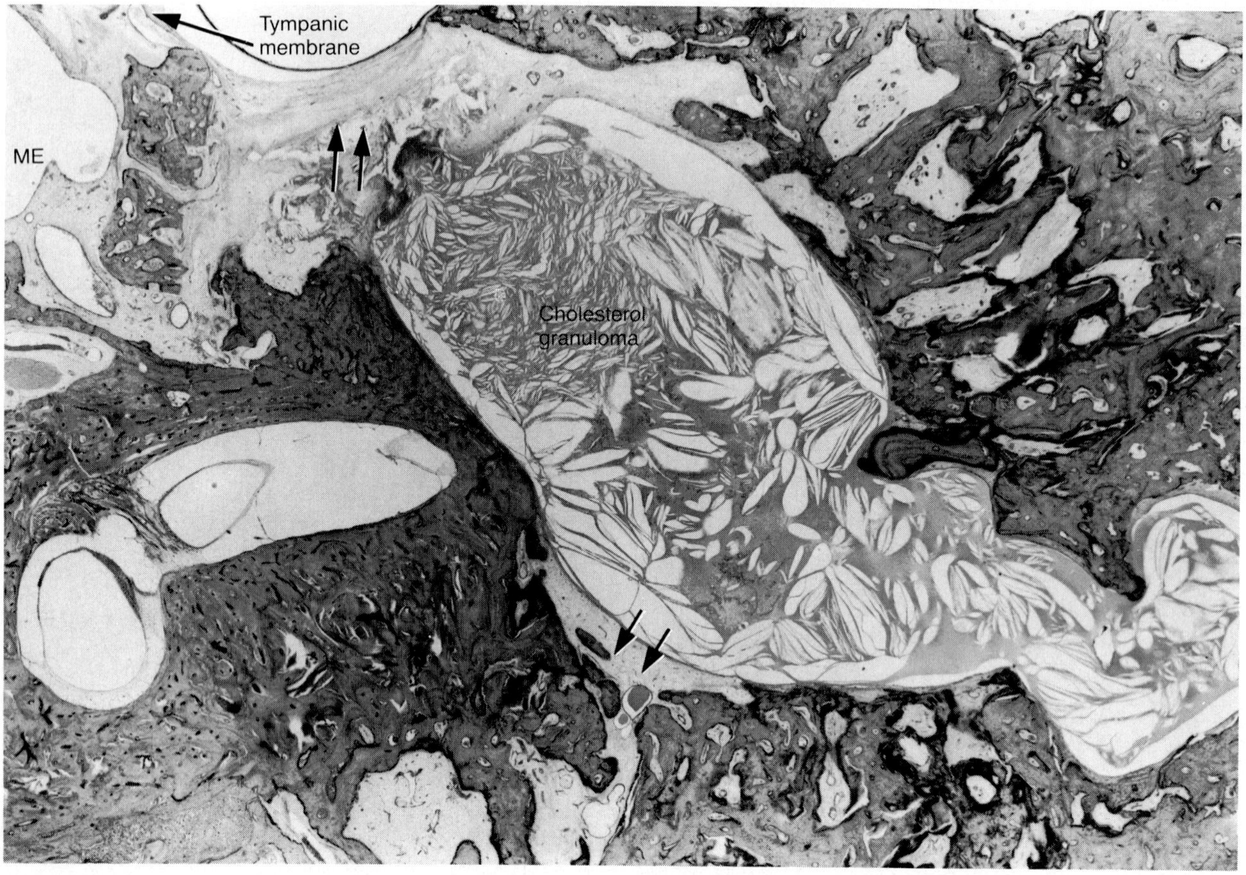

FIGURE 10–31.

FIGURES 10–31, 10–32

These two sections are from an individual who had chronic otitis media behind an intact tympanic membrane, with a large cholesterol granuloma and inflammatory tissue (*parallel arrows*) occupying the mastoid and antrum. ME = middle ear. The cholesterol granuloma and granulation tissue eroded the bone, and the mass shown in Figure 10–32 was found in the middle cranial fossa. This was not the cause of death.

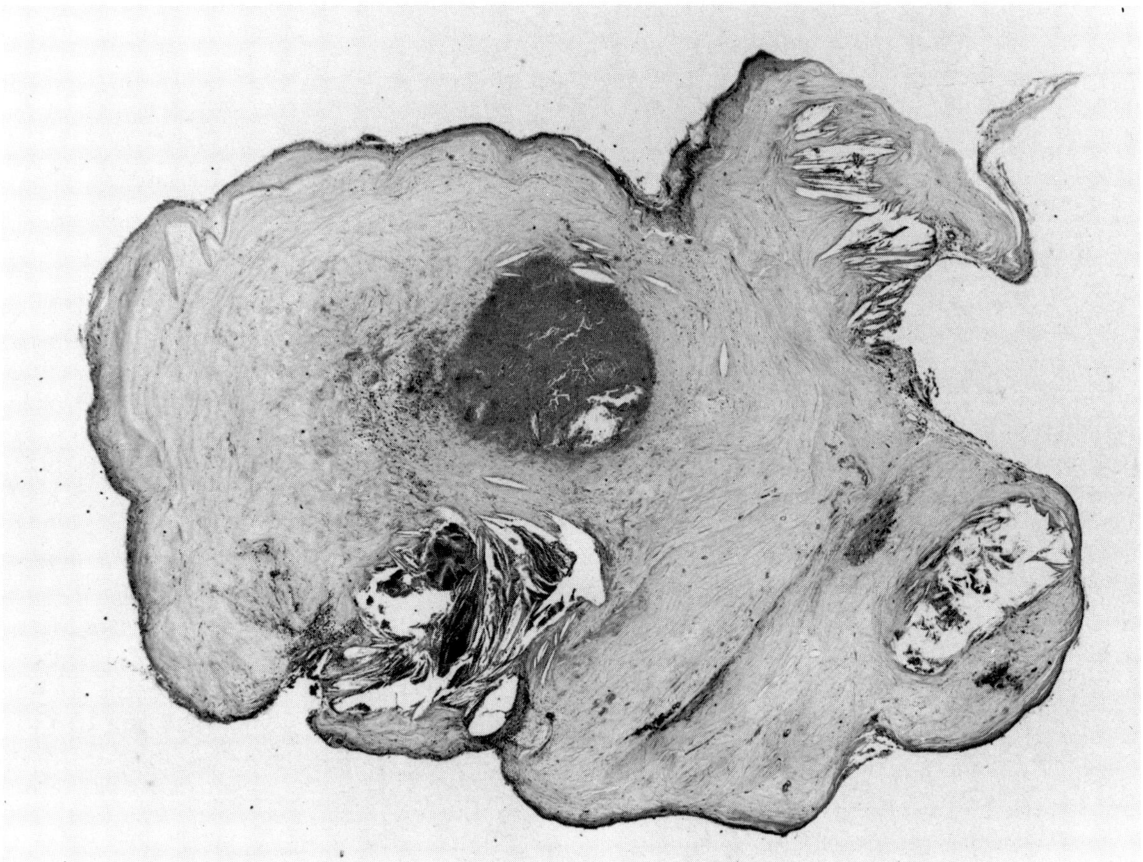

FIGURE 10–32.

CHAPTER 11

Exploratory Tympanotomy

The exploratory tympanotomy (exploration of the middle ear cavity) is highlighted in this chapter as an extremely helpful and innocuous diagnostic and, often, therapeutic procedure. As an integral part of a tympanoplasty, it is therapeutic; used in the presence of an intact tympanic membrane when a diagnosis of ear disease is in doubt, it is diagnostic. This exploration can be performed as a transcanal procedure (when suspected disease is limited to the middle ear) or as an endaural procedure (when suspected disease involves the attic or mastoid, or both). The tympanotomy can be done under local or general anesthesia (depending on the case), and can be used under many different clinical circumstances, such as in cases of unexplained conductive hearing loss and occasional sensorineural hearing losses (for example, if there is suspicion of perilymphatic fistulae), or when the presence of adhesions or a loculated middle ear effusion is suspected. This chapter discusses the use of the exploratory tympanotomy for possible perilymphatic fistulae and for tympanic neurectomy; these topics do not fit into other chapters. The essential concept is that exploratory tympanotomy, which can be used routinely as a safe and simple diagnostic procedure for a variety of middle ear conditions, is also potentially therapeutic.

Exploratory Tympanotomy for Perilymphatic Fistula

Perilymphatic fistulae have no consistent pathognomonic signs. Although some patients may have clearly suggestive symptoms, such as hearing fluctuations associated with vestibular disturbances, tinnitus, and a positive fistula test, more often than not the symptoms are isolated and require a high degree of suspicion on the part of the surgeon.

Fistulae can involve the round window or oval window, or both, and at times even the lateral semicircular canal. They can be caused by implosive or explosive forces; thus they are not entities by themselves but manifestations of an underlying or causative problem. Fistulae caused by granulation tissue, cholesteatoma, and other factors constitute different clinical entities from those discussed here; they are described in different chapters and can involve structures other than the oval and round windows.

Round window fistulae do not necessarily imply a flow of perilymph as an essential element for the diagnosis. Since the approximate average volumes of perilymph and endolymph are 78.3 and 2.76 cu mm respectively, "a free flow of perilymph from the round window" or "a free flow of endolymph after opening the endolymphatic sac" can only be accounted for by other explanations. Free "fluid" gushing from the round window is not perilymph but cerebrospinal fluid and requires a patent cochlear aqueduct and modiolus. At the same time, when this anatomic pathway is not present there is no "free flow," although a fistula still exists.

Procedure

Local or general anesthesia can be used. Exploratory tympanotomy flaps and entrance into the middle ear beneath the annulus have been described in previous chapters. The posterior canal is lowered with curettes in order to clearly visualize the round and oval windows. (If involvement of the lateral semicircular canal is suspected, an endaural approach is preferred.)

The middle ear cavity, including both windows, is completely inspected. It should be noted whether the round window membrane is visible or in a covered position in the niche. It is also important to distinguish the membrane itself from mucosal folds in the niche (the so-called "false membrane").

A fistula may be obvious at this point (Fig. 11–1*A*). If not, the ossicular chain is mobilized and gently palpated and the windows are observed for leaks. The presence or absence of a round window reflex (when mobilizing the ossicular chain) is to be noted; if the window is not visible, a few drops of saline solution can be placed in the niche in order to observe such a reflex.

In the presence of obvious leaks or if the reflex is absent, a patch of connective tissue (collagen) is placed over the window and reinforced with Gelfoam (Fig. 11–1*B*). (The round window membrane is three-layered, with a central layer of connective tissue.) In unclear cases, small pieces of Gelfoam are used to

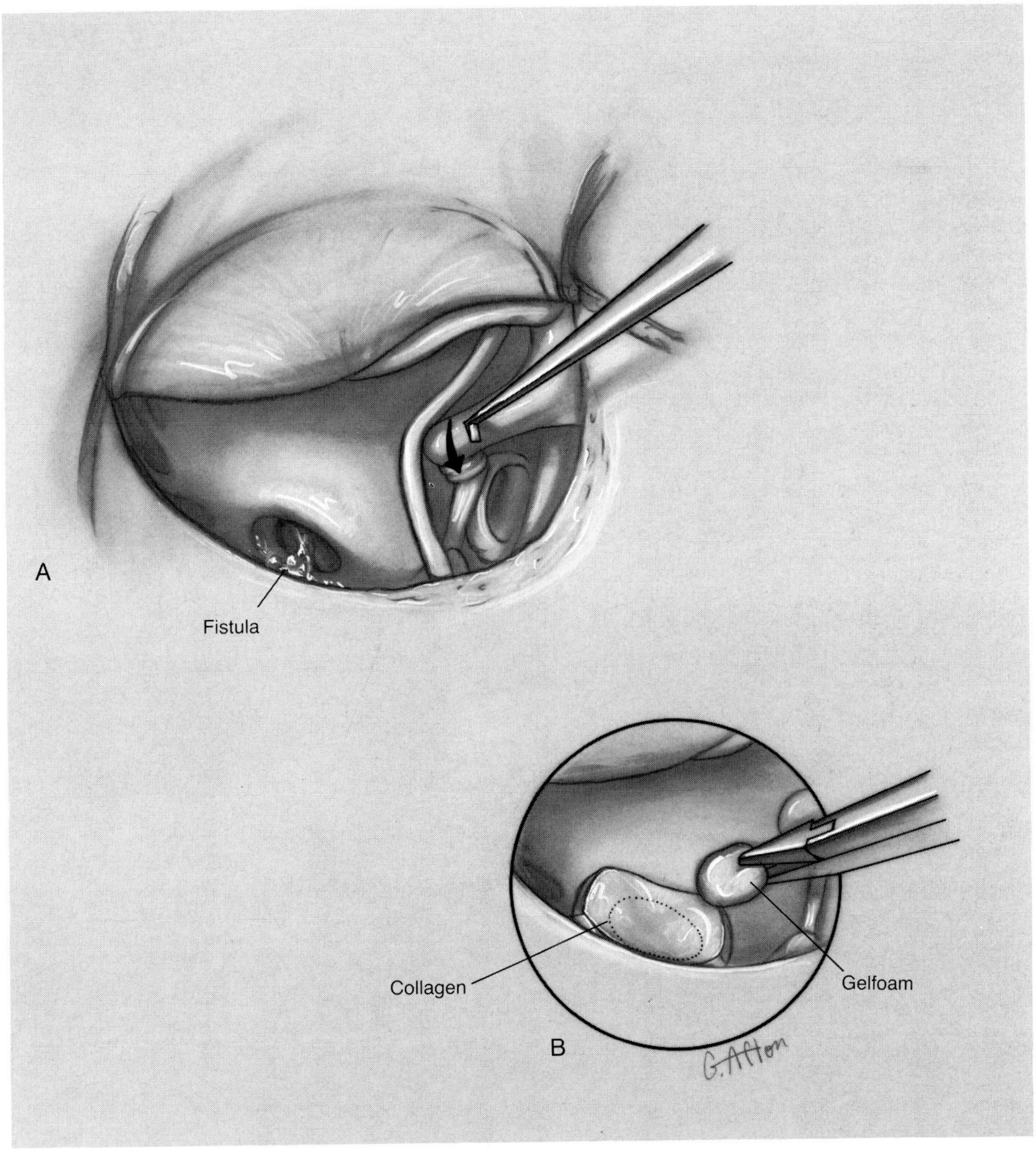

FIGURE 11–1.

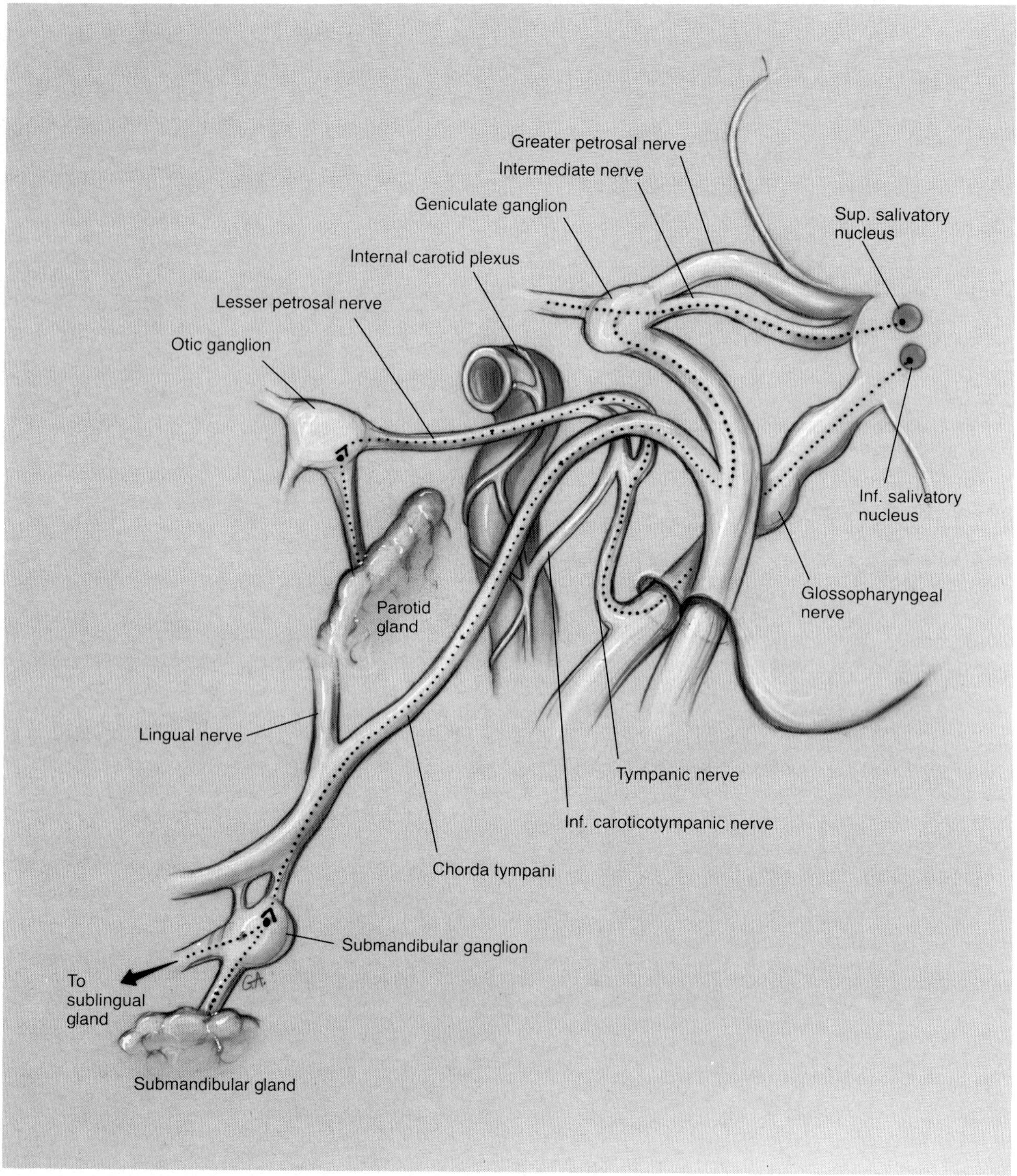
Greater petrosal nerve
Intermediate nerve
Geniculate ganglion
Sup. salivatory nucleus
Internal carotid plexus
Lesser petrosal nerve
Otic ganglion
Inf. salivatory nucleus
Parotid gland
Glossopharyngeal nerve
Lingual nerve
Tympanic nerve
Inf. caroticotympanic nerve
Chorda tympani
Submandibular ganglion
To sublingual gland
Submandibular gland

FIGURE 11–2.

cover such areas since small fistulae may not be visually evident. (If the procedure is being done under local anesthesia the patient can be asked to perform Valsalva's maneuver.)

The flaps are repositioned, the ear canal is packed, and a dressing is applied.

Tympanic Neurectomy

A tympanic neurectomy implies transection of the tympanic plexus with or without division of the chorda tympani. It is used mainly for cases of drooling and chronic parotitis. Some surgeons have used this procedure to treat certain forms of aural pain and even tinnitus. The rationale for its primary uses is founded on the parasympathetic innervation of the sublingual and submandibular glands (via the chorda tympani) and of the parotid gland (via the tympanic plexus). Other indications are based on the multiple sites of interconnection of these nerve endings with other nerves in this small anatomic area (which is not clearly defined) (Fig. 11–2).

Procedure

Exploratory tympanotomy flaps and entrance of the middle ear beneath the annulus have already been described. Initially, the chorda tympani is isolated and a piece sharply removed. This is followed by a careful search of the branches of the tympanic plexus traversing inferiorly to superiorly from the hypotympanum via the promontory prominence (Fig. 11–3*A*). For easier visualization, Gelfoam pledgets saturated with epinephrine solution can be applied to the hypotympanum and promontory (blood vessels may obscure visualization of these thin fibers). *Pieces* of the nerves (at least 3 mm in length) should be removed (Fig. 11–3*B*). It is important to remember that some nerves traverse the promontory through bony grooves and need to be curetted carefully. Drilling should be avoided. On occasion, accompanying vessels can be relatively large (for the area); minor localized bleeding might require application of Gelfoam saturated in epinephrine solution. It is also important to visualize the hypotympanum; in about 50% of cases a larger hypotympanic branch is present (Fig. 11–3C). This branch, which sometimes has an anterior direction, should be located.

The area is packed with small pieces of compressed Gelfoam, the flap is repositioned, and the ear is packed.

Results are consistently satisfactory in the short term, but after a year reinnervation seems to occur in *at least* 30% of cases (usually more). The explanation for this, as well as for the recovery of taste after sectioning of the chorda tympani, is unclear. A discussion of this phenomenon is outside the scope of this book.

Pertinent Histopathology

FIGURES 11–4 TO 11–6

These three photomicrographs of horizontal sections of temporal bones show the nerves of the tympanic plexus (TP), accompanied by their corresponding blood vessels (BV) in bony canals within the promontory. These are important anatomic factors to be considered for a proper neurectomy. Additionally, Figures 11–5 and 11–6 show a thickened mucoperiosteum overlying the promontory, making identification of these grooves very difficult. The surgeon must "peel" this mucoperiosteum.

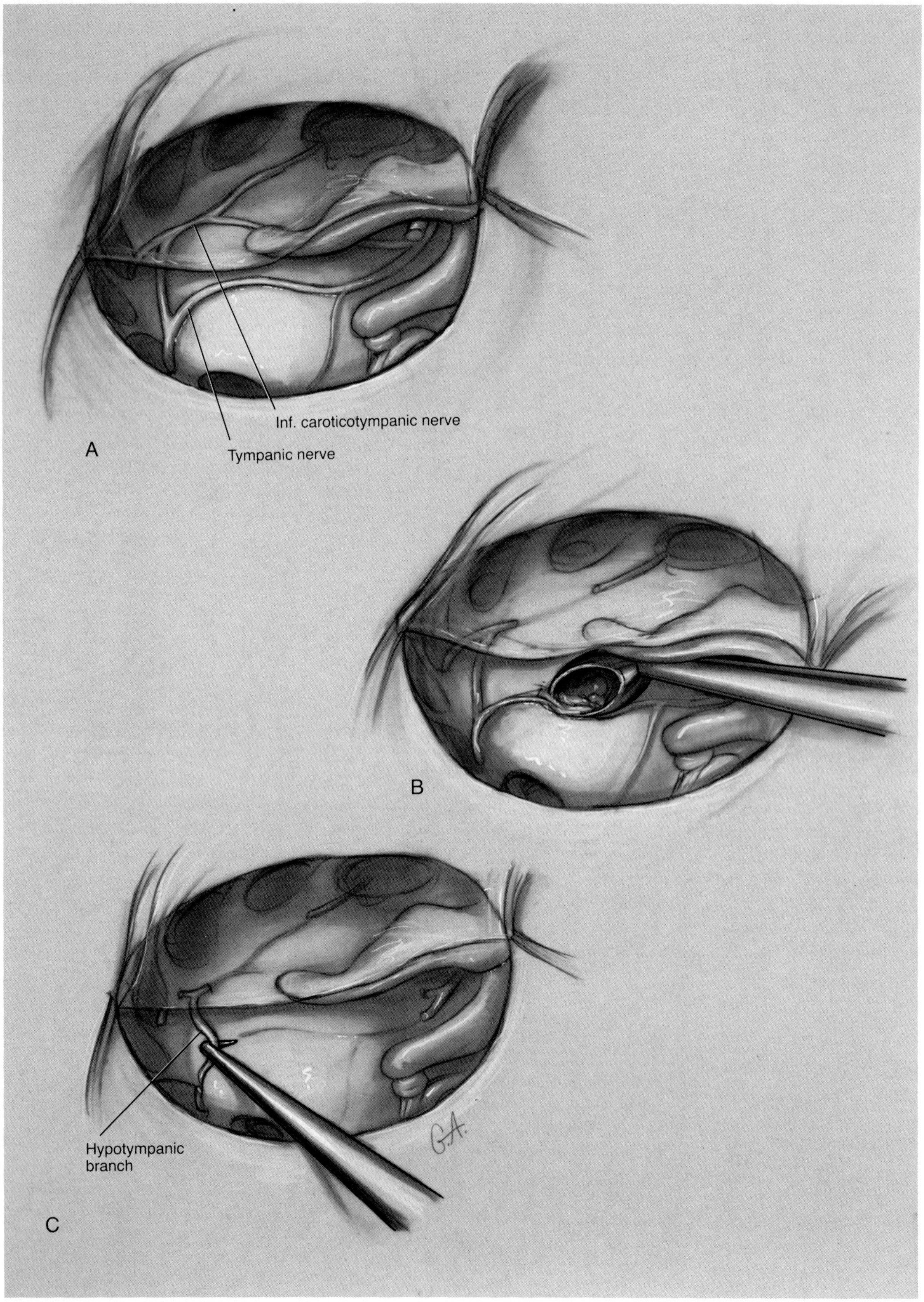
Inf. caroticotympanic nerve
A
Tympanic nerve
B
Hypotympanic
branch
C

FIGURE 11–3.

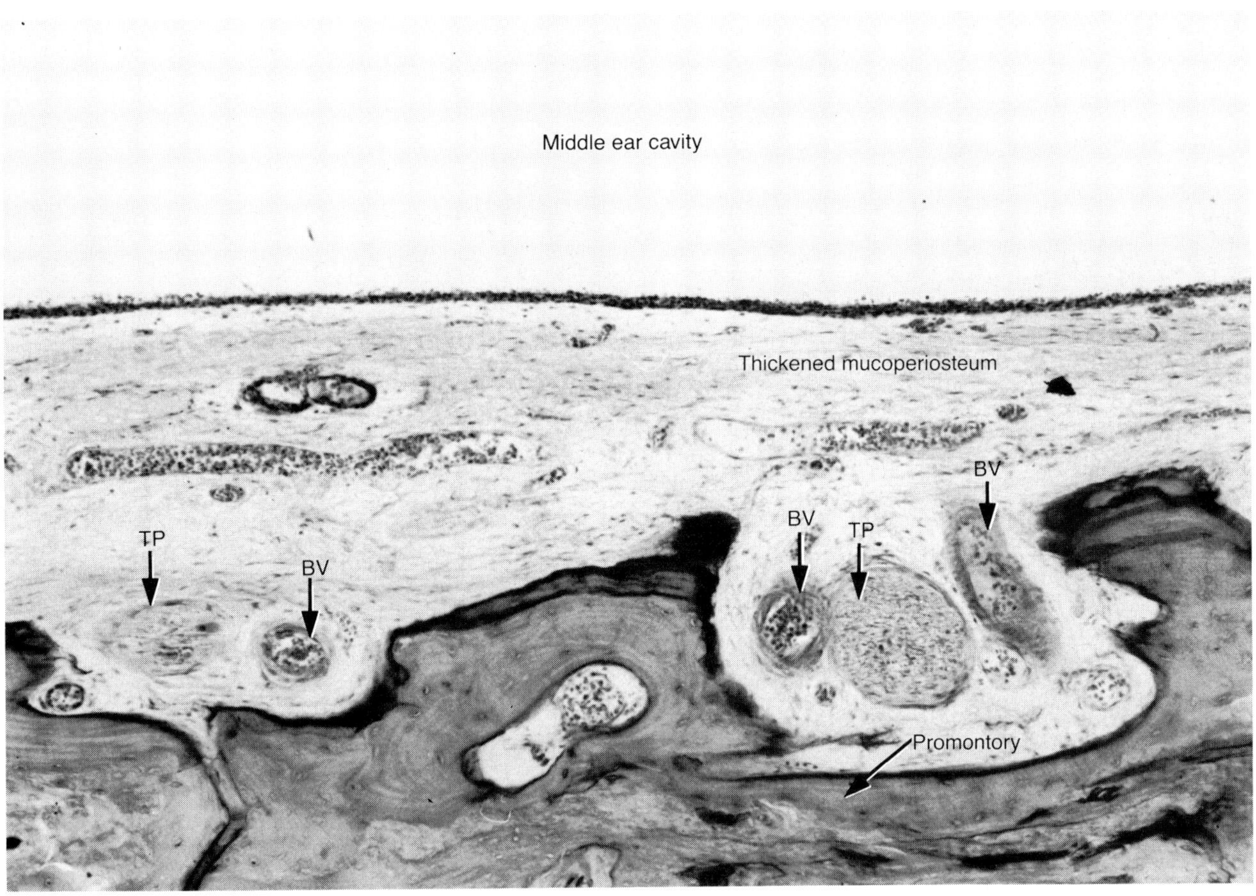
Middle ear cavity
Thickened mucoperiosteum
BV
BV
TP
TP
BV
Promontory

FIGURE 11–4.

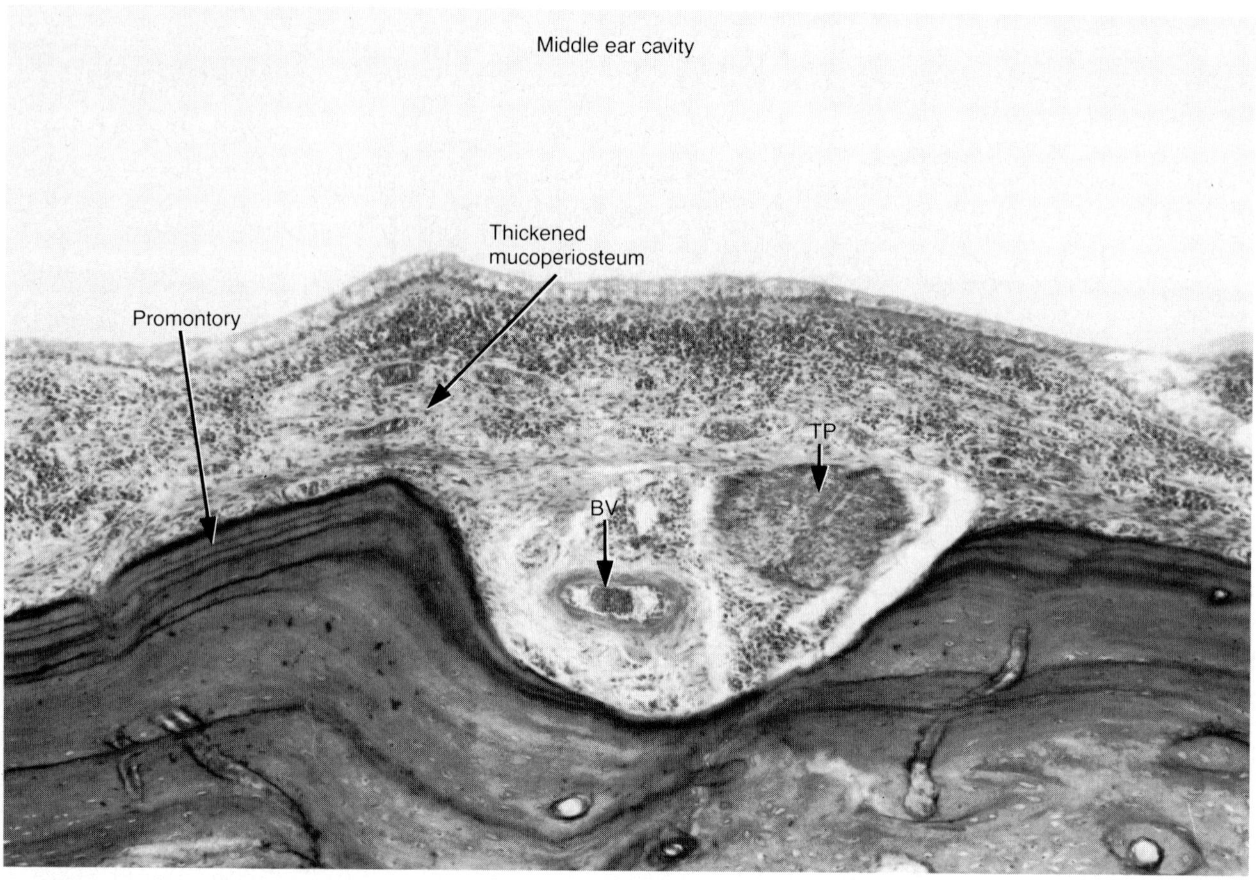
Middle ear cavity
Thickened mucoperiosteum
Promontory
TP
BV

FIGURE 11–5.

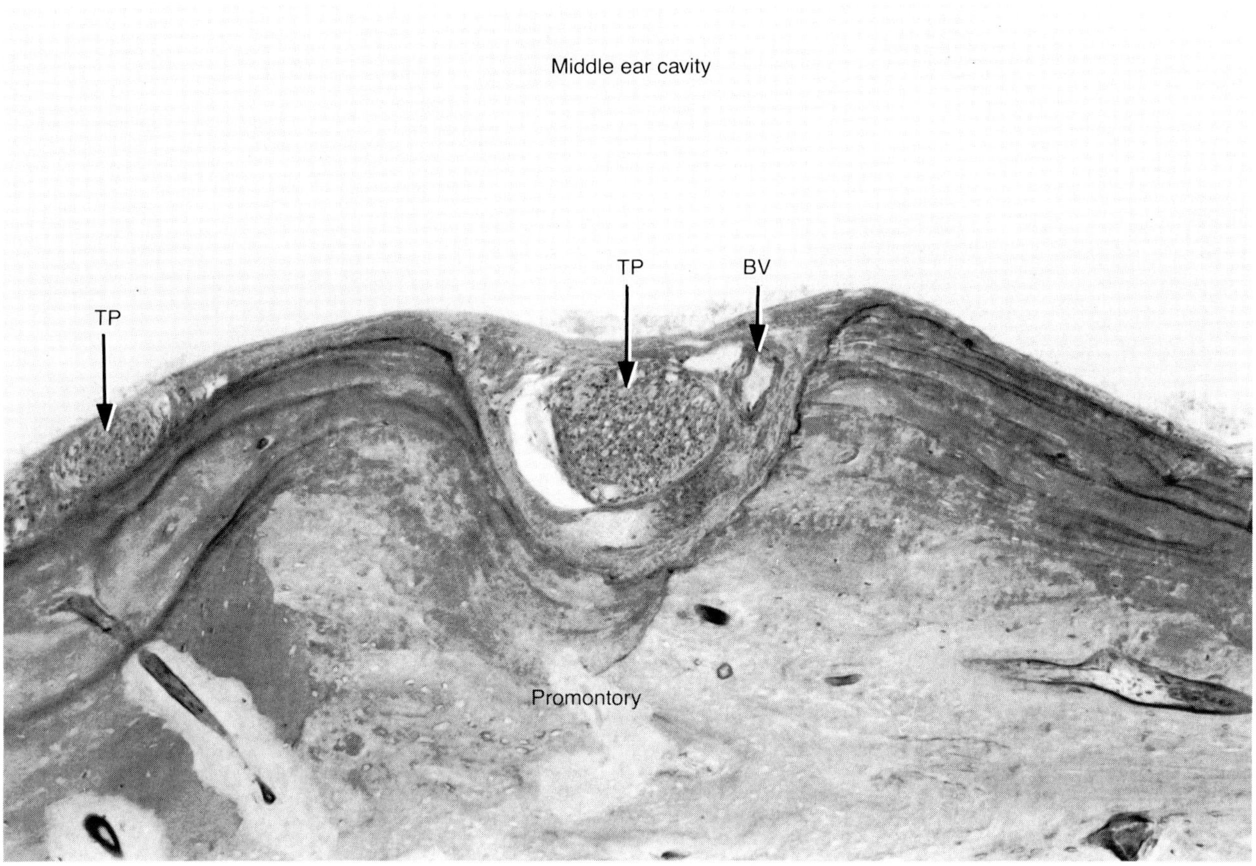

FIGURE 11–6.

CHAPTER 12

Tympanoplasty

Overview

The aim of a tympanoplasty is surgical reconstruction of the damaged tympano-ossicular chain. The basic principles involved are eradication of disease, reconstruction of the tympanic membrane and the sound transformer mechanism, and re-establishment of an aerated cavity. Ideally, the operations discussed in this chapter are performed solely to restore function, with the originating or underlying disease well under control. They are also performed when there are several indications (for example, a tympanomastoidectomy).

These procedures involve the following steps:

1. Thorough evaluation of the status of the patient and the affected ear as a whole.
2. A surgical approach based on the patient's needs.
3. Complete visualization and exploration of the ear.
4. Assessment.
5. Reconstruction (only after steps 1 through 4 are done).
6. Closure and methodical postoperative follow-up.

In order to succeed, tympanoplasty must be approached as a rational method of reconstruction and not as a mere surgical technique. Thorough knowledge of all interdependent factors and available alternatives is essential.

Evaluation entails knowledge of the originating disease, its pathogenesis, and its current status at the time of surgery. The disease can be inflammatory, traumatic, congenital, or neoplastic, and its status can be active, progressive, regressive, latent, or resolved. In large part, the results will depend upon this evaluation and consequent decisions. Adequate planning can lead to a good "recipient" ear for reconstruction and a so-called "dry ear" for surgery. This can make the practical difference between performing a tympanoplasty or a tympanomastoidectomy.

In addition to the status of the middle ear mucosa and the underlying disease, certain important anatomic elements must be considered.

1. A wide ear canal. (A wide, well-aerated canal provides sound transmission, promotes healing, and facilitates cleansing and inspection.)
2. A vibrating, intact tympanic membrane.
3. Properly functioning oval and round windows.
4. A well-aerated middle ear cavity:
   A. Eustachian tube.
   B. Mastoid air cells.
   C. Proper mastoid–middle ear communication.

Classifications of Tympanoplasty

There are many systems of classifications that, in one sense or another, contribute to an overall understanding of these procedures. For purposes of orientation two useful ones are described here, with the expectation that the reader will rationalize them based on his or her own understanding of the problem. This necessarily will lead to agreement or challenge, and not to a "have to learn it" attitude.

Zöllner and Wullstein classified tympanoplasties into the following five types:

Type I. The tympanic membrane is perforated; the ossicular chain is intact and mobile. The graft is placed against the malleus.

Type II. The ossicular chain is partially destroyed, but its continuity is preserved. Either the malleus is damaged (anatomic type II) or an atticoantrotomy has been done, and the graft is placed against the incus or malleus, or both (physiologic type II).

Type III. The malleus and incus are missing, and there is an intact and mobile stapes. The graft is placed against the stapes.

Type IV. The malleus, incus, head, and crura of the stapes are missing. There is a mobile footplate. The graft is placed against the footplate.

Type V. This is similar to type IV, but there is a fixed footplate. The horizontal semicircular canal is fenestrated, and the graft is placed against it and the fixed footplate. Paparella differentiates between types V*a,* which refers to the classic type described, and V*b,* which refers to a purposeful, complete stapedectomy in selected cases, with the graft invaginated into the open window.

Farrior classified tympanoplasty according to the basic pathologic anatomy at the completion of the surgery. He identified the following types:

Type I. Tympanic membrane reconstruction with an intact ossicular chain.

Type II. Reconstruction of a new tympanic membrane in its natural position.

Type III. Reconstruction of a new tympanic membrane on top of a mobile stapes. This is divided into the following subcategories:

III—Classic.
III IG—Incus graft.
III IGM—Incus graft to malleus.
III MG—Malleus head graft.
III BG—Bone graft.
III PORP—Partial ossicular replacement prosthesis.

Type IV. Reconstruction of a new tympanic membrane and columella or footplate of stapes. This is divided into the following subcategories:

IV—Classic.
IV IG—Incus graft.
IV MG—Malleus graft.
IV BG—Bone graft.
IV CG—Cartilage graft.
IV TORP—Total ossicular replacement prosthesis.

Type V. Reconstruction of the tympanic membrane, either over a fistula in the horizontal semicircular canal or with secondary fenestration of the horizontal semicircular canal.

Procedures to be performed, either alone or in combination, include the following:

1. Tympanic membranes—myringoplasty/tympanoplasty.
2. Ossicular chain—tympanoplasty/ossiculoplasty.
3. Labyrinthine windows—tympanoplasty with stapedectomy.
4. Aeration factors—eustachian tube (PE tube), mastoid air cells, mastoid middle ear communication (mastoidotomy/mastoidectomy).
5. Tympanomastoid cavity—tympanomastoidectomy.

A number of grafts and materials can be used in a tympanoplasty. For the purposes of an overall concept, some basic aspects are described here. Knowledge of these elements is essential and further study is recommended, especially in these days when the surgeon must "swim in a sea of gadgets." It is of paramount importance to remember at all times that the surgeon is responsible to the patient. Manufacturers (no matter how dedicated and ethical) are responsible to a board of directors and ultimately to the stockholders. Although it is essential to work side by side with industry for the good of the patient, the decision of what to use and how to use it belongs to the surgeon.

Grafts

Grafts are classified by the relationship between the donor and the recipient into the following categories:

1. Autograft (adjective, autologous). Donor and recipient are of the same organism.
2. Isograft (isogeneic). Donor and recipient are twins (with the same genotype).
3. Allograft or homograft (allogeneic, homologous). Donor and recipient have different genotypes.
4. Xenograft or heterograft (xenogeneic, heterologous). Donor and recipient are different species.

In addition to tissues, other sources and materials are available. They include plastic, metals, and ceramics (alloplastic materials); and denatured animal skin gelatin, film (Gelfilm), and sponge (Gelfoam). In order to achieve a safe, long-term graft, additional criteria must be considered.

1. Biocompatibility—the reaction of the implant in the body (such as presence or absence of cytotoxicity), and influence of the body on the implant (for example, degradation).
2. Biofunctionality—symbiosis of the implant with the implant site.

In terms of its interaction with the body, a material can be:

1. Bioinert—no reaction of the surface to the body (at most a small, fibrous capsule is seen).
2. Biotolerant—good capsule around it without signs of marked cellular activity (such as giant cells).
3. Bioactive—bonding of the material with the surrounding tissue.

Grafting of the Tympanic Membrane

The tympanic membrane has three layers: (1) an outer (lateral) stratified squamous epithelium (continuous with that of the ear canal); (2) a middle connective tissue core containing collagen and elastic fibers (plus the vascular elements); and (3) an inner layer (continuous with that of the middle ear mucoperiosteum).

Perforations that heal spontaneously tend to exclude the connective tissue layer (monomeric membrane). Those membranes that do not heal tend to have ingrowth of the outer squamous epithelium covering the edges of the perforation. The aim of grafting is a truly anatomic reconstruction. The collagen layer placed as a graft reinstates the middle layer, allows epithelial cells to migrate, re-establishes continuity, and permits the membrane to recover its vibratory characteristics. This supports the concepts of reinforcing monomeric membranes and peeling the edges of a perforation before grafting.

Tissues and Materials

Skin. Skin is very useful for covering raw areas in mastoid bowls and meatoplasty. It also provides coverage and, at times, vascularity (in pedicled grafts) over collagen grafts; this gives additional thickness and, more importantly, protects the graft from infection and granulation tissue. It must be remembered that a free collagen graft (for example, fascia) has no blood supply of its own (when originally placed), and is an easy prey for infection and granulation tissue. As useful as skin may be, however, it does not replace collagen grafts. Placed by itself as sole coverage of a perforation, it is doomed to failure. Skin can be obtained as a split-thickness graft (0.003 to 0.004 cm) from a non–hair-bearing area from the upper arm, forearm, thigh, or abdomen, by using a dermatome (DaSilva-Doval-Silver) or a plain razor blade on a straight clamp (Fig. 12–1*A*). It can also be a full-thickness graft from the postauricular region (Fig. 12–1*B*) or the posterior canal skin (for example, via a Lempert II incision [Fig. 12–1C]), or from the medial canal skin as a free or pedicled graft. Pedicled skin grafts have the disadvantage of being thick and cumbersome to work with, but they have their own blood supply.

Collagen. Sources of collagen are mainly the fascia, the perichondrium, and the veins. The most commonly used fascia is the temporal, which is available via the same approach incision or a small separate incision, but in the same operative field (Fig. 12–1*D*, *E*). It is important to obtain fascia proper and not the layer of aerolar connective tissue overlying it, the so-called "fool's fascia" (the latter also has collagen and can be used for grafting). Perichondrium can also be obtained easily from the tragus as such, or as a cartilage-perichondrium graft (see Chapter 10). It can also come from conchal cartilage.

A vein from the dorsum of the hand also is easily obtainable (see Chapter 13). In addition, allogeneic (homologous) perichondrium from the tibia, septum, costochondral cartilage, and so on can be used, as well as allogeneic dura mater, amniotic membrane, and cornea. The authors have no experience with the last three; reports on their use, as well as on other tissues (such as heart valves), are not definitive.

Allogeneic tympanic membrane grafts are very successful (under the proper circumstances), and represent a good anatomic and functional alternative. A long-term drawback is that of viruses living in donor tissue; this might compromise the use of allogeneic grafts in the future.

The ideal graft material would be pure collagen and elastic fibers capable of providing the middle layer, becoming incorporated to the membrane, and allowing and favoring epithelial migration.

Xenogeneic (heterologous) materials, such as bovine dura mater, are currently being evaluated by some groups and, if successful, could eventually become available.

Grafting of the Ossicular Chain

These three interlocked ossicles (under the protective influence of two middle ear muscles), which transmit sound waves as a unit from the tympanic membrane to the oval window, can be partly or totally fixated, dislocated, or destroyed. The purpose of grafting is to re-establish functional continuity from the tympanic membrane to the oval window. Ideally, grafts and materials should be easily positioned and shaped; be readily available; cause minimal tissue reaction; remain stable with infection; and remain in position, not extruding or damaging the tympanic membrane. Common complications include resorption, rejection, fixation, displacement, and extrusion. A brief overall assessment follows; a comprehensive description is outside the scope of this book.

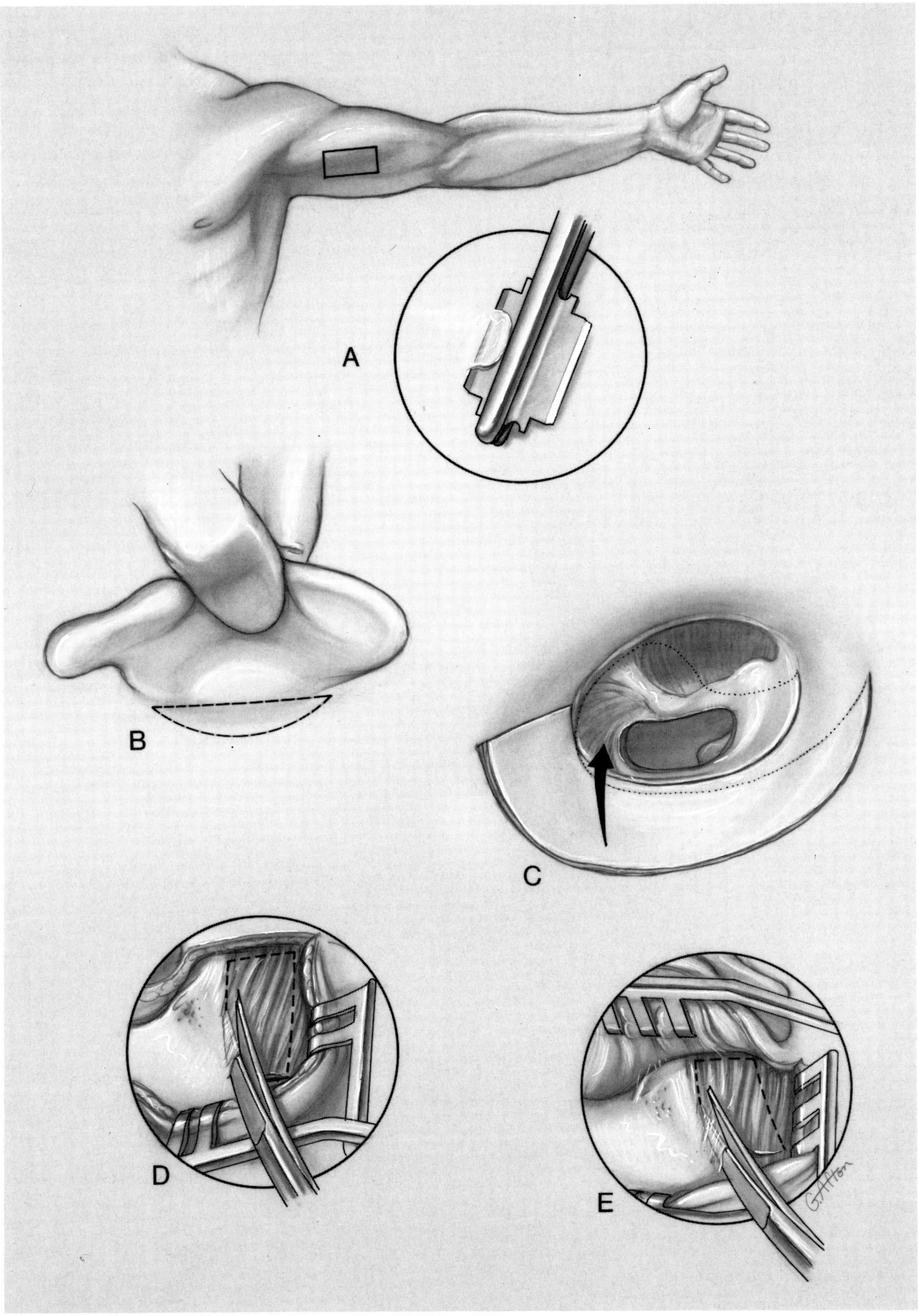

FIGURE 12–1.

Tissues and Materials

Ossicles and Cortical Bone. Ossicular and cortical bone (autologous or allogeneic) grafts are available, are easily sculptured, are the best tolerated, and are least likely to extrude. Their drawbacks include displacement, refixation, and a tendency to adhere to the margins of the oval window, to extrude or displace if there is no malleus (the latter is common to all prostheses), and to atrophy.

Cartilage. Cartilage (autologous or allogeneic) grafts are available, are easily shaped and well tolerated, and show very little extrusion. However, cartilage lacks stiffness, working well at the onset but tending to lose rigidity and "fall apart" after a few years (this is supported by some reports but denied by others). In addition, cartilage tolerates infection poorly.

Plastics. Teflon is used primarily as a piston for a stapedectomy. Although this solid plastic has smooth surfaces, it has no long-term inflammatory reaction. An excellent material when properly used, it is not efficient as a TORP (total ossicular replacement prosthesis). Teflon is a good material for PE tubes.

Plastipore (high-density polyethylene), which has been used in TORPs and PORPs, is still a subject of controversy. Its initially impressive success was followed by an equally unimpressive and disappointing failure in terms of extrusion rate. Plastipore is easily available; is not so rigid as ossicles or ceramics; can be easily shaped according to need; is biomechanically sound; is relatively easy to position and sterilize (this requires skill to do properly); does not adhere to the margins of the oval window; and is an efficient sound conductor. Its drawbacks are that it causes a foreign body reaction in the middle ear, and can extrude and slip. The high extrusion rate is significantly diminished by placing cartilage over the prosthesis (beneath the tympanic membrane or tympanic membrane graft, ideally under the malleus). Slippage at the oval window (when placed over intact, mobile footplates) can be reduced by creating a small opening in the footplate, through which a TORP with a peg in its distal end is inserted (described below). PORPs can be stabilized by making a slit that allows a more stable contact with the stapes head. In spite of these drawbacks, TORPs and PORPs made of Plastipore work very well in properly selected cases and remain a first choice under the proper conditions.

Ceramics. Ceramics, inorganic crystal materials produced at high temperatures, are the "in" materials in ossiculoplasty and reconstructive ear surgery. They have been used successfully in orthopedics and dentistry. Glass-ceramics are produced by thermally treating glass, obtaining a polycrystalline microstructure. The advantages of these dense materials are that they are biocompatible, biofunctional, easy to place and manipulate, and, reportedly, easy to shape. The authors have found, however, that they are hard to reshape and sometimes break, even when shaped with a diamond drill under constant irrigation. Although promising, these materials have still to withstand the test of time in otology. Evidence suggests that they probably will; time and experience should tell us (not the manufacturers). In prosthetics, the most commonly used ceramic is the bioactive, porous, crystalline form of calcium phosphate. Bioglass is an example of glass and ceravital, a form of calcium phosphate with the same calcium-to-phosphate ratio as the natural bone mineral hydroxyapatite, which is perhaps the most biocompatible material available. The essential aim in prosthetics is to obtain materials that are as close to natural as possible, fulfilling the concept of "replacing with same."

Plastics. Silastic is commonly used in middle ear surgery as thin sheets and as PE tubes. It is bioinert (that is, it elicits no long-term inflammatory reaction); its uses are (1) to prevent adhesions when placed over rough, lacerated surfaces or surrounding prostheses or grafts, thus allowing an aerated open space; and (2) to avoid adhesions between different middle ear structures that could compromise their function. If not positioned properly or trimmed smoothly at the edges, it can extrude. Specific uses are described in various chapters of this book.

Gelfoam. Gelfoam (denatured animal skin gelatin) is used universally in otologic surgery. This absorbable gelatin is available as a sterile powder, sponge, or film (0.075 mm thick). Only the last two forms are used. The sterile sponge form, which is capable of absorbing and holding within its meshes many times its weight in whole blood, is absorbed completely in four to six weeks. It is used as a hemostatic agent, to pack the middle ear cavity, to apply pressure between the graft and the tympanic membrane, to promote a mild inflammatory reaction needed at certain points, and as a vehicle for antibiotic-steroid solutions. Gelfilm is an apparently brittle film that becomes soft and rubbery when moistened in saline. It is used to discourage adhesions, such as in separation of the incudostapedial joint from the tympanic membrane. In its dry form, Gelfoam should be decompressed; when saturated, it should be squeezed in order to remove air bubbles. Gelfilm is not useful as a graft for tympanic membrane perforations.

Gelfoam swells as it absorbs fluid. As it expands, it impinges on neighboring structures (which is why it works well in filling the middle ear cavity when an underlay graft is placed). Gelfoam potentially may become a focus of infection.

Tissue Adhesions ("Glues"). Glues have been the dream of many otologists for years. Histoacryl (cyanobutyl acrylate) and Fibrin, the two types that are available, work fairly acceptably but are far from ideal. Either they must await the test of time or we must await a better adhesive. The description of them is beyond the scope of this book.

Myringoplasty–Type I Tympanoplasty

A myringoplasty and a type I tympanoplasty involve repair of the tympanic membrane alone. "Myringoplasty" is the term used when the operation does not include raising flaps to enter the middle ear cavity, whereas a type I tympanoplasty implies the opposite. Different types of tympanoplasties and ossiculoplasties involve procedures in the different structures of the middle ear at or beyond (medial to) the tympanic membrane. The broad term "tympanoplasty" is used for any procedure whose purpose is to eradicate disease and reconstruct the hearing mechanism with or without tympanic membrane grafting. Provided that all the interdependent factors previously described are under control, an overall analysis of the required procedure involves several aspects.

The anatomy of the tympanic membrane must be considered. This includes not only the site and extent of the perforation but also the status of the membrane (atrophic, atelectatic, with tympanosclerotic plaques, and so on). Based on this information, an approach is selected, types of skin flaps (if any) and grafting material to be used are chosen, and positioning of the graft is decided (underlay under the membrane or overlay over the membrane).

A tympanic membrane perforation may be restricted to one quadrant alone—the posterosuperior, posteroinferior, anterosuperior, or anteroinferior. A perforation of Shrapnell's membrane constitutes an exception to this; exploration is advised in all cases. Because of the anatomic position of Shrapnell's membrane, epithelial ingrowth is always a possibility, even with a normal audiogram (for example, a "conductive" cholesteatoma). A perforation also can involve more than one quadrant (Fig. 12–2*A, B*), or it may involve the annulus. It can be total (Fig. 12–2C), central, or marginal. If there are several perforations, underlying disease (such as tuberculosis) should be looked for (Fig. 12–2*D, E*). The tympanic membrane itself may be normal, atrophic, sclerotic, thick, retracted, or adhesive.

These conditions give an index of such factors as the underlying cause, eustachian tube function, aeration, vascularity of the membrane, and so on. All of these will affect the graft take and influence the selection of the type of repair.

Approach

There are no fixed rules for achieving the final purpose, which is adequate visualization through an open canal, allowing a good assessment and repair. The approach should provide a clear visualization around the borders of the perforation and, ideally, clear visualization of the entire annulus. Otologists should be capable of adapting the approach to the needs of the case and not vice versa. There are a number of situations in which one approach has certain advantages over others. They will be highlighted with the understanding that all guidelines are relative.

The alternative approaches are the transcanal, the endaural, and the postauricular. A transcanal approach is used in general for small perforations, or for medium posterior perforations in a wide canal that allows a clear visualization of the anterior border of the perforation. It is inadequate for perforations that are large or that involve the annulus, or for cases that might need an associated mastoid procedure. An endaural approach provides good visibility, especially of the posterior quadrants. For anterior perforations, an associated canalplasty is necessary. This approach allows a meatoplasty in cases of a small, thick meatus. A postauricular approach also provides good visibility, especially of the anterior margin of the tympanic membrane: it allows this view without a canalplasty. It is useful for medium to large perforations as well as anteroinferior perforations, with or without alteration of the annulus. Regardless of the approach, preservation of the annulus maintains the middle ear space, provides support, and reduces the risk of retraction.

Revision surgery in general is done via an alternate incision that allows a graft to be obtained. The main questions in revisions are (1) Why did the procedure fail initially? (2) Was failure caused by exposure, clinical error, or underlying disease?

Whichever approach is chosen, the canal should be smooth and there should be no bony overhangs. If the annulus is missing, a sulcus (if necessary)

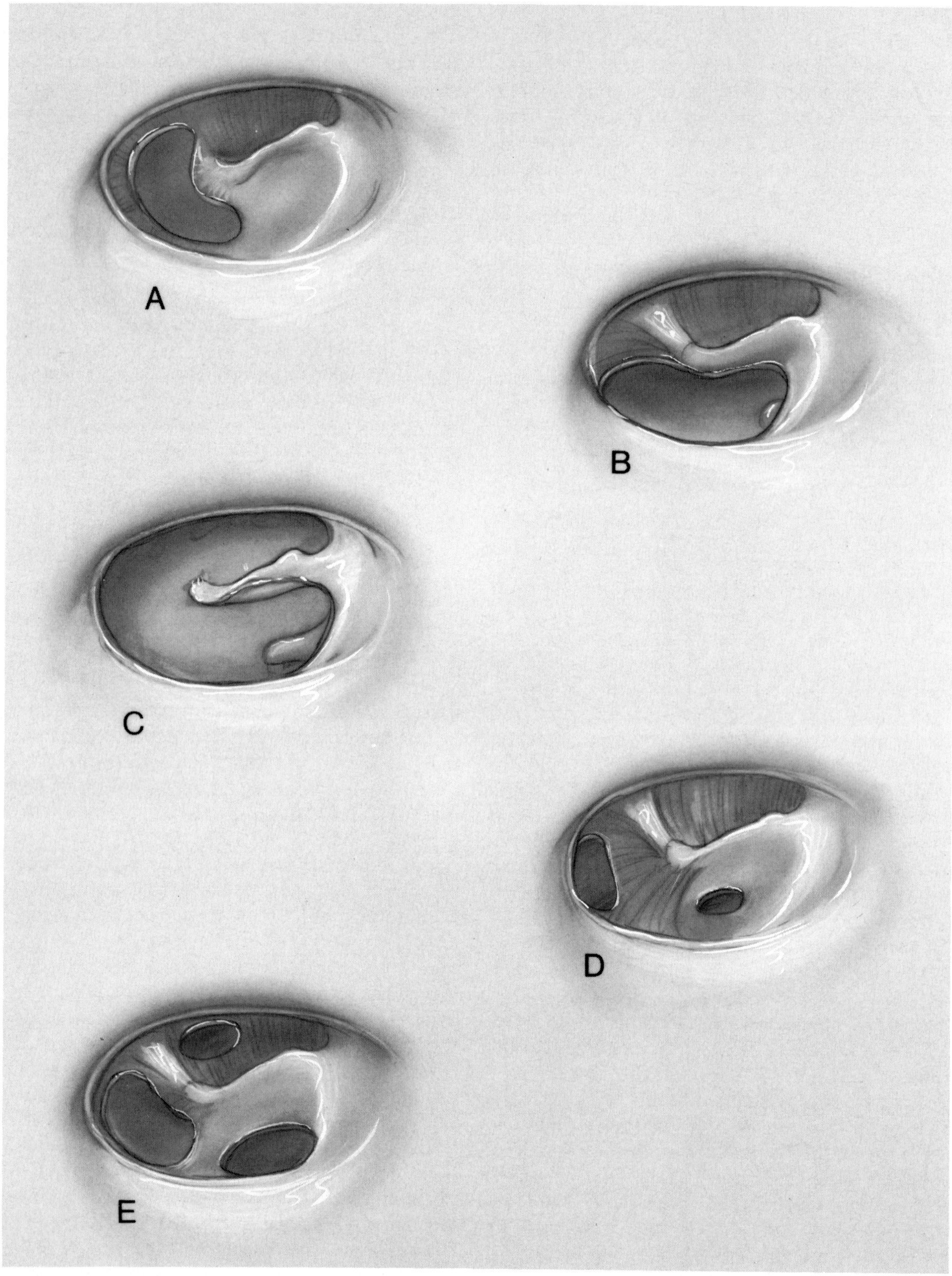

FIGURE 12–2.

should be created (to prevent blunting). If an atticotomy is performed, the attic must be reinforced. If the eustachian tube is dysfunctional a PE tube should be considered.

Once the approach has been selected and performed and the tympanic membrane is visualized, the next decision is the canal incisions to use. (Before elevating the flaps, any tympanic membrane work [such as trimming the edges] should be performed, since it is simpler at this time and the membrane is in its natural position.) The basic principle is to enter the middle ear cavity (type I tympanoplasty) in a way that allows adequate inspection of the cavity and efficient placement of a graft. The alternatives are many and vary according to need and preference, as well as the imagination of the surgeon. A classic posterior canal flap (1 and 6 o'clock vertical incisions) offers adequate exposure in most (if not all) cases and is a good alternative. An anterior or an inferior flap might suffice (Fig. 12–3*A–C*), or a "swinging door" technique can be used (Fig. 12–3*D, E*). If skin reinforcement is needed, a pedicled flap can be utilized. Some of the most commonly used flaps will be described in the discussion of specific procedures. They are simply alternatives and are not necessarily the only choices.

Small Central Perforation

The edges of the perforation are touched with a blunt pick moistened in trichloroacetic acid (Fig. 12–4*A*). Upon contact with the acid, the edges acquire a white appearance. A paper patch (cigarette paper) is applied overlying the perforation (Fig. 12–4*B*). It is important to prevent any acid from falling into the middle ear cavity since this is extremely painful; the instrument should be barely moistened. If this complication occurs, neutral pH otic drops should be used in conjunction with an anti-inflammatory medication. This does not work all the time and can only be used for a small perforation in a healthy membrane.

For tiny central perforations, the edges can be trimmed (Fig. 12–4*C, D*); a small triangle wedge with its base in the annulus is then created (Fig. 12–4*E*). The annulus is elevated (anteroposterior edge) and slid toward the proximal (nonelevated) edge, allowing the edges of the tympanic membrane to come together (Fig. 12–4*F*). Small pieces of Gelfoam are applied over the approximated edges.

For a very small central perforation that requires grafting, the edges are trimmed and the undersurface of the membrane is gently scraped. Instead of raising a flap, an incision is made in the middle of the perforation and toward the annulus (Fig. 12–5*A, B*) The tympanic membrane is carefully reflected, allowing enough space to apply Gelfoam in the middle ear and a medial (underlay) graft (Fig. 12–5*C*). The tympanic membrane is repositioned and Gelfoam is applied over it (Fig. 12–5*D*).

For a small central perforation, an underlay graft is placed through the perforation (Fig. 12–5*E*). The edges of the perforation are trimmed meticulously, and the undersurface of the membrane is gently scraped (freshened); this includes cleansing (if needed) of the manubrium. The middle ear cavity is filled with compressed Gelfoam (Fig. 12–5*F*) and a fascia graft is placed through the perforation, making sure that the edges of the perforation are overlapped by the graft by more than 30%. If needed, a piece of fascia is placed between the tympanic membrane and the long process of the malleus. The malleus handle can be de-epithelialized and a piece of fascia placed laterally.

These procedures require a healthy, well-vascularized tympanic membrane.

Overlay Technique in Central Perforation

Critical Points

1. Complete de-epithelialization.
2. A well-defined, well-placed anterior tympanomeatal angle junction.
3. Attachment of graft to handle of malleus.

Procedure

A postauricular approach has been selected and a temporal fascial graft obtained. The incision of the posterior canal is made at the junction of the lateral and middle thirds of the canal. This procedure involves removal of the canal skin from this junction down to 2 mm lateral to the annulus (excepting the area of skin containing the vascular strip). Vertical incisions are made at 10 and 1 o'clock (Fig. 12–6*A*). Two circumferential incisions are made, the first 2 mm lateral to the annulus (excepting the area between 10 and 1 o'clock) and the second at the junction of the lateral and middle thirds of the canal. (This is an extension of the canal incision along the whole circumference.) The skin is carefully elevated in one piece and preserved. A canalplasty is done if needed. The tympanic membrane is meticulously de-epithe-

Text continued on page 230

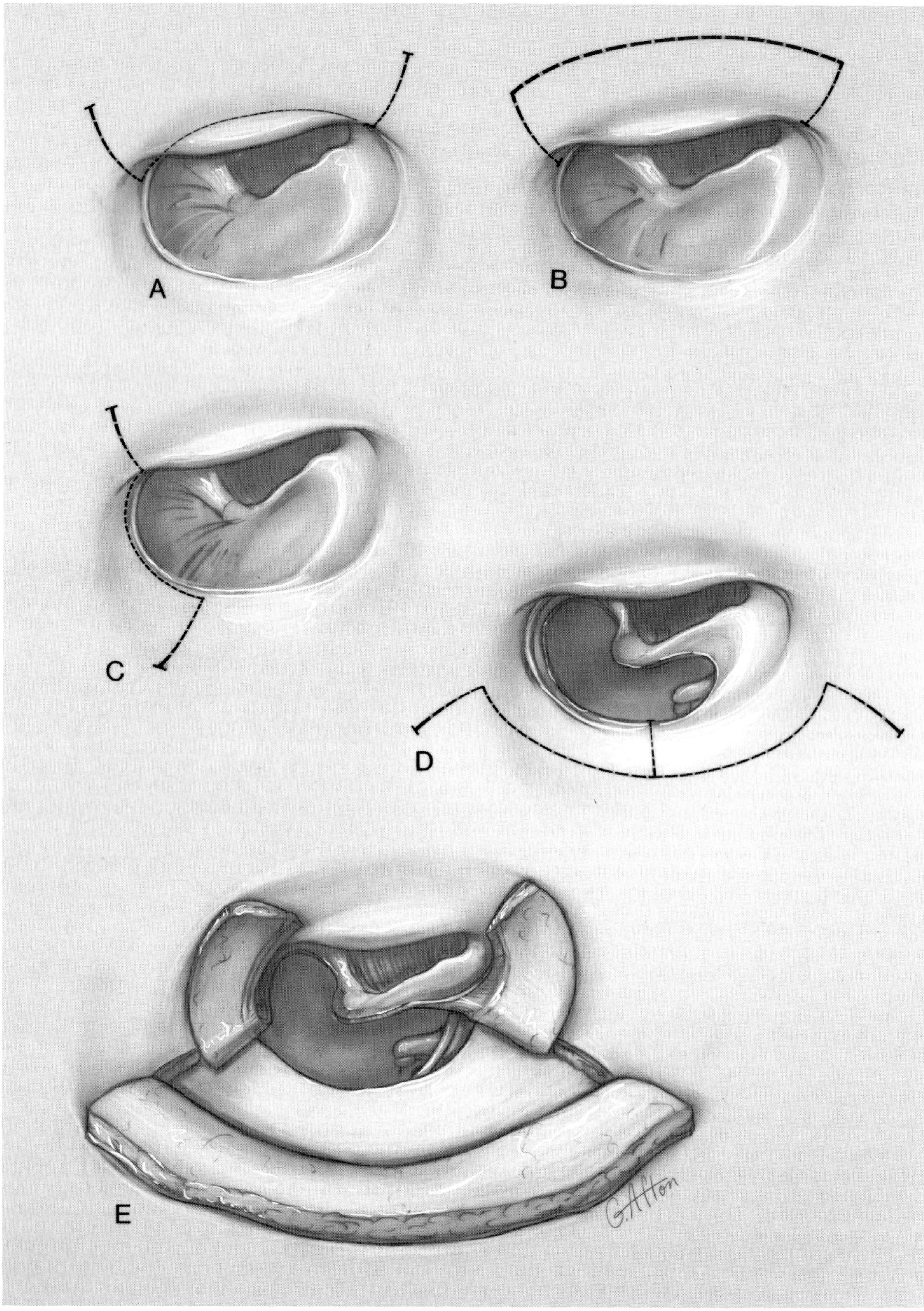

FIGURE 12–3.

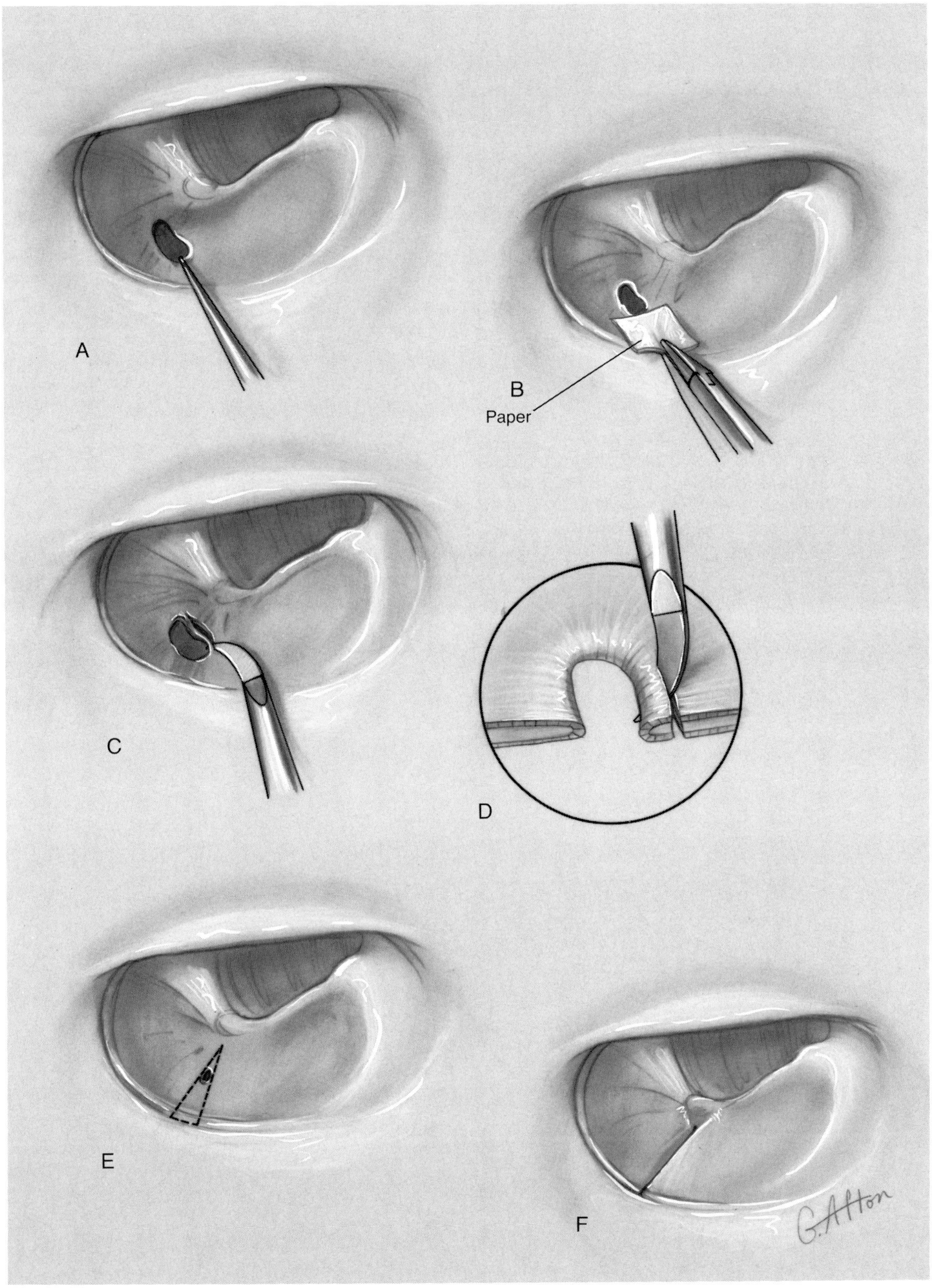

FIGURE 12–4.

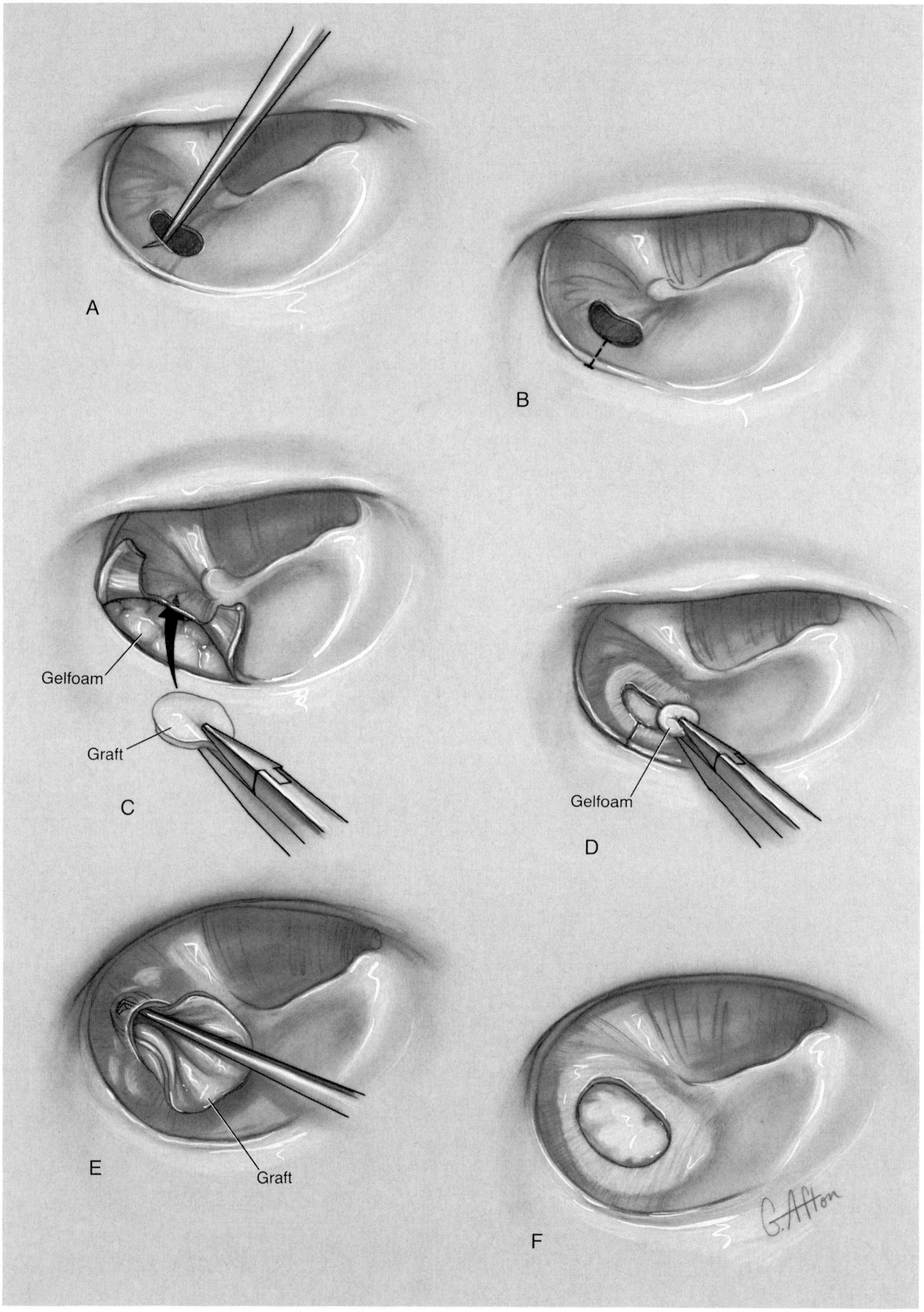

FIGURE 12–5.

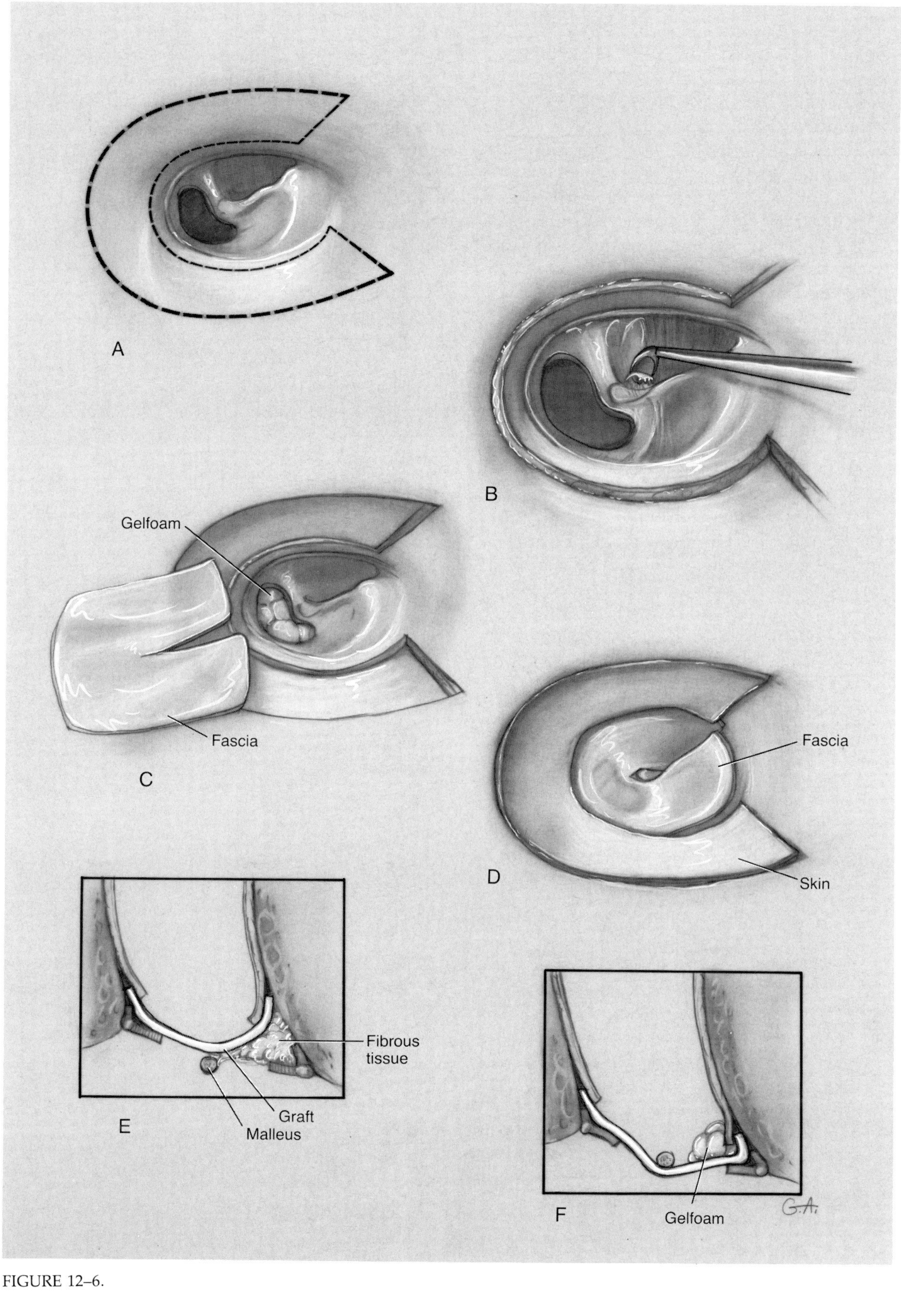
A
B
Gelfoam
Fascia
C
Fascia
D
Skin
Fibrous tissue
Graft
Malleus
E
F
Gelfoam
G.A.

FIGURE 12–6.

lialized with a joint or No. 2 canal knife or small curets (Fig. 12–6*B*). The middle ear is filled with compressed Gelfoam, and the graft is notched to fit around the manubrium (Fig. 12–6*C*). (The manubrium is de-epithelialized and cleansed.) The graft is placed embracing the manubrium; if needed, a piece of fascia is placed over the malleus handle (Fig. 12–6*D*). The skin graft is then returned, overlapping the fascia for a few millimeters. Special care must be observed anteriorly in order to avoid blunting of the graft in the anterior tympanomeatal angle. The canal is packed, usually with Gelfoam in the medial two thirds (Fig. 12–6*F*). In cases where there is no fibrous annulus, the sulcus should be checked; if shallow, it can be drilled with a small bur. Incisions are closed with appropriate sutures and a dressing is applied.

Problems and Complications

Blunting of the anterior tympanomeatal angle is the most feared complication, and usually occurs when there is no annulus and no sulcus. Drilling of the sulcus is helpful. Tight packing at this angle is important (rosebud packing with Owen's silk works quite well for this purpose). Lateralization of the graft (lateral displacement) happens less frequently if the tip of the malleus handle is placed over the fascia. Residual cholesteatoma occurs when de-epithelialization of the tympanic membrane is incomplete. Reperforation anteriorly is especially common if there is no annulus. This is involved with support of the graft (by the annulus) and vascularization in the area.

Underlay Graft for Posterior Perforation in Atrophic Membrane

Using an endaural approach, a temporal fascia graft (by Lempert I incision) and a small skin graft (by a Lempert II incision) have been obtained. The tympanic membrane is visualized; if necessary, a canalplasty is done. The edges of the perforation are trimmed, the undersurface of the membrane is gently scraped, and the membrane is de-epithelialized. Complete de-epithelialization must be done if a skin graft is to be used. If the membrane is atrophic, however, complete de-epithelialization might be more harmful than useful (an underlay graft is being used) because of the potential for tears.

If a PE tube is being considered, this is the time to select an area and place it.

In this example, a classic posterior canal flap with vertical incisions at 1 and 6 o'clock is used (Fig. 12–7*A*); this is a good choice but not the only one. The flap is raised, and the middle ear cavity is entered beneath the annulus. Remember that the annulus provides support and allows for maintenance of the middle ear space. The middle ear space is inspected. (For inspection and evaluation, see Tympanoplasty for Atelectatic Tympanic Membrane in Chapter 10.) For this procedure (repair of a perforation and reinforcement of the membrane) it is assumed to be normal.

A piece of thin Silastic sheeting is placed from the sinus tympanic area to the eustachian tube. The middle ear cavity is filled with compressed Gelfoam, and a piece of Gelfilm is placed over the incudostapedial joint (not under the annulus), between the joint and the membrane, in order to avoid adhesions from the graft to the joint (Fig. 12–7*B*).

The fascia graft is positioned over an area 30% greater than the extent of the perforation, since it will retract by about 30% (Fig. 12–7*C*). One concern with grafts is the possibility of lack of adequate contact with the overlying tympanic membrane. By this "falling into the middle ear cavity" the bridging function might be lost. Although compressed Gelfoam provides adequate contact (if placed correctly), a sound alternative (with proven good results) is the use of microclips to secure the graft against the overlying membrane. If the tympanic membrane is well de-epithelialized the clips will not cause a problem; eventually they will be extruded. (This technique is not described in this atlas.) It is useful to leave a tail (of the fascia) toward the posterior bony canal to be removed. This should be done very conservatively (if at all possible) in order to avoid having the graft rest over the incudostapedial joint (which by now is covered with Gelfilm). The graft is placed embracing the handle of the malleus. A small piece of fascia can then be placed over the handle. The piece of skin harvested via the Lempert II incision is placed over the fascia (covering the perforation) (Fig. 12–7*D*). The ear is packed (Fig. 12–7*E*). Endaural incisions are closed with the appropriate sutures, and a dressing is applied.

Underlay Graft for Large Anterior Perforation

A temporal fascia graft has been obtained via the postauricular approach. A posterior canal incision is made at the bony cartilaginous junction. The tympanic membrane is visualized, the edges of the perforation are trimmed, the undersurface is scraped,

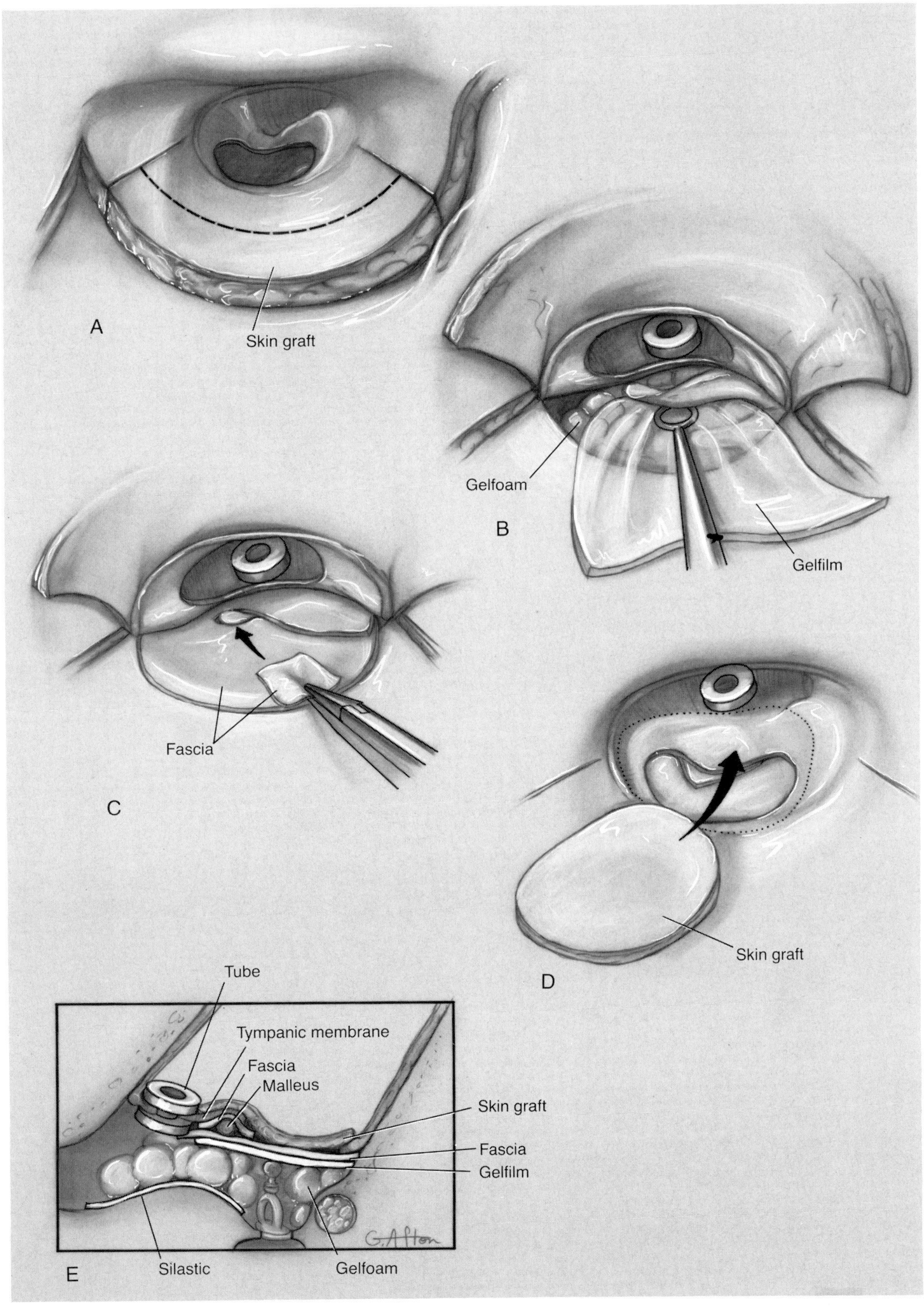
A
Skin graft
Gelfoam
B
Gelfilm
Fascia
C
Skin graft
D
Tube
Tympanic membrane
Fascia
Malleus
Skin graft
Fascia
Gelfilm
Silastic
Gelfoam
E

FIGURE 12–7.

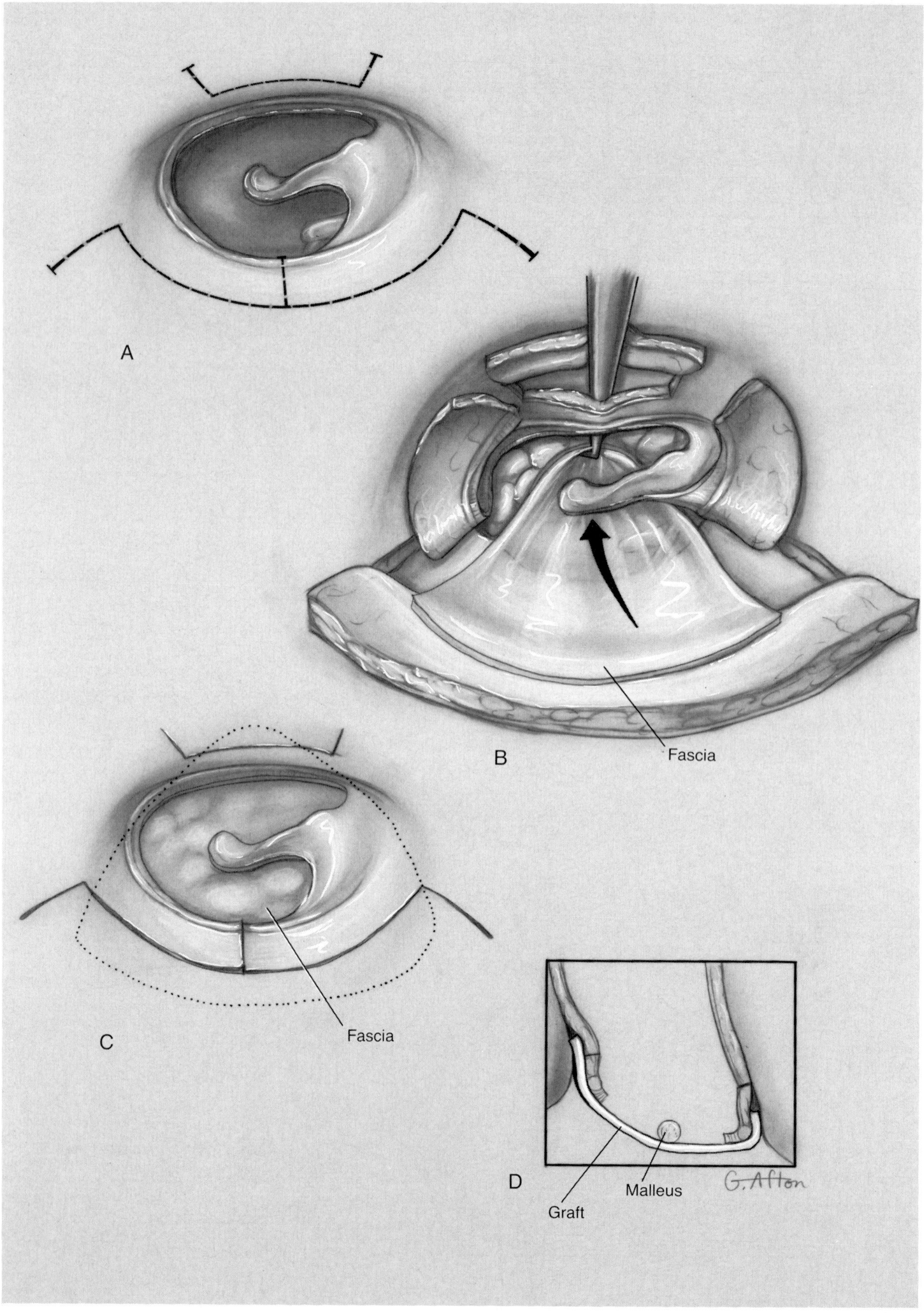

FIGURE 12–8.

and the membrane is de-epithelialized. (It is assumed that a canalplasty is not needed.)

Incisions are made for the flap (a classic posterior canal tympanoplasty incision, although others could have been made as well) (Fig. 12–8*A*). The "swinging doors" imply the elevation of superiorly and inferiorly based skin flaps. The horizontal incision is made 5 to 7 mm lateral to the annulus. The flap is divided with a vertical incision at 9 o'clock (it could also be at 11 o'clock); this incision involves both the tympanic membrane and the annulus. This results in two flaps (one superiorly and one inferiorly based), which are elevated anteriorly up to (and beyond if necessary) the malleus superiorly, and to 6 o'clock (or further) inferiorly.

The middle ear cavity is entered and examined. (It is assumed that all that is needed is placement of a graft.)

If only the annulus is left anteriorly, the problem of graft support becomes an issue. Abundant Gelfoam packing should be planned. A good choice is to de-epithelialize the annulus anteriorly and to make small incisions 3 to 4 mm in length (or longer if needed) and raise a small anterior flap. The annulus is gently elevated anteriorly for the same extent as the incision (made in the skin of the canal), and the fascia graft is pulled beneath the annulus onto the anterior canal and covered with the small anterior flap (Fig. 12–8*B*, *C*). This avoids retraction of the graft in such a critical area. (The rest of the graft positioning is similar to that in the endaural approach described above.) A piece of thin Silastic sheeting is placed from the sinus tympani to the eustachian tube. The cavity is filled with compressed Gelfoam; a piece of Gelfilm is placed over the incudostapedial joint. The graft is placed posteriorly as well, and the flaps are repositioned (Fig. 12–8*D*). (Note the distinct advantage of leaving the vascular strip untouched.) Packing is done. Incisions are closed with appropriate sutures, and a dressing is applied.

Allograft for Total Perforation

The use of an allogeneic tympanic membrane allograft constitutes one more effective means of restoring continuity of the membrane. Its indications are similar to others, but this graft is especially used for failures of standard tympanoplasty (such as recurrent perforations or lateralization of grafts), and in cases in which there is a high risk of failure with standard tympanoplasty. An allograft is not a panacea and is not easy to position adequately; however, it allows the use of the tympanic membrane or ossicles, or a tympanic membrane with ossicles. A donor membrane must be selected of the proper size and side to fit well in the recipient.

Assuming either an endaural or a postauricular approach, enough bone is removed (by canalplasty) to completely visualize the annulus (or the sulcus, if the annulus is not present). The malleus handle is meticulously cleansed, and the tympanic membrane remnants are de-epithelialized. If the annulus is absent, the sulcus is carefully drilled in order to seat the allograft in good position.

Incisions are made at 11, 2, and 7 o'clock and include the annulus, unless the annulus is complete (Fig. 12–9*A*). The flaps expose the middle ear cavity. Some Gelfoam is placed, and allograft is positioned first over the malleus (Fig. 12–9*B*). The flaps are then repositioned. Packing is done, the incisions are closed (Fig. 12–9*C*), and a dressing is applied.

An allogeneic tympanic membrane graft has certain drawbacks. Different sides (right or left) and sizes must be available in the operating room. It is not easy to position the graft properly. Allografts tend to form adhesions and are associated with granulation tissue in the middle ear cavity. (Silastic should be used, as well as Gelfoam [conservatively]). Immunologic rejection sometimes occurs. (This is fairly well controlled, however.) In addition, there is a potential for transmitting viral particles from the donor to the recipient, since some viruses are not easily eliminated by sterilization processes. The source of the allograft obviously is critical.

Tympanoplasty–Ossiculoplasty

The title of this section is chosen for didactic purposes. However, the reader should be aware that an ossiculoplasty is part of a tympanoplasty. These procedures involve restoring the sound conduction capabilities of the ossicular chain with or without a tympanic membrane graft. The end result should be continuity in vibration of the new chain, with a solid contact with the tympanic membrane and a mobile oval window membrane or plate.

The ossicular chain or its components can be affected by fixation, dislocation, fracture, or dissolution (resorption). These conditions may be congenital, or they can be caused by trauma, neoplasm, or infection. The choice of procedure will depend upon the type of ossicular problem, the anatomic environment, the space available (intact post wall, canal wall down, and so on), and the status of the mucosa (which in turn depends upon the status of the

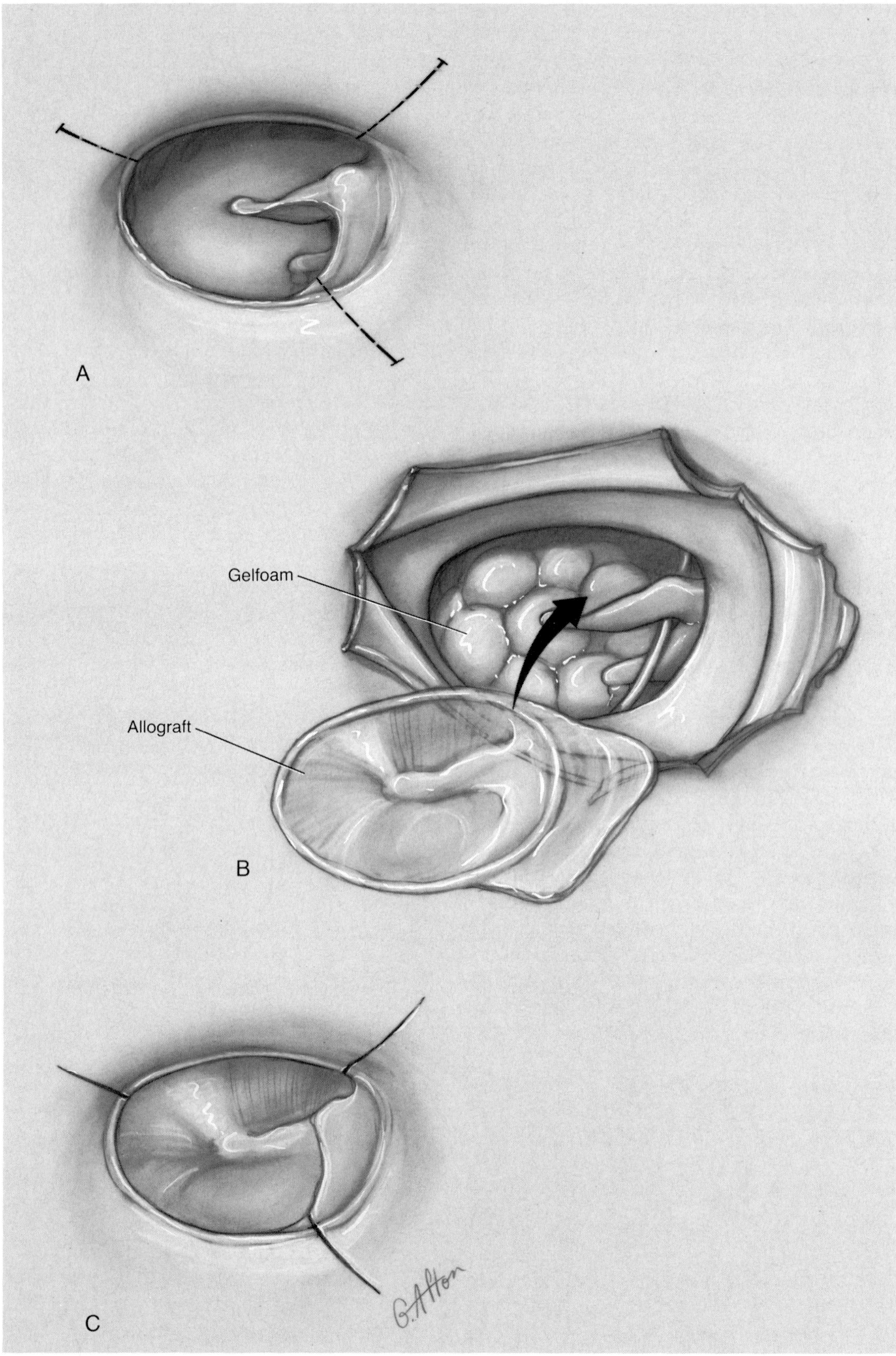

FIGURE 12–9.

underlying disease). For practical purposes, it is assumed that the underlying disease is under control and that the middle ear space is adequate. All possible ossicular changes and examples of surgical repair in selected situations will be discussed, with the understanding that there are other choices available.

Isolated Ossicular Lesions

Malleus (Fig. 12–10*A*)

This is an essential bone in ossiculoplasty repair. The presence or absence of the handle of the malleus, together with the presence or absence of an intact and mobile stapes, will determine in great part the type of procedure to be performed.

The malleus is rarely affected alone; if it is, the problem usually is an anterior fixation of the head. (It may also be a traumatic dislocation.) If it is associated with a mobile stapes, an atticotomy is done with exposure of the incudomalleal joint (Fig. 12–10*B, C*) (see Chapter 13). The fixation is verified, and the joint is separated with a joint knife.

Points to remember: Disarticulate the incudostapedial joint before drilling in the attic. This will help to avoid inner ear damage. Reinforcing the posterosuperior canal quadrant (atticotomy site) before closure will discourage retraction pockets and other complications.

The head of the malleus is amputated with a malleus nipper (Fig. 12–10*D*). The incus also is removed, since it has lost its articulation to the head of the malleus. Reconstruction will be based toward the head of the stapes. There are two alternatives: laying the tympanic membrane (intact or grafted) over the head of the stapes (classic type III tympanoplasty) (Fig. 12–10*E*), and placing a graft or prosthesis between the mobile handle of the malleus (the fixed head has been amputated) and the head of the stapes. The latter course is better in terms of reestablishing continuity in an adequate middle ear space. This can be done in a number of ways:

1. Using the head of the malleus. Holding the head of the malleus with an ossicle holder, shape it to fit between the head of the stapes and handle of the malleus. Drill a hole in it to receive the head of the stapes. Then flatten it (notch it a little, making a groove) to fit under the handle (Fig. 12–10*F*).

2. Using the incus. The short process of the incus is clipped. An acetabulum is drilled in the long process for fitting over the head of the stapes. This is followed by drilling a groove over the remaining body for fitting under the malleus handle (Fig. 12–11*A, B*).

3. Using cortical bone. A graft that is shaped similar to a sculptured incus or malleus head can be drilled, creating a concave hole to fit over the head of the stapes and a notch or a groove to fit under the malleus handle (Fig. 12–11*C, D*). (If desired, a T-shaped cortical bone can be used.)

4. Using a partial ossicular replacement prosthesis (PORP). The larger surface area of a PORP provides more stability; however, it must be covered with a thin piece of cartilage (such as tragal cartilage) that exceeds the edges of the PORP. When placed, it must provide a slight tension over the tympanic membrane (Fig. 12–12*A*). The cartilage is between the PORP and the malleus handle. If there is no malleus handle, the cartilage is placed directly under the tympanic membrane or tympanic membrane graft; in these cases, a large piece of cartilage is preferred. Some surgeons even suture the cartilage to the head of the PORP. In the distal portion of the PORP, an opening or notch is made for better contact with the head of the stapes and stapedial tendon. In some cases a PORP can be carved from cartilage, and this type of graft fits quite well (Fig. 12–12*B*). It also allows trimming of the head of the cartilage PORP to fit the angled position of the membrane (Fig. 12–12*C*). In positioning PORPs (and TORPs), abundant Gelfoam is placed in the middle ear cavity in order to provide support and maintain position after repositioning the flaps and tympanic membrane. Ceramic PORPs are also available (Fig. 12–12*D*).

Incus (Fig. 12–13*A*)

The incus problems and repairs discussed here assume an intact malleus handle and stapes. The incus is the ossicle most commonly affected by ear infections (erosion of the lenticular process) and trauma (fracture-dislocation). It may also be absent (owing to trauma or previous surgery) or fixed (usually in association with the malleus head).

If erosion involves a small portion of the distal end of the lenticular process, continuity can be reestablished by any of the following methods:

1. Using a cortical bone chip. A square of bone is delineated in the cortex, removed, and shaped. A small acetabulum is drilled for the head of the stapes, and a groove for the remaining long process of the incus (Fig. 12–13*B–E*).

2. Using a cartilage chip. A piece of cartilage shaped similarly to the cortical bone chip can be used.

3. Using a prosthesis that embraces both the remaining lenticular process and the head of the stapes.

Text continued on page 241

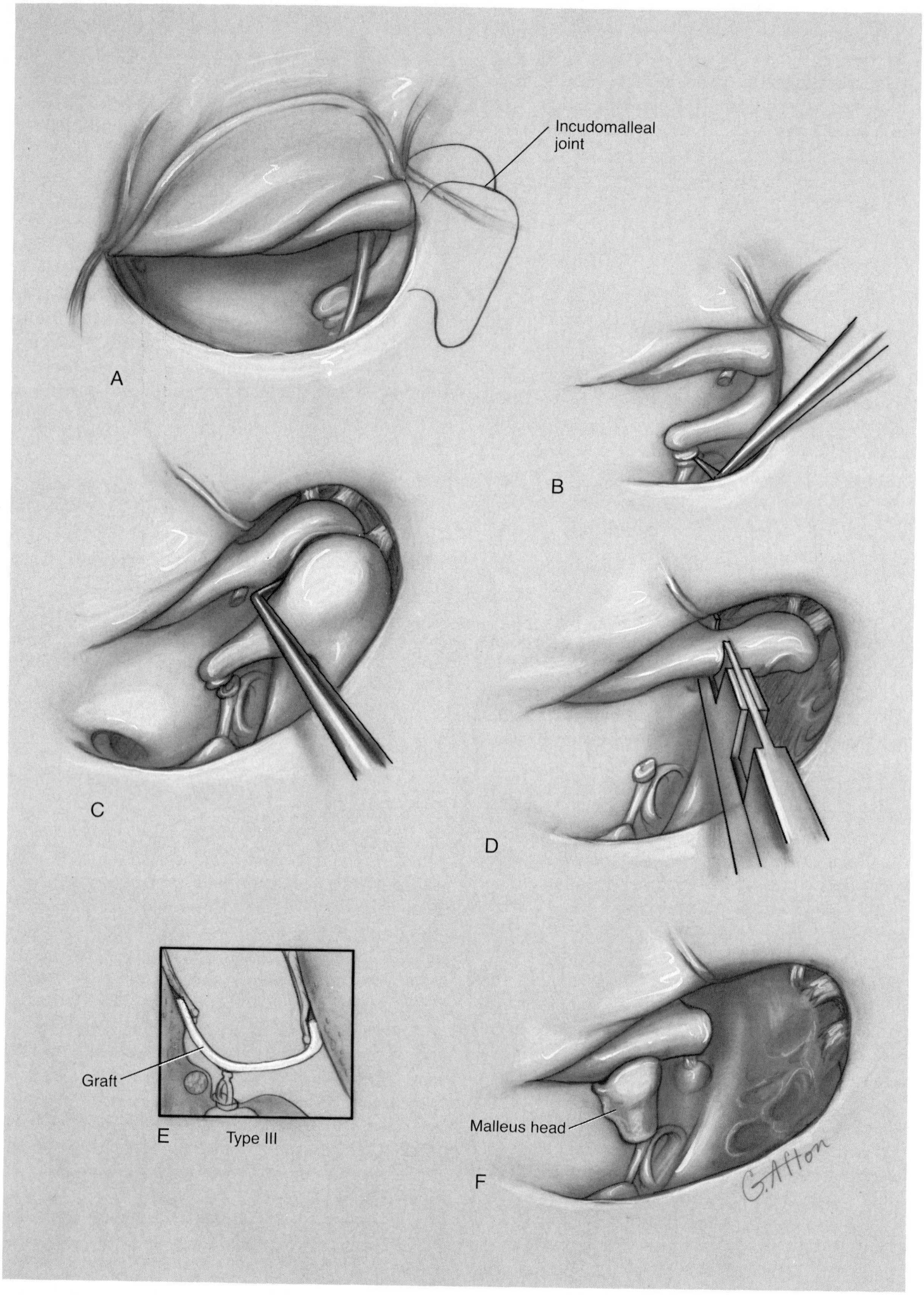
Incudomalleal
joint
A
B
C
D
Graft
E
Type III
Malleus head
F
G.Afton

FIGURE 12–10.

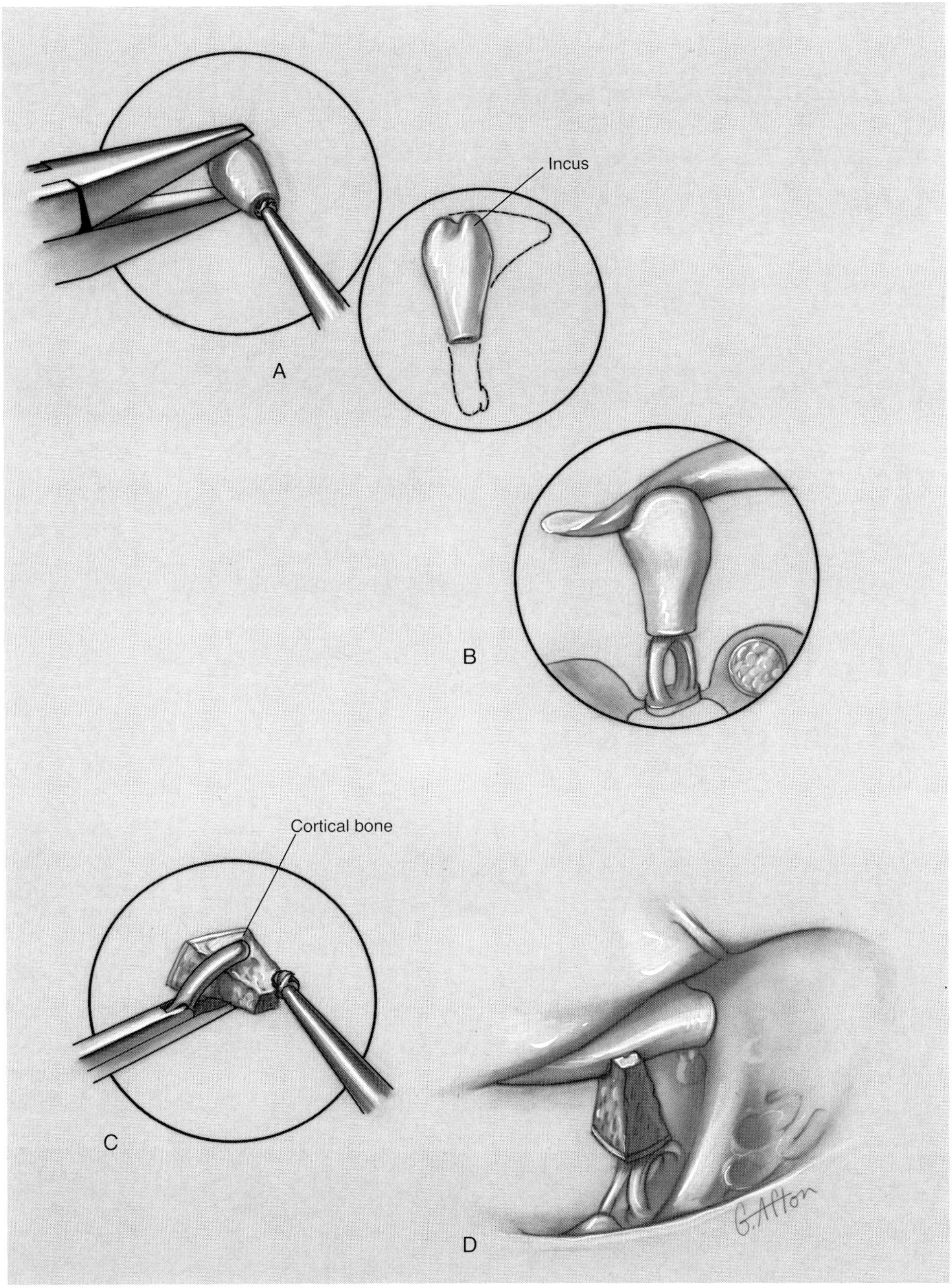

FIGURE 12–11.

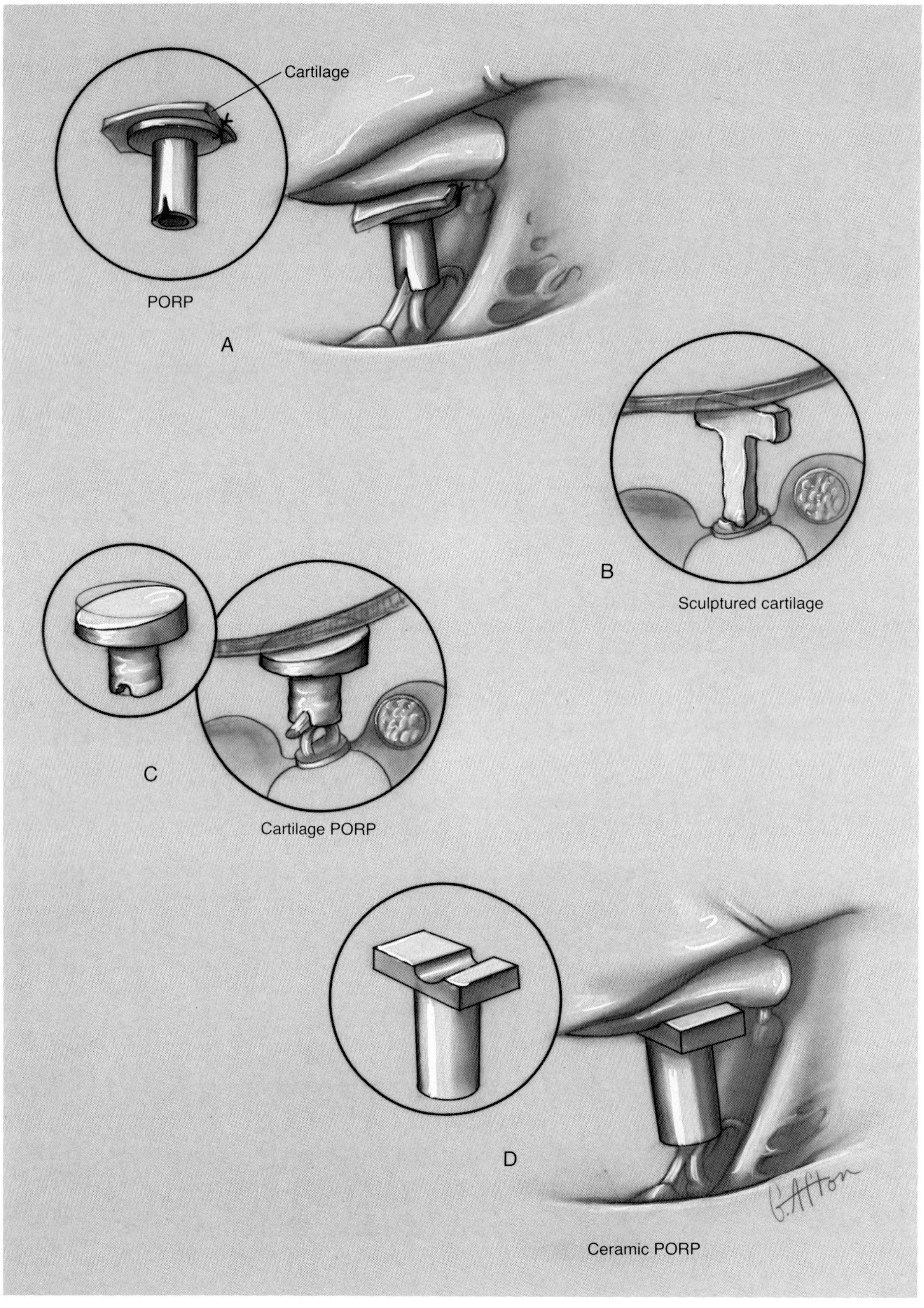
Cartilage
PORP
A
B
Sculptured cartilage
C
Cartilage PORP
D
Ceramic PORP

FIGURE 12–12.

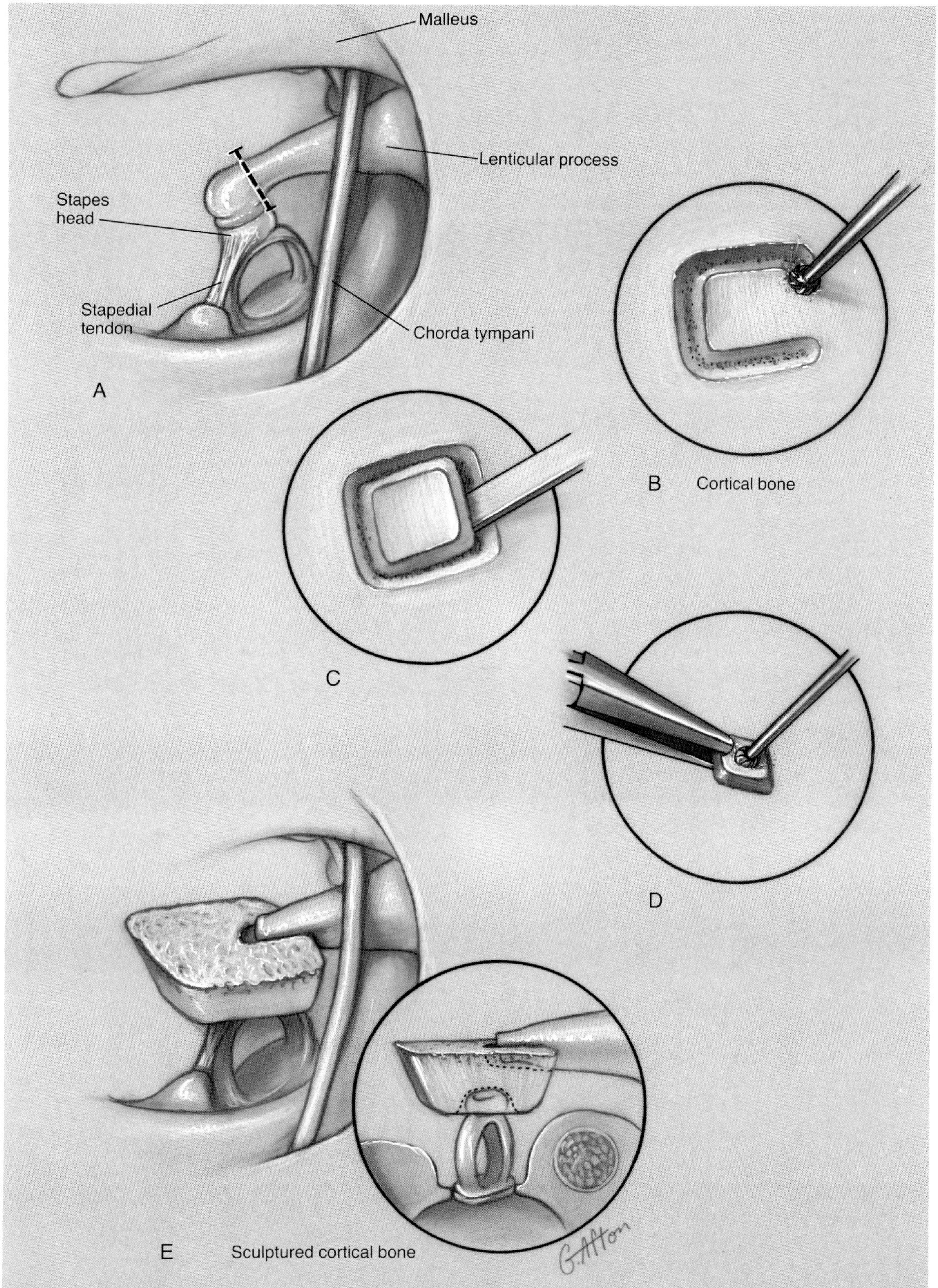
Malleus
Lenticular process
Stapes head
Stapedial tendon
Chorda tympani
A
B Cortical bone
C
D
E Sculptured cortical bone
G. Alton

FIGURE 12–13.

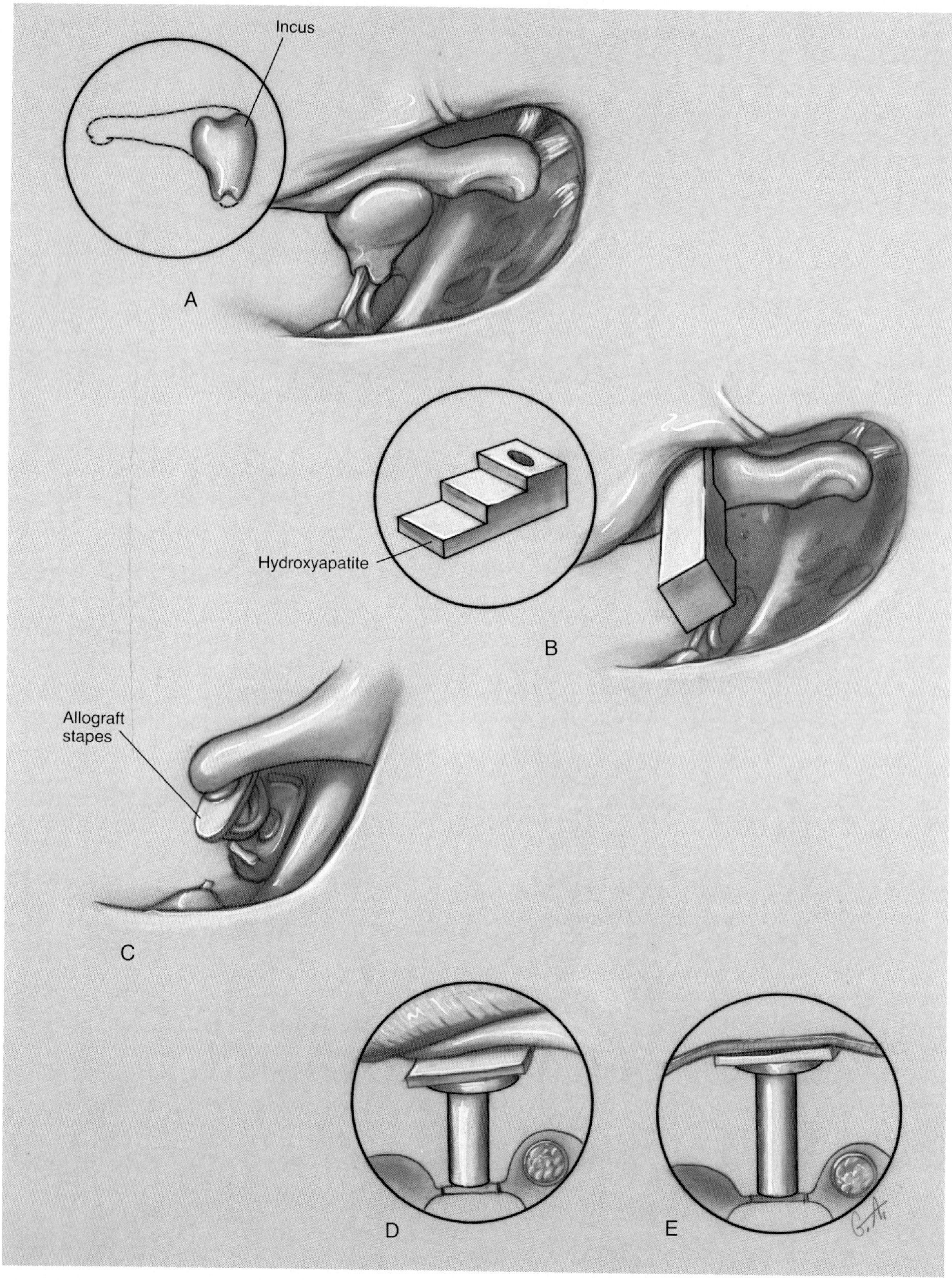

FIGURE 12–14.

If there is dislocation, the ideal procedure is reapproximation and repositioning using Gelfoam or "glue" (Fibrin or Histoacryl), or both. However, this is seldom possible. In traumatic dislocations, adhesions and fixations are very common.

If reapproximation is not possible, or interposing bone or cartilage in lenticular erosion does not suffice, there are alternatives:

1. Incus transposition. A small atticotomy is done, and the incus is carefully separated from the malleus. It is shaped by removing the long process, and a notch for the stapes head is made at the end of the short process. The articulating surface is enlarged to accept the malleus handle (Fig. 12–14*A*).
2. Use of the malleus head. Once the head is removed, the situation is as described for fixation of the head of the malleus. The same procedures apply, except that if the malleus is mobile and the head itself is not used (and any of the other alternatives are not preferred), the malleus head is left in place and only the incus is removed.

In the case of a missing incus, the second alternative remains valid. In all of these procedures, allogeneic (allograft) ossicles and cartilage are also a good alternative.

Another method is to use an interposition prosthesis made of hydroxyapatite. A pocket is created between the malleus and the overlying membrane. The large end of the prosthesis is placed over the head of the stapes and the distal (thin) end in this newly created pocket (Fig. 12–14*B*). The advantage is that stability is provided by utilizing both the tympanic membrane and malleus handle, with no connection to the bony annulus or facial ridge. This is a clever prosthesis (which still must stand the test of time, however). It must be mentioned, however, that drilling in it is not so simple as suggested. Patience, carefulness, and copious irrigation are recommended. An additional prosthesis of this same material (the Wehrs incus prosthesis) fulfills very nicely the function of a sculptured incus between the malleus and stapes head without the drilling and sculpturing of the incus. This too must be evaluated over time.

Stapes

Fixation of the stapes by otosclerosis is dealt with in Chapter 13. Fixation related to inflammation (fibrosis) or tympanosclerosis is rare in an isolated form (that is, not affecting other ossicles at the same time). In these exceptional cases, a stapedectomy will suffice and the results should be as good as in otosclerosis. However, it is essential to do this stapedectomy in a "dry ear" and as a single procedure. It should not be performed in conjunction with a tympanoplasty because of a high risk of sensory hearing loss. If a tympanoplasty is performed, the stapedectomy is delayed. Careful staging is crucial.

Fractures of the crura are treated with a piston prosthesis from the incus to the oval window, unless the fracture is the rare one that allows a crurotomy. Again, these procedures are done in a "dry ear." In cases of fractured crura and footplate, it is safer to remove the footplate and use connective tissue to seal the window. (A wire connective tissue prosthesis is preferred but it is not essential.) An alternative in fractured crura and intact mobile footplate is the use of an inverted allograft stapes (Fig. 12–14*C*).

Combined Ossicular Problems

Repairs become more troublesome if the malleus handle or stapes (or both) are absent. This means that the prosthesis must be supported by the grafted tympanic membrane, which carries a higher risk of failure, or a longer prosthesis must be used from the tympanic membrane to the oval window.

Fixation of the head of the malleus associated with a fixed stapes footplate has been shown to be repaired with a malleus-to-oval-window wire connective tissue prosthesis. While this is a good alternative, it has the drawbacks of lateralization and loss of adequate conductivity. It must be remembered that whenever the stapes footplate is removed, a fistula of the oval window is a potential complication. Regardless of the graft or prosthesis, an adequate seal is essential. Alternatives include the use of a TORP, a TORP-shaped cortical bone ossicle, cartilage, or ceramic prosthesis, or a sculptured ossicle (autologous or allogeneic).

In cases of fixation of the ossicular chain by tympanosclerosis, the first stage implies mobilization, completion of the malleus, disarticulation of the incus, and so on. This prepares for a second procedure in which the stapedectomy is done. Surgical repair involves the alternatives described below.

When both the malleus and incus are absent (usually seen in chronic otitis media cases, and not uncommonly in tympanomastoidectomy procedures), or when both ossicles are a single, congenital, nonfunctional "mass," the alternatives are a classic type III tympanoplasty or use of a short prosthesis or graft (described above), if the stapes is intact and mobile. If the stapes is fixed or damaged, a long prosthesis (tympanic membrane to footplate or oval window graft) is necessary.

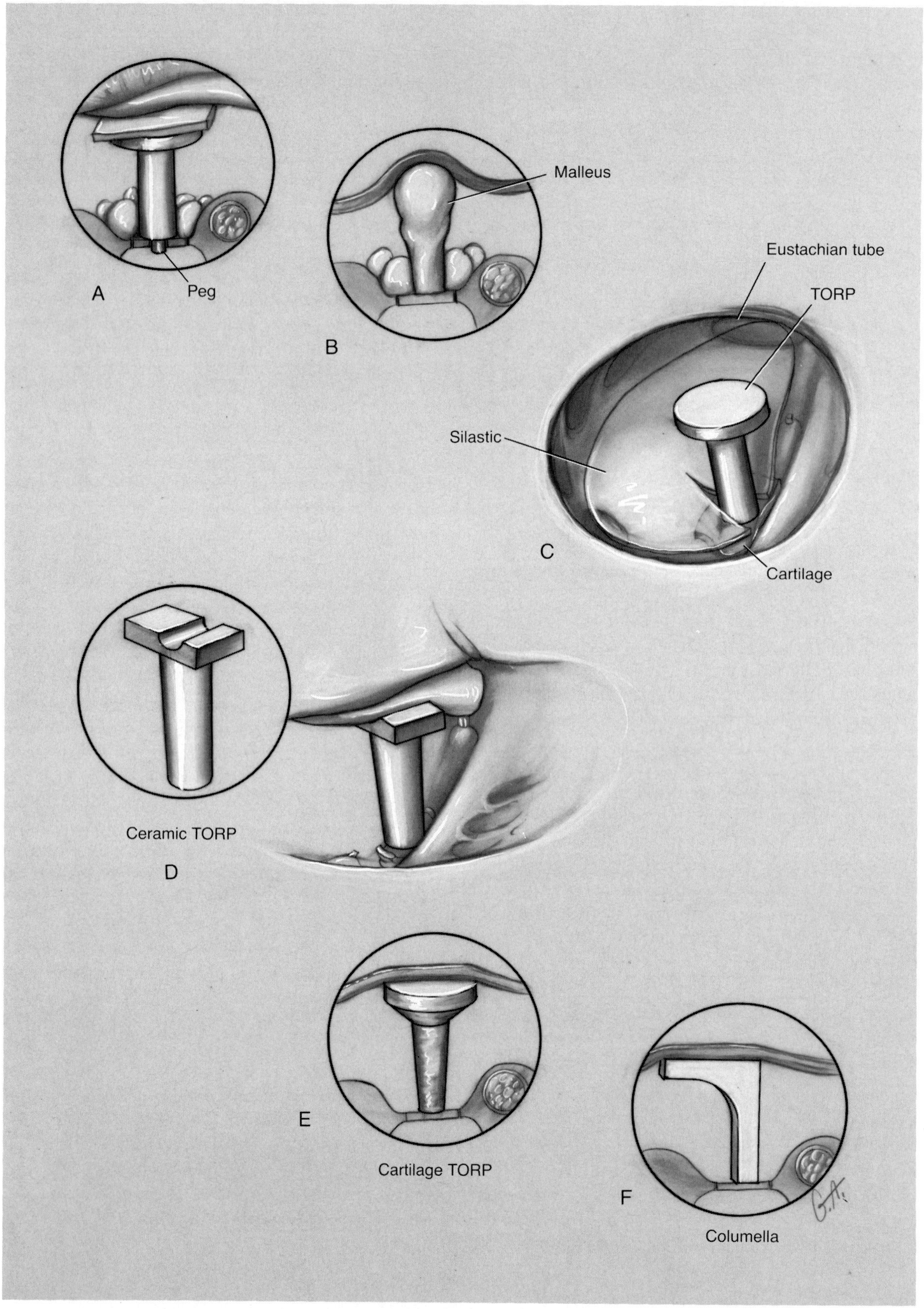
A
Peg
Malleus
B
Eustachian tube
TORP
Silastic
C
Cartilage
Ceramic TORP
D
E
Cartilage TORP
F
Columella

FIGURE 12–15.

If the malleus is absent and there is an intact and mobile stapes, a short prosthesis is used. However, a long prosthesis is indicated if the stapes is damaged (Fig. 12–14*E*).

In cases of tympanomastoidectomy, the concept of space becomes relevant in terms of reconstruction. At this point and with this type of disease, an intact-bridge tympanomastoidectomy makes good sense (if needed, of course; if possible, an intact-wall procedure is preferred).

As mentioned earlier, a critical factor is the presence or absence of the malleus handle. An equally important factor (sometimes overlooked) is the presence or absence of a mobile footplate. For practical purposes, the use of a TORP will be described, followed by other alternatives.

Placement of a TORP

Two points of contact are crucial. The usual tendency is to think in terms of extrusion and forget the distal end of the TORP (over the footplate or oval window graft).

The TORP is cut to the necessary length. This may be 3.5 mm for an open cavity, 4 mm if the malleus handle is present, or 5 mm if it is absent.

A thin but large piece of cartilage is placed over the TORP (beneath the malleus or tympanic membrane graft) to provide protection from extrusion (some surgeons suture it to the TORP). If there is a footplate or membrane, the TORP is placed over it and is supported with abundant Gelfoam to secure it in position. A TORP with a peg can be used to provide more stability at the footplate and prevent slipping (Fig. 12–15*A*). Once the TORP is placed, it should impart some tension to the tympanic membrane. A TORP-shaped piece of cartilage or cortical bone can be used, as well. A small piece of Silastic can be placed, surrounding the prosthesis at the oval window area, in order to prevent adhesions (Fig. 12–15*C*). A ceramic TORP can also be used (Fig. 12–15*D*), as well as a sculptured incus. The latter should be flattened toward the tympanic membrane in order to provide a smooth and wide contact. If the malleus handle is present, drilling a groove in the TORP provides better stability. Whenever a long prosthesis (TORP type) is placed over an oval window without a footplate, there is a possibility of a fistula and good seal is needed. If there is a potential for retraction (for example, eustachian tube dysfunction), these prostheses may lead to fistulization by sliding into the oval window.

Pertinent Histopathology

FIGURES 12–16 TO 12–18

Chronic otitis media with perforation of the tympanic membrane. The lower magnification (Fig. 12–16) shows the three layers of the tympanic membrane: (1) the outer epithelium (stratified squamous epithelium), continuous with that of the external ear canal; (2) the middle ear connective tissue layer, continuous with both the connective tissue layer of the external ear canal and middle ear; and (3) the inner mucosal layer, continuous with that of the middle ear. The higher magnifications (Figs. 12–17, 12–18) clearly show the ingrowth of outer stratified squamous epithelium (*arrows*). This epithelium is removed before placement of a connective tissue graft; otherwise there will be no migration of epithelial cells over the graft. The purpose of the graft is to "replace" the lost connective tissue and to serve as a bridge for migration of epithelial cells to close the gap (perforation). These photomicrographs illustrate the concepts of perforation and grafting; they are not meant to imply or to suggest grafting a perforation during an acute episode of otitis media, even if superimposed over a chronic process.

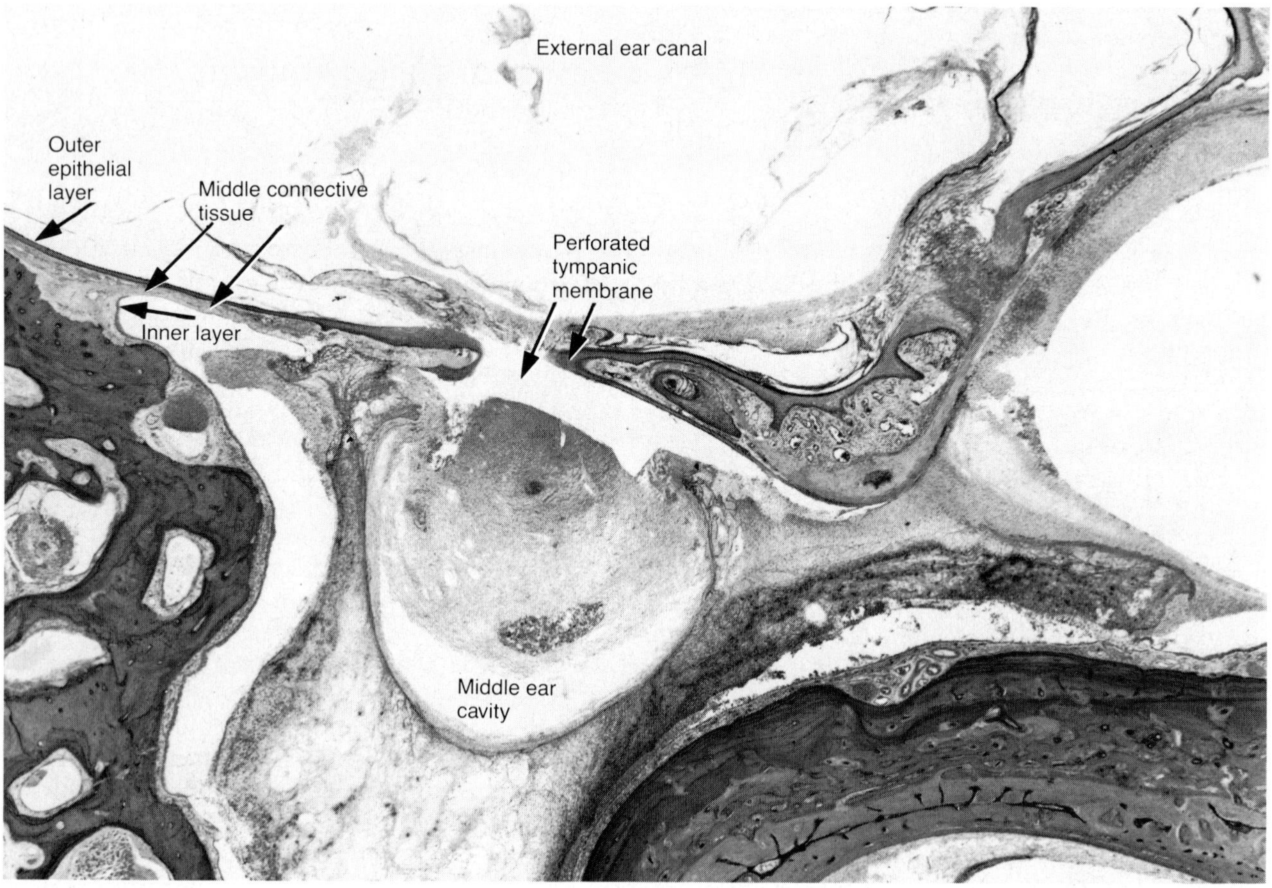
External ear canal
Outer epithelial layer
Middle connective tissue
Inner layer
Perforated tympanic membrane
Middle ear cavity

FIGURE 12–16.

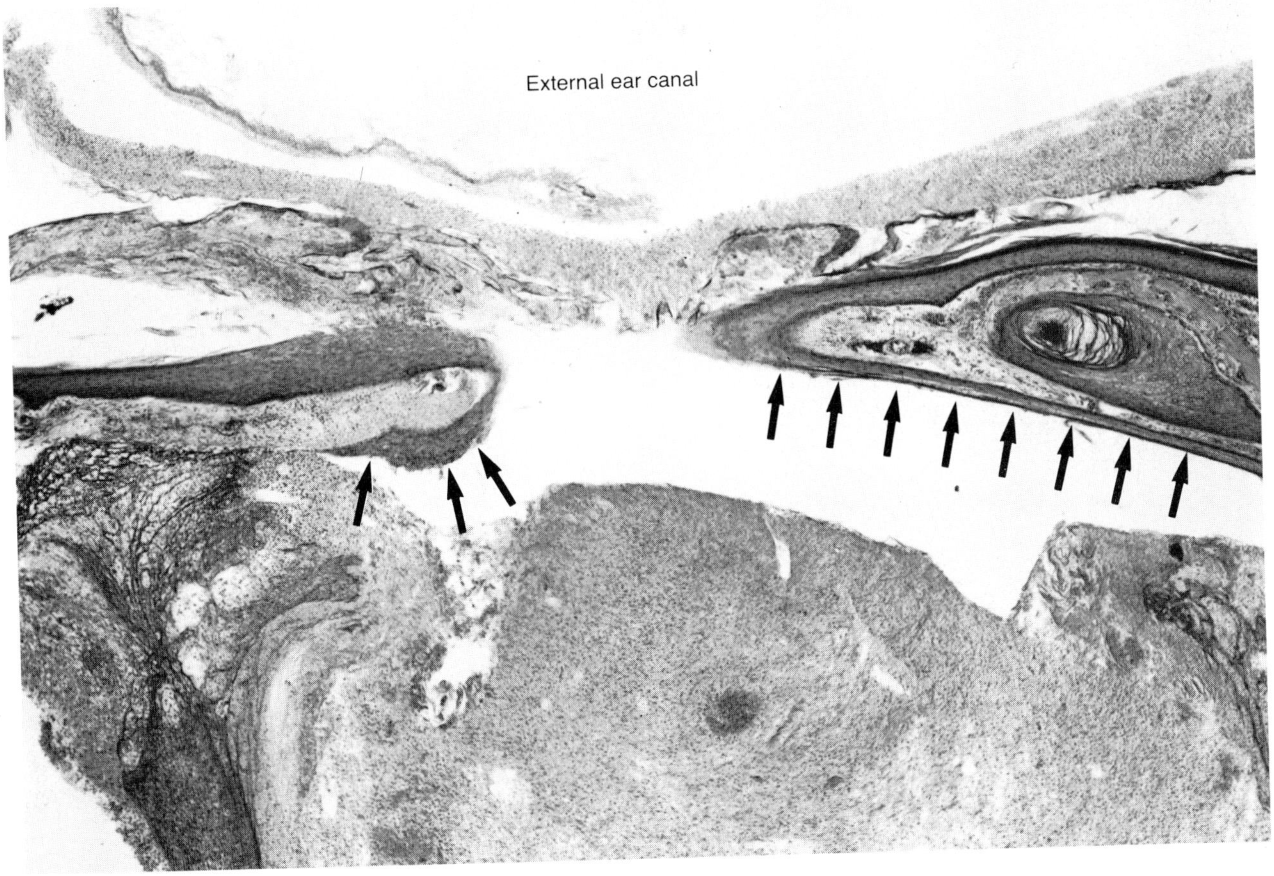

FIGURE 12–17.

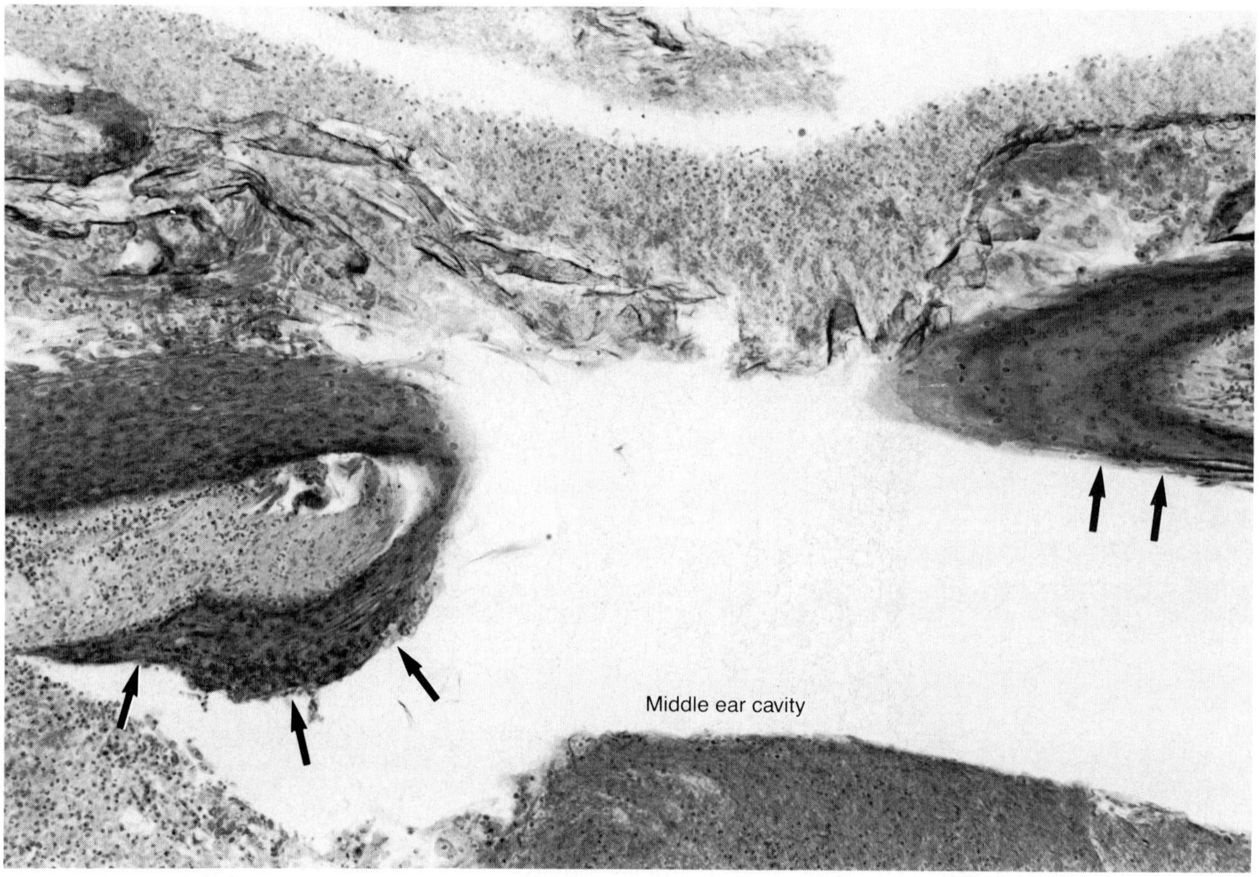

FIGURE 12–18.

CHAPTER 13

Surgery for Stapes Fixation

Stapes procedures aim to re-establish sound transmission through a stiffened ossicular chain, secondary to fixation of the stapes. These procedures involve partial or total removal of this ossicle and replacement with mobile portions of it or with a prosthesis.

Two surgical procedures that have been used successfully for stapes fixation will not be discussed at length here. Although a detailed description is beyond the scope of this atlas, the reader should be aware of them. They are (1) fenestration of the lateral semicircular canal, and (2) sonoinversion. Fenestration of the lateral semicircular canal allows vibrations to reach the hair cells through the scala vestibuli, bypassing the ossicular chain, with a resultant mild air–bone gap of 25 to 30 dB. Although this procedure has been replaced by stapedectomy, it should be kept in mind. It can be of use in some unusual cases of otosclerosis, as an interval operation in some forms of tympanoplasty, and could eventually re-emerge as a surgical technique for delivery of drugs to the inner ear. Sonoinversion (technique of Garcia-Ibánez) delivers vibratory stimulation through the round window membrane by utilizing a prosthesis from the incus or malleus to the round window. The normal mechanism of sound transmission via the ossicular chain to the oval window is successfully "inverted."

The basic head position with slight hypertension and the transcanal approach have already been described; the discussion will focus on procedures after the annulus has been elevated.

Stapes procedures generally are done under local anesthesia with sedation. General anesthesia also can be used; however, it has the disadvantage of preventing the surgeon from monitoring vestibular symptoms or hearing gains in the operating room.

Some surgeons prefer a small endaural approach, since it provides good exposure and allows bimanual surgery without the need for speculum holders; however, speculum holders are used by a majority of surgeons. The authors prefer a transcanal approach, using an ear speculum without a holder. A well-fitted ear speculum holds in place quite well. It is not hard to stabilize the speculum with the left hand (for a right-handed surgeon), while using an insrument (such as a suction tip) at the same time. The procedure can be started with a smaller speculum; once the incisions have been made, a tightly fitting one is used.

Small exostoses of the canal (if any) are removed. (If they are large or if a canalplasty is necessary, this should be done as a separate procedure and the stapedectomy delayed until complete healing has been achieved, which could be a matter of months.) It should be remembered that entrance to the middle ear must be made in a dry field and beneath the annulus. From this point on, the microscope is used at a magnification of at least 10 ×. In general terms there are three basic types of stapedectomy—partial, total, and piston. The procedure here will be a general approach, and the different types will be described on the basis of the findings and their indications.

Once the annulus is elevated, the first objective is to obtain adequate exposure and then to explore the ear. Work on the stapes is the final step, and is only begun after all other work is completed. A useful rule of thumb for exposure of the oval window is to achieve clear visualization of the pyramidal eminence and the superior aspect of the facial nerve. Most of the time, this requires removal of bone from the posterior canal; in doing so, the chorda tympani

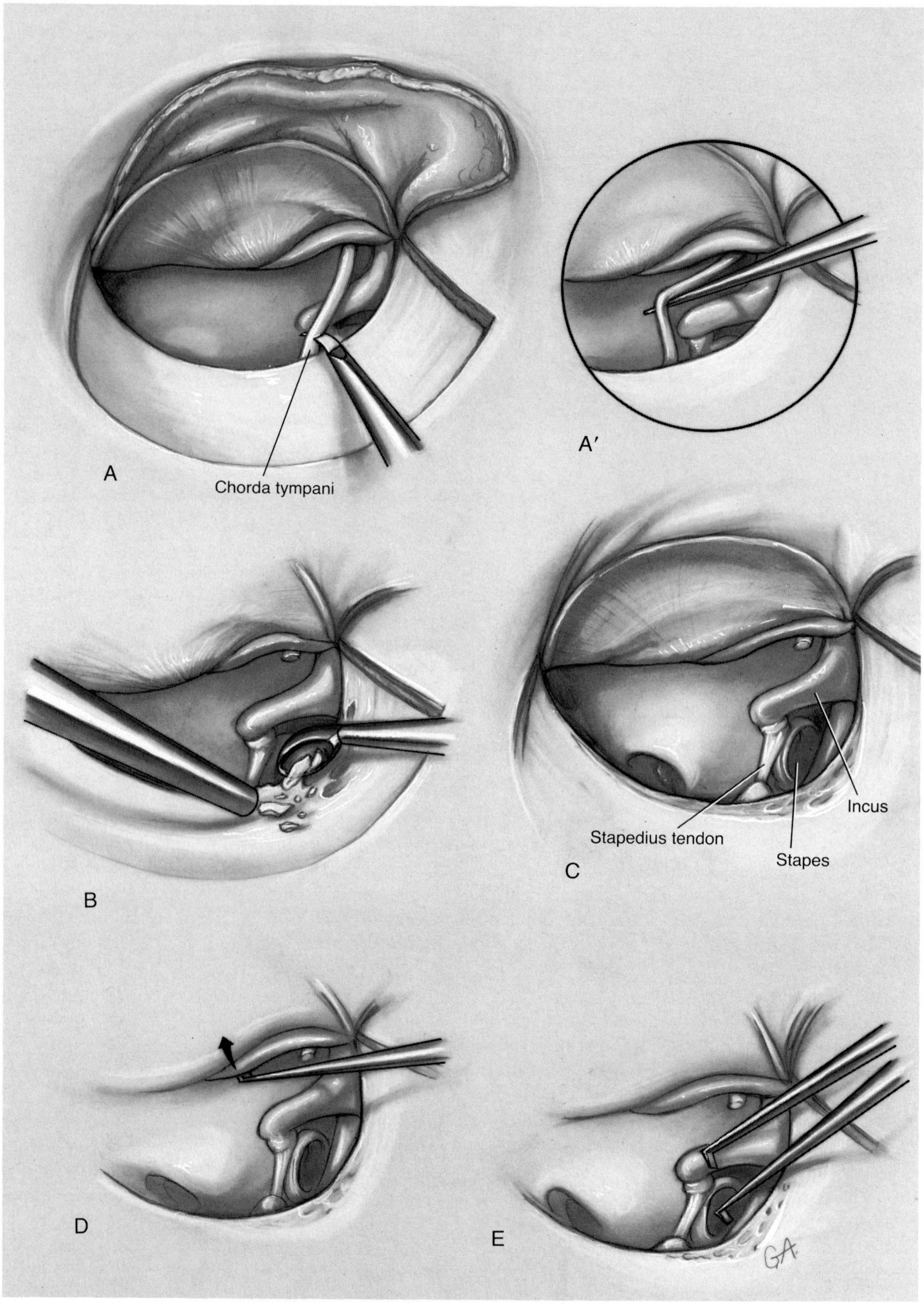

FIGURE 13–1.

must be freed. Usually a fine needle can be used to mobilize the chorda anteriorly toward the incus (Fig. 13–1*A′*). If the chorda will be stretched by this maneuver, it is better to section it sharply with a knife or a Bellucci scissors (Fig. 13–1*A*).

Bone of the posterior canal can be drilled or curetted. The authors prefer to curet it with large stapes curets in strokes away from the ossicles (avoiding luxation of the ossicles). Meticulous removal of bone chips should be done (Fig. 13–1*B*). Once visualization has been achieved, all anatomic landmarks are inspected (Fig. 13–1*C*).

The presence of an open round window is important. Total obliteration will lead to a poorer result. Drilling a round window also leads to poor results and complications and is not recommended. A very small opening (*not* surgically induced) in the window should suffice for a satisfactory outcome; this should be kept in mind. However, in some patients with obliterated round windows some gain in hearing can be obtained; since such an improvement might make a significant difference in their lives, a stapedectomy should be attempted.

The ossicular chain is then palpated (using an angled hook or Hough hoe) in order to locate points of ossicular fixation (Fig. 13–1*D*, *E*). Special attention is paid to cases of unilateral hearing loss, in which nonotosclerotic fixations are more frequent. Fixation of the malleus most often is congenital, and the fixation is at the head. This finding requires an atticotomy (previously described) and exposure of the head of the malleus (Fig. 13–2*A*). The authors prefer to use curets, but if a drill is used, the incus should be separated from the head of the stapes with a joint knife in order to avoid acoustic trauma. Attachments can sometimes be released, and small pieces of Silastic can be placed to avoid fixation (Fig. 13–2*B*); however, unless the attachments are minimal, this is usually followed by refixation. A solid fixation requires removal of the head of the malleus with malleus nippers (Fig. 13–2*C*) and placement of a malleus to oval window prosthesis, a bone strut, or a total ossicular replacement prosthesis (TORP) (Fig. 13–2*D*–*F*). (See also Chapter 14 for alternative procedures utilizing a laser.)

Under 10 × or 16 × magnification, the oval window and stapes are inspected (Fig. 13–3). Is there a normal-sized oval window, a promontory overhang, or a dehiscent facial nerve? Is the facial nerve over the footplate? Is there a persistent stapedial artery? Is the stapes fixed anteriorly or posteriorly? Is the footplate of normal size (on average, 1.4 mm wide and 3.0 mm long)? Is part, half, or all of the footplate involved? Is there obliteration of the footplate and window by otosclerotic foci?

On the basis of these observations and the preference and experience of the surgeon, the specific surgical procedure is selected. Regardless of the procedure, the underlying idea is that all or part of the footplate is to be removed, and a membrane (preferably collagenous) used in its place for a seal. If a prosthesis will be employed, a firm and lasting contact must be established with the long process of the incus (or the malleus handle).

Total Stapedectomy with Prosthesis

The classic total stapedectomy is used here as the primary procedure to describe general principles and problems encountered during surgery. The description assumes that there is nonobliterative fixation of the stapes, the rest of the ossicles are mobile, the round window is patent, and the oval window is of normal size. The distance between the incus and the footplate is measured. The average measurement from the head of the stapes to the footplate is 3.29 mm ± 0.15 mm, to which is added 1 mm of the lenticular process. The average length of a prosthesis is 4.0 mm in women and 4.25 to 4.50 mm in men. If a wire connective tissue prosthesis is to be used, it should be made at this time. Connective tissue should be harvested at this point as well.

Harvesting a Graft

Once the stapes has been removed, the vestibule is exposed and a new membrane is needed to seal the opening. Connective tissue, specifically collagen, allows the formation of a stable seal that becomes part of the window. While Gelfoam stimulates tissue growth and is used satisfactorily by many surgeons, these membranes tend to be thin and carry a higher risk of fistula formation and perilymph leakage. Different sources are used, such as fat and connective tissue from the earlobe or postauricular area, tragal perichondrium, or a vein. Tissue from the earlobe and postauricular area is used for wire connective tissue prostheses, and from perichondrium or vein as sealing membranes with simple wires or pistons. Type of prosthesis, ease of handling, and individual preferences will determine such choices.

A small incision suffices for harvesting tissue from the earlobe or postauricular area (Fig. 13–4*A*, *B*). The incision is closed with one or two appropriate sutures

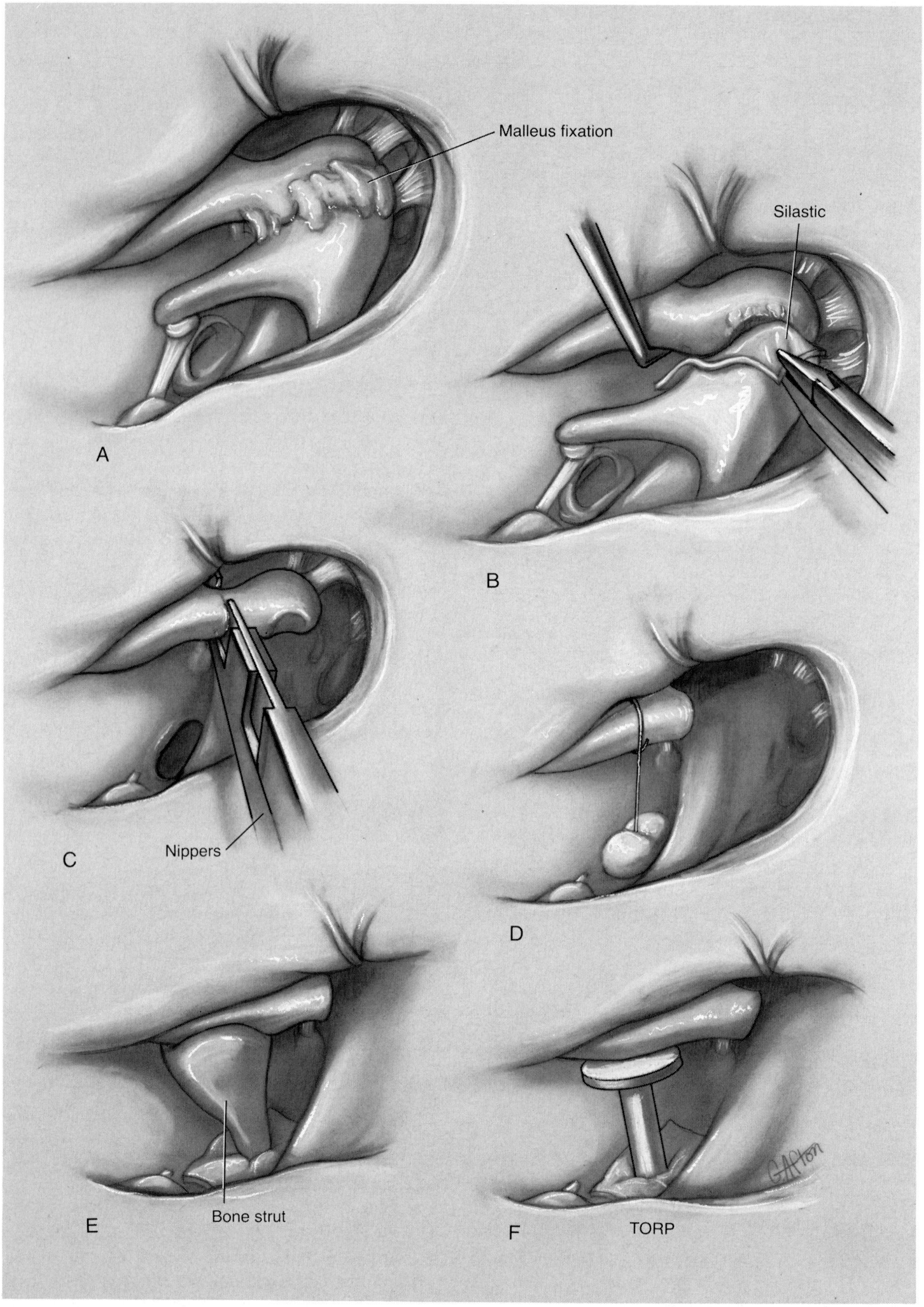
Malleus fixation
A
Silastic
B
C
Nippers
D
E
Bone strut
F
TORP
GAlton

FIGURE 13–2.

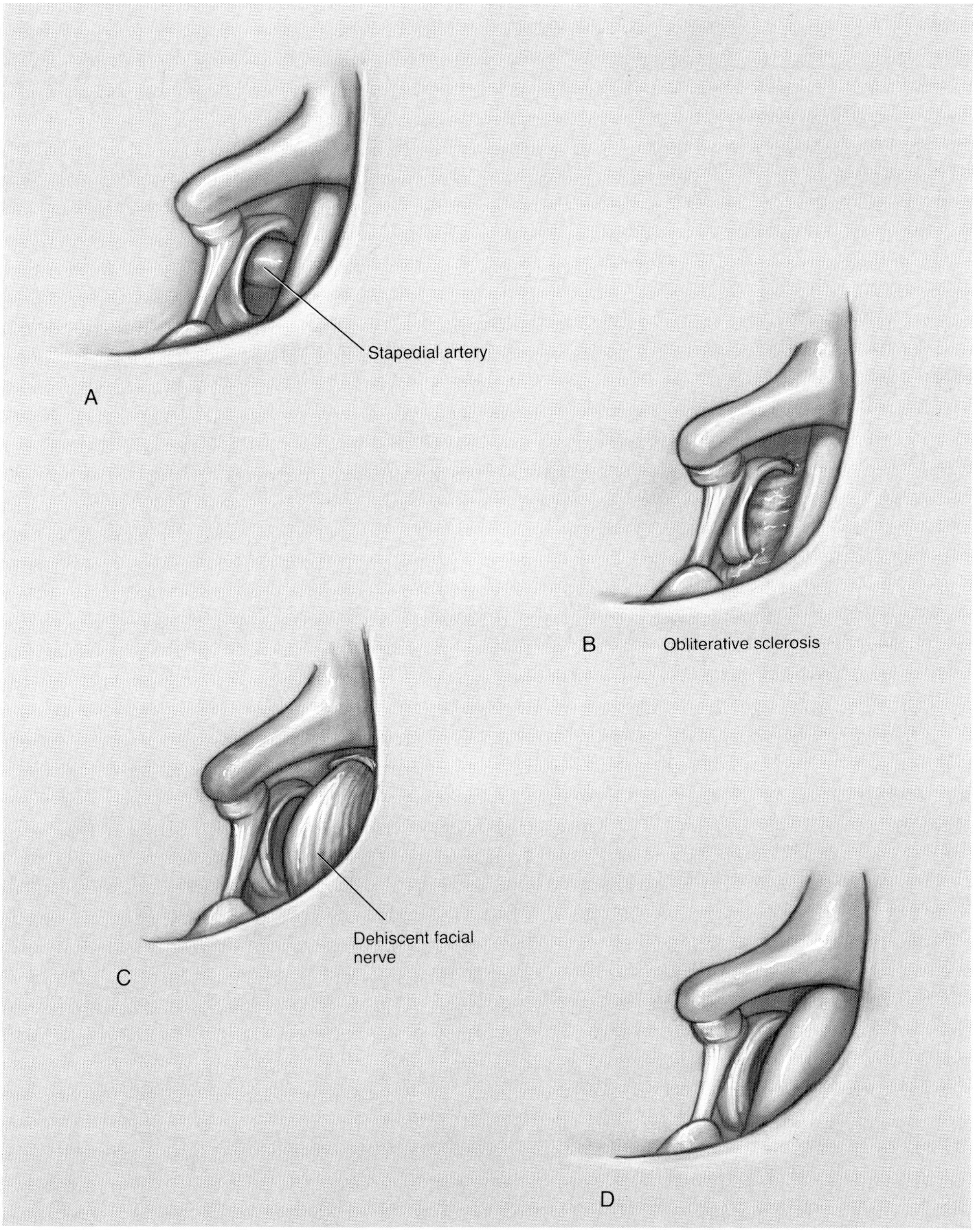
Stapedial artery
A
B
Obliterative sclerosis
Dehiscent facial
nerve
C
D

FIGURE 13–3.

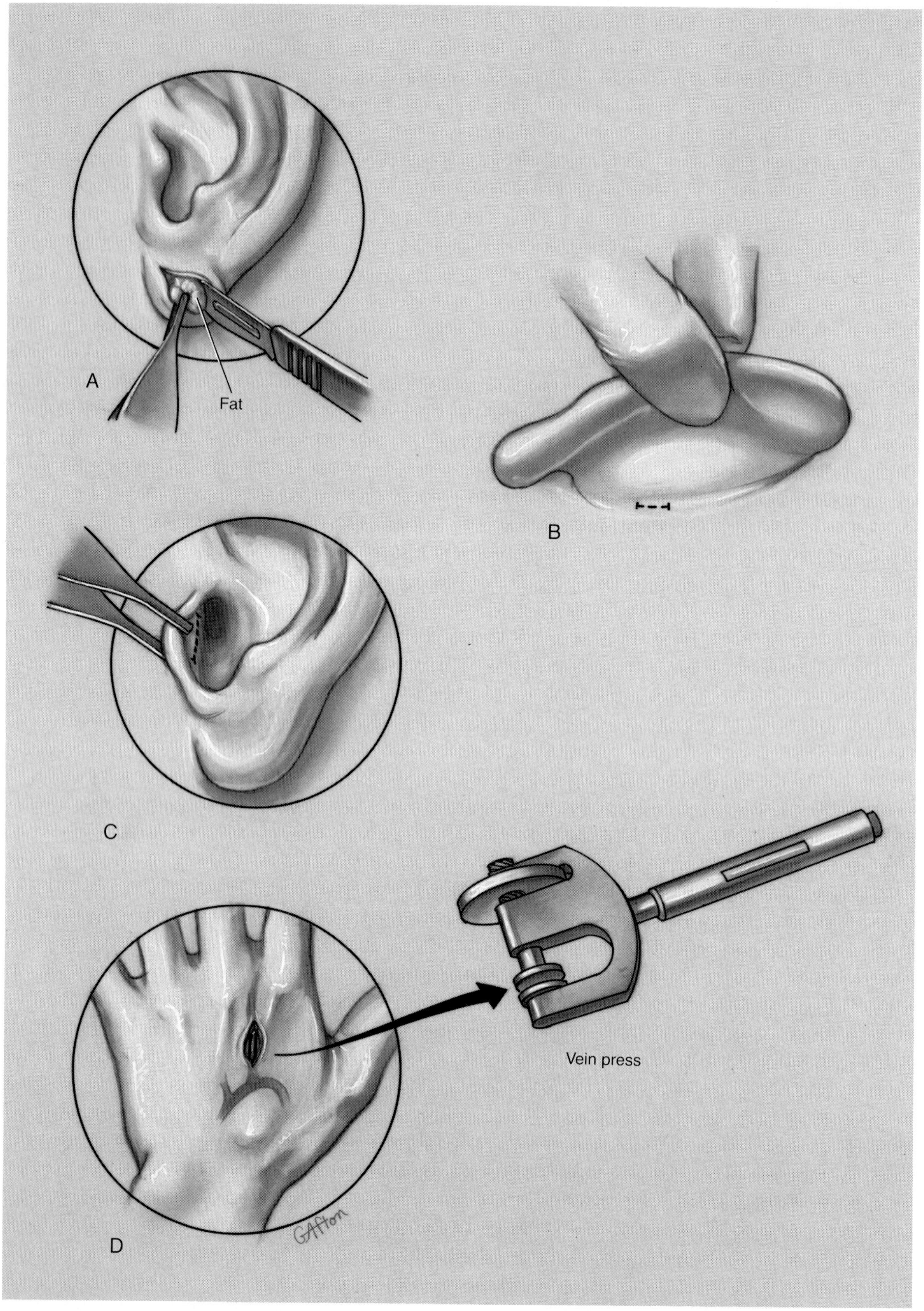

FIGURE 13–4.

and the tissue is left in saline solution. Tragal perichondrium is obtained via a small incision in the undersurface of the tragus, exposing the perichondrium, which can be peeled off the underlying cartilage (Fig. 13–4C). Meticulous hemostasis is done, the incision is closed with two or three appropriate sutures, and the perichondrium is gently pressed and rinsed in saline. All instruments and materials used in this area should be rinsed in order to remove any particles from their surfaces.

Vein can be harvested from the dorsum of the hand by a small incision. Both ends are carefully tied; the midsection of the vein (size as needed) is removed and split open, the endothelial layer is removed, and the vein is pressed and rinsed in saline (Fig. 13–4*D*). In general, the adventitial layer is placed facing the vestibule. With perichondrium, the side in direct contact with the cartilage is placed facing the middle ear; otherwise small cartilage remnants may fall into the vestibule, potentially causing complications.

Making the Prosthesis

Many satisfactory prostheses are commercially available. Except for polyethylene struts and wire Gelfoam prostheses (which tend to have a higher incidence of fistulae) and Plastipore pistons (which tend to cause local reactions), the vast majority of prostheses are satisfactory if properly used. Their use will depend on surgical findings and the surgeon's preference and experience. Both wire and connective tissue and wire Teflon pistons can be made at surgery. These are the classic prostheses that have stood the test of time. The wire and connective tissue prosthesis can be tailored to the needed length or bent or curved in narrow windows or prominent facial nerves; it also provides an excellent seal.

The technique for making an incus-to-oval window prosthesis is depicted in Figure 13–5. A piece of connective tissue is cut to a size of 2 × 3 mm. This is placed on the edge of the die and is tied at its midportion with a 0.005-mm stainless steel wire (Fig. 13–5*A*). A drop of saline helps handling and placing of the tissue in the desired position. With an alligator forceps holding both ends, the knot is tightened until it disappears into the connective tissue. The wire is looped around the larger post of the die with the bottom of the connective tissue at 4 mm (Fig. 13–5*B*). The connective tissue end is rotated around the smaller post (Fig. 13–5C). Wire-cutting scissors are used to cut the loop (to hook into the incus) larger or shorter, according to the size of the long process of the incus. The wire-cutting scissors are slid up to the knot in the middle of the graft and the wire is sectioned. No sharp ends should be left unless the patient has otosclerosis associated with endolymphatic hydrops; in this case, an end purposely left sharp might work as a "conservative tack." The prosthesis is left in saline until use. A 5-mm malleus-to-oval window prosthesis is shown in Figure 13–5*D*.

The making of a wire piston is shown in Figure 13–6; the technique (after Rosales) is self-explanatory.

Procedure

The footplate is fractured at the midline with a needle (Fig. 13–7*A*). Creating a hole in the footplate is frequently described, but for a total stapedectomy an actual fracture is better and prevents a floating footplate. The mucosa is not elevated at the footplate; this avoids bleeding and helps to prevent small, loose fragments from falling into the vestibule. If there is bleeding, small pieces of Gelfoam saturated with a solution of 1:1000 epinephrine are applied topically. A No. 24 suction tip with the finger off the hole is used. It cannot be emphasized enough that the suction tip must stay away from the oval window at all times. Suctioning perilymph in the oval window can cause a "dead ear."

The incudostapedial joint is gently separated with a joint knife (Fig. 13–7*B*); the knife is slid between the incus and the head of the stapes to ensure that separation is total. The stapedial tendon is sectioned with the joint knife or a Bellucci scissors (Fig. 13–7*C*, *D*). Sometimes it is possible to gently peel it along with the mucoperiosteum and leave it attached to the long process of the incus (Fig. 13–7*E*, *F*). This allows perhaps some protection from sound and permits better vascularity to the long process of the incus. In the unusual event of a prominent pyramidal eminence, the tendon is sectioned and the eminence curetted. The head and crura of the stapes (stapedial arch) are mobilized with an angled hook toward the promontory and *not* in an anteroposterior direction (which can cause part of the footplate to drop into the oval window). Usually the arch fractures at the junctions of the crura with the footplate, and is removed with the angled hook or a baby alligator forceps (Fig. 13–7G). Measurements are now made (Fig. 13–7*H*).

At this point, the patient is instructed not to move or talk. Similar recommendations apply to those in the operating room. The footplate is removed with a Hough hoe or a right-angled hook (Fig. 13–8*A*). It is

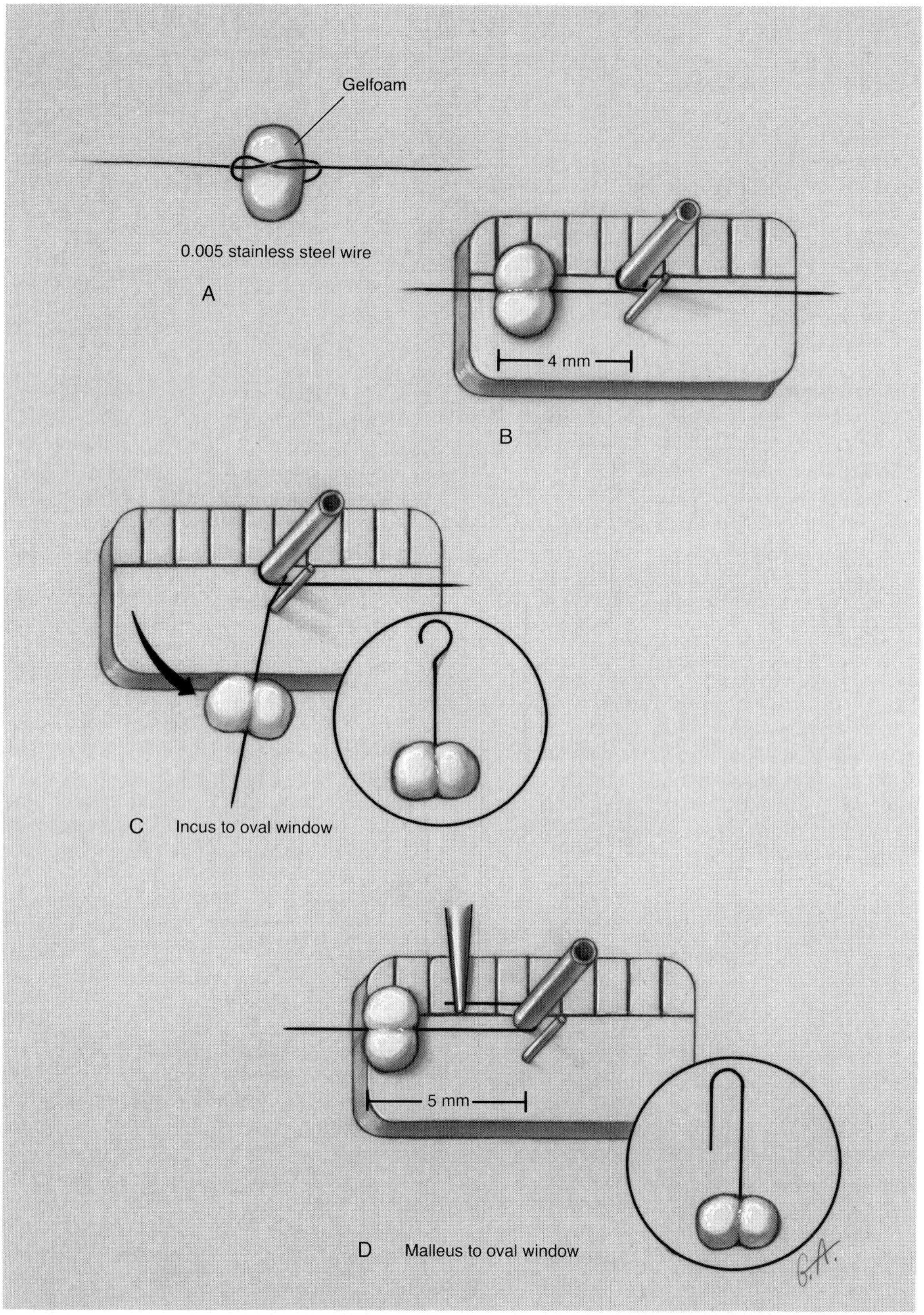
Gelfoam
0.005 stainless steel wire
A
4 mm
B
C
Incus to oval window
5 mm
D
Malleus to oval window

FIGURE 13–5.

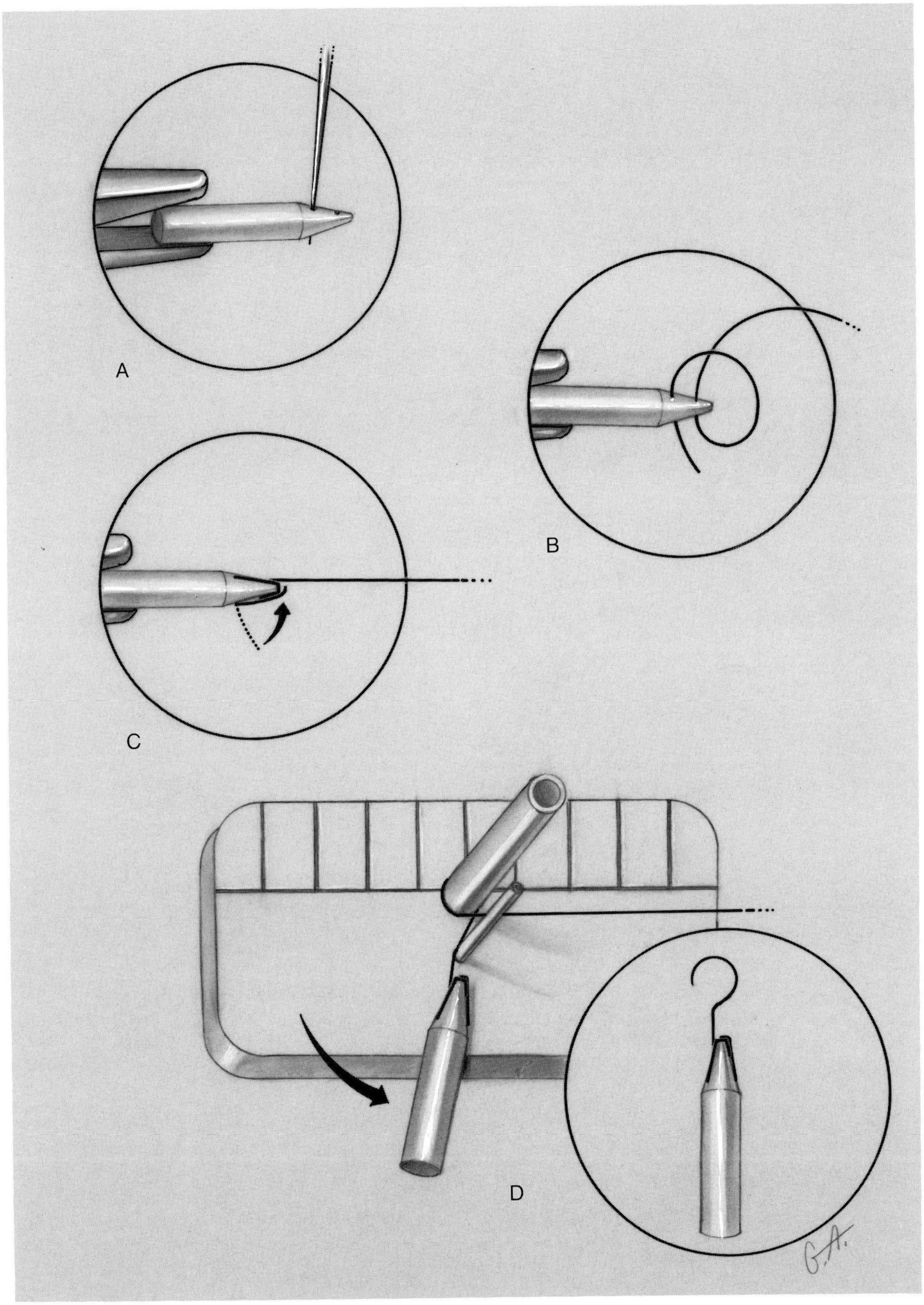

FIGURE 13–6.

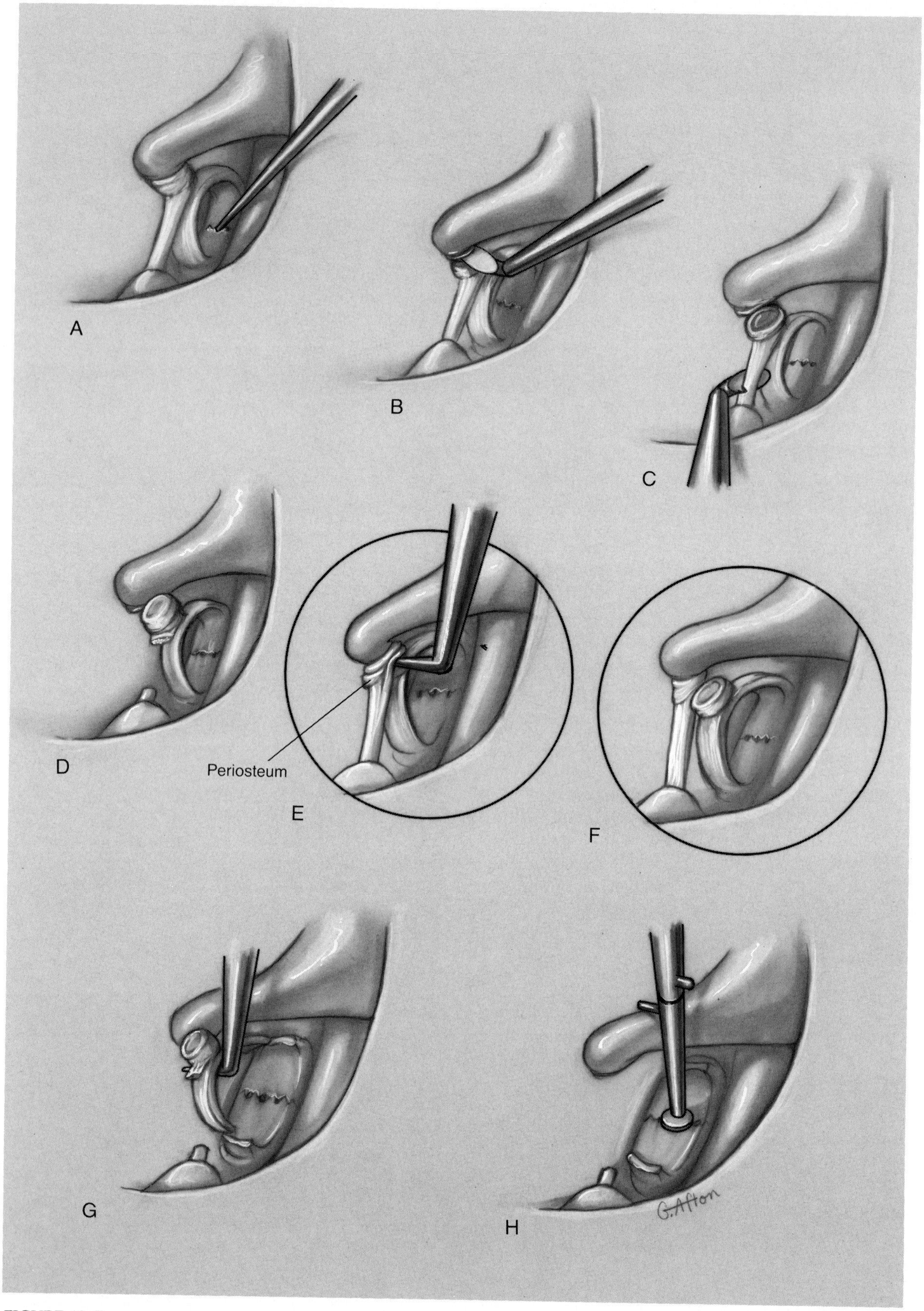

FIGURE 13–7.

important to place the instrument just barely beneath the fragments to be removed in order to avoid damaging the underlying vestibular structures. Bone fragments are either totally or partially removed (usually by removing the posterior two thirds of the footplate), depending upon the procedure to be done (Fig. 13–8*A*).

With an alligator forceps or a horizontal opening forceps (which allows better visualization) holding the bare edge of the wire, the prosthesis is placed (Fig. 13–8*B*). If it cannot be placed easily in position, it is released and mobilized bimanually (for example, with the suction tip and a Hough hoe). If the wire is bent during positioning, it is better to use a new prosthesis than to fix it. The oval window should be left open for the shortest time possible; excessive time of exposure is directly related to effects on hearing. Once the wire connective tissue is well centered, additional connective tissue can be used to seal the window. If a prosthesis without connective tissue is used, the oval window graft is placed before the prosthesis (Fig. 13–8*C*). Such a graft ideally should fit precisely; it cannot be too small or too large. If a piston is used, connective tissue is wrapped around it. Small pieces of Gelfoam can then be placed over the connective tissue and around the prosthesis. Piston width in a stapedectomy is from 0.6 to 0.8 mm, whereas in a stapedotomy (described below), it is 0.4 mm.

The prosthesis is crimped with a McGee crimper or an alligator forceps. The crimper has the advantage of not closing completely; thus there is less chance of fracturing the long process of the incus (Fig. 13–8*D*). It is also light and thin and does not obstruct vision. Crimping is done in an anteroposterior direction and involves only the ring around the incus; otherwise, the prosthesis will be bent and will have to be changed. Teflon wire pistons bend very easily if not crimped properly. The round window reflex, the mobility of the ossicular chain, and the adequacy of the prosthesis position are checked at this point, after which the flap is repositioned. The patient is then asked if there is any improvement in hearing. Finally, the ear canal is packed (described below).

Problems and Variations During Surgery

Bleeding. Small vessels respond very well to topical application of cotton balls or Gelfoam saturated with epinephrine. In the footplate it is preferable to use Gelfoam in order to avoid cotton strands. Lidocaine (Xylocaine) with epinephrine should *not* be used in the open vestibule since it can cause marked vestibular disturbances. The presence of an abnormal jugular bulb has been described in another chapter; if its location allows a safe exploration and stapes procedure, it should not be a contraindication. A persistent stapedial artery (running over the footplate) is a very unusual finding. This artery is fairly large and should not be confused with small but prominent mucoperiosteal vessels in the footplate. If a small opening on the footplate can be made and a small piston placed, the procedure can be done; otherwise, the operation should not take place.

Obliteration of the round window and fixation of the malleus have been described.

Accidental Dislocation of the Incus. The incus should be palpated. If the dislocation is partial and the incus moves with the malleus, the prosthesis is placed as usual. If it is totally luxated, a malleus-to-oval window prosthesis (or an equivalent prosthesis, as described in Chapter 12) is substituted.

Fracture of the long process of the incus while crimping the prosthesis is rare; if it happens, the prosthesis can be crimped on the remaining strut (Fig. 13–9*A*). If this is impossible, a malleus-to-oval window prosthesis (or its equivalent) can be used instead.

Pain. An occasional patient might complain of pain when the middle ear mucosa is touched. Topical application of 2% lidocaine in cotton or Gelfoam pledgets suffices.

Prominent Promontory. This can be drilled carefully in order to provide adequate visualization (Fig. 13–9*C*). Depending upon the visualization obtained, a small piston or a wire connective tissue prosthesis is placed. An abnormal (open or redundant) seventh nerve in itself is not a contraindication. It may be possible to mobilize it gently with a blunt hook, allowing an opening to be made in the footplate for placement of a prosthesis. Sometimes, depending upon the anatomic conditions, a wire connective tissue prosthesis can be bent to fit. On occasion, an offset Robinson prosthesis fits precisely. Flexibility and use of a prosthesis to fit the need are paramount; the course of action should reflect the anatomic and functional needs of the patient and the rational and safe approach of the surgeon.

Narrow Oval Window. A narrow window can be secondary to a prominent overlying promontory; it can also represent a congenital defect, which not uncommonly leads to a perilymph "gusher." It is also very important to assess the facial nerve and its relationship to the footplate (Fig. 13–9*D*). If the window itself is quite narrow and a congenital defect is suspected, a small opening can be made with a

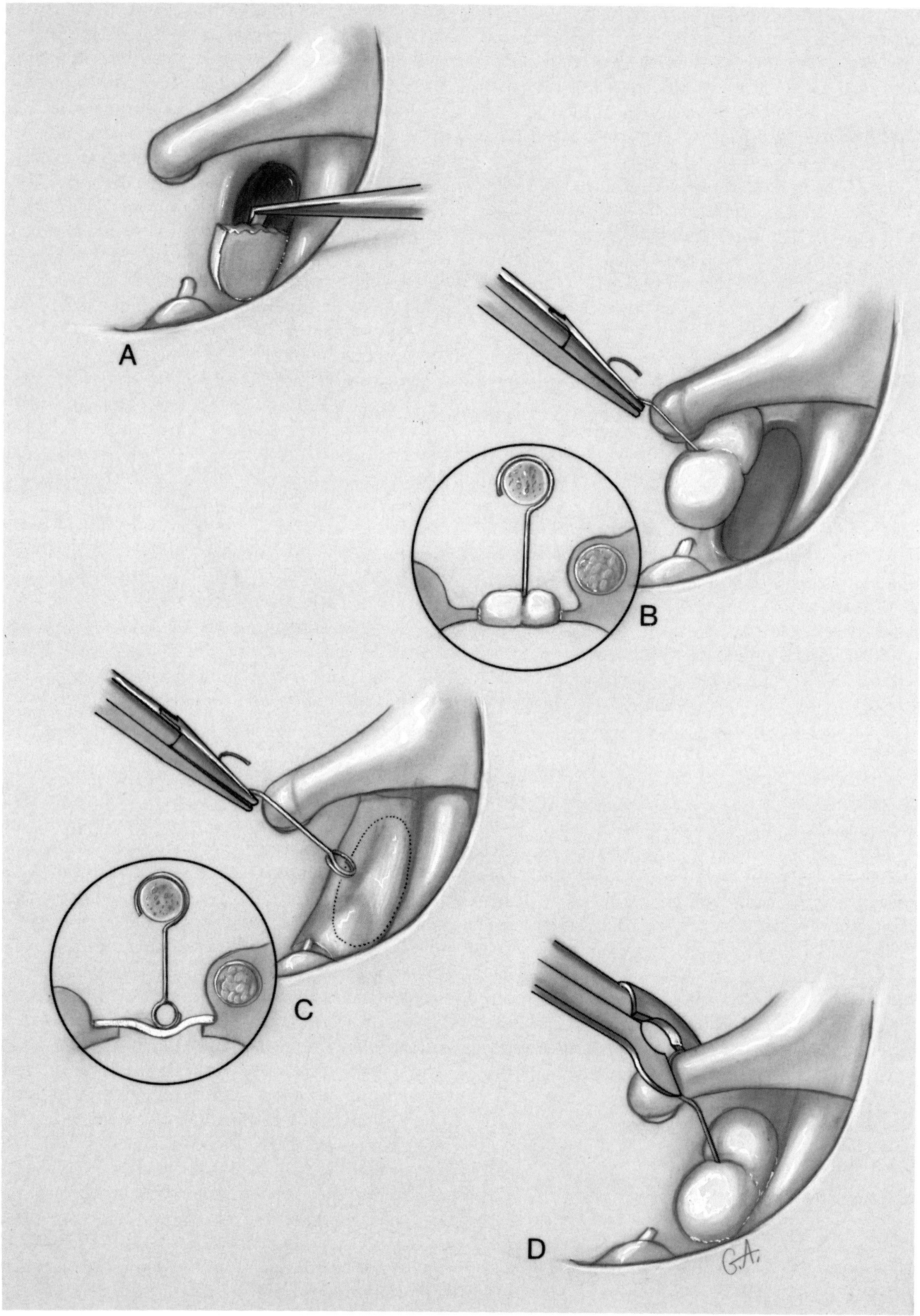

FIGURE 13–8.

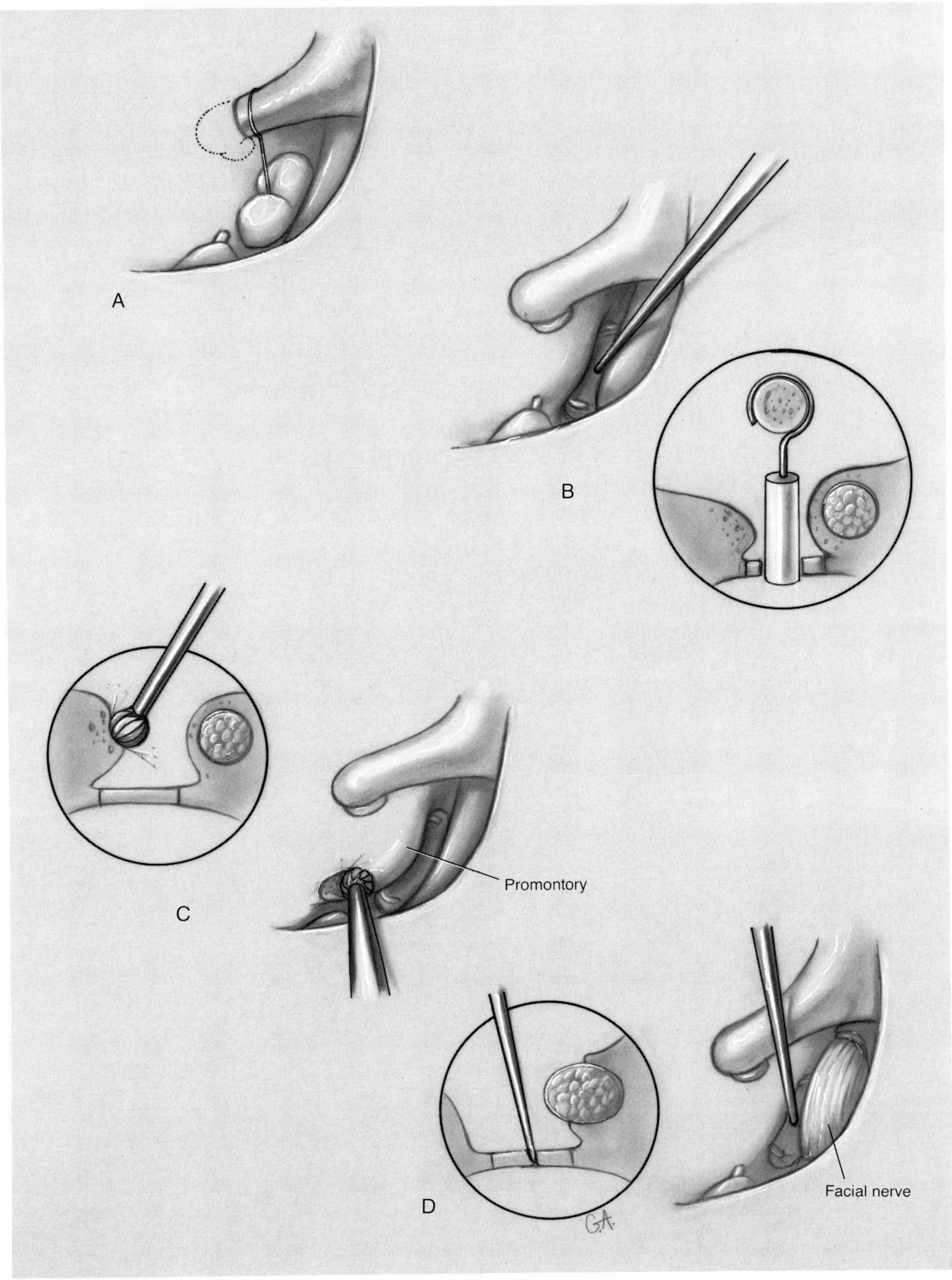

FIGURE 13–9.

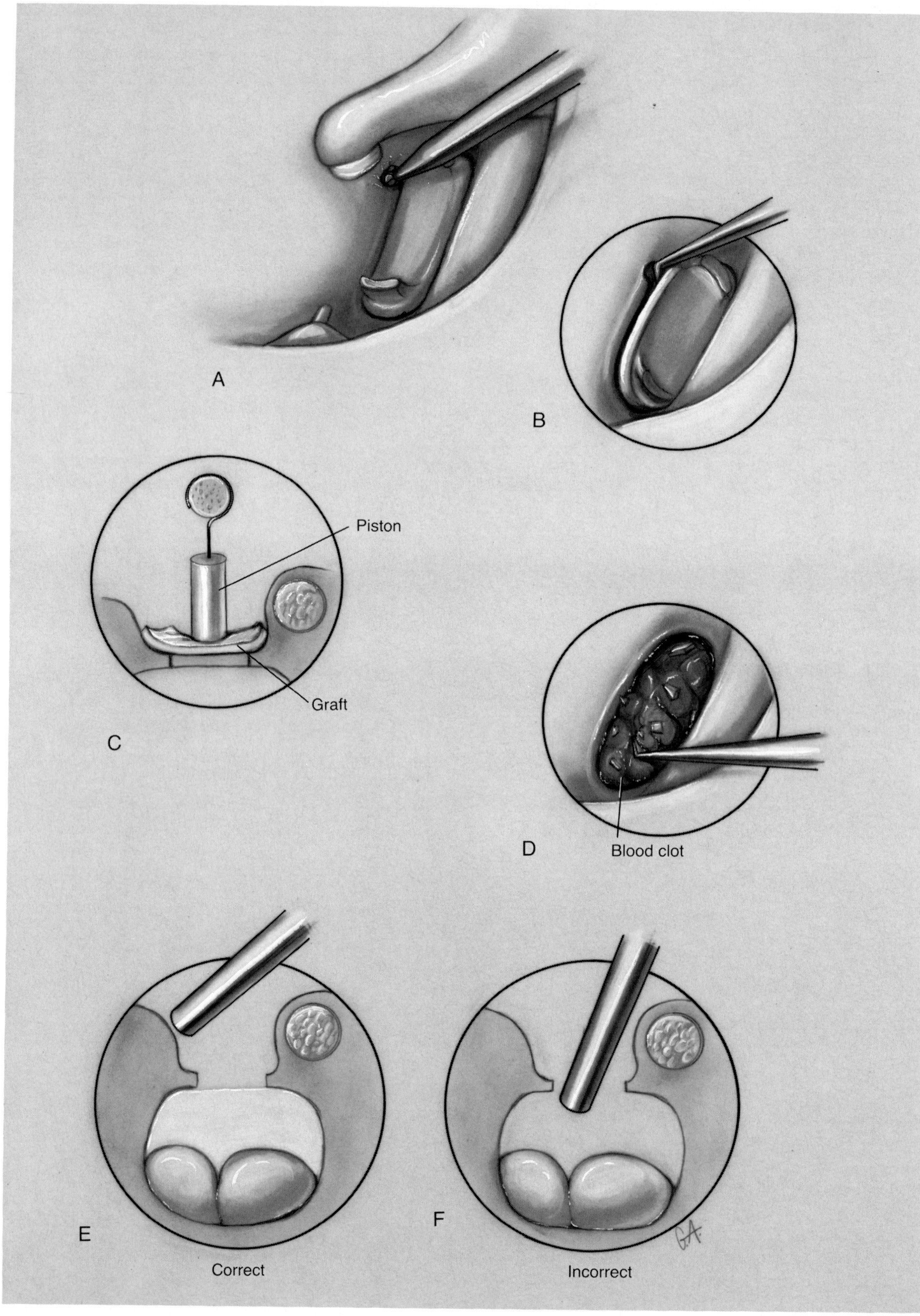

FIGURE 13–10.

small, sharp needle; if a gusher is found, it is covered with connective tissue and Gelfoam. The head of the patient is raised and the procedure is terminated. If there is no gusher, the small opening can be enlarged to place a 0.4-mm piston or a thin prosthesis.

Cerebrospinal Fluid Leak. A "gusher" is uncommon, and is generally (but not exclusively) seen in cases of a congenitally fixed stapes (and a patent cochlear aqueduct). The patient's head is elevated and a large connective tissue wire prosthesis used for a seal, with additional connective tissue.

Dry Vestibule. If the perilymph is accidentally suctioned out of the oval window (the suction tip should *never* be put into the oval window [Fig. 13–10*E, F*]), the window will refill. If it does not, a few drops of saline are used to fill it. Blood might stimulate an inflammatory reaction in the vestibule.

Floating Footplate. This refers to a footplate that becomes mobile before an opening is made in it and after removal of the arch (the superstructure consisting of the head and crura). This is a difficult challenge. One way to avoid it is to fracture the footplate before removing the arch. A floating footplate tends to occur in a stapes that has been previously mobilized or in one with poor fixation.

Sometimes the footplate can be carefully removed with an angled hook. If this is impossible, an opening can be made with a diamond bur or small bur in the anteroinferior margin, and the footplate removed with a hook (Fig. 13–10*A, B*). If this too is impossible and the footplate is not depressed, fascia can be placed over it and a shorter piston placed. If refixation occurs (which is likely), the footplate can be revised with better chances of success (Fig. 13–10C).

Depressed Fragments. Depressed fragments can be removed carefully with a hook, but "fishing" in the vestibule should be avoided; it is better to leave the fragments in the vestibule and use ample amounts of steroids, topically and parenterally. Some authors recommend placing a few drops of blood in the vestibule and allowing them to clot; when the clot is removed the fragments may come out with it (Fig. 13–10*D*).

Obliterative Otosclerosis

If an obliterative focus is found—for example, if the oval window has no discernible footplate owing to otosclerotic change (Fig. 13–11*A*)—the procedure is different. If the patient is a child with an active focus, it is better to delay this procedure. (The question of operating on children with otosclerosis is not an easy one; in general, it seems better to delay such procedures but some surgeons do perform them, reportedly with good results.)

A thick footplate must be thinned with a 0.6- to 1-mm cutting or diamond bur with slow rotation (Fig. 13–11*B*). This is done anteroposteriorly, saucerizing evenly and applying just enough pressure over the footplate to be effective. Bone dust is meticulously removed. If the footplate is thinned evenly (to a thin bluish plate), a small (0.5-mm) opening is made and a piston surrounded by connective tissue is placed (Fig. 13–11*C–E*). Less commonly, the footplate is fractured and removed, and a graft is placed.

Stapedotomy

This procedure has gained many advocates in recent years because it has been suggested that it involves less risk of inner ear damage, less chance of adhesions between the graft and vestibular contents, and less mobility of the oval window as a whole. As with all surgical innovations, time and experience will tell. The procedure also can be done with a laser (see Chapter 14). The operation is similar to a classic stapedectomy, up to the point of opening the footplate. Then the footplate is perforated with a sharp needle (or special microdrill) in three different spots. Enlargement of these openings is done very carefully with angled hooks, trying to leave a single central opening that is slightly larger than 0.4 mm. The size can be measured with a 0.4-mm measuring rod. This step can be done without removing the stapes arch, avoiding mobilization of the stapes. Once this is done, the incudostapedial joint is separated and the crura are *sectioned* with crurotomy scissors; the prosthesis is then placed over the incus and into the footplate opening and surrounded with connective tissue.

Stapes Interposition

In the presence of a wide niche, an anterior fixation, and a healthy posterior crus, an interposition procedure is a rational alternative. It represents a safe and logical approach but is difficult to perform properly, requiring ability and experience. The procedure involves removing a portion of the footplate (fixed) and mobilizing the posterior crus (as a "prosthesis") over an underlying graft, thus re-establishing the continuity and mobility of the ossicular chain.

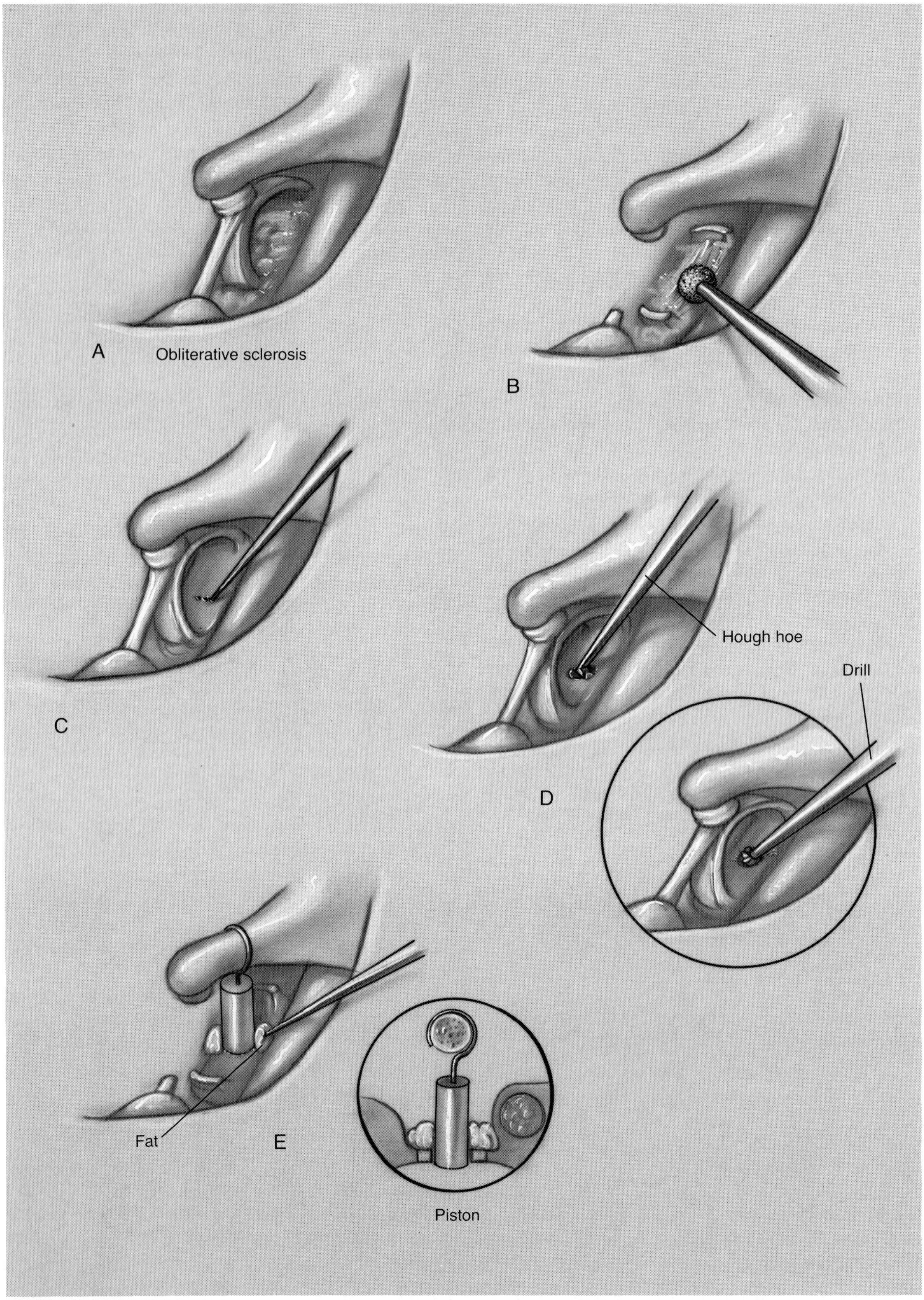

FIGURE 13–11.

Initially the anterior crus is sectioned with angled crurotomy scissors (Fig. 13–12*A*). Portmann (an advocate of this procedure) recommends sectioning in the main axis of the stapes, introducing the scissors between the malleus and the incus, since the simpler approach through the promontory carries the risk of fracturing the stapes at another site. This is followed by sectioning of the stapedial tendon. The posterior crus is then carefully fractured with a microhook at its junction with the footplate. When the posterior crus is free (from mucosal adhesions as well), it is mobilized anteriorly while the incus is lifted with a Hough hoe (thus avoiding fractures in the posterior crus) (Fig. 13–12*B*). The footplate is fractured and the posterior two thirds are removed (Fig. 13–12*C* and Fig. 13–13*A*). A graft is placed and the posterior crus is repositioned over the graft (while the incus is lifted), re-establishing ossicular continuity and mobility (Fig. 13–13*B–D*).

Some surgeons perform this procedure by removing part of the anterior crus and the anterior half of the footplate (an anterior crurotomy). The remaining mobile posterior crus and underlying mobile footplate are mobilized toward the center of the oval window (over the graft). The stapedial tendon might or might not be sectioned, according to need. A posterior crurotomy also can be done in reverse fashion, but usually the point of footplate fixation is anterior.

Malleus-to-Oval Window Prosthesis

The aim of this procedure is to place a wire prosthesis from the handle of the malleus to the oval window. It is important to place the wire under a subperiosteal pocket in the handle of the malleus, as close to the short process as possible.

Such prostheses are commercially available, but a wire connective tissue can be made. Stapes prosthesis wire and a bending die are used to manufacture a prosthesis; only the large post of the die is used to shape the "crook" or "handle" (see Fig. 13–5).

With a joint knife, an incision is made through the mucoperiosteum on the undersurface of the handle of the malleus, creating a subperiosteal pocket (Fig. 13–14*A*). On occasion it is necessary (because of contact with the overlying tympanic membrane) to place the prosthesis at the neck of the malleus. The stapes arch is removed first, and the prosthesis is placed to ensure correct length. Initially the prosthesis is held in a manner similar to a stapes prosthesis, but it is placed at a right angle to the malleus handle (Fig. 13–14*B*). Once it is over the malleus handle (under the periosteal pocket), it is turned down so that it is perpendicular to the handle; this maneuver makes positioning easier. If the length is satisfactory, the prosthesis is displaced anteriorly, the footplate is removed, and a connective tissue graft is placed over the oval window. The prosthesis is positioned and then tightened bimanually (with an angled hook and suction tip or blunt instrument) along the undersurface of the malleus (Fig. 13–14*C*). It should be remembered that, regardless of how well the prosthesis might fit, it is anatomically and functionally less efficient than a stapedectomy prosthesis; at the same time, the oval window is subjected to more trauma (the mobility of the malleus is greater than that of the incus and has less dampening effect).

Closure and Packing

The flap is carefully repositioned. If a small tear is present, the edges are carefully approximated. If necessary, small pieces of Gelfoam or connective tissue can be used, and the flap left somewhat loose. For larger perforations, a graft is placed and ample amounts of antibiotics and anti-inflammatory medications are used. Packing techniques have been described. The patient must lie with the operated ear up and is closely followed postoperatively; the need to avoid straining, lifting, or undue effort cannot be emphasized enough. Complications continue to be very possible until complete healing has occurred (at four to six weeks) and may still occur thereafter. Some failures can be traced to overconfidence in the operative procedure. It has been argued that prophylactic antibiotics are unnecessary; however, the authors strongly recommend the use of intraoperative and postoperative antibiotics.

Complications

As in any surgical procedure, awareness and prevention of possible complications are the keys. Adequate preoperative evaluation, a well-defined diagnosis, and rational surgical plans are of paramount importance. The patient on the operating table is assumed to have had a thorough overall check (including cardiovascular status, allergies, endocrinologic problems, and so on).

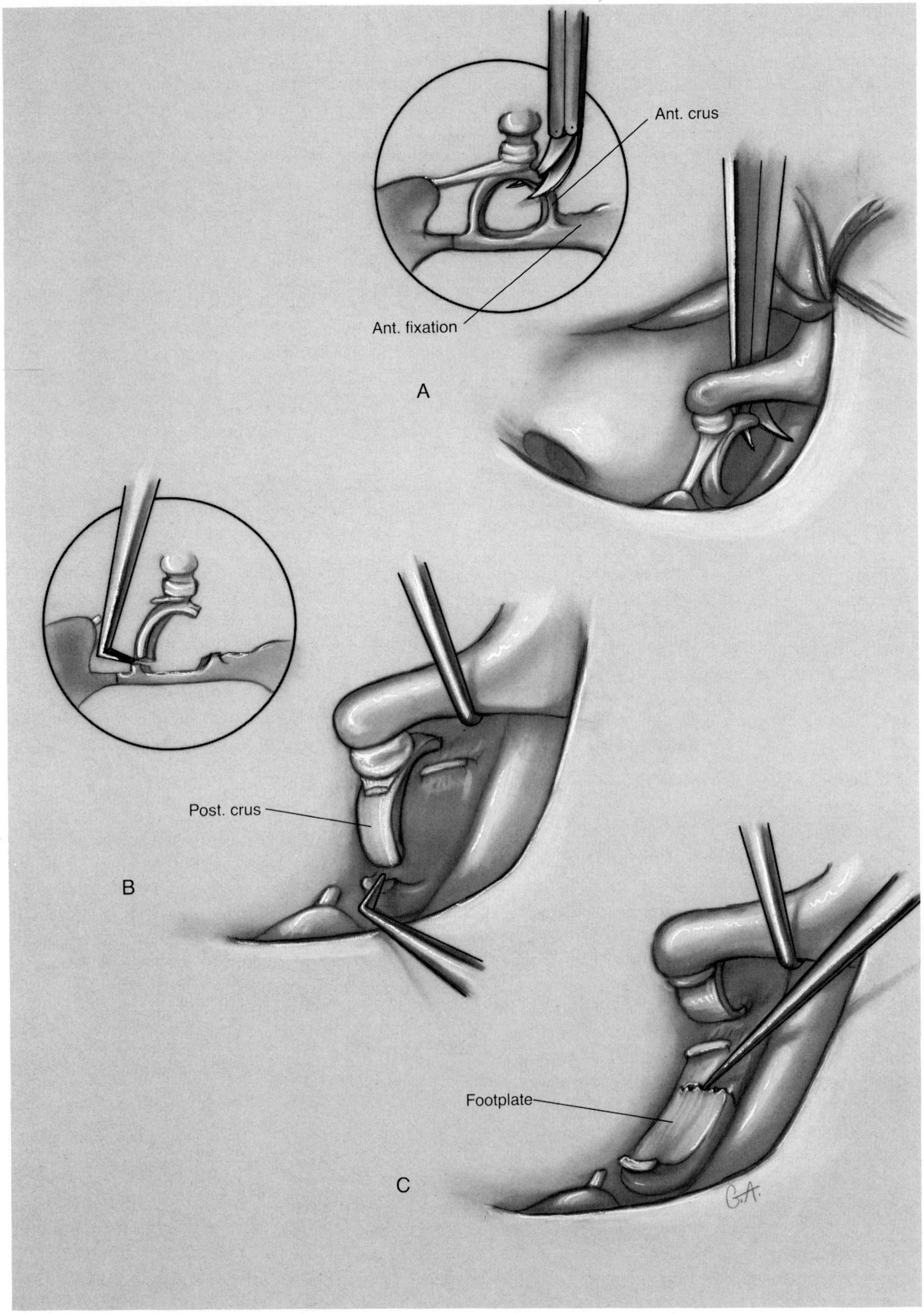

FIGURE 13–12.

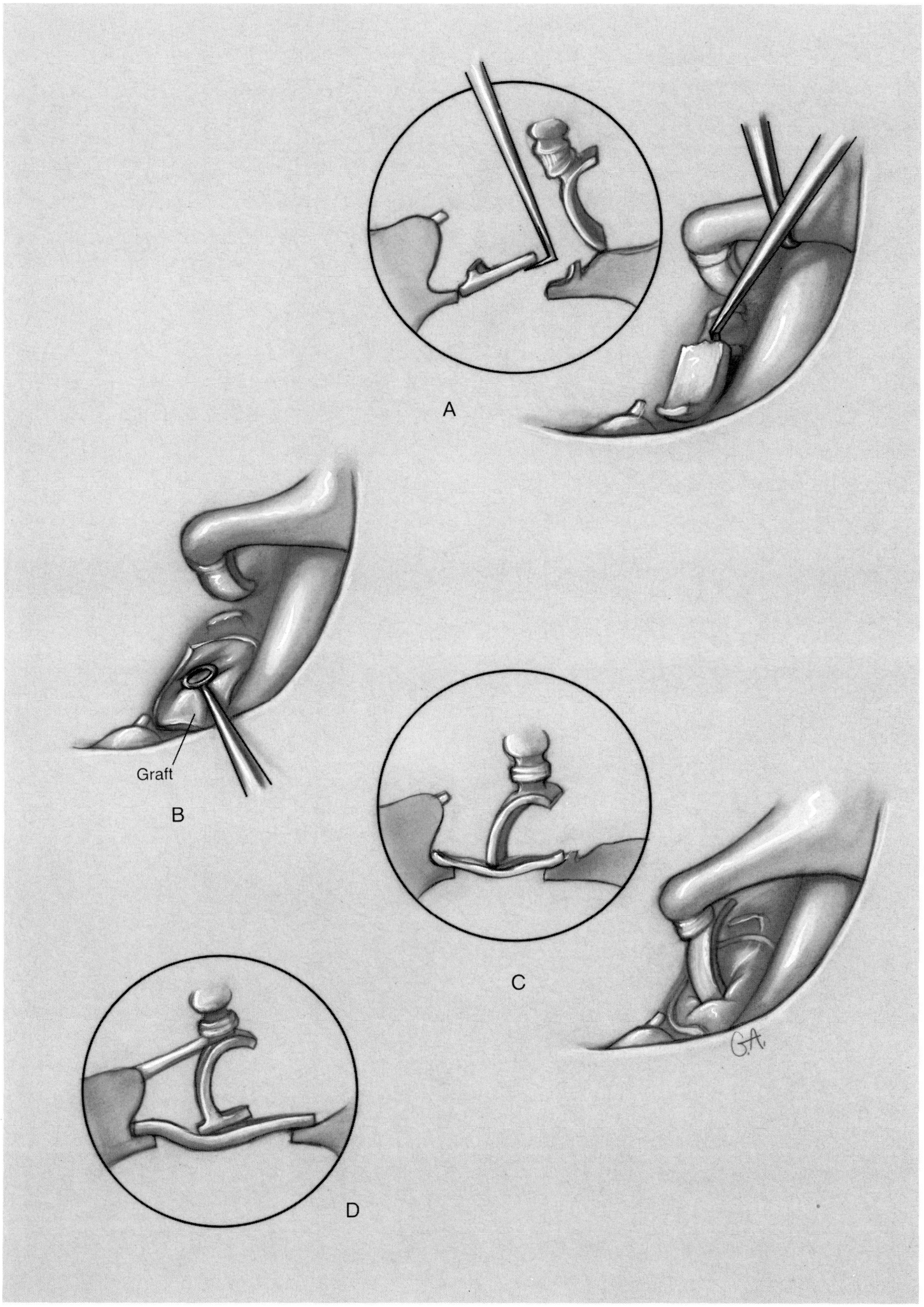

FIGURE 13–13.

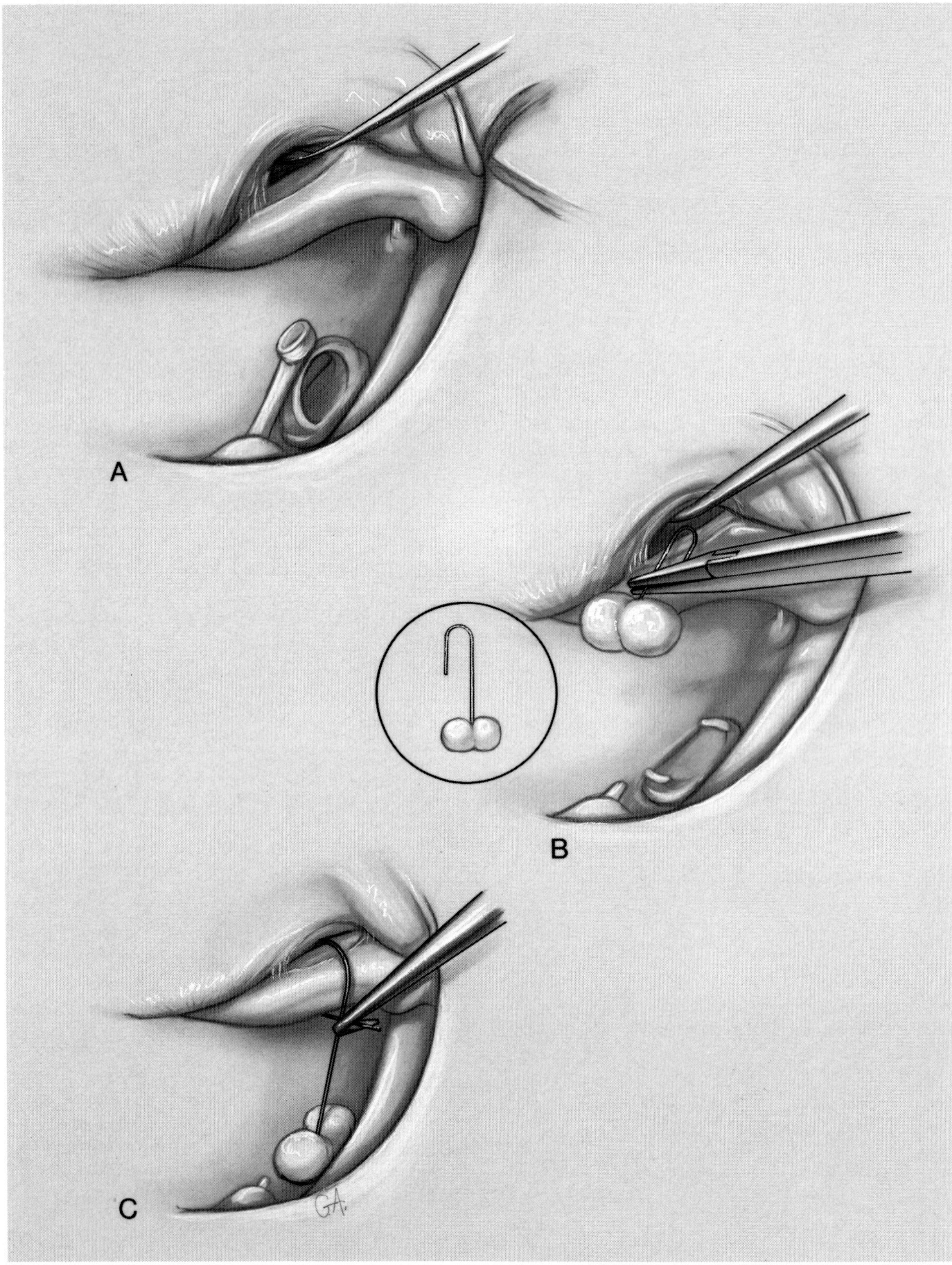

FIGURE 13–14.

Dysgeusia following injury to the chorda tympani is characterized by tingling or a metallic taste on the tongue on the operated side, or both. This always improves, but the reason for the improvement is unclear.

Infection is rare, especially if adequate prophylaxis (including meticulous cleansing of the ear canal) has been undertaken. If it occurs, the packing should be removed, cultures obtained (if possible), and antibiotics given (or changed) topically and parenterally. Infection may lead to labyrinthitis and should be treated aggressively.

Facial palsy may follow injection of local anesthetics, but should be only temporary. Palsy immediately following stapedectomy probably signals damage to an exposed nerve in the oval window during the procedure. Surgical re-exploration is indicated. It should be kept in mind that damage probably is restricted to local edema or puncturing of the nerve; sectioning of the nerve is extremely rare. Delayed paralysis must be evaluated, and is treated in the same manner as Bell's palsy.

Vertigo is fairly common during the first few postoperative days; however, symptoms should be mild, short lived, and responsive to rest and vestibular sedatives. Vertiginous symptoms should not be taken lightly; they could be a warning sign, which left unattended might lead to irreversible sensory deafness. Persistence of vertigo or severe vertigo might be indicative of a perilymph fistula, a thin or leaky graft, periprosthesis leak around a Teflon piston (associated with fluctuating hearing loss), a prosthesis that is too long, labyrinthitis, or reparative granuloma. Operative causes include trauma during the operation or loose bone fragments in the vestibule. Early trauma or barotrauma may displace a prosthesis, leading to a fistula.

If these symptoms persist in spite of therapeutic measures and clinical judgment suggests a complication, or if there is a sensory hearing involvement, exploration is indicated. When revising a stapedectomy (or any ear procedure), special care must be taken in lifting a thin skin flap. Overlooking this important point might lead to serious and unnecessary tears in the flap or tympanic membrane. In general, not much graft is removed when revising, and connective tissue is placed around the oval window graft. The round window is evaluated for tears; if it is questionable, a small piece of Gelfoam can be used to obliterate the niche. If the prosthesis is found to be too long, the wire can be gently bent bimanually and the prosthesis shortened. If this is impossible or inadequate, the prosthesis should be replaced. Replacement carries the risk of pulling vestibular adhesions. Vertigo leading to sensory deafness is rare after one month, but can occur up to three to six years later. On occasion, vertigo might persist for years, even with good hearing; it may eventually require surgical correction.

Patients usually have a mild sensation of echoing along with tinnitus of no significance, but tinnitus and a feeling of resonance may indicate fistulae or labyrinthitis, especially if accompanied by vertigo.

Reparative granuloma is one of the few emergencies following stapedectomy. It occurs one to two weeks after surgery and is characterized by diminished hearing following an initial gain. Additional symptoms include aural fullness, loss of discrimination, and disequilibrium. The tympanic membrane may be dull, red, and thickened, with a hypervascular flap and inflammation in the posterosuperior quadrant. Removal of the granuloma is done in a piecemeal fashion, and fascia is placed over the graft. The prosthesis can be replaced by a new connective tissue wire prosthesis. Granulomas have not been shown to recur.

Conductive hearing losses occurring after initial gains are indications for revision. A prudent waiting period is suggested. A perforated tympanic membrane will require a myringoplasty. A delayed conductive hearing loss with an intact tympanic membrane suggests problems with the prosthesis. If there are adhesions around the prosthesis, they should be sharply excised and Gelfilm or Silastic placed. If necessary, the prosthesis is replaced. Prostheses that are displaced can be either repositioned or replaced; if the latter, they are gently loosened from the long process of the incus with angled hooks bimanually. If this is impossible, they can be sectioned with small scissors and replaced. If necrosis of the long process of the incus is present, the prosthesis is placed in the remnant. If this is impossible, a malleus-to-oval window prosthesis (or placement of a bone graft or TORP) is indicated.

A piston is used if there is recurrent bone deposition with closure of the oval window. If the focus is active and risk is involved, things should be left as they are for the time being. It should be kept in mind that the results of revision stapedectomy are not so good as in primary procedures; at the same time, vestibular involvement with secondary sensory hearing loss is more likely.

Pertinent Histopathology

FIGURE 13–15

This horizontal section shows a large otosclerotic focus fixing the stapes anteriorly and posteriorly. The stapes footplate is thickened. Note that the branches of Jacobson's nerve on the promontory (*parallel arrows*) are almost entirely surrounded by otosclerotic bone.

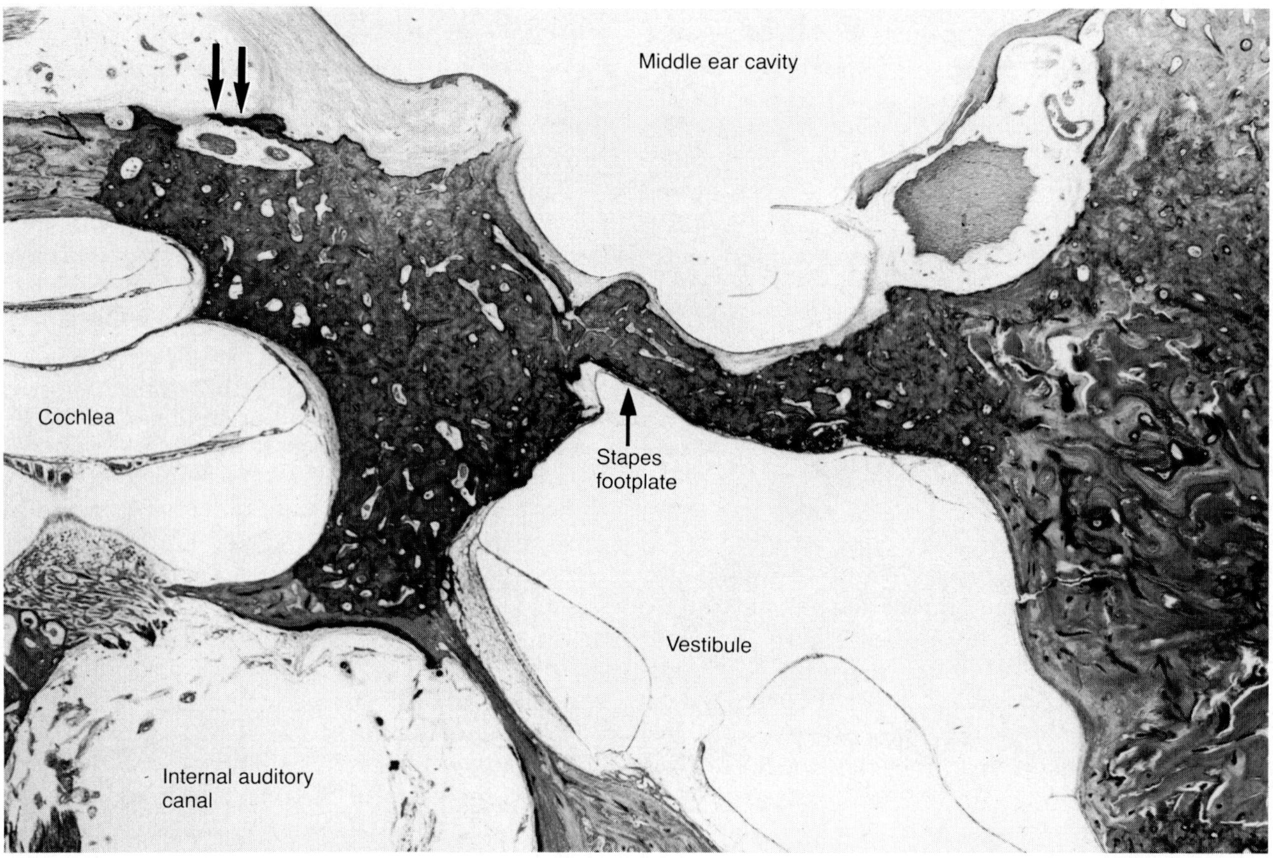

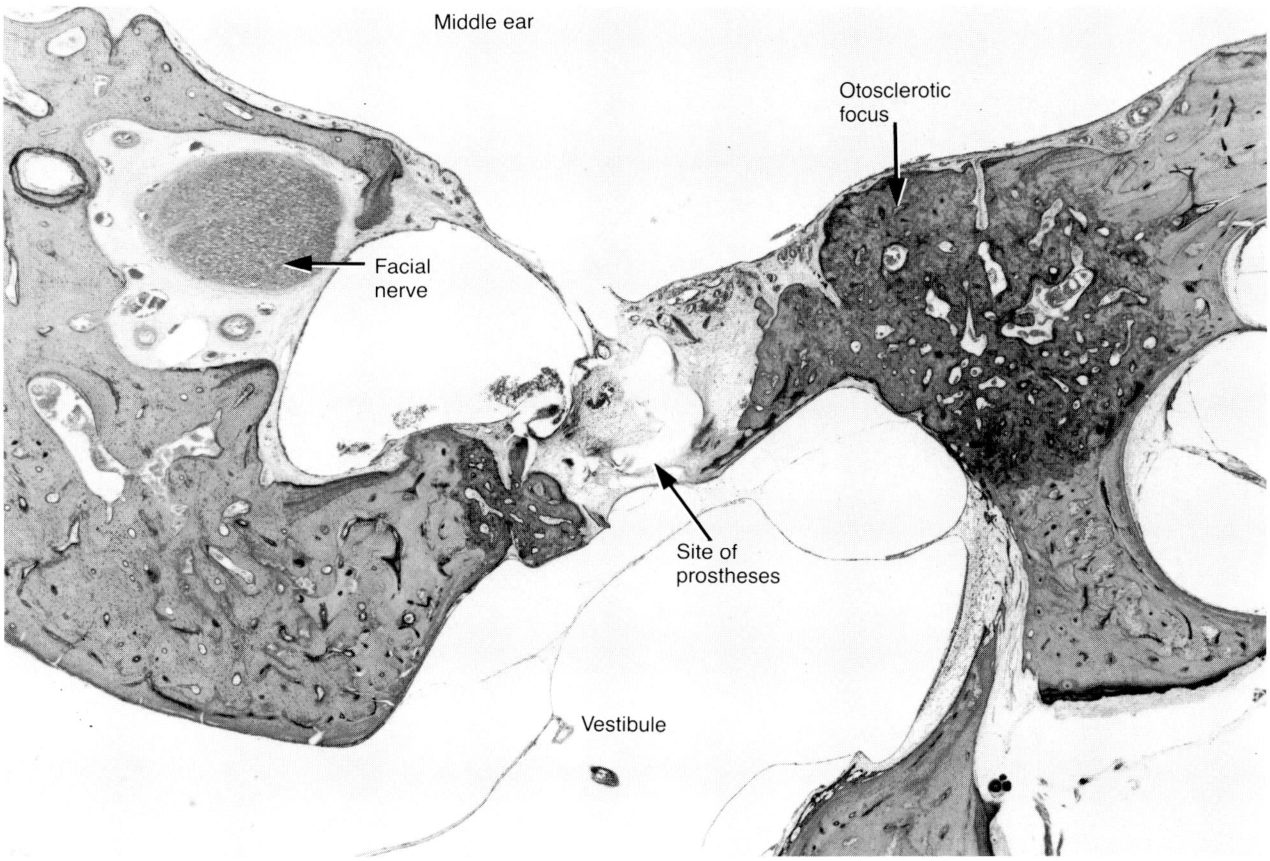

FIGURE 13–16

This section at the level of the oval window area is from the temporal bone of an individual who had a successful stapedectomy. Part of the otosclerotic footplate has been excised; the site is evident. The vestibule is intact. Note the close proximity of the vestibular contents.

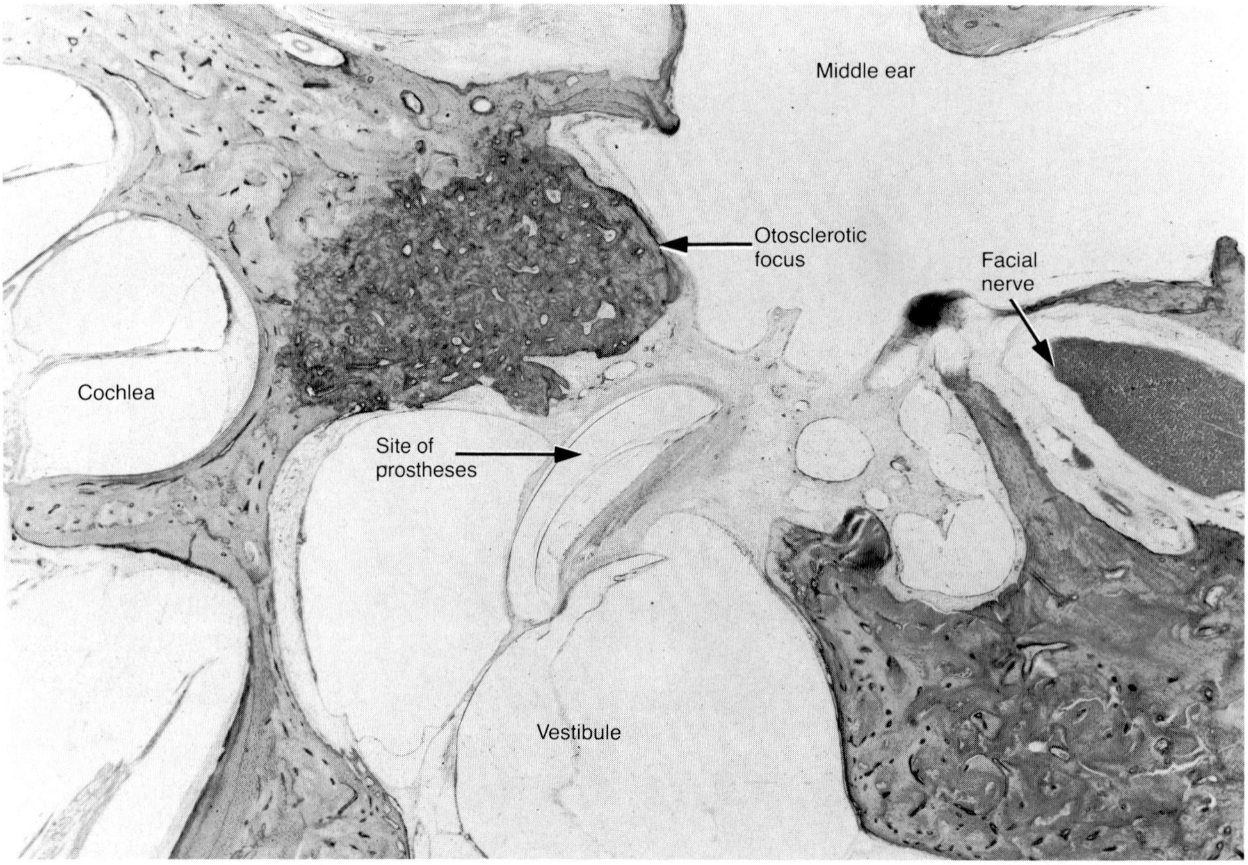

FIGURE 13–17

This section is from the temporal bone of an individual who underwent a stapedectomy with a piston prosthesis. The site of placement is evident; it can be seen that the piston was too deep and impinged on the vestibular structures. The surgical result was not ideal, and the patient had two pistons placed subsequently.

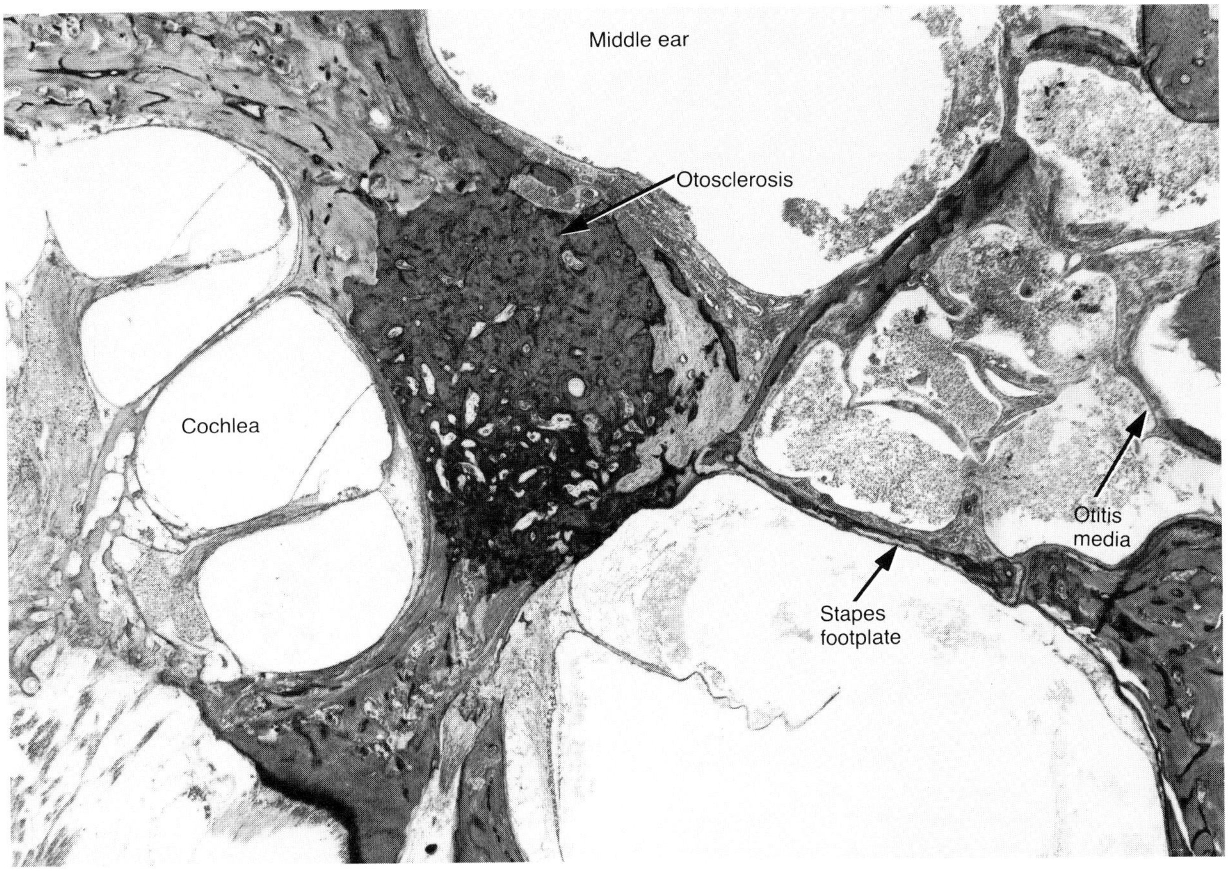

FIGURE 13–18

This horizontal section shows a stapes fixed by otosclerosis and a middle ear cavity with changes caused by otitis media. The section shows very clearly that if the footplate were removed under these conditions, the middle ear process would immediately penetrate the vestibule, with disastrous potential complications. (Some inflammation of the vestibule is evident.)

CHAPTER 14

Lasers in Otologic Surgery

The word laser is an acronym for *l*ight *a*mplification by *s*timulated *e*mission of *r*adiation. In the early 20th century Albert Einstein predicted that this form of energy existed. It was not until 1960 that Theodore Maimon developed the first working laser, made of a ruby crystal. Next, the gas laser was developed by Alec Javon in 1961. From these early lasers have come the many advanced models in medical use today.

A number of laser systems are currently available for use in the head and neck area. The authors feel that the visible-wavelength lasers—the argon and the KTP-532—are best suited for otologic work.

These visible-wavelength lasers are most useful for a number of reasons:

1. They allow for energy transmission through fiberoptic cables. Therefore, no articulating, bulky arms are needed and delivery of the beam to the intricate spaces of the middle ear is more easily accomplished.

2. The visible-spectrum lasers do not need a carrier beam to be seen by the naked eye. With the CO_2 beam, which uses an invisible wavelength, a carrier beam is needed in order to focus the beam on the surgical site; if these beams are not *exactly* coaxial, or if the mirrors of the articulating arm are imperfectly aligned, the surgical beam may not be delivered precisely where it is needed.

3. The visible-wavelength beams are readily absorbed by pigment and not by clear fluids, so hemostasis can be accomplished.

4. Along with fiberoptic capability a number of hand pieces have been developed, allowing the beam to be delivered by an alternate method. The hand piece is held like a scalpel, and the beam is focused by moving it up and down.

The development of the laser in otologic surgery has been a remarkable advance; like any surgical tool, however, it must be used correctly. Understanding the laser is absolutely essential, and proper training through a "hands-on" course is necessary before one can efficiently and safely use this new tool.

In discussing the surgical applications of the laser, three terms must be defined: *power, spot size,* and *pulse duration.* The power of the beam is its energy output and is measured in watts. Spot size refers to the diameter of the beam, and can vary from microns to millimeters. Pulse duration is the amount of time in which the beam actively performs its surgical function; it may be measured in milliseconds or it may be continuous. All of these functions can be varied at any time for different surgical needs.

Power density is another concept that must be understood. It is defined as the power per unit volume (Fig. 14–1*A*). The power of the laser beam is constant, but by varying the spot size of the beam at the focal point, the power density can be significantly altered. Focusing the beam to a very small spot size greatly increases the power density; with a large spot size the power density is decreased. This is a crucial concept in laser surgery and is vital in understanding the surgical ramifications of the laser.

The surgical effects of the laser beam are tissue cutting, tissue coagulation, and tissue vaporization (Fig. 14–1*B*). They can be achieved by manipulating the spot size of the beam and varying the power. Cutting of tissue requires the highest power density, so a very small spot size and large amounts of power are used. For vaporization of tissue, full power is used with a larger spot size; the depth of vaporization can be controlled. Coagulation requires a large spot

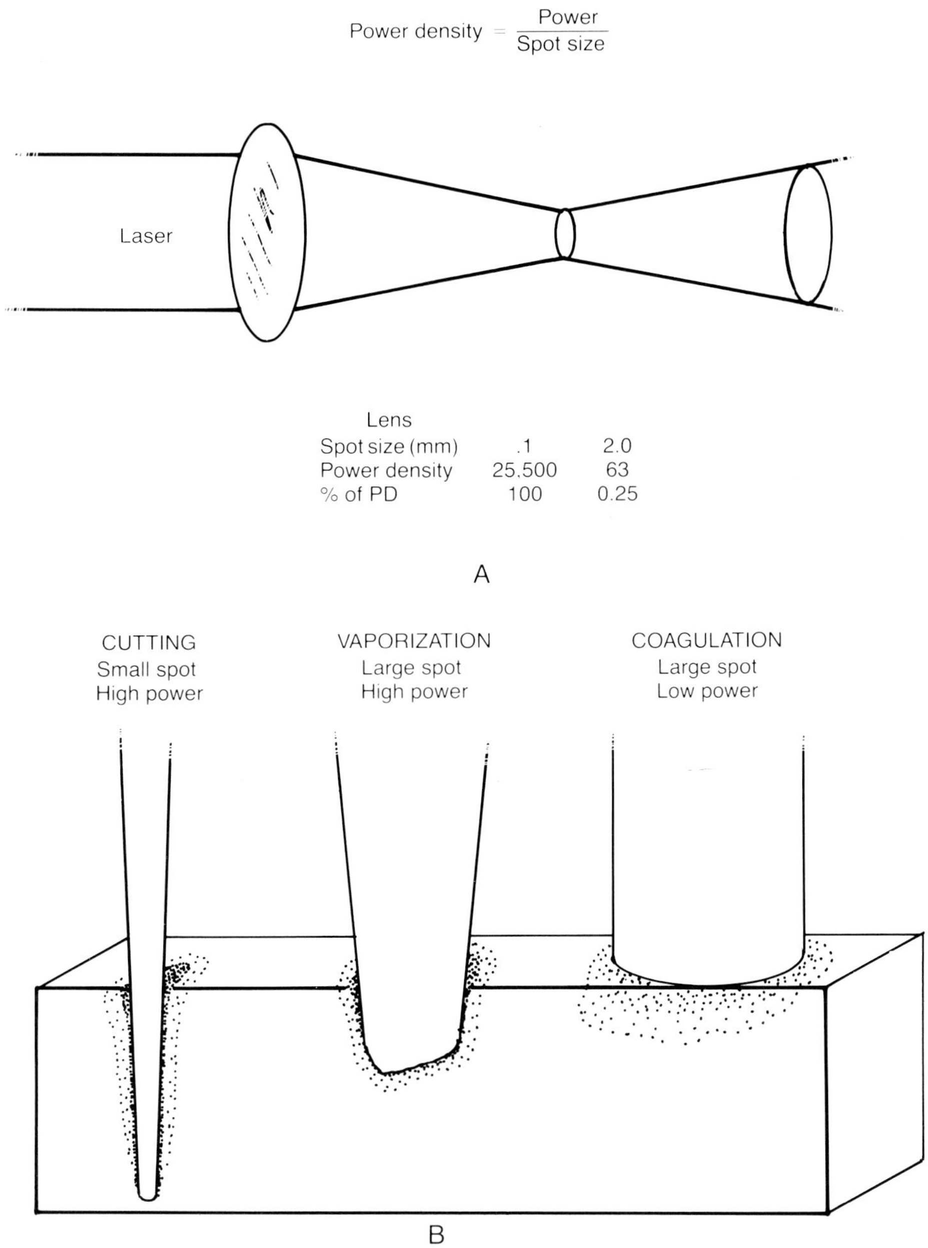

FIGURE 14–1.

size and a low power setting. Coagulation of vessels can only be accomplished with visible-wavelength lasers (argon and KTP-532) and not with the CO_2 laser.

Actual manipulation of the beam is done by the surgeon. The spot size can be altered in two ways. With the beam delivery device attached directly to the microscope, the spot size is changed by a rheostat-type device on the microscope; while directly visualizing the beam, the surgeon can vary the diameter of the beam as needed. The hand-held delivery system focuses as the hand piece is moved up and down while the beam is watched at the surgical site. Pulse duration and power are set on the machine itself or by a remote control at the operating table. The beam is activated by a foot pedal.

Laser Stapedotomy

This section describes applications of the laser in the middle ear, but the principles and techniques also apply to mastoid work. Specific approaches to the surgical site (incisions, flaps, and so on) have been described elsewhere. The discussion will focus only on laser applications to tissues; any specific approaches that are called for are explained.

Highlights

1. Good local anesthesia.
2. Good hemostasis.
3. Removal of the scutum.
4. Knowledgeable nursing assistants.
5. Superior instrumentation.
6. Use of a stapes holder.
7. Preservation of the chorda tympani.
8. Visualization of the pyramidal process and the facial nerve.
9. Understanding of laser techniques and use.
10. Complete visualization of the ossicles.

Pitfalls

1. Forming blebs in the external auditory canal while injecting.
2. Tearing the tympanic membrane during elevation.
3. Inadequate exposure.
4. Tearing the chorda tympani.
5. Inexperienced scrub nurse.
6. Injuring the facial nerve.
7. Placing the prosthesis too deep in the oval window.

Procedure

The laser stapedotomy is a very successful and efficient procedure. Initially the ear is prepared and draped in the usual fashion. All stapedotomies are done under local anesthesia; the authors use 2% lidocaine with 1:20,000 epinephrine. A standard four-quadrant injection is made with a 27-gauge needle. The ear is then irrigated with povidone-iodine (Betadine) through a bulb syringe.

A standard stapes flap is elevated with a round knife. A semicircular incision is made starting at the 6 o'clock position, traveling up the posterior canal wall, and ending at the 12 o'clock position just above the short process of the malleus. The flap is elevated to the annulus and the middle ear is entered in the usual fashion. The chorda tympani nerve is identified and preserved.

The stapes flap is rotated anteriorly until the posterior border of the malleus is directly visualized. The bony scutum is then removed until the facial nerve is visualized above the stapes and the pyramidal process of the stapedial tendon is identified posteriorly. It is very important to visualize these two structures to ensure adequate working room.

Manipulation of the malleus and incus is then done to rule out fixation of either structure as the cause of the conductive hearing loss. Attention is now focused on the stapes; again, manipulation with a small right-angled hook is done to confirm fixation. The incus-stapes joint is separated. The stapes holder is then brought into the field.

With adjustment of the laser spot size and beam parameters done preoperatively, the actual laser work begins. The stapedial tendon is focused on and vaporized, using the laser at 2.0 watts of power and a pulsed beam of 0.1 second. The beam is sharply focused on the tendon by a "joy stick" mounted on the microscope, and is fired by a foot control when the operator is ready. The smoke plume is drawn away by a No. 22 suction tip held in the operator's left hand (Fig. 14–2*A*).

Once the tendon has been vaporized, a measurement is taken from the lateral surface of the incus to the footplate of the stapes. Adding 0.5 mm to this measurement gives the proper length for the prosthesis. This length will vary with the type of prosthesis, point of measurement, and other factors. The laser beam is then focused on the posterior crus of the stapes. Again, with a pulsed beam and the same power settings, the crus is lased away (Fig. 14–2*B*).

Two suggestions may be helpful at this stage:

1. If the bone is very white, vaporization may be slow because the beam is absorbed by pigment. A drop of blood, bone char, or even gentian violet will help greatly. Once the initial dark bony char develops, vaporization proceeds very quickly.

2. When excess char builds up around the bone, vaporization may again be slow. The char should be gently chipped away with a small right-angled pick.

Once the posterior crus has been vaporized, the anterior crus is addressed. Often it can be seen directly and removed in the same way as the posterior crus. When the anterior crus cannot be directly visualized because of the body of the incus, a specially designed mirror is needed to reflect the beam onto it. The beam is first focused on the promontory just anterior to the anterior crus. The mirror is introduced until the anterior crus is reflected. The beam is then bounced off the mirror onto the anterior crus until it is vaporized (Fig. 14–2*C*).

Attention is then turned to the footplate of the stapes. The authors use either a 0.8-mm or a 0.6-mm

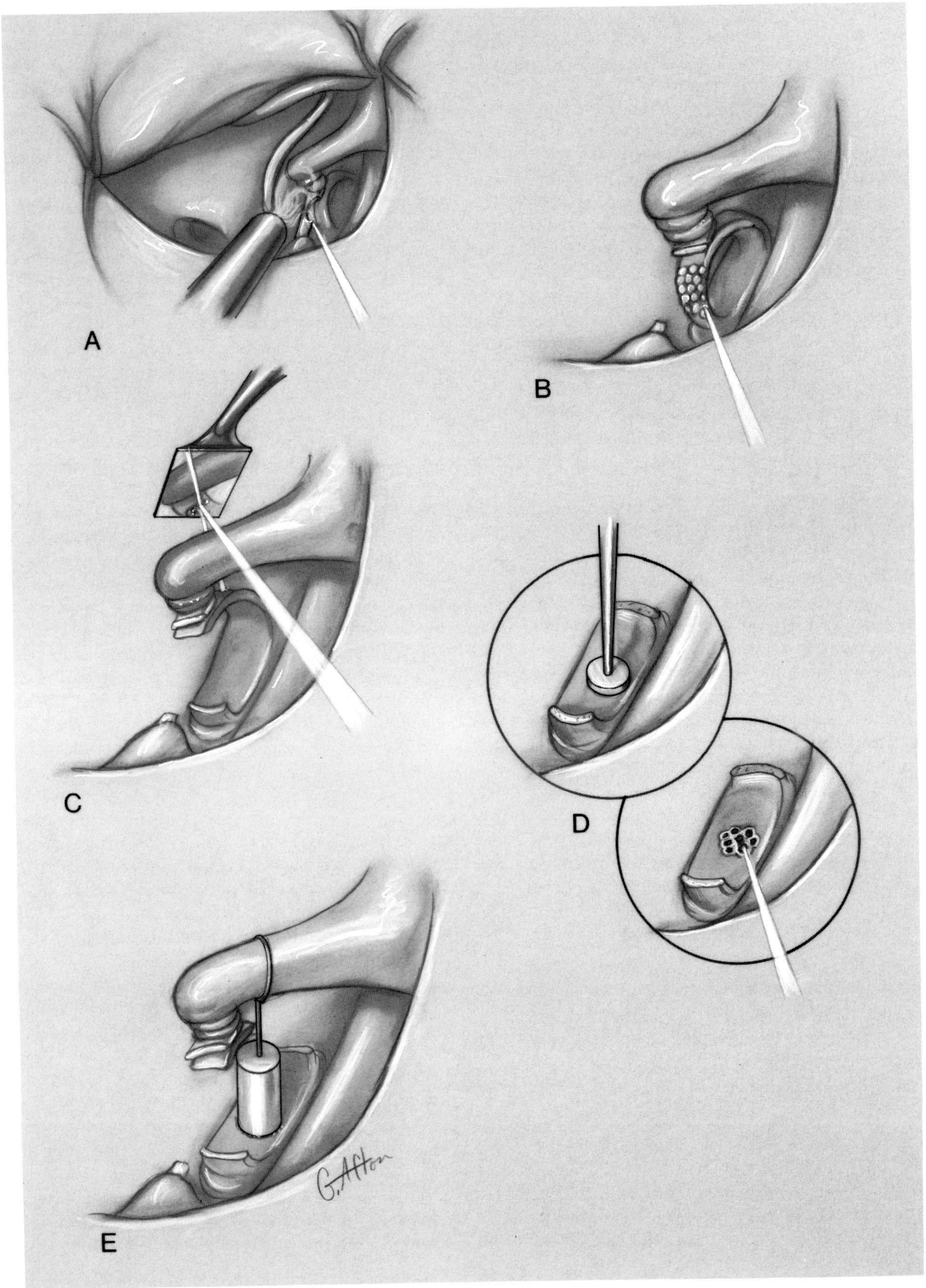

FIGURE 14–2.

opening into the inner ear; the former is preferred unless there is not enough room. A template is placed on the footplate, making a visual image of the 0.8-mm site (Fig. 14–2*D*). The laser is turned to 1.8 watts and a 0.1-second pulsed beam. A rosette pattern is made on the footplate, corresponding to the 0.8-mm stapedotomy opening. Usually one pulse will open the footplate. It is important to overlap these laser "hits," because the char from each previous hit will absorb the heat and allow for better vaporization. The template is reintroduced to ensure that the opening is the proper size.

The prosthesis is then positioned over the incus and into the stapedotomy opening and crimped into position (Fig. 14–2*E*). The part of the prosthesis that fits into the vestibule is exactly 1 mm in length; when properly positioned, half of it, or 0.5 mm, sits in the vestibule. Since this section of the prosthesis is only 1 mm long, it is easy to judge the correct depth.

Two additional suggestions are relevant here:

1. If some of the laser hits do not cause perilymph to flow and do not extend all the way through the footplate bone, this is not cause for alarm. If most of the hits go through the bone, the prosthesis will easily break through the remaining ones.

2. Sometimes a small amount of residual char from the vaporization is left on the footplate. It is not necessary to remove this.

Once the prosthesis is correctly positioned and crimped, the tympanic membrane is repositioned. All sound in the operating suite (monitors, fans, lasers, and so on) is reduced, and the patient is asked to count numbers to obtain a subjective hearing level. When the surgeon is satisfied with the hearing level, the footplate is revisualized. If the prosthesis is firmly fixed in position, one or two small drops of autogenous blood are instilled in the oval window to act as a seal. The flap is then repositioned and packed with Gelfoam, a mastoid dressing is placed, and the patient is taken to the recovery room.

Laser Applications in the Middle Ear

Initially restricted to stapedotomy procedures, use of the laser has been expanded to include every case in the authors' otologic practice. It has proved to be extremely useful in reconstruction and cholesteatoma work in the middle ear and mastoid.

Ossicles

The laser has been very beneficial in work around the ossicles. Since manipulation of the ossicles and corresponding trauma potentially may cause sensorineural hearing loss and ossicular disarticulation, it is desirable to minimize this manipulation. The highly focused beam of the laser can virtually eliminate manual trauma involving the ossicles.

The laser is especially useful in the presence of cholesteatoma or adhesions around the stapes or in the oval window niche. With very adherent disease, disarticulation with resultant perilymph leak is always a hazard. Using a finely focused beam of short pulse duration (0.1 to 0.3 seconds) and low power (2 to 3 watts), disease can be vaporized without trauma to the nearby ossicles.

Another use for the laser is in the ear filled with adhesions and polypoid material. Setting the beam for coagulation parameters, surface coagulation of these small vessels can be accomplished. Eliminating or reducing this nuisance bleeding permits a safer and faster procedure. In addition, vaporization of the adhesions can be accomplished with adjustment of the beam parameters. Again, this eliminates much of the vibratory trauma, reduces bleeding, and allows the surgeon to remove the adhesions layer by layer (Fig. 14–3*B*). This precision, especially in the depths of the oval window with disease around the stapes, greatly enhances the ability to remove tissue without trauma to the surrounding normal anatomic structures.

Another ideal situation for laser work is erosion of the lenticular process of the incus. Although eroded and lacking a bony connection with the stapes, the lenticular process often has enough bone left to make reconstruction difficult. Using the laser, the surgeon can vaporize the bone quickly, sharply, and atraumatically to allow more room for the reconstructive procedure (Fig. 14–3*A*).

The laser also is quite useful in tympanic membrane work. Freshening the edges of a perforation in preparation for a graft can be done easily and quickly. A pulsed or continuous beam focused on the periphery of the perforation can be used to remove the rolled edges of the perforation (Fig. 14–3*C*).

When elevation of the periosteum of the malleus is required in grafting techniques, the area around the umbo is always very adherent. Tugging and pulling of this tissue causes considerable vibratory trauma throughout the ossicular chain. Once again, tissue can be lased away without trauma (Fig. 14–3*D*).

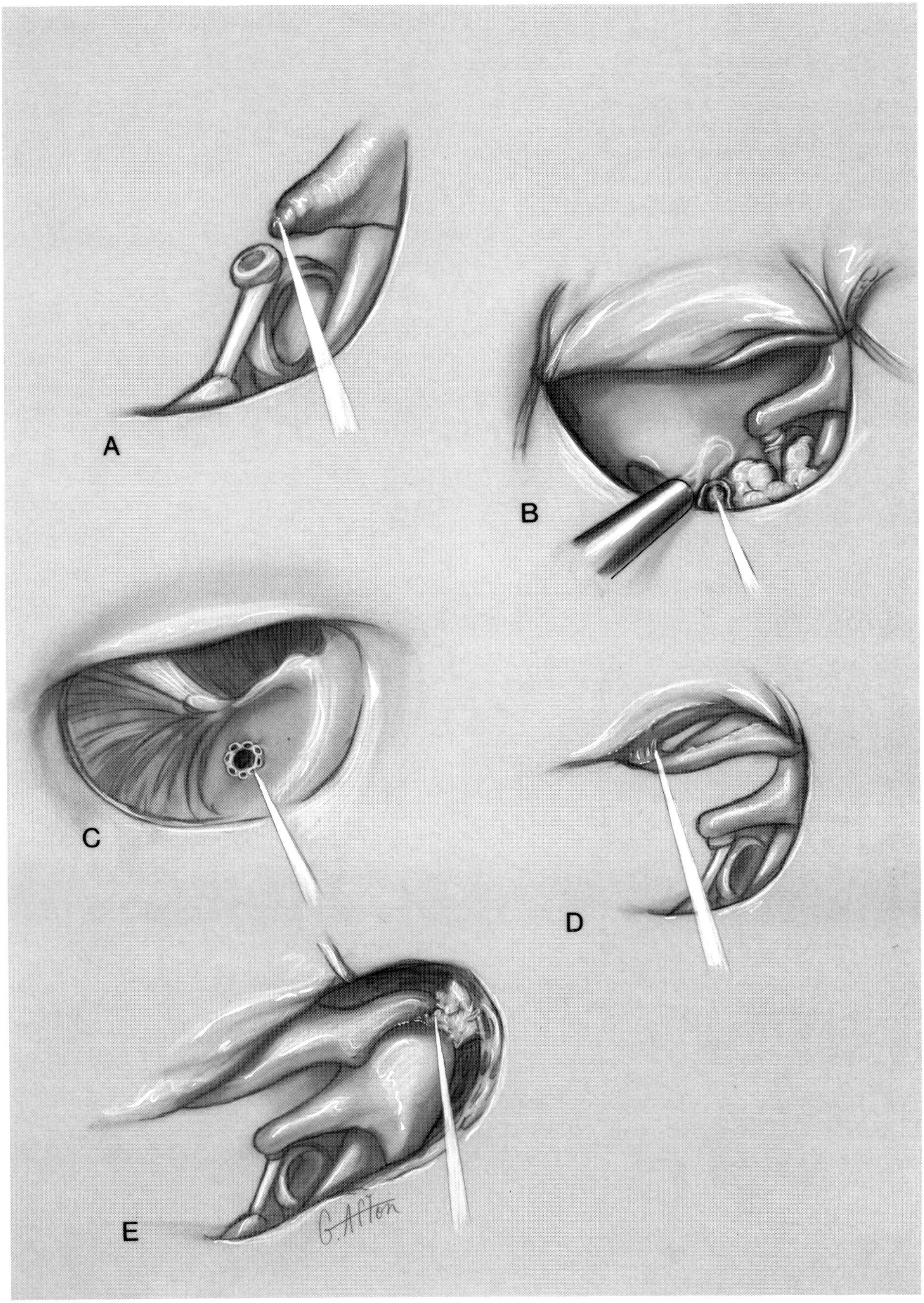

FIGURE 14–3.

As mentioned previously, the argon and KTP-532 lasers are readily absorbed by pigment and hemoglobin. Because of this affinity, hemostasis of small middle ear cleft bleeding can often be accomplished. With a large spot size, pulsed beam, and low power, nuisance bleeding from mucosal areas can be controlled. Again, the speed and precision of the laser in hemostasis lends itself greatly to the enhancement of reconstructive work.

The laser is ideally suited for repair of a fixed malleus. The difficulty in drilling around the ossicles in the attic is greatly reduced. Also, disarticulation of the incus-stapes joint is not needed because of the atraumatic bone vaporization. A standard postauricular incision is made and an atticotomy is performed (described elsewhere in this book). Drilling is done until the fixed ossicles are identified. In the authors' experience, the difficulty lies in freeing the fixation, which is usually anterior and medial to the malleus and incus. It is extremely difficult to drill this bone away; curetting also is crude and difficult. Once the fixation is visualized, the laser provides an ideal way to remove the bone without trauma to the ossicles. A pulsed or continuous beam sharply focused on the bony fixation vaporizes the bone, allowing free mobility of the chain (Fig. 14–3*E*). A small piece of Silastic is then inserted between the ossicles and the area of fixation to help prevent bone regrowth.

Summary

The laser has markedly reduced the degree of vibratory trauma to the ossicles and thus to the inner ear fluids. By minimizing trauma, the surgeon reduces the chances of iatrogenic sensorineural hearing loss. The precision of the beam allows the surgeon to reach areas of the middle ear cleft safely, quickly, and with less potential for injury to the patient. A second major advantage lies in the hemostatic properties of the visible-spectrum laser. The confines of the middle ear have always been difficult to reach for conventional coagulation. The pigment-absorptive properties of the visible-spectrum beams have greatly enhanced this procedure. These two features of the laser have added a new dimension to otologic surgery.

Neurotology and the Laser

The laser also is used extensively in neurotologic practice, and has been an invaluable addition to acoustic neuroma work. It is used for three functions: (1) hemostasis, (2) vaporization of the tumor, and (3) tumor cutting for removal.

Procedure

Tumor exposure is accomplished by the standard approaches to the posterior and middle fossa, which have been described elsewhere. In the translabyrinthine approach, the internal auditory canal bone is thinned on its superior, posterior, and inferior borders. Once the eggshell-thin bone is left, the laser is used initially for surface coagulation (Fig. 14–4*A*). The area over the facial nerve in the anterosuperior quadrant is covered with Cottonoid for protection. The laser is used at approximately 4 to 6 watts of power with a pulsed beam and a large spot size. Because of the beam's affinity for pigment, it is absorbed by the hemoglobin. Coagulation is accomplished over the surface of the tumor and through the eggshell-thin bone. Surface coagulation of the small capillaries before opening the dura of the internal auditory canal reduces and sometimes completely prevents nuisance bleeding from small dural tumor vessels. Once surface coagulation is accomplished, the facial nerve is identified in the internal auditory canal. Dissection is accomplished in the canal in the standard fashion. After the facial nerve is identified and Cottonoid is packed around it for protection, the tumor bulk in the canal is vaporized away (Fig. 14–4*B*). By manipulating the power settings and beam spot size, tumor can be vaporized safely and quickly, often with minimal bleeding.

Standard posterior fossa procedures—protection of other cranial nerves, the cerebellum, and the brainstem with Cottonoid—are followed once tumor removal in the angle is begun. The facial nerve is always kept in view but is protected with Cottonoid. Tumor removal by vaporization is done almost exclusively with the laser in the cerebellopontine angle. The authors use full power (8 to 10 watts) with a

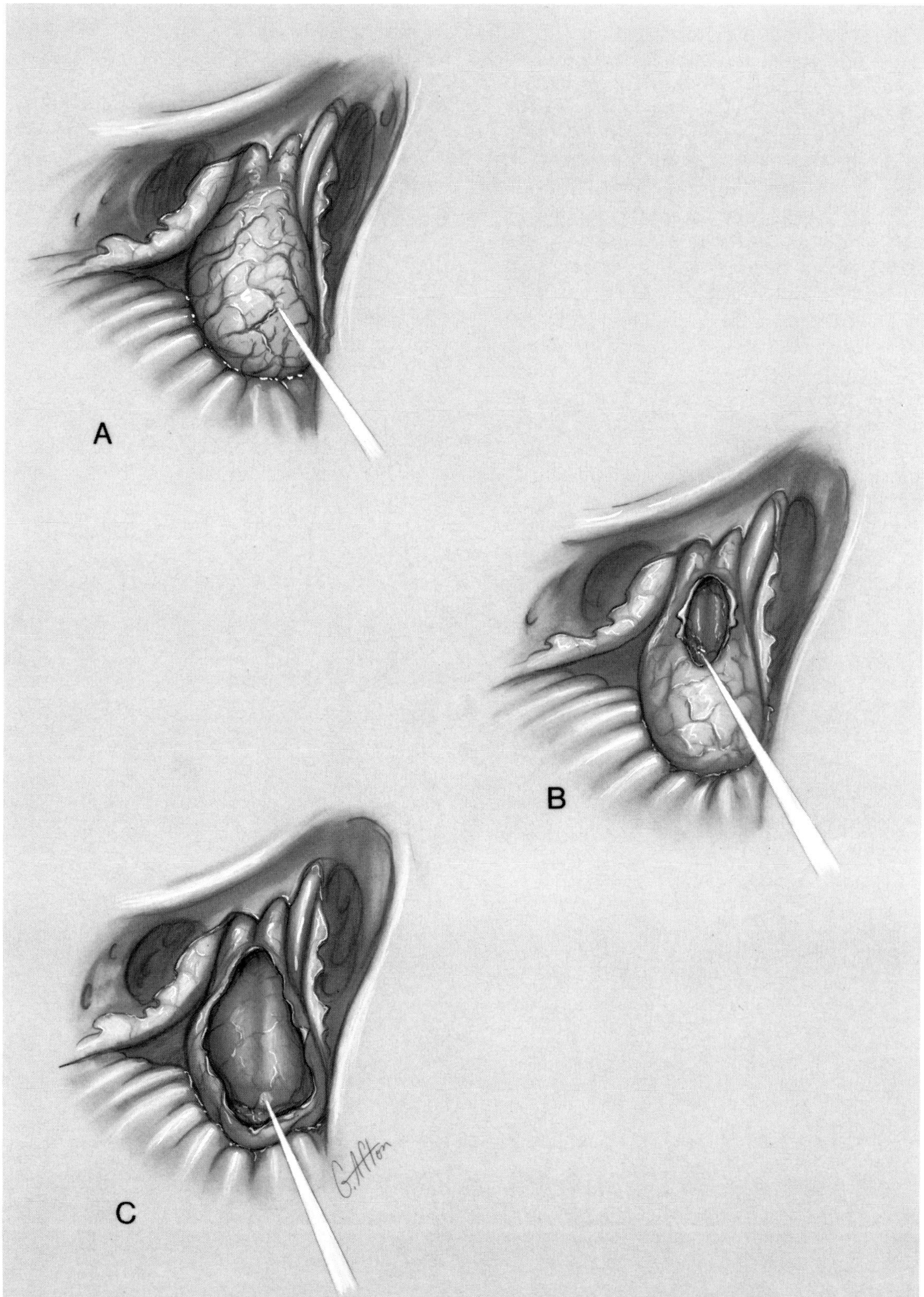

FIGURE 14–4.

continuous beam and a medium spot size. Tumor removal is done from the interior of the tumor, initially keeping the capsule intact. Suction is used to draw away the smoke plume from the vaporization process. As its interior is vaporized, the tumor capsule collapses and further dissection of the capsule from surrounding structures can be accomplished. With very large tumors, the tumor itself can be cut away with the laser. The beam parameters are changed to a very sharp focus with full power and continuous duration. Using this beam, tumor bulk is cut away easily with minimal bleeding (Fig. 14–4C).

The techniques and uses of the laser in the suboccipital approach are similar. An additional step is that the dura over the posterior lip of the internal auditory canal is lased away; again, it can be removed quickly and without bleeding, and less time is needed for bipolar cautery or drilling.

Sectioning of the vestibular nerve can also be done with the laser. The nerve is isolated by standard techniques, and the cochlear and facial nerves are protected with Cottonoid; the vestibular nerve is then vaporized away. In this case, however, the authors feel that conventional sectioning with scissors is just as effective.

Vascular lesions, especially small glomus tympanicum tumors, also can be debulked with the laser. Small feeder vessels are easily coagulated with the visible-spectrum beam. The capsule of the tumor is cauterized with low power settings and a diffused beam. This use of the laser "toughens" the capsule, allowing for easier and safer manipulation of the tumor. Large vessels cannot be coagulated with the beam, but by reducing the feeder vessels, tumor removal is facilitated.

In summary, the laser has proved to be an invaluable tool in otologic and neurotologic work. Standard techniques are greatly facilitated by the laser; it is precise, fast, safe, and very efficient, and will probably become standard in the near future. The next hurdle in otology is the inner ear, and the laser may be of benefit in the not too distant future.

CHAPTER 15

Surgical Approach for Bone Conduction Hearing Devices

Bone conduction hearing devices are in an early phase of development, but a first generation is now available for clinical use. This area of otology should witness significant positive changes in future years.

Conductors are available in two types, percutaneous and transcutaneous. This chapter describes the surgical technique (Hough's technique) for implantation of the Xomed audiant bone conductor.

This bone conductor is a transcutaneous device consisting of an external and an internal component. Externally (outside the patient), a microphone receives sound and channels it to a sound processor; this directs an amplified signal across the skin to the implant (the internal component), which is screwed into the skull. The amplified signal is transmitted by skull vibration into the inner ear and sound is perceived. The external and internal parts of the device are held together electromagnetically. The system is battery operated.

This device currently is used in patients with external or middle ear impairments with good bone conduction and speech discrimination who cannot benefit from conventional hearing aids (owing to congenital malformations, chronic external otitis or other factors). Indications for the device will be expanded. Some basic instruments (Xomed kit) are required in order to position the internal receiver in the skull; they are shown in Figure 15–1.

Aim

To expose a site in the area of the linea temporalis for safe placement of the receiver, while allowing adequate skin coverage and a position for the external device that is comfortable and harmless.

Procedure

After preparation and shaving of the postauricular area, the ear is sterilely draped. A postauricular line is traced horizontally at a level immediately superior to the tragus. The receiver (implant) is to be placed behind the posterior edge of the pinna. Approximately 15 to 18 mm from this posterior edge and immediately above the horizontal line, the bur hole template is positioned and the site of the receiver delineated (Fig. 15–2*A*).

An incision site is traced at least 1 cm posterior to the edge of the receiver and injected with 2% lidocaine (Xylocaine) with 1:100,000 epinephrine. The incision is deepened down to the periosteum, a flap is elevated, and the linea temporalis is identified. If the subcutaneous tissues are thick, the area that will

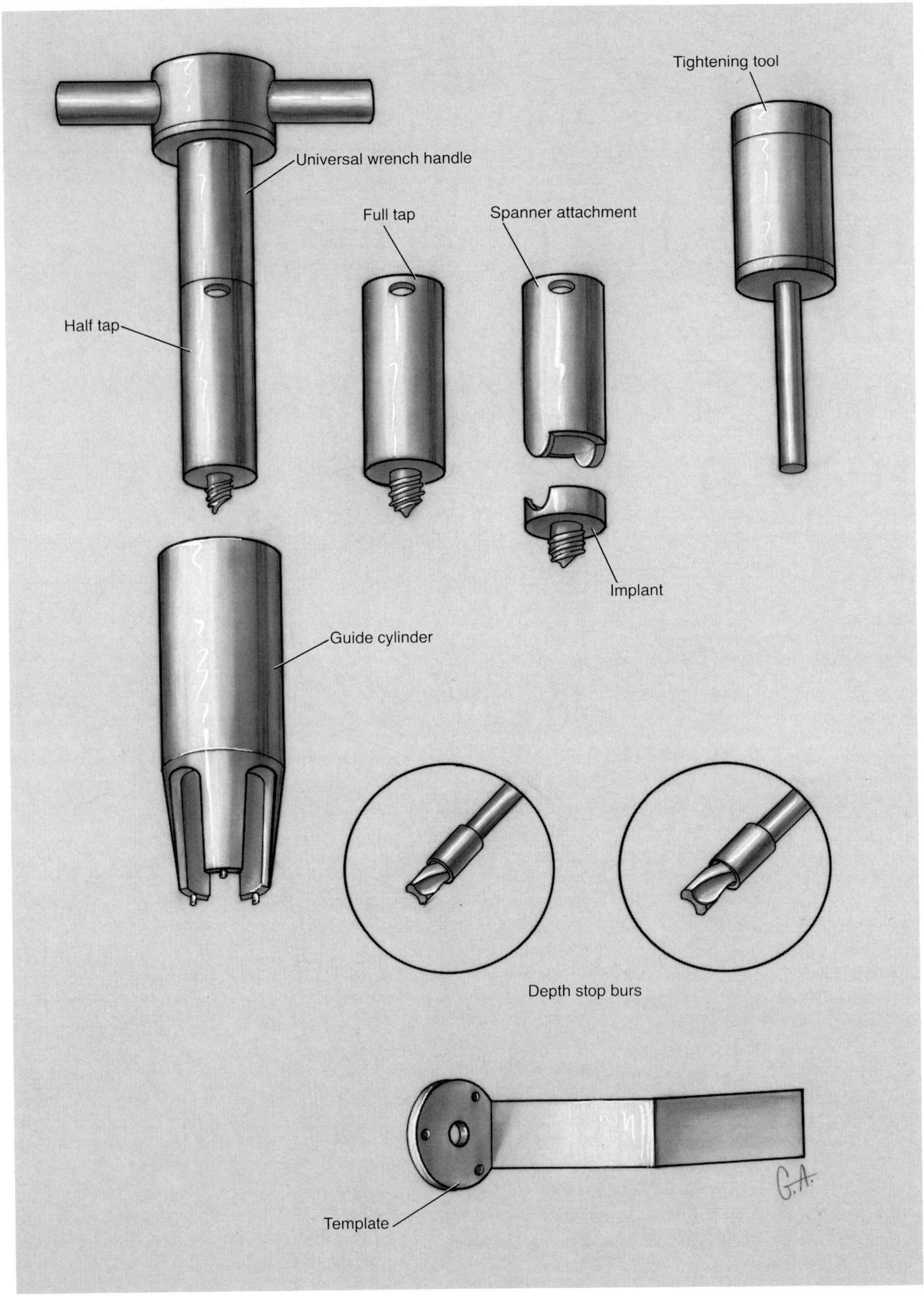
Tightening tool
Universal wrench handle
Full tap
Spanner attachment
Half tap
Implant
Guide cylinder
Depth stop burs
Template
G.A.

FIGURE 15–1.

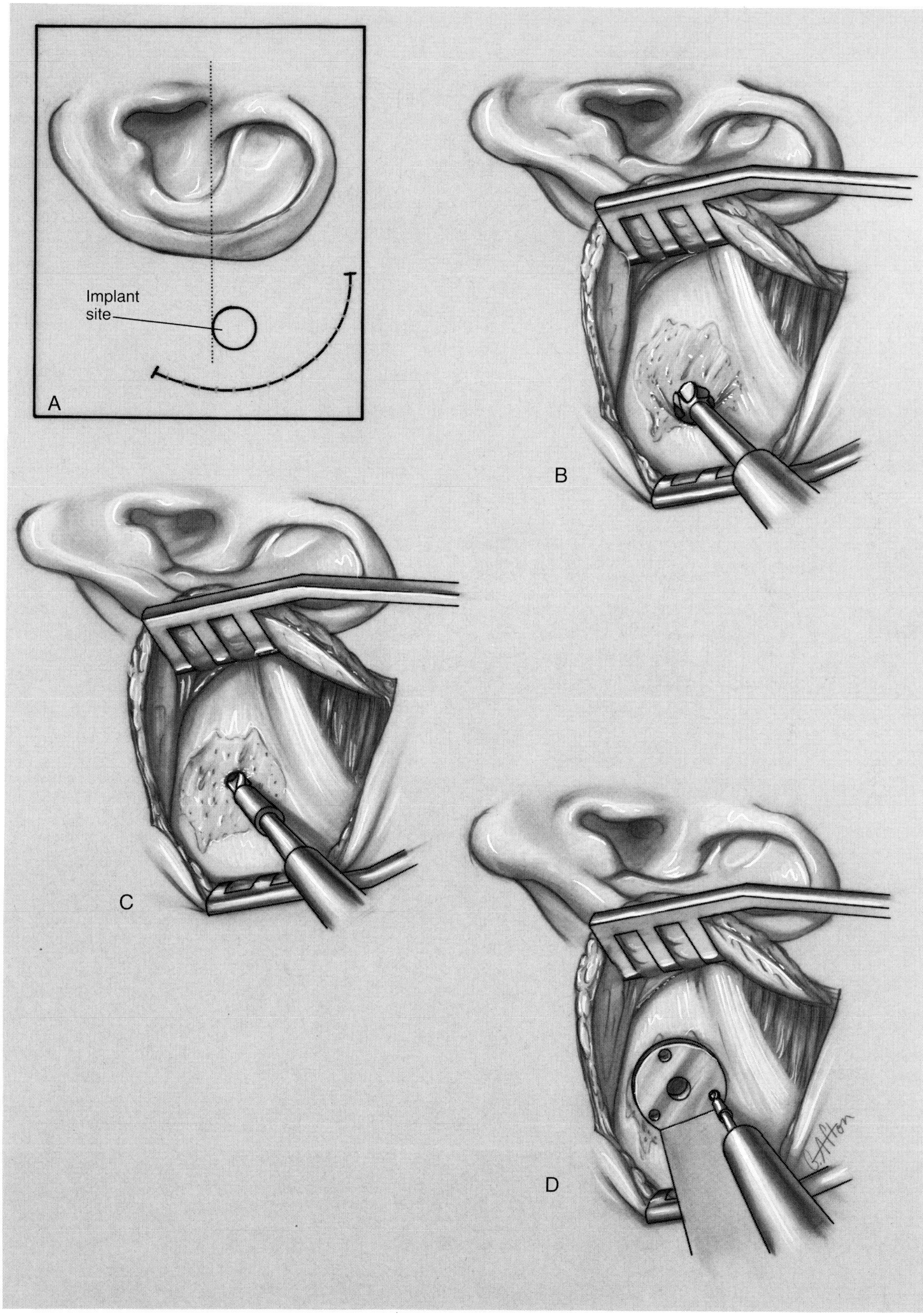

FIGURE 15–2.

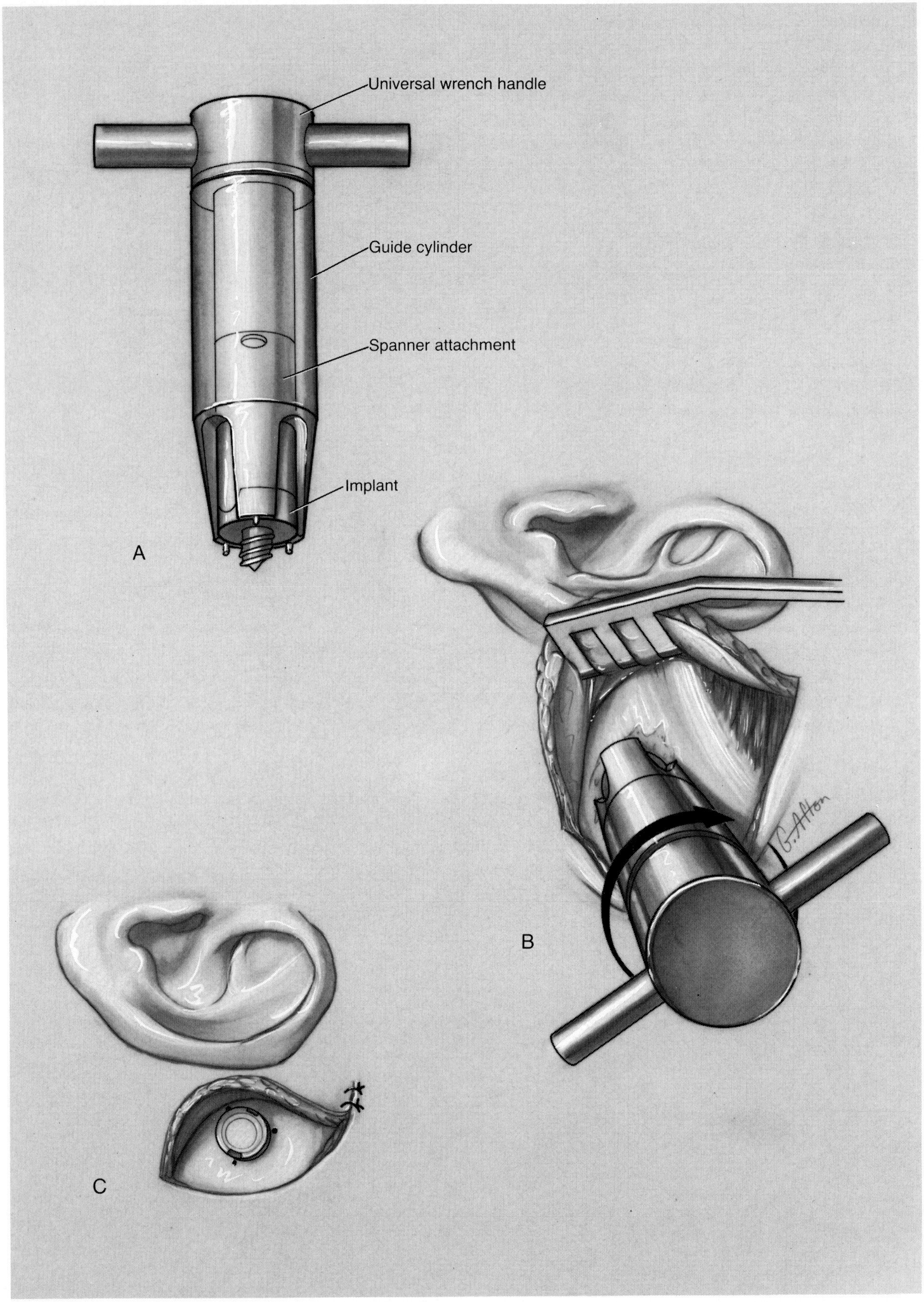
Universal wrench handle
Guide cylinder
Spanner attachment
Implant
A
B
C

FIGURE 15–3.

cover the receiver is thinned in order to permit adequate transcutaneous transmission and magnetic coupling between the external and internal devices.

The area where the receiver will be placed is reidentified, marked, and evened with a bur kit without drilling deep into the bone (Fig. 15–2*B*). (This area needs depth to receive the screw of the implant.)

Using the larger bur in the kit (the burs have a depth stop), the center hole is drilled (Fig. 15–2*C*). If a cerebrospinal fluid leak occurs, the site is sealed with bone wax and an adjacent site is used.

Using the small bur in the set and the bur hole template as a guide, three small control holes are drilled (Fig. 15–2*D*). The larger central hole is destined for the central screw of the implant. The three adjacent control holes will receive the three pegs of the guide cylinder and impart stability to it.

The next step is to develop a thread in the center hole for the screw of the implant. This is done in two stages, using the "half tap" and "full tap" instruments.

The guide cylinder is placed upright. The three pegs are inserted in the corresponding three holes to keep the cylinder perpendicular to the bone surface.

The first tap to be used is the half tap; this is tightened to the universal wrench handle with the tightening tool. The universal wrench (with the half tap tightened to it) is then slid through the guide cylinder and rotated clockwise, firmly pressing against the skull. Rotation continues for ¾ of a turn, until the gap between the wrench handle and guide cylinder is closed.

The half tap is removed from the skull, then loosened and removed from the universal wrench. The full tap is now tightened to the universal wrench, slid through the guide cylinder, and placed over the center of the screw hole. First, it is gently turned ½-turn counterclockwise (in order not to alter the thread previously made by the half tap) and then clockwise until the gap between the wrench handle and guide cylinder is closed. The full tap is then removed from the screw hole. The thread in the center hole is now ready for the screw of the implant.

The full tap is removed from the universal wrench handle and replaced with the spanner attachment, which is designed to hold the implant both mechanically and electromagnetically. The implant is placed in the spanner and inserted through the guide cylinder until it faces the center hole (Fig. 15–3*A*). The implant (with the screw facing the hole) is gently turned ½-turn counterclockwise (again, in order not to alter the thread in the hole), and then clockwise until the gap between the wrench handle and guide cylinder is closed and there is a feeling of resistance (Fig. 15–3*B*). The wrench and the guide cylinder are removed. The implant is gently checked for tightness (Fig. 15–3*C*). The flap is repositioned, the incision is closed in layers with appropriate sutures, and a mastoid dressing is applied.

Testing and use of the external device begins at 8 to 12 weeks, depending upon the healing process.

Complications

This is a simple procedure in terms of surgical trauma; it can be done under local anesthesia and has few complications. Other than those inherent in raising a postauricular flap (discussed elsewhere), the main potential problem is that of cerebrospinal fluid leak. Burs with a "stop" (such as those in the kit) do not allow a deep penetration; if a leak does occur, sealing the opening with bone wax should suffice. Prophylactic antibiotics could be useful in these cases. An initial high dose of intraoperative intravenous antibiotics is recommended. Other complications are caused by failure to follow careful surgical techniques.

CHAPTER 16

Surgical Approaches for Cochlear Implants

Although there are marked differences among the different types of cochlear implants, the basic principles of and surgical approaches for these devices are similar. This chapter will describe only the basic surgical approaches that apply to implants in widespread use.

Cochlear implants consist of an external and an internal component. Externally, a microphone picks up the sound stimulation and sends it to the sound processor, transforming it into a coded electrical stimulus that is carried to the internal component. An internal receiver channels this stimulus through one or more active electrodes to the cochlea, for the purpose of stimulating the auditory nerve. An "indifferent" or ground electrode is placed close to or away from the active electrode; if the latter, it is usually placed in the temporal muscle. Different types of implant devices require different types of ground electrodes.

The internal receiver can be placed either under the skin (transcutaneous stimulation) or with a plug protruding from the skin (percutaneous stimulation). In most cases, the active electrode is placed on or through the round window of the cochlea. Two surgical approaches for placement of the electrode will be described.

Three basic approaches can be used: (1) the posterior tympanotomy (facial recess); (2) the mastoidotomy/tympanotomy; and (3) the external auditory canal groove. The approach via the external auditory canal groove has been used for some of the Storz-San Francisco devices; it will not be described in detail. As in the facial recess approach, a large postauricular flap is elevated in continuity with the skin of the posterior canal and tympanic membrane, directly exposing the middle ear cavity. A groove is created in the posterior canal, extending from the region of the round window to the anterior margin of the mastoid cortex. The groove is covered with cortical bone and temporal fascia or with acrylic bone cement, in order to prevent skin from dipping into the groove and contacting the electrode lead. Surgical preparation and positioning is similar to that for mastoidectomy, except that the area to be shaved and prepared is more extensive than in a regular mastoidectomy. An important point concerns the use of cautery. When the electrodes are in the surgical field, the use of cautery might lead to the transmission of electrical currents into the cochlea, with potentially devastating effects. Judicious use of bipolar cautery, or no cautery at all, is indicated once the electrodes are in the surgical field.

Posterior Tympanotomy (Facial Recess)

Surgical Steps

1. Positioning of the internal receiver site.
2. Postauricular incision.
3. Elevation of a postauricular flap.

4. Removal of temporal muscle.
5. Drilling of a seat for the internal receiver.
6. Simple mastoidectomy.
7. Opening of the facial recess.
8. Exposure of the round window.
9. Placement of the internal receiver.
10. Insertion of the electrode via the round window opening.
11. Securing of the internal receiver.
12. Closure, packing, and a mastoid dressing.

Procedure

A dummy electrode is used to determine the postauricular position of the internal receiver. It should be at or above the linea temporalis, allowing enough space without interfering with the use of eyeglasses. Some surgeons prefer to place the receiver more inferiorly. The receiver site can be traced with a marking pen or a circular impression can be left by pressing a dummy receiver against the skin.

Infiltration of the postauricular incision site is the same as in a mastoidectomy; however, it is more extensive because of the posterior extent of the incision. The incision is made 1 cm behind the outer edge of the internal receiver and extends down to the level of the mastoid process without bending toward it, in order to avoid compromise of the occipital artery. The flap is developed anteriorly between the scalp and the temporal muscle until the spine of Henle is exposed.

A piece of temporal muscle over the squamous portion of the temporal bone is removed, as well as temporal fascia. This allows for an adequate seat for the receiver, and for a thinner scalp if a transcutaneous device is to be used. A seat for the internal receiver is drilled (Fig. 16–1*B*). It is important to do this in a plane parallel to the scalp surface. With a transcutaneous device, it is useful to secure the receiver with permanent sutures (Fig. 16–2*A*, *B*). With a 2-mm pilot drill, two holes 2 mm apart are drilled on both sides of the seat, at a distance of 0.5 to 0.75 cm from the outer edge; a passage between the holes is made with a 0.5-mm cutting bur at a 30-degree angle. For a percutaneous device, additional holes can be drilled for placement of screws (Fig. 16–2*A'*).

A simple mastoidectomy and opening of the facial recess is done (Fig. 16–1*A*) (see Chapter 7); the only difference is that the edges of the cavity are not saucerized in order to allow for a groove for the electrode. Two additional holes can be drilled in the border of the mastoid cavity for the purpose of securing the electrode at this level with permanent sutures.

The round window niche is visualized through the facial recess (Fig. 16–2*D*). Using a small bur, the anterosuperior lip of the niche is removed and the round window membrane is brought directly into view. If the window cannot be visualized, drilling toward the promontory will help to provide a straight view of the basal turn, bypassing the "hook." This should be done cautiously, in a step-by-step fashion. If bone growth is present in this area, a "straight position" is reached and drilling is done anteriorly (forward) into the scala tympani. This will lead to an open scala or provide a space for placing the electrode.

The electrode is then introduced and the round window niche is sealed with fascia (Fig. 16–3). A nonserrated or specially coated alligator forceps should be used for electrode insertion, helped by blunt wire guides or hoes. Extreme care must be used when handling the electrode in order to avoid damaging it. With the 3M House type, only the noninsulated portion is introduced.

Once the electrode has been placed, the internal receiver is secured. For a transcutaneous device, 4-0 silk sutures are passed through the 2-mm holes drilled around the seat (Fig. 16–4*A*). For a percutaneous plug, an opening is created just above the plug, avoiding skin tension at all costs. The opening is made with a skin punch of the same size as the plug provided in the manufacturer's surgical kit.

The postauricular incision is closed with 3-0 absorbable sutures for the subcutaneous tissues and 4-0 silk for the skin. A Penrose drain can be used. This is followed by application of a mastoid dressing.

Mastoidotomy/Tympanotomy Approach

Advantages

1. Technical simplicity.
2. Involves less bone drilling and tissue removal.
3. Carries almost no risk to the facial nerve.
4. Allows for direct view of and work in the round window niches.
5. Active electrode is covered by a thick layer of tissue along its entire course (not just subcutaneously).
6. Provides a better angle in the basal turn of the cochlea for sliding the electrode, making full insertion easier.

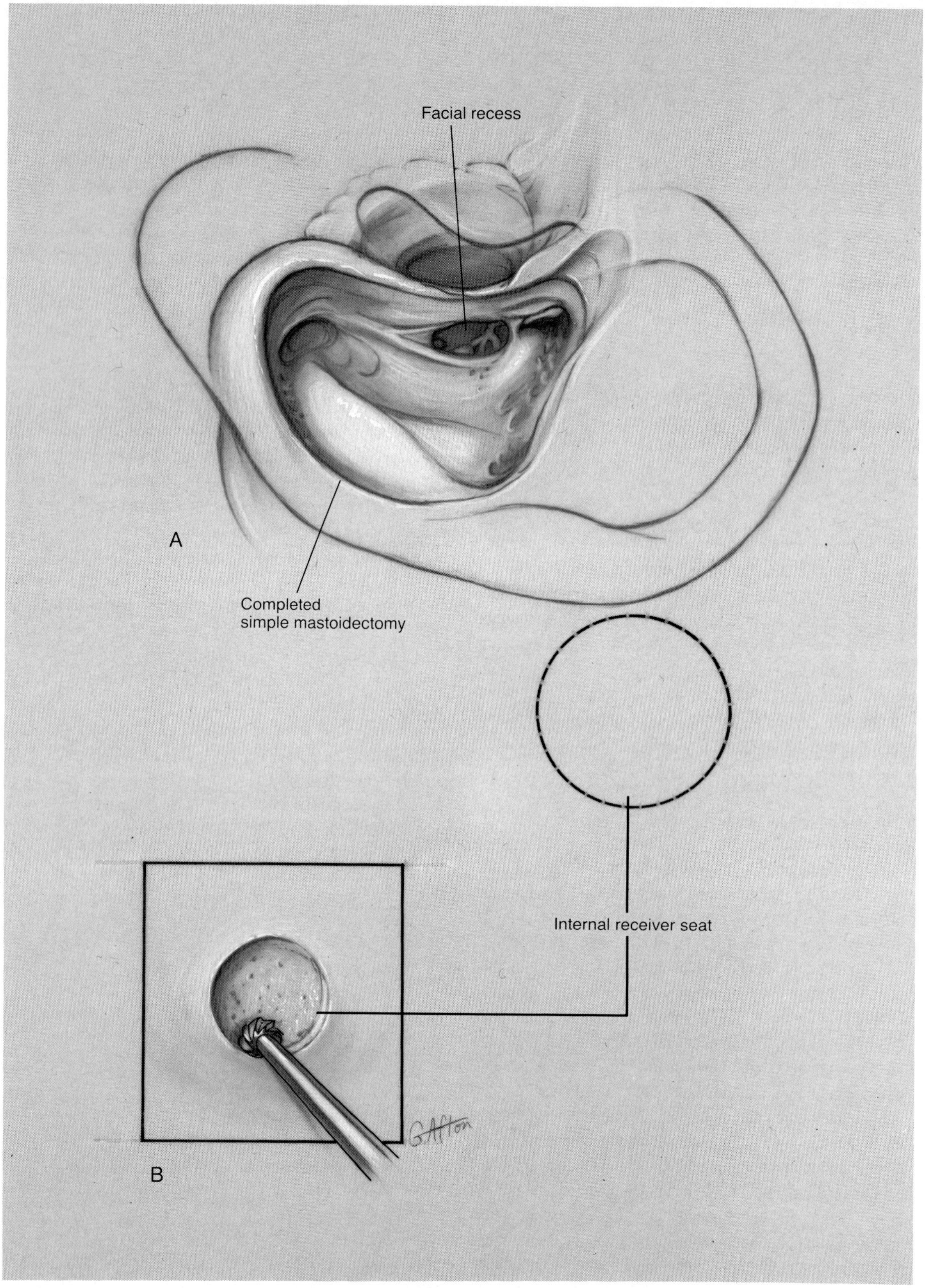
Facial recess
A
Completed
simple mastoidectomy
Internal receiver seat
B

FIGURE 16–1.

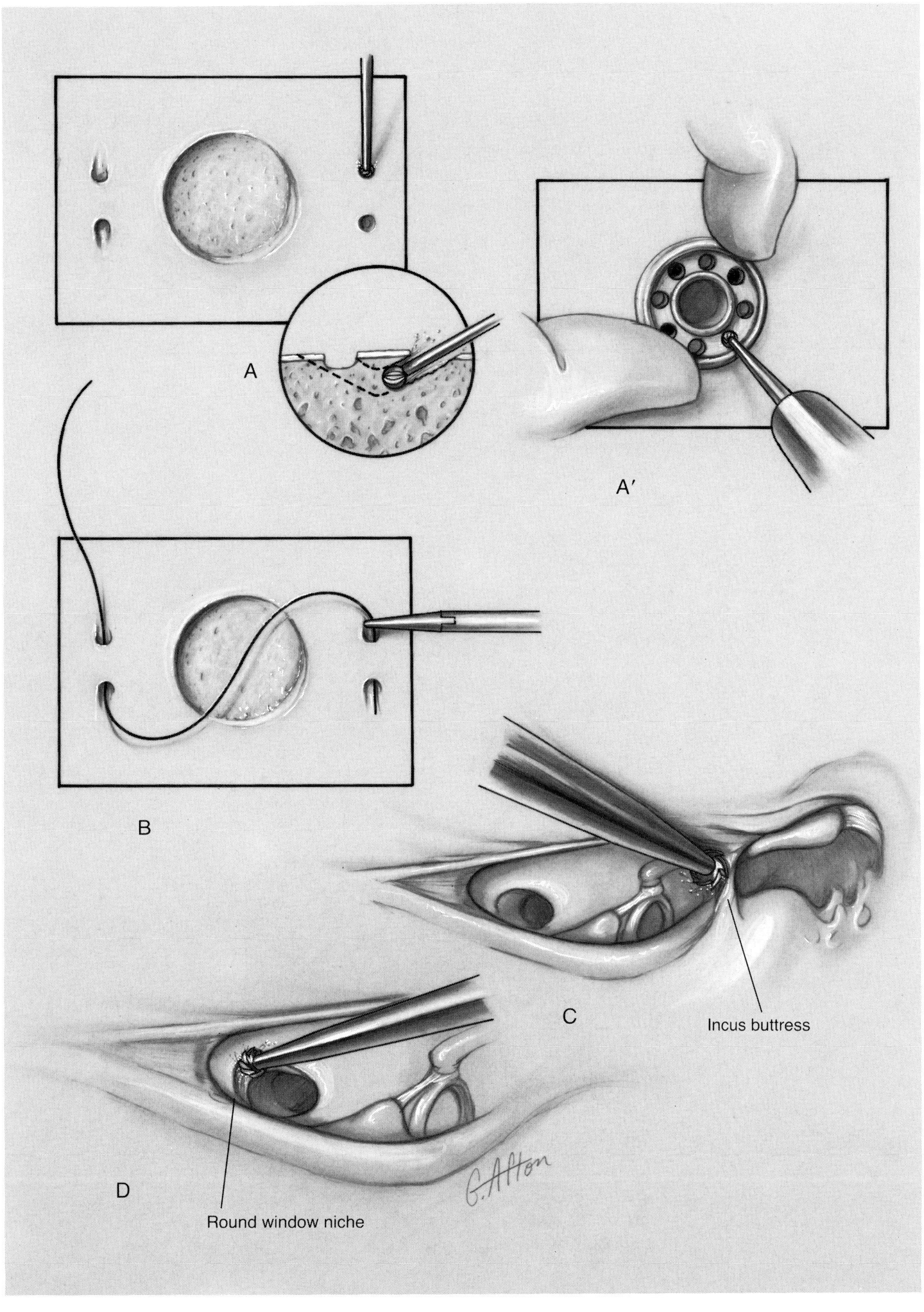

FIGURE 16–2.

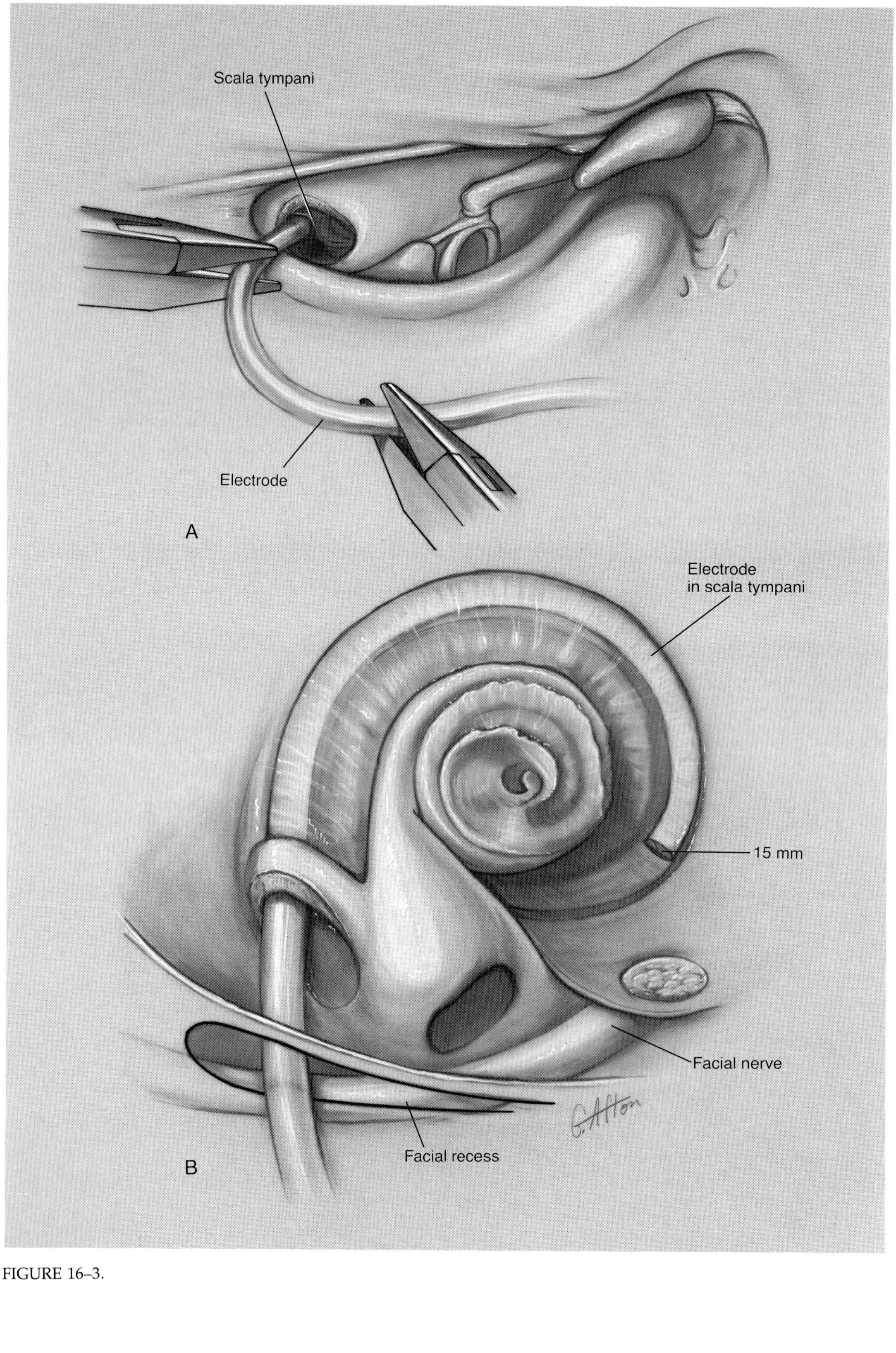
Scala tympani
Electrode
A
Electrode
in scala tympani
15 mm
Facial nerve
Facial recess
B

FIGURE 16–3.

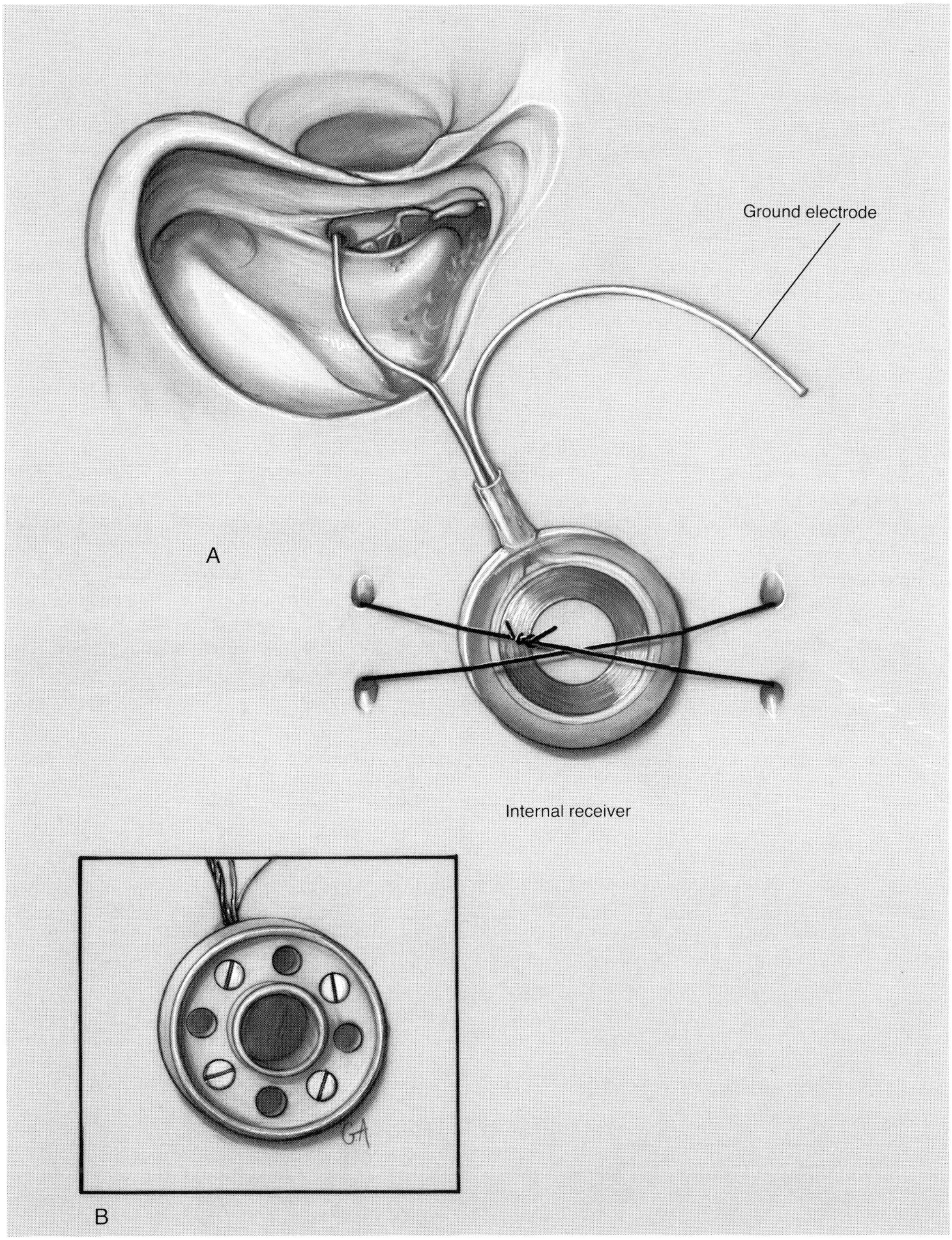

FIGURE 16–4.

7. Small postauricular flap carries less risk of hematoma or infection; requires no drains; makes healing easier; and allows no tension of the skin with percutaneous plugs.
8. Allows faster recovery and shorter hospitalization.

Surgical Steps

1. Endaural incisions (Lempert I and II).
2. Canal incisions at 6 and 2 o'clock.
3. Exposure of the middle ear.
4. Drilling of the round window niche and visualization of the round window membrane.
5. Small atticotomy.
6. Mastoidotomy.
7. Postauricular incision.
8. Removal of temporal muscle and periosteum.
9. Drilling of a seat for the internal receiver.
10. Tunneling of the electrode from the postauricular incision into the mastoidotomy opening.
11. Introduction of the electrode into the antrum and middle ear.
12. Insertion of the electrode into the cochlea.
13. Securing of the internal receiver.
14. Creation of a skin opening (for percutaneous receivers).
15. Closure, packing, and a mastoid dressing.

Procedure

The first incision (Lempert I) is made semicircumferentially between 6 and 12 o'clock on the posterior wall at the bony cartilaginous junction. The second incision (Lempert II) runs between the tragus and helix (at the incisura). The extension of this incision is approximately 0.75 cm. The posterior canal skin (cartilaginous portion) is preserved and gently elevated with a small periosteal elevator, clearly exposing the entire posterior bony canal (Fig. 16–5*A*). Two-prong retractors are used for exposure; occasionally three-prong retractors are needed.

With a scalpel, vertical incisions are made at 6 and 2 o'clock. In a completely dry field, a flap is elevated and the middle ear cavity is entered beneath the annulus. All anatomic structures and landmarks are visualized. Using stapes curets, the posterior canal wall is enlarged and a small atticotomy is done (Fig. 16–5*B*). Special attention is paid to the round window niche. The anterosuperior portion is removed with a small bur and the round window membrane is brought directly into view (Fig. 16–5*C*). Any additional drilling needed for exposure is delayed until the electrode is inserted (see Posterior Tympanotomy [Facial Recess] Approach).

A piece of Gelfoam is used to cover the round window and a large piece of cotton is placed over the ear canal. This avoids contamination by bone dust and debris from the mastoidotomy drilling.

A mastoidotomy is done by drilling in the fossa mastoidea toward the antrum (Fig. 16–5*D*). The opening should be large enough to visualize the antrum. The posterior edge is beveled and all sharp bony edges are smoothed. The incus is disarticulated from its stapes and malleus attachments with a joint knife and totally removed. If desired, a dummy electrode can be inserted through the mastoidotomy opening and into the niche to verify the adequacy of the exposure. The middle ear and mastoid are then filled with an antibiotic solution.

A postauricular incision is needed for the sole purpose of placing the internal receiver; it should be made at or above the linea temporalis, allowing enough space without interfering with the use of eyeglasses. Lidocaine (Xylocaine) 2% with 1:100,000 epinephrine is injected. The circumferential incision measures 3 to 3.5 cm and is deepened through the subcutaneous tissues until the temporal muscle is reached (Fig. 16–5*E*, *F*). The seat size for the internal receiver is measured, and the corresponding underlying temporal muscle and periosteum are removed. The periosteum is saved for grafting the round window niche. The bone seat is drilled down to accommodate the receiver (Fig. 16–6*A*) and, depending upon the type of receiver, additional holes are drilled either for sutures or for screw placement (see Posterior Tympanotomy [Facial Recess] Approach).

An electrode guide is passed from the endaural to the postauricular incision by tunneling it beneath the temporal muscle. An electrode guide, which is similar to an antrum trocar, is specially curved and has a blunt distal opening to avoid damaging the electrode (Fig. 16–6*B*). The obturator is removed and the electrode introduced into the guide (Fig. 16–6*C*); the guide is then withdrawn and, with it, the electrode is carried into the mastoidotomy opening. It is then passed to the antrum and into the middle ear. The exposed round window membrane is detached with an angled pick, and the electrode is introduced with a nonserrated baby alligator forceps in an angle pointing toward the basal turn of the cochlea, immediately past the hook (Fig. 16–6*D*). The opening of the round window is sealed with periosteum wrapped around the electrode (Fig. 16–7*A*). Small pieces of Gelfoam are then placed lateral to the

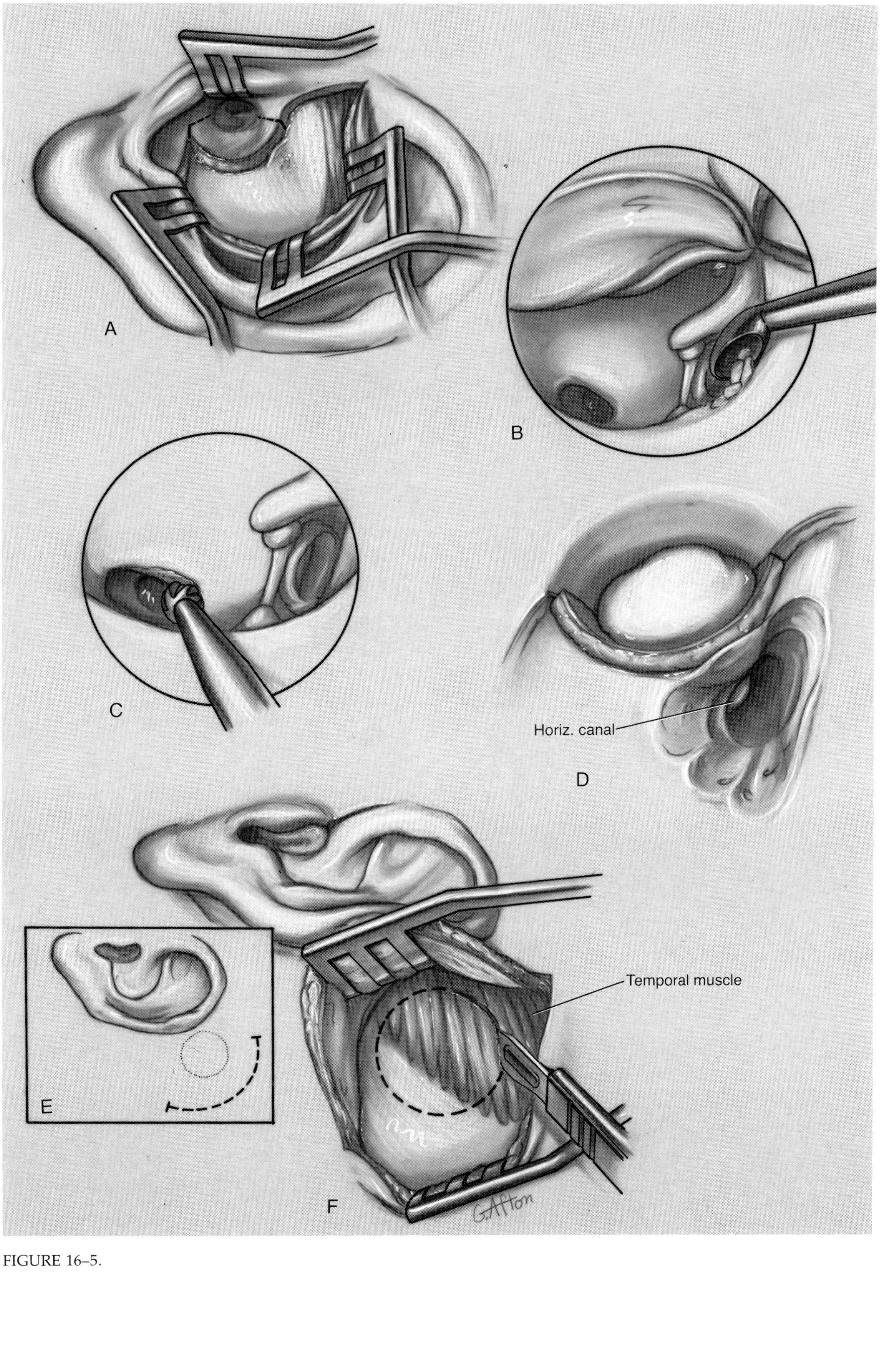

FIGURE 16–5.

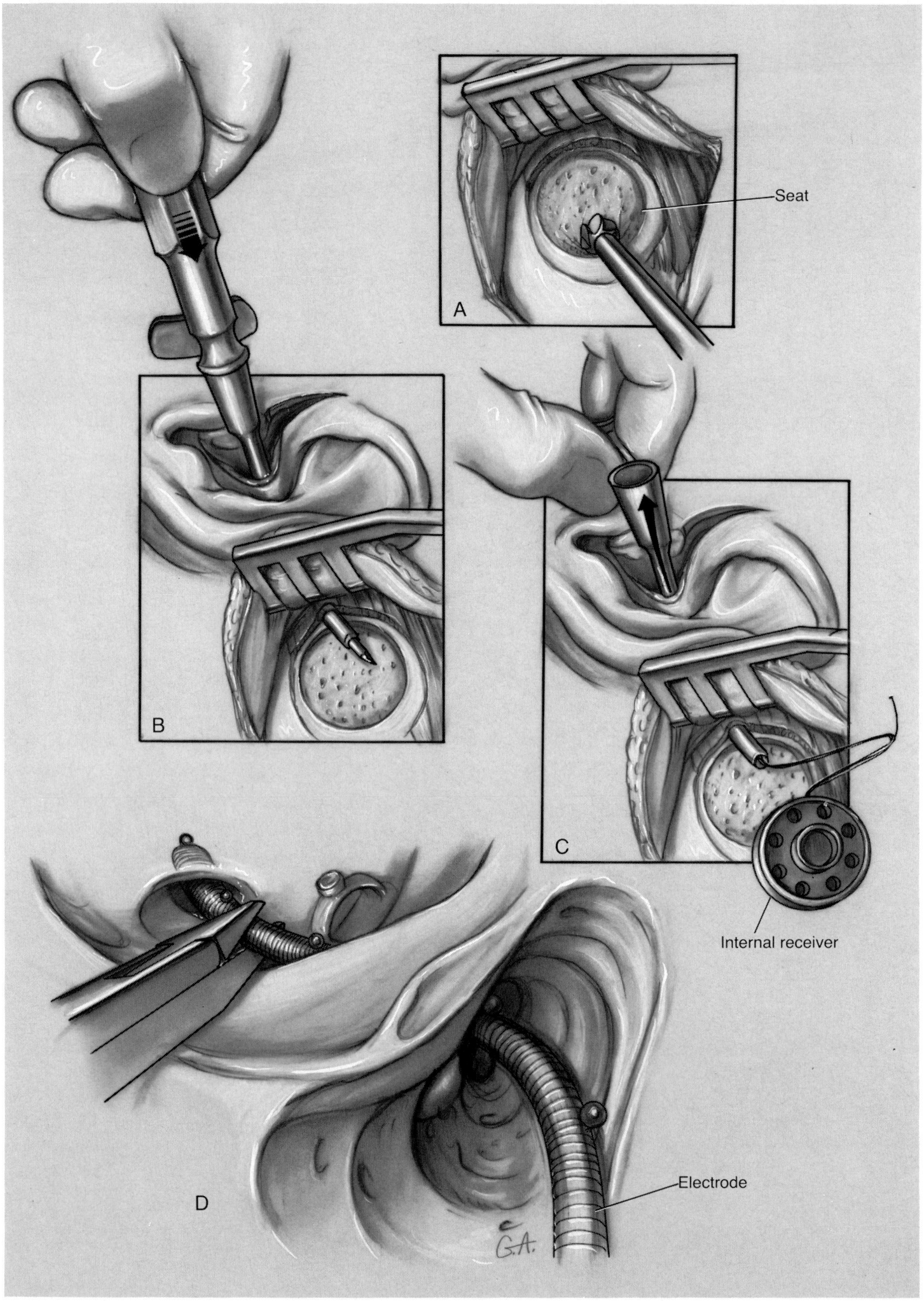

FIGURE 16–6.

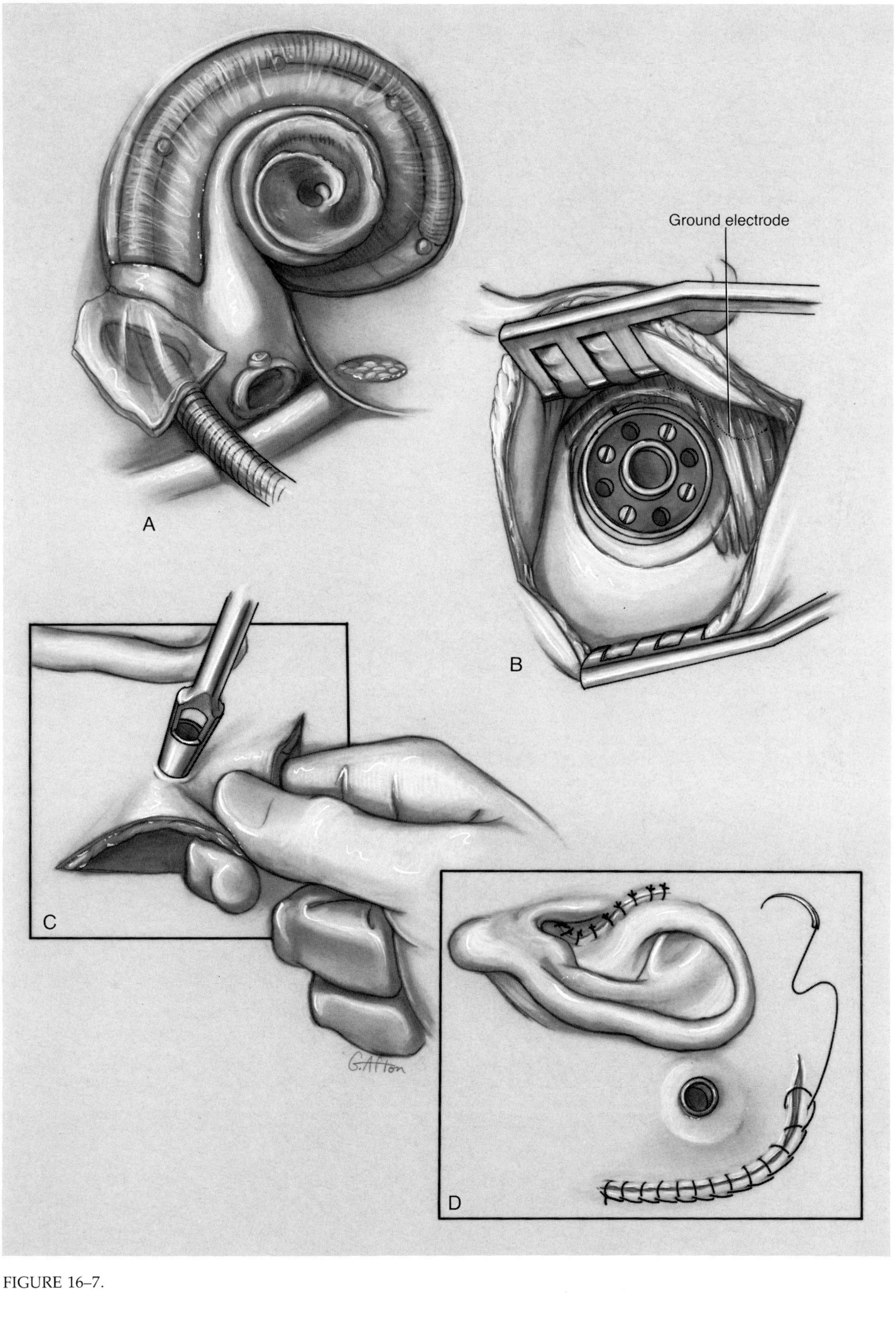

FIGURE 16–7.

periosteum graft. With a Symbion implant, the promontory electrode is positioned over the promontory and secured with a covering of periosteum graft as well.

The internal receiver is then secured in place with sutures or screws (Fig. 16–7*B*), the ground electrode (if separate) is placed in the temporal muscle fibers, and the rest of the periosteum is used to seal the antrum. If a percutaneous plug is being used, impedance is checked at this point. An opening for the plug is made anterior to the postauricular incision with a skin punch of the same size as the plug (Fig. 16–7*C*). Skin tension should be avoided.

The canal flap is repositioned. Gelfoam and an antibiotic ointment are used in the distal two thirds of the canal, and gauze is embedded in antibiotic ointment in the distal one third. Incisions are closed with subcutaneous 3-0 chromic catgut and skin sutures of 4-0 silk (Fig. 16–7*D*), and a mastoid dressing is applied.

CHAPTER 17

Surgery for Incapacitating Peripheral Vertigo

The title of this chapter has been purposely selected to indicate that the surgical procedures described here are designed for treatment of vertigo of labyrinthine origin. At the same time, the term "incapacitating" implies that symptoms are still present after adequate medical evaluation and treatment. It is understood, therefore, that these procedures are performed in a small percentage of patients, since in the majority of cases medical treatment alone will suffice. (Evaluation and medical treatment are outside the scope of this book.) In addition, it should be kept in mind that vertigo is a manifestation of an underlying problem that must be assessed and (if possible) defined; depending on the cause, different surgical alternatives will be selected. This is one of the areas in otology where our lack of true knowledge is most evident; therefore, careful and nondestructive choices are recommended if at all possible.

Surgical procedures can be destructive or conservative in nature. They may be aimed at draining an assumed endolymphatic hydrops, whether at the endolymphatic sac level or at the saccule, they may involve destruction of the labyrinth (labyrinthectomy) and/or sectioning of the vestibular nerve or other nerves, such as the singular nerve of the posterior semicircular canal. None of the many surgical procedures available are universally accepted or provide 100% relief. These are factors to keep in mind when selecting a specific approach. This chapter will describe those that are used or discussed most commonly, without implying that those not described are useless or unimportant.

Endolymphatic Sac Procedures

These procedures constitute a conservative, usually efficient approach for vertigo, and are the initial choice (not uncommonly the only choice necessary) of many surgeons. Despite the location of the sac in the posterior fossa dura, knowledge of its anatomy and adequate surgical technique usually permit a safe operation. In the event of failure, any other procedure can be done without added difficulty.

Aim

To identify and expose the endolymphatic sac overlying the dura mater of the posterior cranial fossa.

Highlights and Surgical Steps

1. Perform a complete simple mastoidectomy.
2. Drill to, but not below, the dome of the horizontal semicircular canal.
3. Identify, preserve, and measure the hard angle containing the posterior semicircular canal.
4. Identify the position of the sigmoid sinus and its relationship to Trautmann's triangle.

5. Decompress the lateral sinus and dissect the infralabyrinthine cell tract.
6. Incise the endolymphatic sac.

Pitfalls

1. Skeletonizing or damaging the posterior semicircular canal.
2. Insufficiently unroofing the dural plate.
3. Failing to identify the endolymphatic sac and its lumen.
4. Damaging the incus.
5. Debris in the middle ear.
6. Bleeding in the lateral sinus.

Procedure

In endolymphatic sac surgery, a thorough simple mastoidectomy (see Chapter 7) is advocated. During this step the bony plate overlying the posterior cranial fossa dura is identified. Trautmann's triangle is defined and the hard bone containing the posterior semicircular canal is identified (Fig. 17–1*A, B*). The sac comes toward the dura from the direction of the posterior semicircular canal and can be identified as it exits the hard angle intact. A good method of preventing damage to the posterior semicircular canal is to measure the area containing this structure and leave it untouched (undrilled). With a fenestrometer, measure 10 mm from the tip of the short process of the incus or fossa incudis, along the axis of the horizontal semicircular canal (30 degrees from the tegmen); then measure 12 mm from the fossa incudis at an angle of 45 degrees from the tegmen (Fig. 17–1*B*). This area is left untouched while the infralabyrinthine cell tract is drilled to expose the sac location (Fig. 17–1*B, C*). Special attention is paid to the position of the sigmoid sinus (Fig. 17–2*A*); on occasion, it partially overlies the dural plate, reducing the size of Trautmann's triangle (interestingly, this is fairly common in patients with Meniere's disease). The plate is thinned down to eggshell thickness, then gently elevated and separated from the underlying dura with a duckbill elevator. The sac is identifiable as a thickened white area of the dura over the thin surrounding dura (Fig. 17–2*B*). The posterior semicircular canal should not be thinned or skeletonized. Drilling is done immediately inferior to this area. If the lateral sinus is in such a position that it tends to partially cover the dura or make access to it difficult, the patient's position should be checked first; the head might be bent too far forward. If after repositioning the head of the patient the sinus is still prominent, it should be decompressed by removing part of its bony covering facing the dura. Infralabyrinthine cells may have to be drilled (leading toward the jugular bulb). The sac is identified.

At this point, there are several alternatives:

1. Decompression of the sac (rèmoval of the bony covering) is all that is done.
2. The sac is incised in its lateral surface with a sharp knife (for example, a sickle knife). This is the original (and current) Portmann procedure (Fig. 17–2*C*).
3. A valve is placed in the lumen (in the expectation that microliters of excessive endolymph will drain).
4. A small incision is made on the medial surface of the sac in order to open up the subarachnoid space. Into this opening a flanged Teflon tube is inserted. The outer surface is tightly packed (a piece of fascia can be used).
5. A thin piece of Silastic sheeting (0.01 cm) is cut in a T-shaped fashion and placed in the lumen. Small pieces of Silastic sheeting (spacers) are used to separate the dura from the floor of the posterior canal. A Silastic "apron" is applied and held in place with Gelfoam (Fig. 17–3*A–D*).

The mastoid cavity is packed with Gelfoam over the decompressed area, and the incision is closed in layers with appropriate sutures. At the end of the procedure, a ventilation tube may be placed in the tympanic membrane (Fig. 17–3*E*). It is important to thoroughly cleanse the mastoid cavity before closure.

The effectiveness of this procedure may be due to decompression of overlying bone, drainage of endolymph by opening of the sac, increased vascularity, or other factors; a discussion is outside the scope of this book. The fact remains that any procedure that involves opening the sac has comparable results.

Complications are those of mastoidectomy (see Chapter 7), opening of the posterior semicircular canal, and cerebrospinal fluid fistulae. The best treatment is prevention. The technique of isolating the hard angle is practical. If the posterior semicircular canal is accidentally opened, the fistula should be grafted immediately; however, a "dead ear" is almost certain. Fistulae that leak cerebrospinal fluid are uncommon and self-limiting; high-dose antibiotics should be used in order to avoid meningitis. It is uncommon to have to re-explore and place a large piece of fascia and muscle (along with tight packing of the mastoid cavity with Gelfoam).

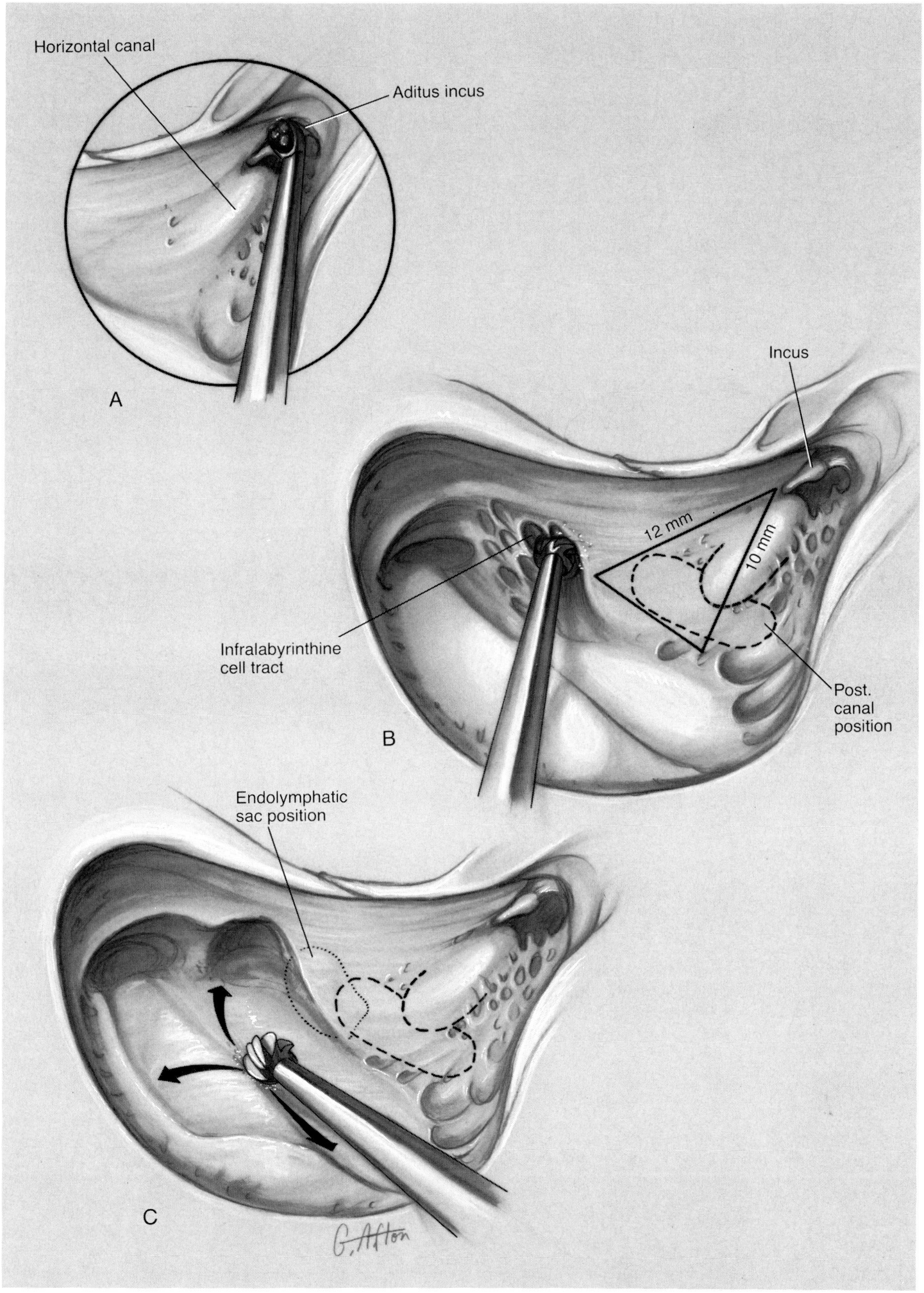
Horizontal canal
Aditus incus
A
Incus
12 mm
10 mm
Infralabyrinthine
cell tract
Post.
canal
position
B
Endolymphatic
sac position
C
G. Afton

FIGURE 17–1.

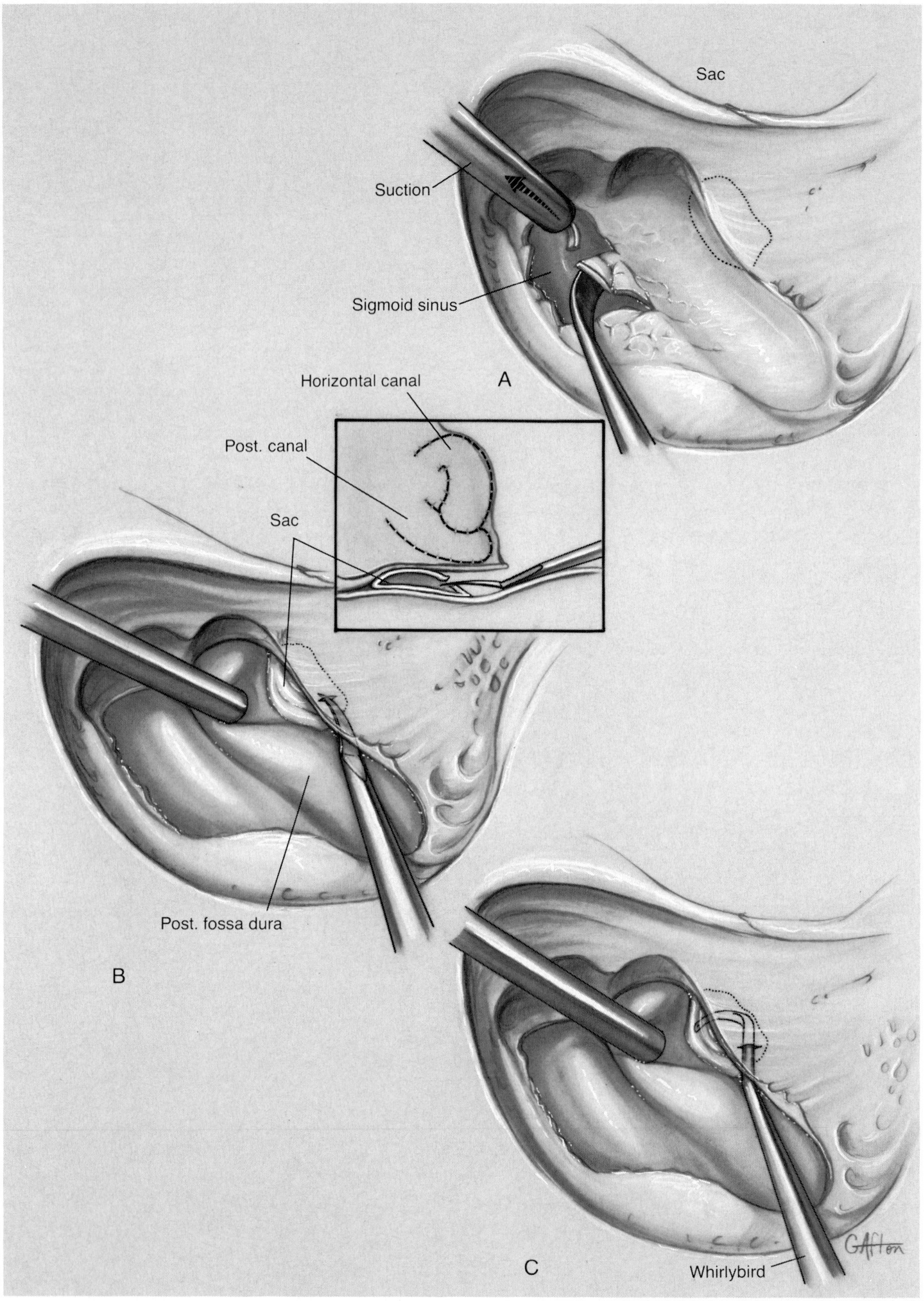
Sac
Suction
Sigmoid sinus
Horizontal canal
A
Post. canal
Sac
Post. fossa dura
B
C
Whirlybird

FIGURE 17–2.

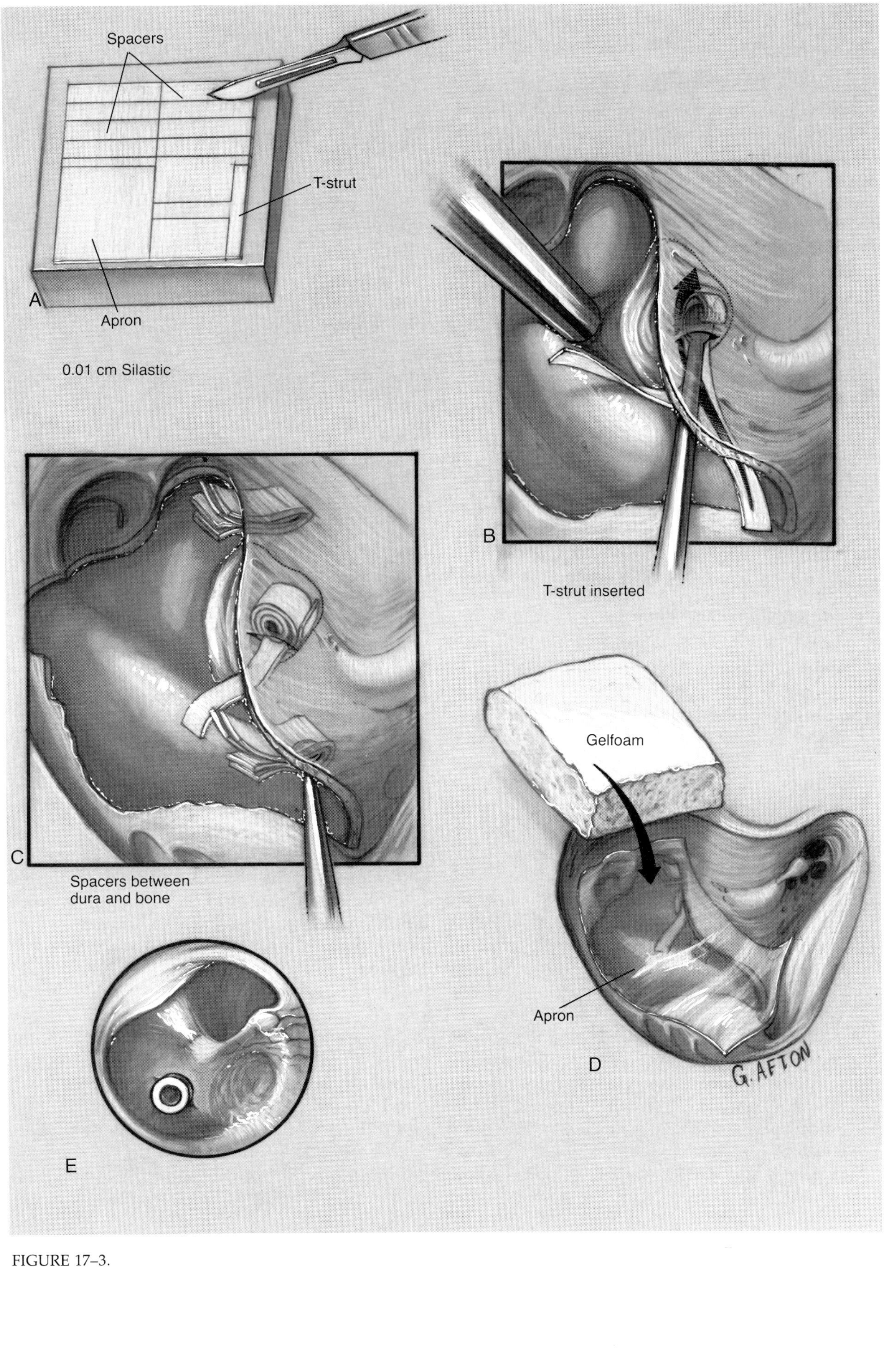
Spacers
T-strut
A
Apron
0.01 cm Silastic
B
T-strut inserted
C
Spacers between
dura and bone
Gelfoam
Apron
D
G. AFTON
E

FIGURE 17–3.

Saccule Procedures

These are mentioned for the sake of completeness and an overall concept. The most common (such as the Fick and tack procedures) are associated with severe, irreversible sensorineural hearing loss and are rarely used. (An intermediate, safer alternative used occasionally in cases of otosclerosis associated with hydrops is a wire connective tissue prosthesis with a small peg [from the wire around the connective tissue] [Fig. 17–4*A*]; this is described in Chapter 13.) Both procedures are intended to decompress a dilated saccule under the anterior portion of the oval window, which is clearly exposed. They are done through a transcanal approach. The Fick operation involves opening the footplate and then the saccule (Fig. 17–4*C*), whereas the tack procedure involves the placement of a sharp tack through the footplate (anterior aspect) (Fig. 17–4*B*). It is important to seal the footplate with connective tissue. The tack "decompresses" the saccule when it becomes dilated. Closure is similar to that for a stapedectomy.

Singular Neurectomy

This selectively destructive procedure entails sectioning the nerve of the posterior semicircular canal (singular nerve) for the treatment of benign peripheral positional vertigo (caused by an alteration in the posterior semicircular canal, such as cupulolithiasis). The nerve runs parallel to the anterosuperior portion of the round window membrane (Fig. 17–5*A*).

The round window niche is exposed via a transcanal approach. If necessary, the posteroinferior canal wall is curetted for better exposure. The bony round window niche is drilled carefully with a small bur and the anterosuperior portion of the round window membrane is exposed (Fig. 17–5*B*). The bone immediately anterior to the membrane is thinned down (without involving the membrane and leaving a piece of bone intact between the membrane and the thinned area). The nerve is 1.5 to 2 mm deep (slightly deeper is the basal turn of the cochlea); it is identified and sectioned with an angled hook (Fig. 17–5*C*), and the area is covered with Gelfoam.

This procedure is more easily described than performed. It is quite difficult to find the nerve (even in a temporal bone in the laboratory). For anybody attempting this procedure, a reasonable number of temporal bone dissections are recommended.

Destruction of the posterior labyrinth by ultrasound (Arslan's procedure) is not described in this book. Its indications are few and can be covered by the other procedures; furthermore, the author has no experience with it. The reader is referred to the literature.

Labyrinthectomy

Labyrinthectomy, a procedure that is fairly commonly employed, entails total destruction of the labyrinth. It should be reserved for patients with no usable hearing; even then, the significance of the procedure must be considered. Is the causative disease bilateral? Could it eventually become bilateral? Is there any chance that the patient needs a cochlear implant?

A labyrinthectomy can be done through a transcanal or a transmastoid approach.

Transcanal Approach

Highlights

1. Clear identification of the facial nerve is essential to avoid any potential lesions while drilling in the oval window.
2. Removal of the oval window contents must be done without deepening the window or pushing the instrument hard into the walls. Only a thin plate separates this area from the internal auditory canal, and a cerebrospinal fluid leak is a potential complication.

Exposure is obtained via an exploratory tympanotomy approach (see Chapter 5). Both the oval and the round windows are exposed. It is important to visualize and identify the position and status of the facial nerve in relationship to the oval window (Fig. 17–6). The stapes is removed and the contents of the oval window are suctioned. With a hook, the rest of the contents are removed (Fig. 17–7*A, B*). The promontory is drilled and both windows are connected (Fig. 17–7*C*). The labyrinth is filled with Gelfoam saturated with streptomycin sulfate.

Text continued on page 307

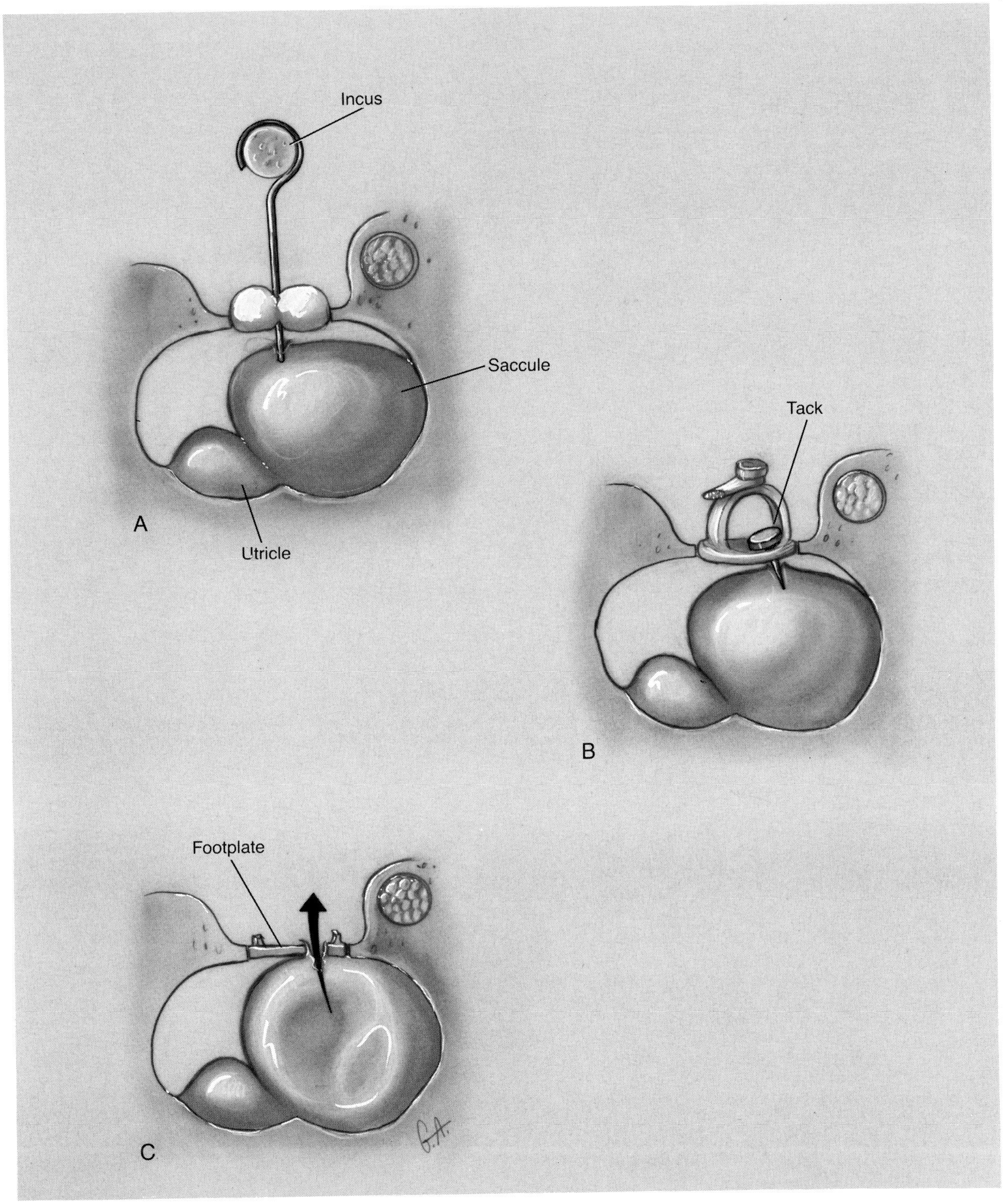

FIGURE 17–4.

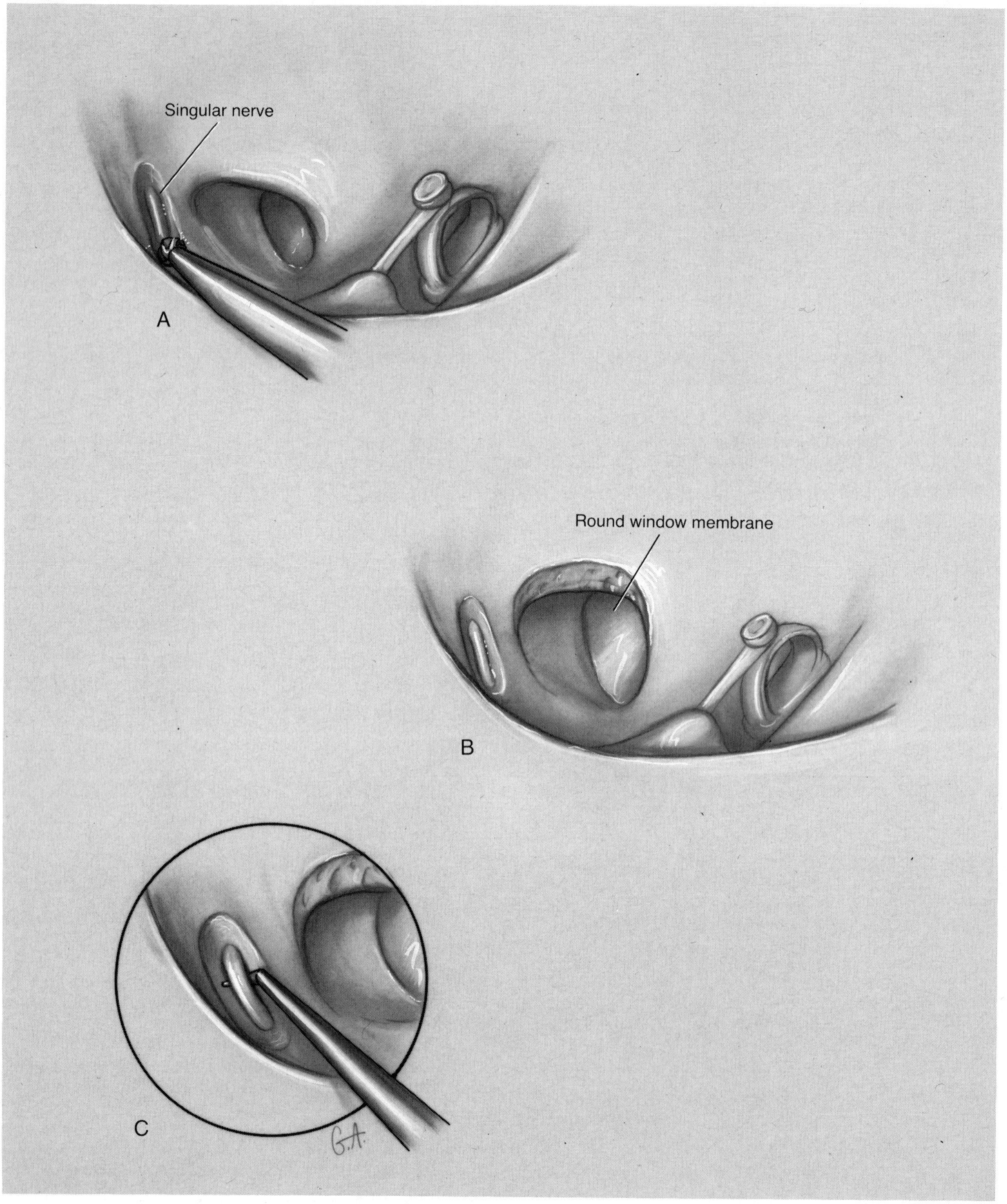

FIGURE 17–5.

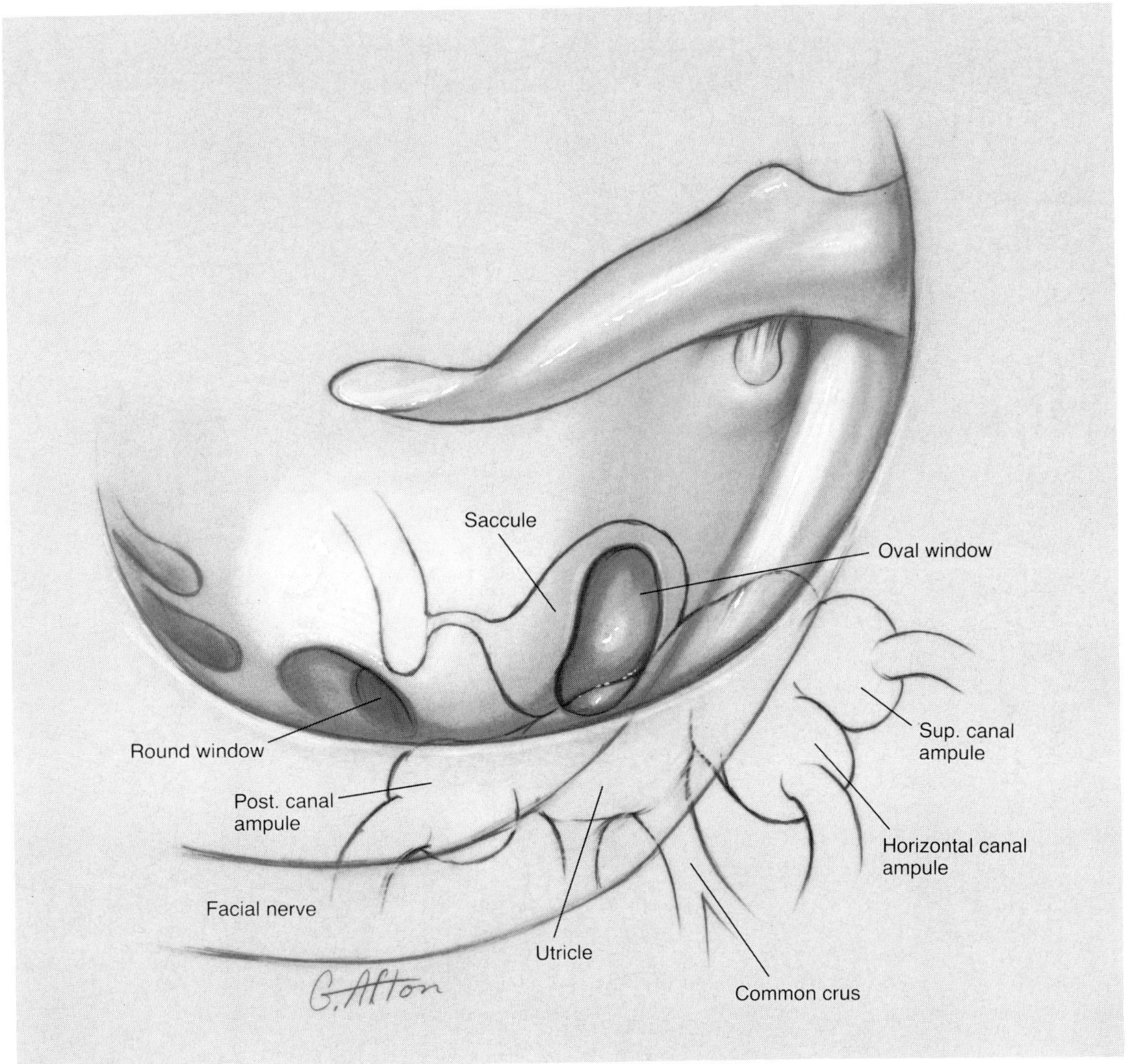
Saccule
Oval window
Round window
Sup. canal ampule
Post. canal ampule
Horizontal canal ampule
Facial nerve
Utricle
Common crus
G. Alton

FIGURE 17–6.

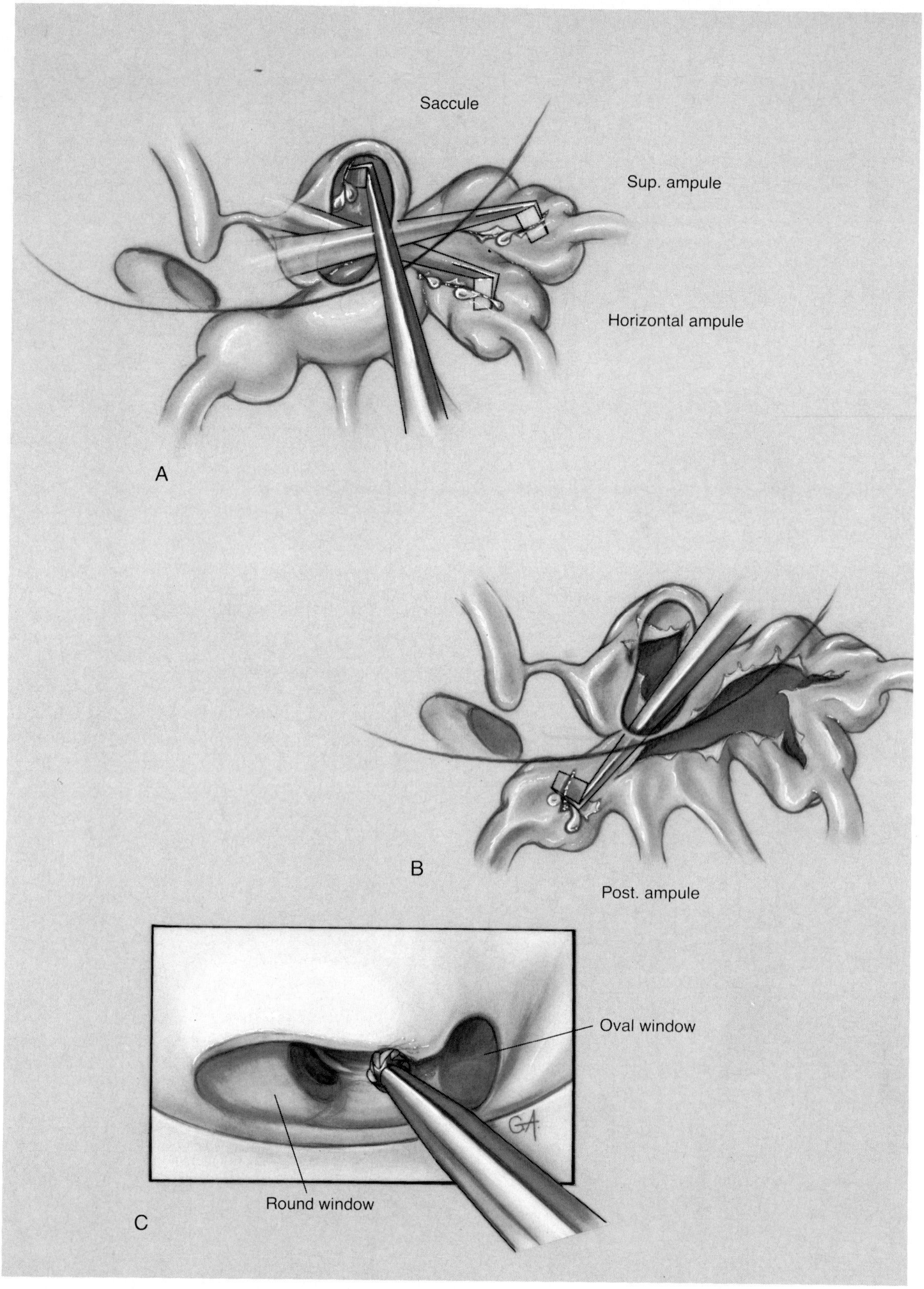
Saccule
Sup. ampule
Horizontal ampule
A
B
Post. ampule
Oval window
Round window
C
GA

FIGURE 17–7.

Transmastoid Approach (Transmastoid Labyrinthine Dissection)

Aim

Complete removal of the semicircular canals and the soft tissue of the vestibule.

Highlights

1. The sinodural angle must be completely thinned for adequate exposure of the vestibule.
2. The tegmen must be thinned for adequate visualization of the superior aspect of the semicircular canals.

A simple mastoidectomy is done. The three semicircular canals are skeletonized until the membranous labyrinth is visible through the bone as a thin blue line (Fig. 17–8*A*). The relationship of the facial nerve to the horizontal semicircular canal is defined (Fig. 17–8*B*). The three canals are drilled (one by one) and their contents carefully removed by suction and the use of hooks (Fig. 17–8*C*). The space is filled with Gelfoam saturated with streptomycin sulfate.

Retrolabyrinthine Approach to the Cerebellopontine Angle and Sectioning of the Vestibular Nerve

Aim

Exposure of the cerebellopontine angle and the eighth cranial nerve with preservation of the labyrinth.

Highlights

1. Mannitol may be given to aid shrinkage of the cerebellum.
2. The anterior limit of the dissection is the posterior semicircular canal.
3. The sigmoid sinus must be adequately decompressed and mobilized.
4. Bone must be completely removed from the sinodural angle and posterior fossa.
5. A dural flap is hinged anteriorly and draped over the posterior semicircular canal.
6. The superior half of the eighth nerve is sectioned.

Pitfalls

1. Failing to remove bone adequately up to the posterior semicircular canal.
2. Inadvertently entering the labyrinth.
3. Failing to decompress the sigmoid sinus adequately, leading to poor visualization.
4. Incompletely sectioning the vestibular nerve.
5. Inadvertently sectioning the cochlear nerve fibers.

Procedure

For this approach, the patient lies supine. The preparation and draping of the patient are the same as for a standard ear procedure, with the exception that a larger area of the head is shaved. The patient's head is positioned at the foot of the table to allow the surgeon's legs ample room beneath the table. The patient must be securely strapped to the table, since frequent side-to-side rotation is needed. The patient's left lower abdomen is also prepared and draped for harvesting of an abdominal fat graft.

The postauricular incision is made as usual but is located further posteriorly—2 to 3 cm (at its most posterior position)—to allow drilling posterior to the sigmoid sinus. This is essential for complete decompression of the sigmoid sinus, which permits proper angulation and visualization into the cerebellopontine angle. The incision runs in a semilunar fashion and is carried through the periosteum of the mastoid cortex, avoiding the temporal muscle superiorly. The periosteum is then elevated and the ear held forward with cerebellar retractors. Retractors placed in a superior-to-inferior direction will hold the temporal muscle out of the surgical field.

Using the largest cutting bur and suction irrigation, drilling is begun. The mastoid cortex is removed as in a routine mastoidectomy. Care is taken to saucerize the edges and to keep the lateralmost opening as wide as possible. Removal of bone is extended behind the sigmoid sinus for a distance of up to 1 cm; the bone is thinned to eggshell thickness,

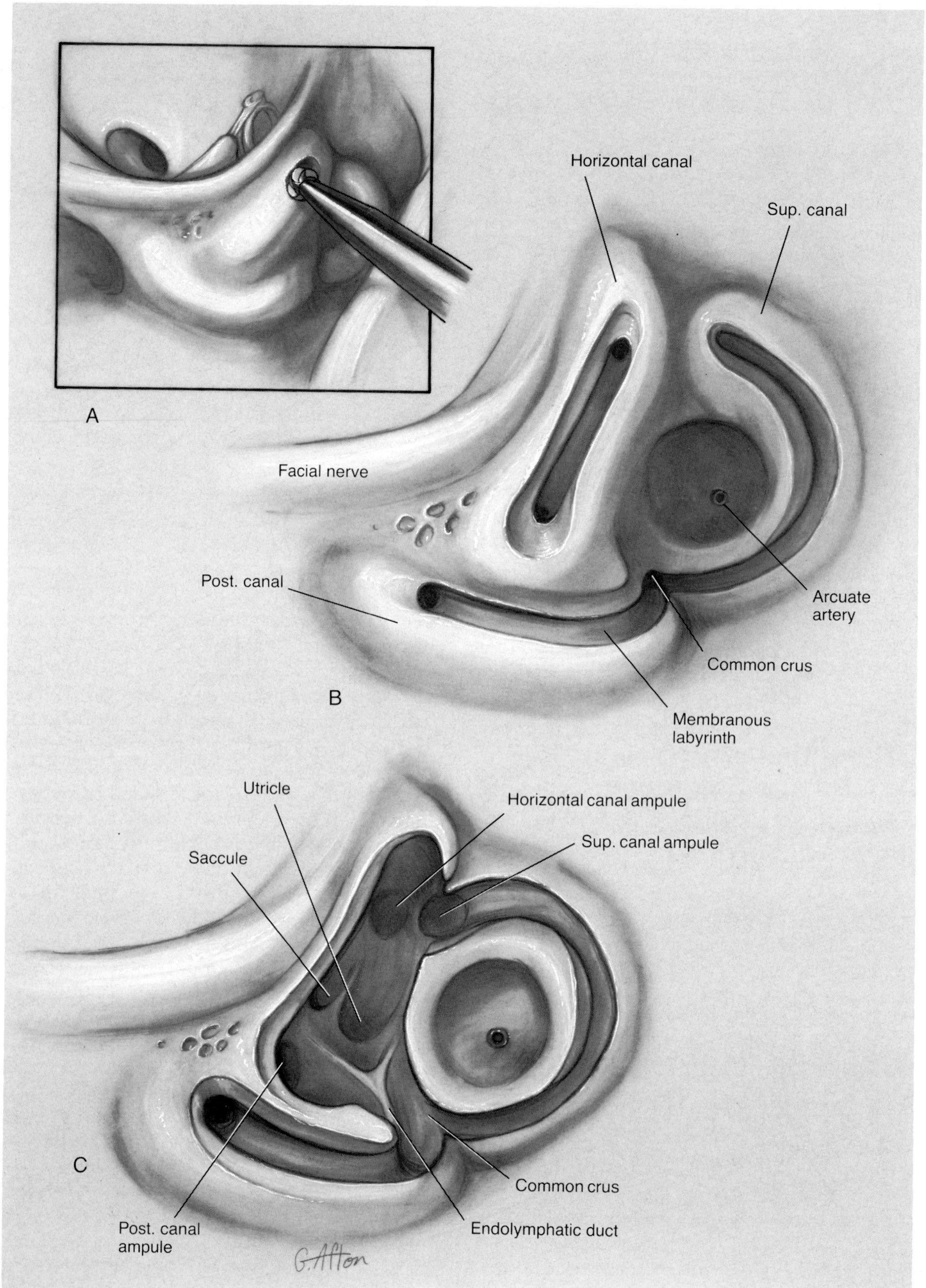
A
Horizontal canal
Sup. canal
Facial nerve
Post. canal
Arcuate
artery
Common crus
B
Membranous
labyrinth
Utricle
Horizontal canal ampule
Sup. canal ampule
Saccule
C
Common crus
Endolymphatic duct
Post. canal
ampule
G. Afton

FIGURE 17–8.

and final removal from the sigmoid and dura is accomplished later with the diamond bur. Be alert for emissary veins that run from the sigmoid sinus to the mastoid cortex.

At this point the operating microscope is brought into the field. The mastoidectomy is completed as described in Chapters 5 and 7, and the basic landmarks (the horizontal semicircular canal, the incus, and the course of the facial nerve) are visualized. With these landmarks, accurate identification of the posterior semicircular canal can be made. This represents the anterior limit for removal of bone and exposure into the cerebellopontine angle; if bone removal is not complete up to the posterior semicircular canal, a troublesome ridge of bone will hinder adequate exposure to the angle. Inferiorly the dissection is continued into the infralabyrinthine and retrofacial cell tracts. Bone removal is also necessary here for adequate exposure of the cerebellopontine angle and the eighth cranial nerve. The posterior fossa dura is followed medially and the jugular bulb, if superiorly located, is exposed. The superior limit within the infralabyrinthine cell tract will be the hard bone of the labyrinth. Although it is not necessary to "blue-line" it, constant awareness of the location of the descending portion of the facial nerve is needed to avoid injury to it. The endolymphatic sac is located within the dura at this level.

Bone removal from the posterior fossa dura is now completed with the large diamond bur and suction irrigation. The diamond bur allows for safer bone removal and avoids tearing of the dura or sinus. Bill's island of bone is often left over the sigmoid sinus to protect it during retraction or further drilling medially.

The dural opening is made with a No. 59S Beaver knife or similar sharp instrument. The first incision parallels the sigmoid sinus and runs between the sinus and the endolymphatic sac inferiorly (Fig. 17–9*A*). The superior incision parallels the superior petrosal sinus and runs in the sinodural angle. (Care must be taken to avoid injury to the vessels and the cerebellum immediately under the dura.) The dural flap created is hinged anteromedially at the level of the posterior semicircular canal (Fig. 17–9*B*); it is draped over the canal and a stay suture is placed if needed. Long Cottonoids are placed over the exposed cerebellum (for protection) and gentle retraction is applied. The cisterna lateralis inferiorly is bluntly probed to provide a profuse cerebrospinal fluid leak if one has not occurred; this allows the cerebellum to relax. Good visualization of the cerebellopontine angle and its structures is then obtained.

The eighth nerve lies near the level of the ampullated end of the posterior semicircular canal and runs in a plane in line with the horizontal semicircular canal. With adequate exposure, the fifth nerve may be seen anterosuperiorly. Inferiorly the ninth, tenth, and eleventh nerves can be seen. The seventh nerve lies medial to the eighth and can be visualized with gentle retraction of the latter. Often the lateral branch of the anteroinferior cerebellar artery is seen between the seventh and eighth cranial nerve rootlets (Fig. 17–10*A*). Arachnoid adhesions may obscure the cerebellopontine angle and its structures. Careful dissection with a sharp hook may be needed to lyse these adhesions.

At this level, the eighth nerve consists of one trunk. The vestibular segment of the nerve lies superior to the cochlear segment. Usually, careful high-power inspection of the nerve trunk will reveal the cleavage plane separating the two segments; it is often highlighted by a small vessel on the surface of the nerve (Fig. 17–10*B*). (In approximately 20% of patients, this plane is difficult to discern.) Using a small hook, the cleavage plane is developed. Sectioning of the vestibular division is done with a sharp hook or microscissors, carefully avoiding injury to the facial or cochlear nerves (Fig. 17–10C). As the vestibular division is sectioned the ends will retract, leaving a 3- to 4-mm gap.

After sectioning of the nerve, the cerebellopontine angle is inspected for good hemostasis. The previously harvested abdominal fat is cut into long strips, which are placed just into the dural opening with the tails brought out to the mastoid cavity. Careful and tight placement of these strips has been found to provide a good seal against postoperative cerebrospinal fluid leakage. The long tails are then folded into the mastoid and antrum, and the postauricular incision is closed. A mastoid pressure dressing is applied and left in place for two days.

Intraoperative Complications or Problems

With good training and expertise, this procedure is remarkably free of intraoperative complications. The most common problems are caused by bleeding from injury to the sinuses; they are treated as discussed in Chapter 5 (Translabyrinthine Approach to the Internal Auditory Canal). With careful preparation and meticulous exposure, other problems listed there should be avoided. Additional potential problems are those accompanying a mastoidectomy.

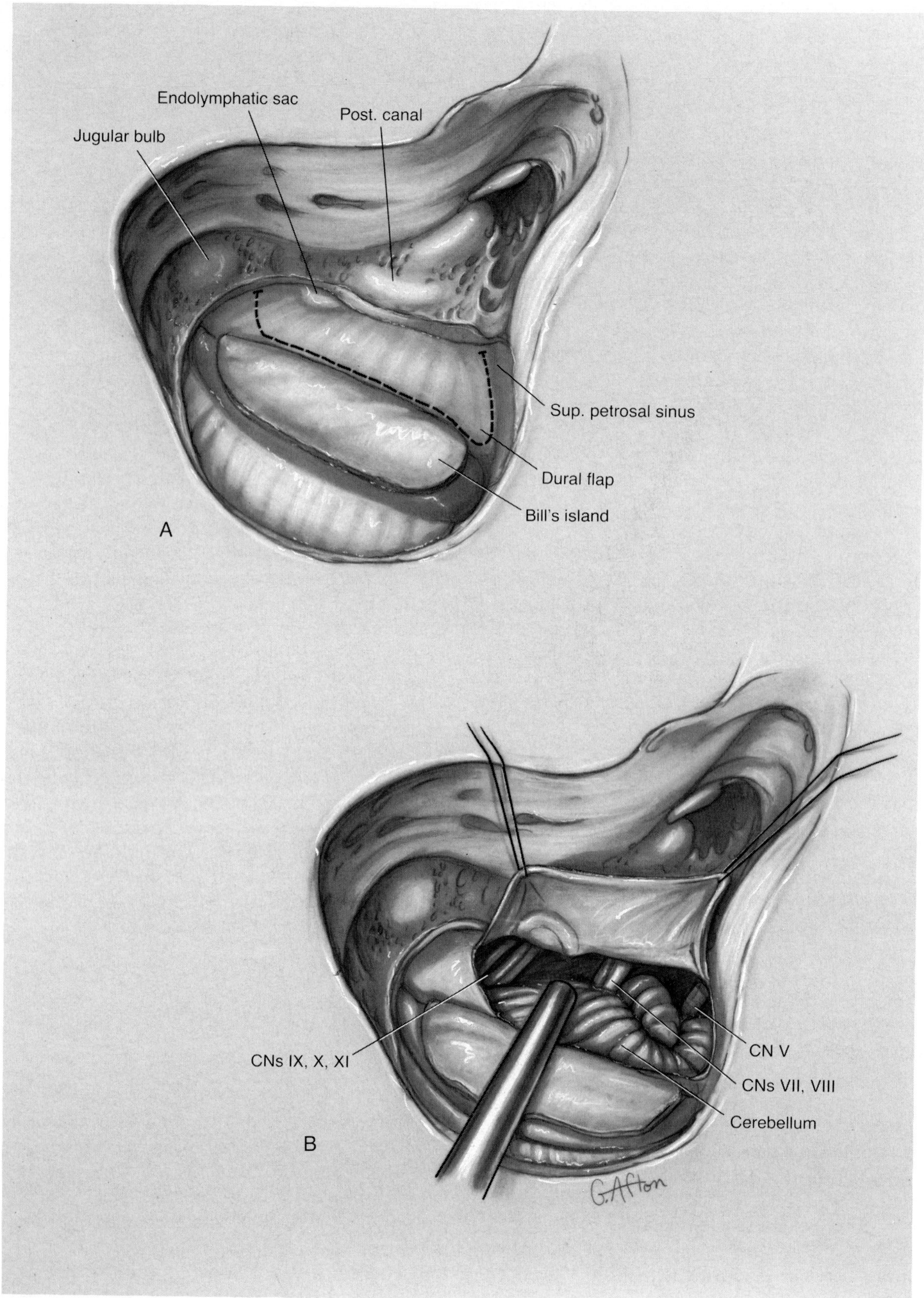

Endolymphatic sac
Post. canal
Jugular bulb
Sup. petrosal sinus
Dural flap
Bill's island
A
CNs IX, X, XI
CN V
CNs VII, VIII
Cerebellum
B
G. Afton

FIGURE 17–9.

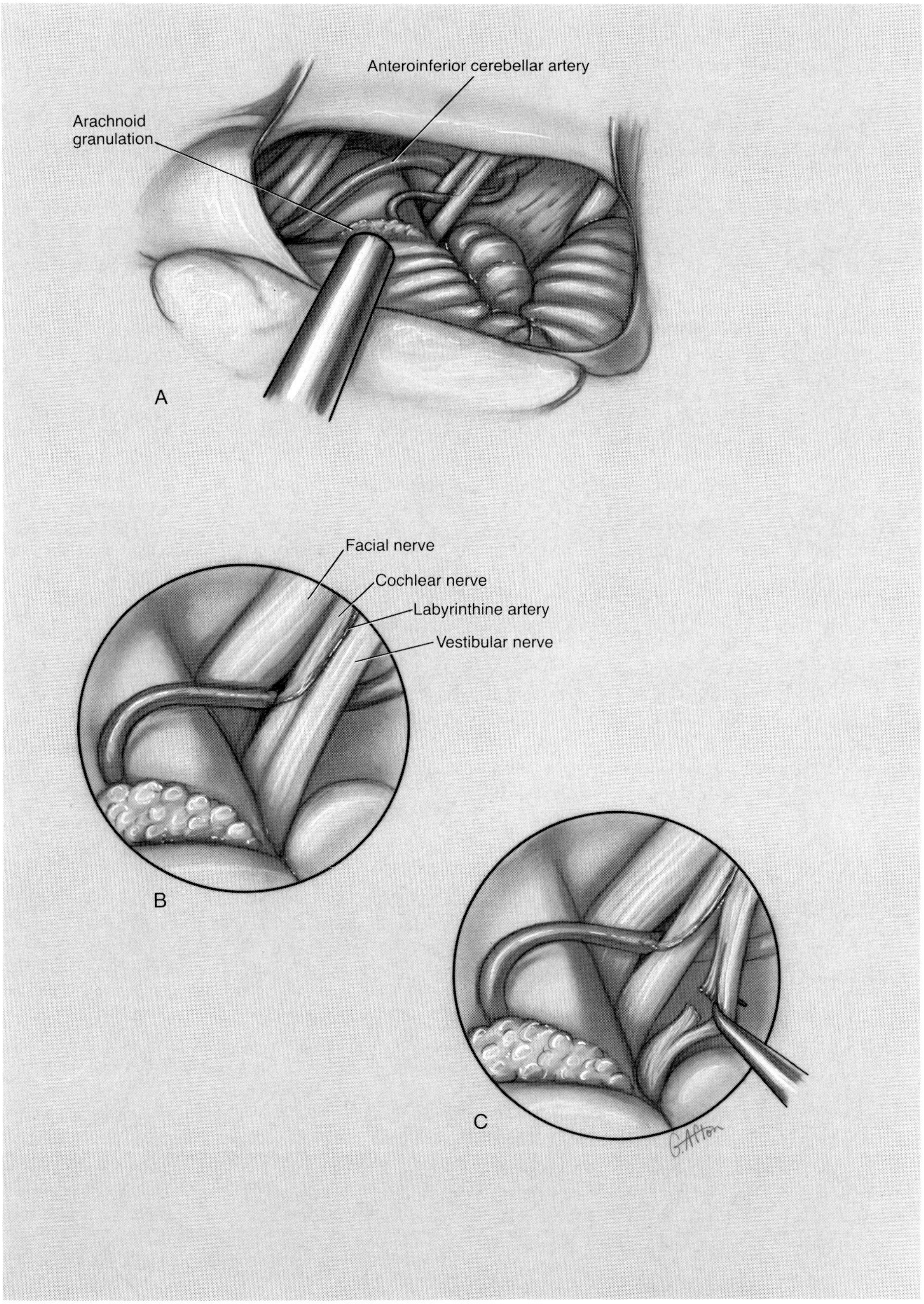
Anteroinferior cerebellar artery
Arachnoid granulation
A
Facial nerve
Cochlear nerve
Labyrinthine artery
Vestibular nerve
B
C

FIGURE 17–10.

Pertinent Histopathology

FIGURE 17–11

This temporal bone was from an individual who underwent fenestration of the horizontal semicircular canal for a vertiginous syndrome. The vertigo subsided temporarily. This section shows that what appear to be simple conservative "fenestrations" result in localized reactions with new bone formation.

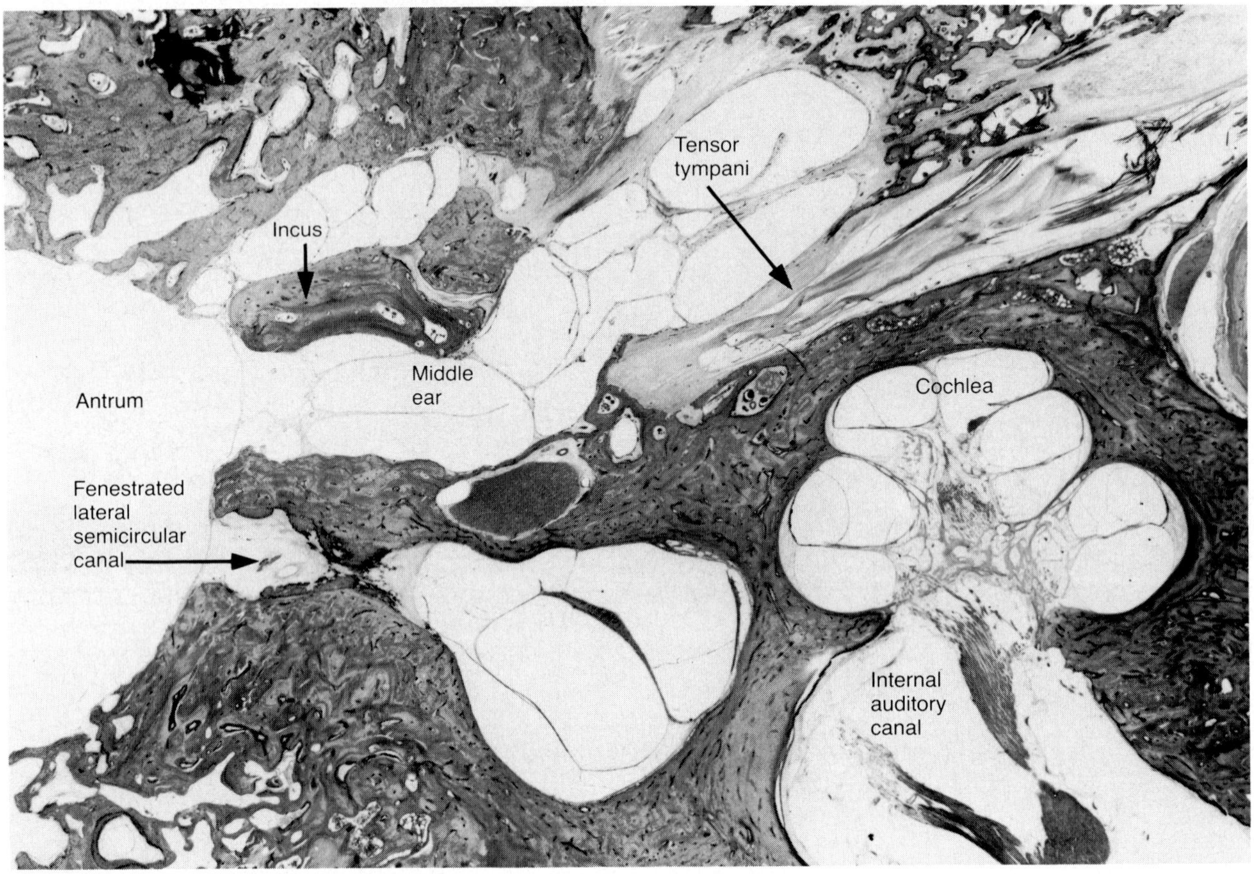

FIGURE 17–11.

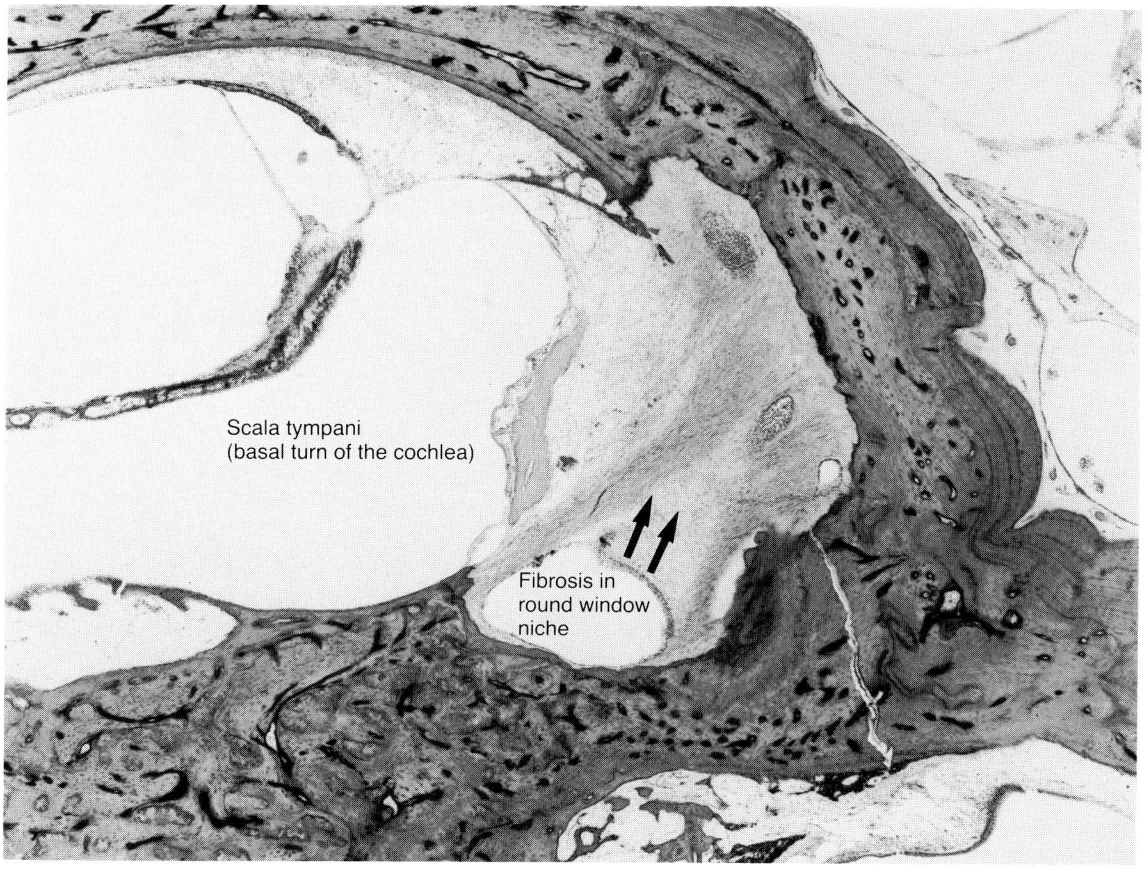

FIGURE 17–12

This patient underwent an unsuccessful "round window labyrinthotomy" for vertigo. A severe sensorineural hearing loss that was present preoperatively did not change postoperatively. This section shows the marked localized inflammatory reaction in the round window niche that is associated with seemingly minor surgical trauma.

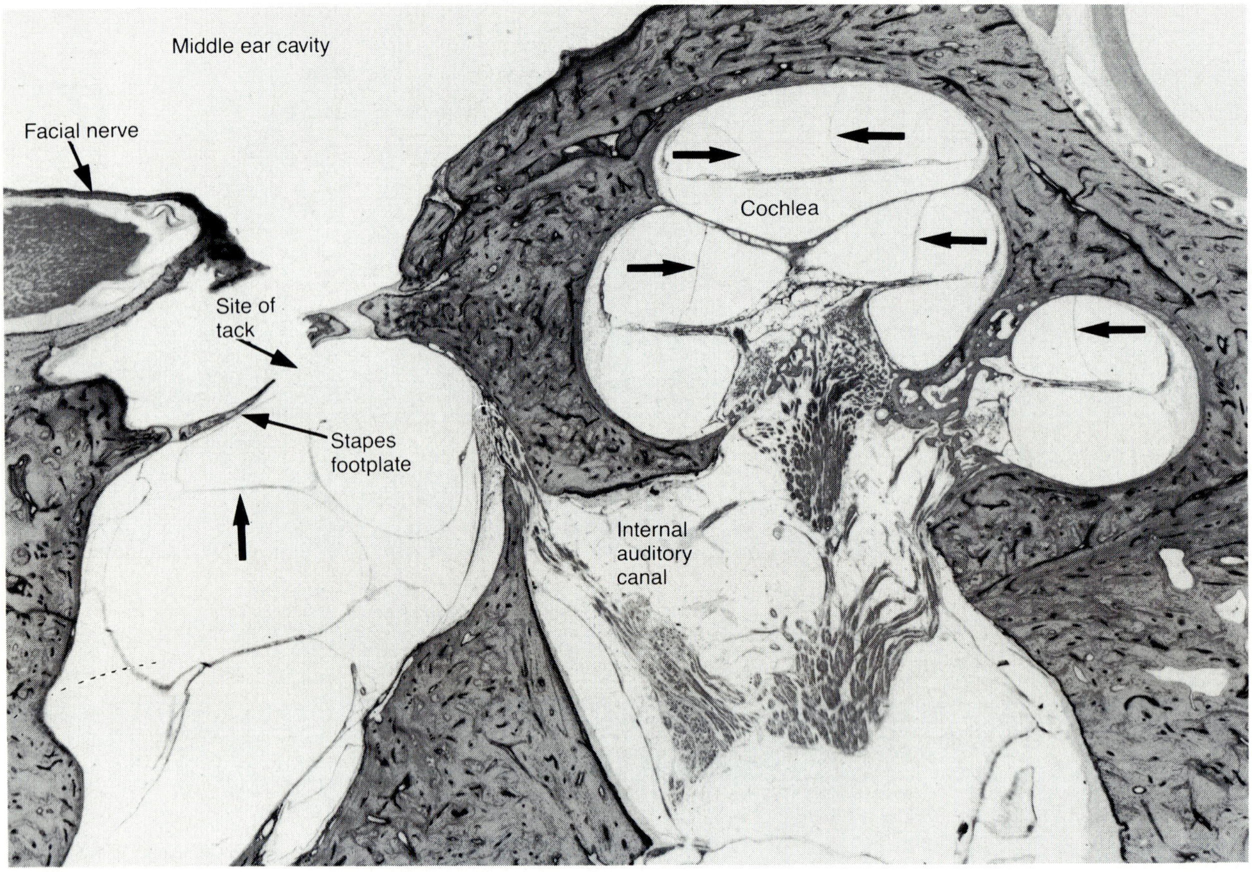

FIGURE 17–13

This patient underwent an unsuccessful tack procedure for a vertiginous syndrome. The opening in the footplate corresponds to the site of the tack. The section shows that in spite of the tack the hydrops persisted (*arrows*). In this particular case the tack did not achieve its purpose, but such failure is infrequent. This section is presented in order to give a visual orientation to endolymphatic hydrops and the rationale for a tack procedure.

CHAPTER 18

Intratemporal Facial Nerve Surgery

The aim of the procedures discussed in this chapter is to re-establish safe continuity of the axons of the facial nerve that have been compromised by trauma or disease. This remains constant whether the procedure involves freeing, decompressing, or reanastomosing. A complete discussion of the indications for surgical exploration of the facial nerve or any of its segments is outside the scope of this atlas; the comments here are intended only to contribute to a thorough understanding of specific procedures. Intratemporal facial nerve paralysis can be caused by different factors and can occur in different segments. Based on adequate preoperative assessment, the required procedure might involve a wide myringotomy, a transcanal or transmastoid approach, an exploration of the first nerve segment at the internal auditory canal, or a total facial nerve exploration.

Myringotomy

Facial paralysis may occur during an acute episode of otitis media. Performing a wide myringotomy for drainage of purulent effusion, obtaining a sample for culture, and placing a large-bore tube (along with adequate medical treatment) will suffice in the majority of cases. It is important to use a large tube. Small type I tubes tend to become plugged, requiring a second drainage procedure.

Transmastoid Approach

Surgical Steps

1. Those of a simple mastoidectomy.
2. Those of a facial recess approach (if needed).
3. Identifying the different segments of the facial nerve and skeletonizing the facial canal.
4. Removing the bony covering.
5. Opening the sheath of the nerve (if indicated).

Procedure

For practical surgical purposes, the facial nerve can be divided into three segments: (1) within the internal auditory canal and labyrinth; (2) the mastoid (vertical); and (3) the tympanic (horizontal middle ear).

The transmastoid approach provides access to the tympanic and mastoid segments of the nerve. Simple mastoidectomy and facial recess approaches have been described up to the point of clearly identifying the facial (fallopian) canal. The anatomy of the canal should now be reassessed (Fig. 18–1*A*).

Mastoid Segment. From the external genu, the nerve proceeds vertically to the stylomastoid foramen at

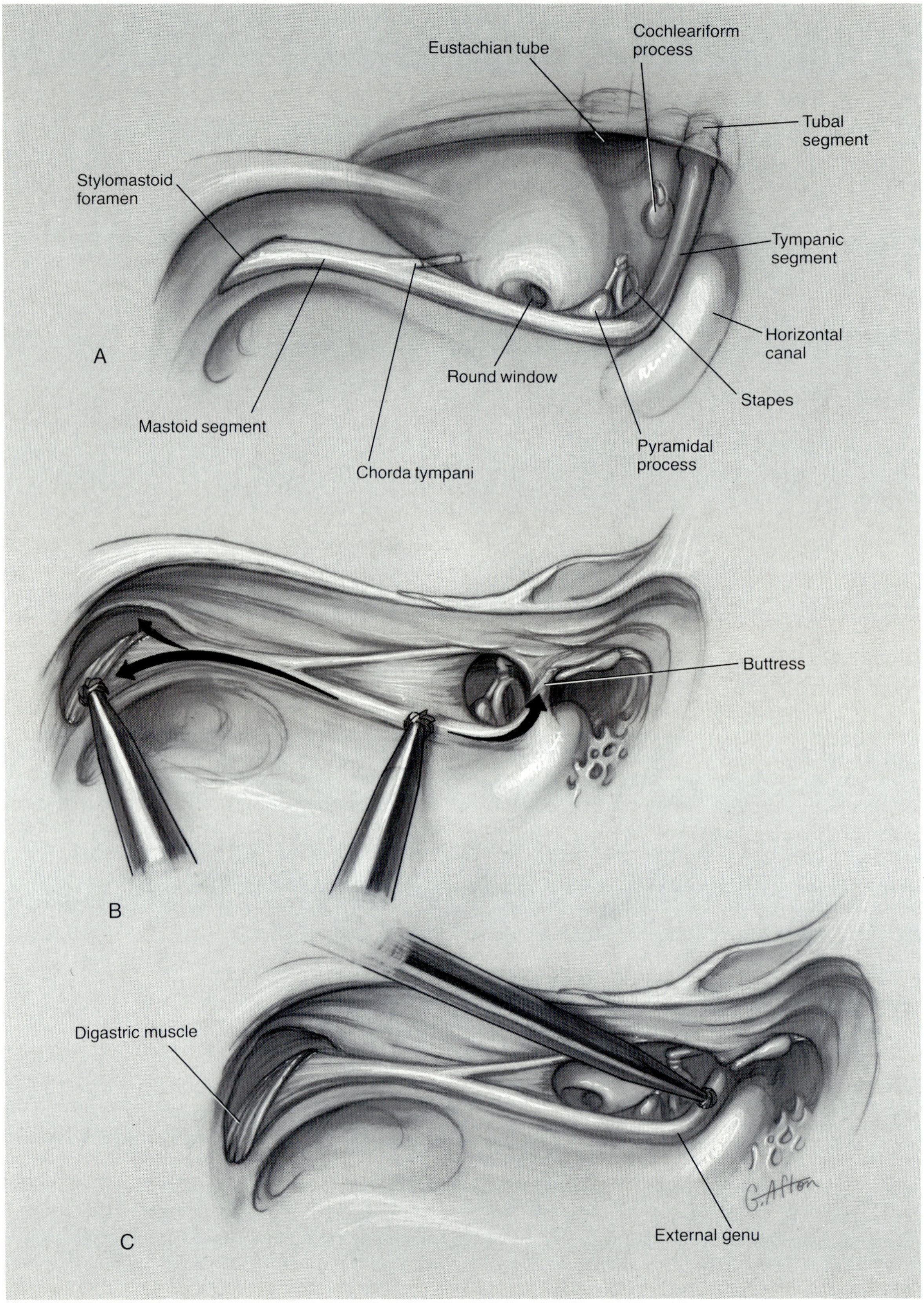
Eustachian tube
Cochleariform process
Tubal segment
Stylomastoid foramen
Tympanic segment
Horizontal canal
A
Round window
Stapes
Mastoid segment
Pyramidal process
Chorda tympani
Buttress
B
Digastric muscle
External genu
C
G. Afton

FIGURE 18–1.

the level of the anterior edge of the digastric ridge (Fig. 18–1*A*, *B*). The nerve usually is medial to the horizontal canal (a good landmark), but at times it may be lateral to it (congenitally or by inflammatory disease) or it may have a posterior projection at the genu, lending itself to potential damage. It is useful to visualize the nerve anterior to the digastric ridge, noting how lateral it becomes as it reaches the mastoid tip.

Tympanic Segment. The nerve appears in the region of the cochleariform process at the geniculate ganglion, then runs posteriorly toward the oval window (not uncommonly, it is dehiscent at this point) to a point just inferior and generally medial (deeper) to the horizontal semicircular canal. Exposure of the tympanic segment is helped by enlarging the aditus ad antrum. This dissection, combined with enlargement of the facial recess approach, allows visualization anteriorly toward the cochleariform process. Drilling with a small bur is done under the incus without damaging or dislocating it; if this is not possible (which usually is the case), the incus can be removed with a joint knife (Fig. 18–2*A*). If necessary, the tendon of the tensor tympani can be sectioned, permitting elevation of the malleus; this will allow complete drilling toward the geniculate ganglion. If required for better exposure, an exploratory tympanotomy flap (previously described) can be elevated and additional transcanal exposure can be obtained. The mastoid segment can be dissected from the level of the fossa incudis or from the digastric ridge. From the ridge, it can be followed superiorly to the external genu; although this approach is perfectly acceptable, the authors tend to follow nerves peripherally rather than centrally and to start at the level of the fossa incudis. Drilling is done with parallel strokes in the direction of the nerve (superior to inferior or vice versa).

The entire facial canal should be thinned to eggshell consistency with a diamond or polishing bur. However, the facial nerve sheath should not be exposed with the bur. The thinned bone is fractured with a pick and the bone fragments are lifted gently with a Whirlybird, without using the facial nerve as a fulcrum (Fig. 18–2*B*). The sheath is split open with a sharp sickle knife or a Beaver knife (Fig. 18–2*C*). Special situations and handling of the nerve itself are described below. When closing, the incus is repositioned and held in place by several small pieces of Gelfoam. Both articulations (with the stapes and the malleus) are carefully repositioned. Closure and packing are done as in a mastoid procedure. The exposed nerve is then covered with gold foil (or a similar material) in order to avoid fibrosis and tissue ingrowth. Fascia should not be used directly over the nerve fibers.

Transcanal Approach

This approach allows access to the tympanic segment of the facial nerve and, if extended inferiorly, makes it possible to expose the mastoid segment down to the stylomastoid foramen. This can be used adequately in a sclerotic mastoid, but in a well-pneumatized mastoid it might result in a large cavity with an underlying exposed nerve. Risks of infection in these cases must be considered. This exposure can also be obtained by an endaural approach.

Procedure

A large tympanomeatal flap is created with vertical incisions at 2 and 6 o'clock, and the middle ear cavity is entered beneath the annulus (see Chapter 7). The posterior and superior walls are enlarged with burs and curets to facilitate exposure. The incus is separated from the stapes with a joint knife. If necessary, the tendon of the tensor tympani is sectioned to allow elevation of the malleus. The fallopian canal is thinned, the sheath is exposed, and the procedure is continued as in the transmastoid approach (including repositioning of the incus). The flap is repositioned and the canal is packed (Fig. 18–3).

Special Situations and Management of the Nerve

The techniques described assume the need for total decompression, which is not necessarily the case at all times. In cases of acute mastoiditis (with an exposed nerve and facial paralysis) with no penetration of the facial nerve sheath by granulation tissue or cholesteatoma, it might be better not to open the sheath. There is a risk that the nerve can be involved by the underlying inflammatory process. A thorough mastoidectomy with a facial recess approach, allowing cleansing and aeration of the cavity and middle ear, might suffice. It is also possible that opening of the sheath, followed by bulging of the nerve until normal nerve areas are exposed at both ends of the bulge, may be sufficient.

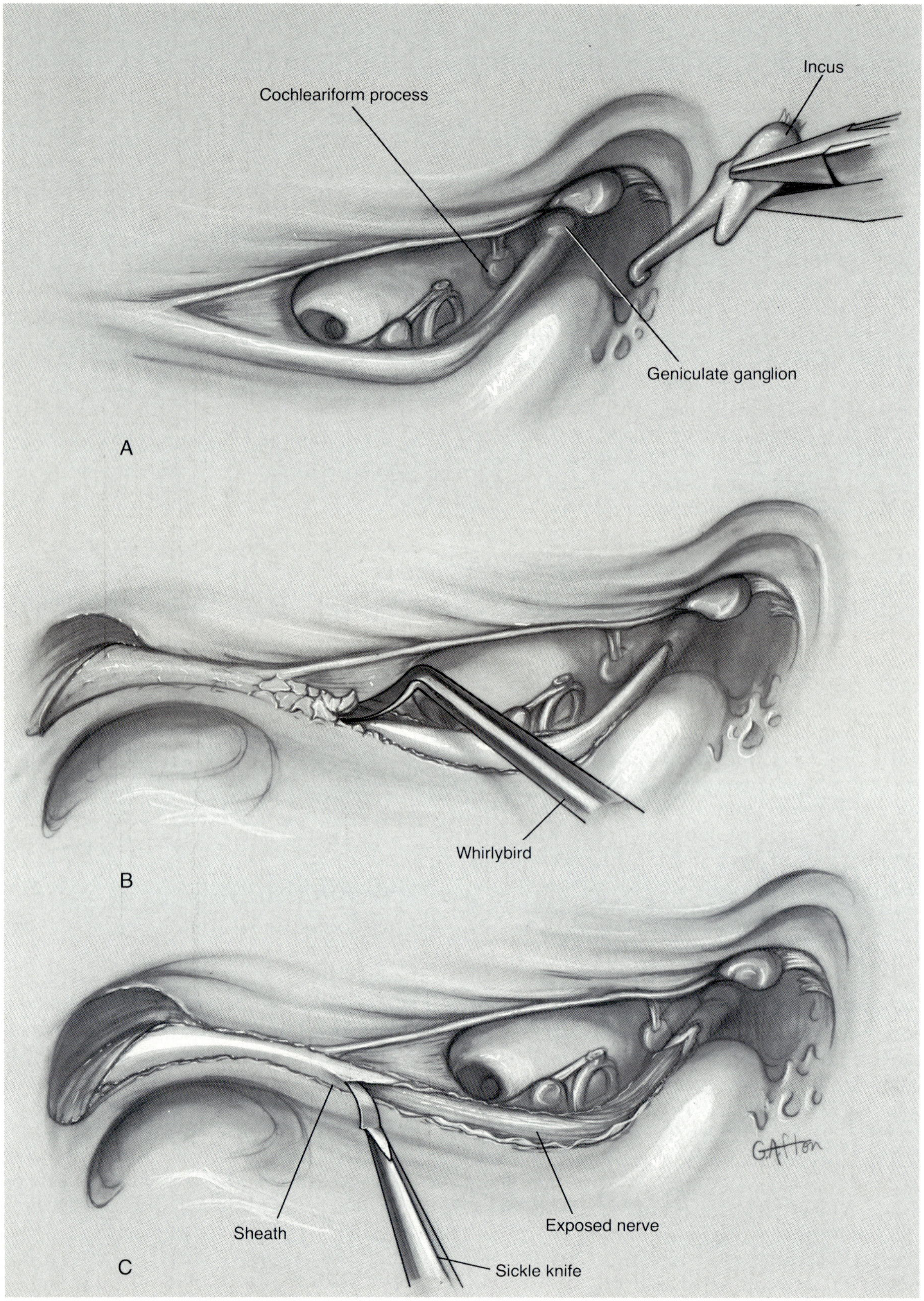
Incus
Cochleariform process
Geniculate ganglion
A
Whirlybird
B
Sheath
Exposed nerve
Sickle knife
C
GAfton

FIGURE 18–2.

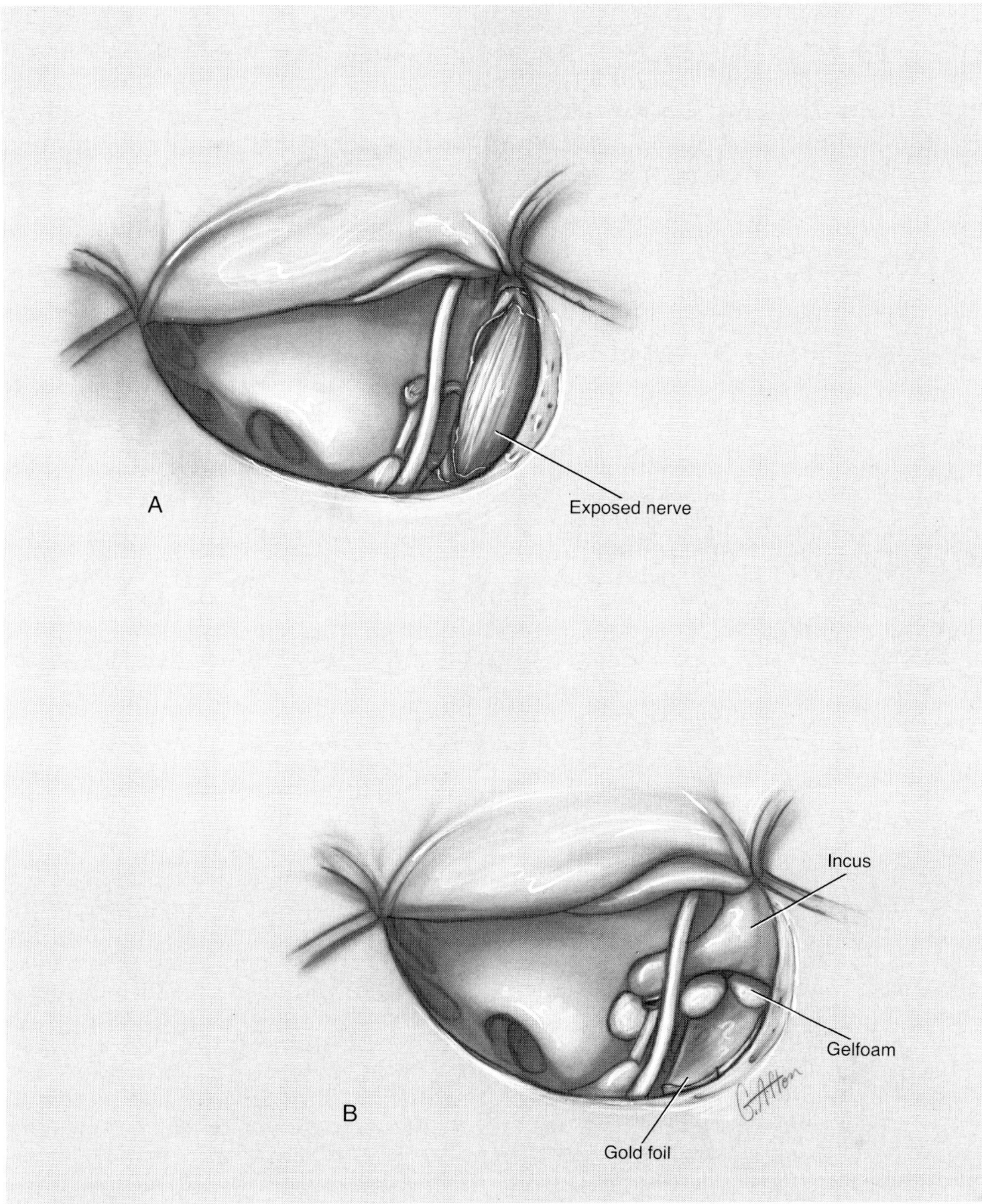

FIGURE 18–3.

In cases of herpes zoster, it is appropriate to decompress up to the geniculate ganglion.

Fractures of the temporal bone involving the facial nerve may be longitudinal or transverse. Transverse fractures tend to occur along the axis of the internal auditory canal and require a middle cranial fossa approach (described below). Longitudinal fractures involve the ossicles and tympanic segment of the facial nerve. Fractures through the mastoid bone will affect the mastoid segment. Along with ossiculoplasty, bone fragments impinging on the nerve should be meticulously removed.

Trauma to the nerve may also be the result of accidental injury by a bur or other instrument, and can occur at any level. This happens more commonly in the tympanic segment on the floor of the facial recess while tissue is being removed. Special care should be observed in cases of previous surgical trauma, which may be the result of an inadequate approach or an uncompleted operation that left residual disease. In these cases, it is necessary to complete the original operation, reassess anatomic landmarks, and then repair the nerve damage.

Management of the affected nerve itself is aimed at re-establishing safe continuity of the nerve axons, either through decompression or by restoring continuity of disrupted nerve fibers. If the area of disruption is small, the edges of the fibers should be sectioned sharply and repositioned in anatomic continuity. (However, macerated edges do not regenerate adequately.) If the nerve has been completely transected, the edges should be sectioned sharply and both extremes brought together anatomically. Suturing is extremely difficult in these cases and is seldom adequate; adhesive glue serves the purpose more effectively.

If the nerve edges cannot be brought together or if part of the nerve must be removed (as in excision of a neuroma), a nerve graft is called for. This graft will serve as a matrix or pathway for the axons that are growing from the proximal portion into the distal end. Although there are many sources of nerve grafts, branches of the superficial cervical plexus (especially the greater auricular nerve) are preferred because they are found in the vicinity of the operative field, they are of adequate size, and they are easily obtained. The greater auricular nerve traverses laterally to the sternocleidomastoid muscle after emerging around its posterior edge as a single nerve trunk.

An infra-auricular incision is deepened through subcutaneous tissues. Anterior and posterior skin flaps are developed, the sternocleidomastoid muscle is exposed, and the greater auricular nerve is identified. The nerve is sectioned sharply (selecting the desired length), and the wound is closed in layers with appropriate sutures. The sheaths of the two nerves are approximated (proximal stump to proximal end of greater auricular nerve, distal to distal) with 9-0 or 10-0 nylon sutures. Adhesive glue also can be used.

Middle Cranial Fossa Approach

Aim

To fully expose the labyrinthine segment of the facial nerve from the geniculate ganglion to the internal auditory canal, and to preserve hearing. (Although described here for facial nerve exploration, this procedure also is used for removal of small intracanalicular acoustic neuromas while preserving good residual hearing, and occasionally for sectioning of the vestibular nerve.)

Highlights

1. If a prior facial nerve exploration through the mastoid and tympanic segments has been accomplished, a tegmental defect is made with a diamond bur at the level of the cochleariform process. This will aid accurate orientation when the middle fossa floor is exposed.
2. The surgeon is seated at the head of the table with the patient supine.
3. The horizontal limb of the craniotomy is two-thirds anterior and one-third posterior to the external auditory canal.
4. The anterior limit of dural elevation is the middle meningeal artery, with the dura elevated in a posterior-to-anterior direction.
5. The most consistent landmark is the greater superficial petrosal nerve; the arcuate eminence is helpful but is often indistinct.
6. Medial to the geniculate, the labyrinthine portion of the fallopian canal is very narrow; only millimeters separate the ampulla of the superior semicircular canal posteriorly from the cochlea anteriorly.
7. Familiarity with the House-Urban retractor is recommended before its use. Its mechanism allows for three adjustments during retraction.

Pitfalls

1. Tearing of the dura with herniation and damage to the temporal lobe.
2. Avulsion of the greater superficial petrosal nerve and injury to the facial nerve.
3. Excessive bleeding from the middle meningeal artery.
4. Injury to the cochlea or superior semicircular canal.

Procedure

For this approach the patient lies supine, and the surgeon sits at the head of the operating table. The incision extends superiorly to the auricle; thus the head shave extends nearly to the top of the skull anteriorly and posteriorly until virtually the entire side of the head is prepared for surgery.

The incision is made approximately 0.5 cm anterior to the tragus and extends posterosuperiorly for approximately 6 to 8 cm; it is carried to the level of the temporal fascia. Often the superficial temporal artery is encountered inferiorly; it is best to tie it with a suture. This plane of dissection is developed bluntly and Weitlaner retractors are placed. The temporal muscle is incised in a T fashion with the horizontal limb extending along the zygomatic arch for 3 to 4 cm; the muscle is then elevated from the squamous portion of the temporal bone and the retractors are reinserted.

A craniotomy is then made by outlining a flap approximately 2.5 cm square with a large cutting bur (Fig. 18–4*A*). The horizontal limb should be located so that two-thirds of it lies anterior to the external auditory canal, and one-third lies posterior. To avoid injury to the dura, the craniotomy cuts are drilled to paper-thin thickness. The "bone flap" is fractured with a joker or similar blunt instrument; it is then carefully elevated, avoiding any tearing of the dura, which would lead to temporal lobe herniation and possible injury. For optimum visualization, the flap must be as close to the floor of the middle cranial fossa as possible; thus the inferior cut is made at the level of the zygomatic root. If a ledge of bone remains after the flap has been elevated, it may be removed sharply with the rongeur to place the opening at the level of the middle fossa floor. Bleeding may occur from bone and from vessels on the dural surface of the temporal lobe; the former are stopped with bone wax and the latter with light cautery. Again, special care must be taken to avoid injuring the dura.

The House-Urban retractor is then placed on the parallel vertical edges of the craniotomy defect (Fig. 18–4*B*). To prevent the dura from being caught in the blades of the retractor, it is reflected with a blunt instrument from the edges of the craniotomy. The dura is then gently elevated from the middle fossa floor in a posterior-to-anterior direction. As the dura and temporal lobe are elevated medially, the retractor blade is slowly advanced to provide the needed retraction. The first landmark to be identified is the middle meningeal artery as it exits from the foramen spinosum (Fig. 18–4*C*); this marks the anterior limit of dural elevation. Brisk bleeding often will be encountered in this area, necessitating packing with Surgicel. The dissection is then continued medially, again in a posterior-to-anterior direction. The greater superficial petrosal nerve is identified; it runs anteriorly on the surface of the middle fossa after exiting the facial hiatus. Careful posterior-to-anterior dural elevation will avoid inadvertent elevation of this nerve, which could place traction upon the geniculate ganglion and cause injury to it, as well as to the facial nerve. In a small percentage of cases the geniculate ganglion itself may be dehiscent. If a defect has been created in the tegmen during a previous mastoidectomy, it is now encountered. The surgeon will know that the geniculate ganglion is just medial to it.

The next landmark to be identified is the arcuate eminence, which marks the dome of the superior semicircular canal. This is not a consistent landmark and is frequently indistinct. It lies slightly posteromedial to the geniculate ganglion. Again the retractor blade is continually advanced to provide needed retraction as the dural elevation continues medially. Important surface landmarks that aid orientation have now been identified.

Removal of bone and exposure of the facial nerve is now begun. A large diamond bur with suction irrigation (to prevent heat transfer to the underlying facial nerve and structures) is used initially. Bone removal is begun at the facial hiatus and continued a short distance posteriorly, following the greater superficial petrosal nerve to the geniculate ganglion (Fig. 18–5*A*). Here the facial nerve runs medially toward the internal auditory meatus. Immediately medial to the geniculate ganglion, a small diamond bur is used, since only a few millimeters separate the ampulla of the superior semicircular canal (posterior) from the cochlea (anterior). The facial nerve runs through this small space. Bone removal is continued medially to fully expose the labyrinthine segment of the facial nerve; this affords more room, since the plane of the superior semicircular canal runs in a 45- to 60-degree angle posteriorly from the ampulla.

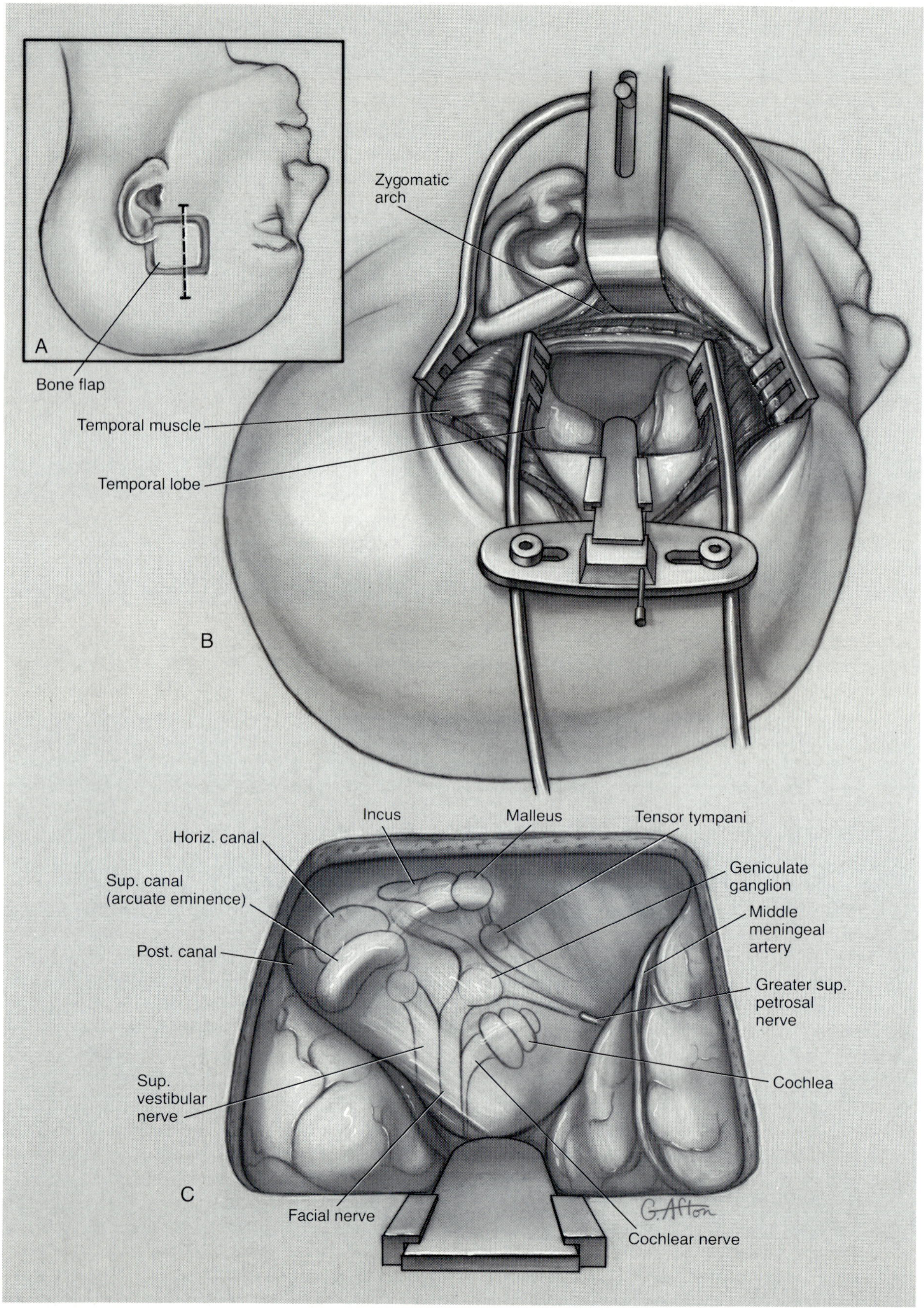
A
Bone flap
Zygomatic arch
Temporal muscle
Temporal lobe
B
Incus
Malleus
Tensor tympani
Horiz. canal
Geniculate ganglion
Sup. canal (arcuate eminence)
Middle meningeal artery
Post. canal
Greater sup. petrosal nerve
Cochlea
Sup. vestibular nerve
C
Facial nerve
G.Afton
Cochlear nerve

FIGURE 18–4.

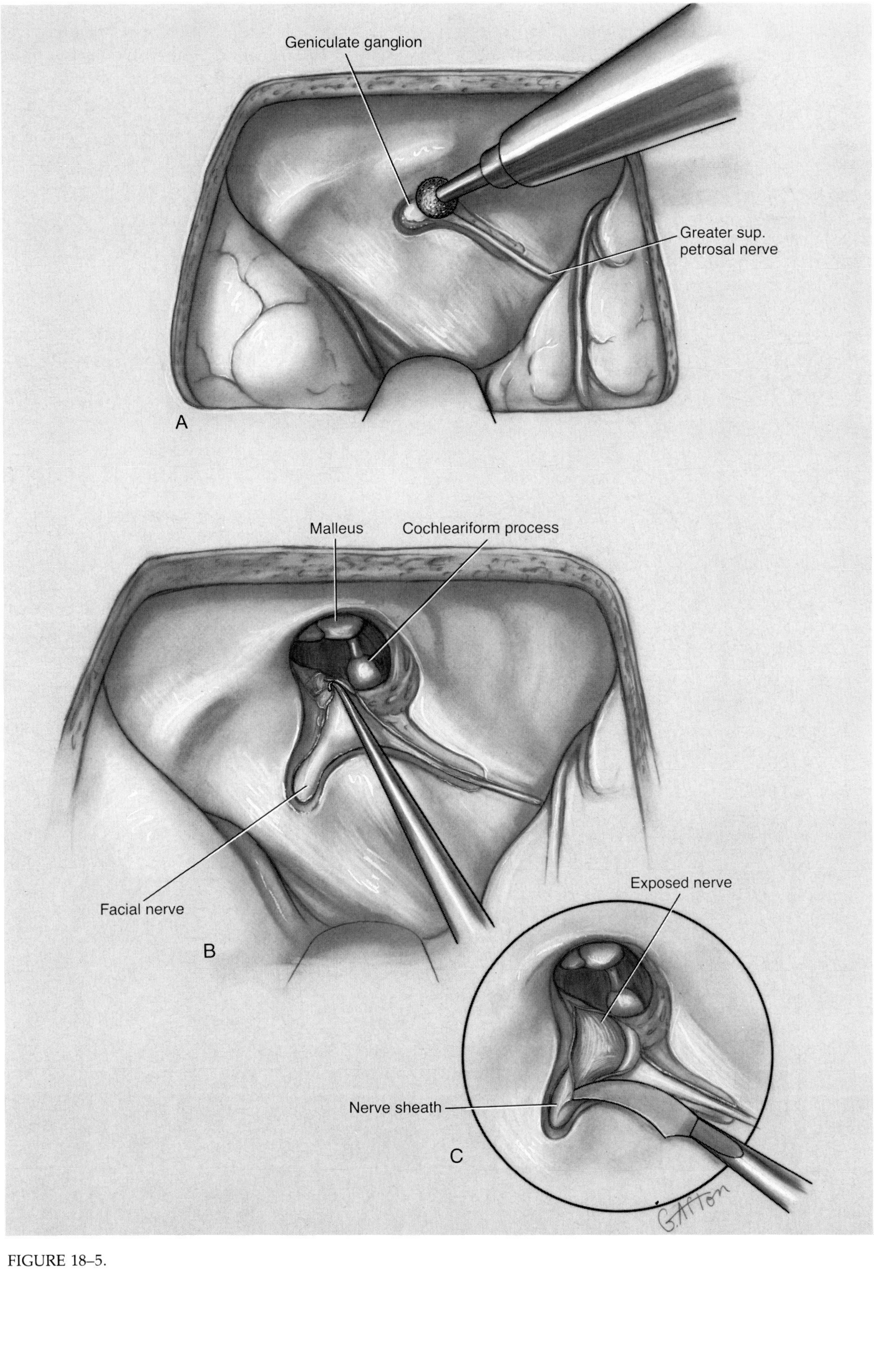
Geniculate ganglion
Greater sup. petrosal nerve
A
Malleus
Cochleariform process
Facial nerve
B
Exposed nerve
Nerve sheath
C
G.Afton

FIGURE 18–5.

Bone is thinned around approximately 50% of the facial nerve. The eggshell-thin bone may then be removed with a hook or blunt instrument. It is not necessary to expose the facial nerve along the entire length of the internal auditory canal. Medial dissection to the narrowest point of the canal usually constitutes adequate decompression. Here cerebrospinal fluid flow will be encountered upon entering the internal auditory canal.

The facial nerve is then fully exposed from the geniculate ganglion distally to the tympanic segment up to the cochleariform process (Fig. 18–5*B*). (This is easily performed through the tegmental defect created previously.) Care must be taken not to injure the malleus head or other ossicles in order to prevent sensorineural hearing loss. Opening the facial nerve sheath (if desired) may be accomplished by extending the opening from the tympanic segment to the labyrinthine segment (Fig. 18–5*C*).

The defect in the internal auditory canal is closed with a temporal muscle plug and the temporal lobe is allowed to re-expand. The bone flap is then repositioned and the wound is closed in layers—temporal muscle, subcutaneous tissue, and skin. Usually no external drainage is used. A sterile dressing is applied.

Pertinent Histopathology

FIGURE 18–6

This patient developed a facial paralysis diagnosed initially as Bell's palsy. An unsuccessful surgical decompression was performed. The section shows tumor involvement of the facial nerve (metastatic carcinoma of the prostate).

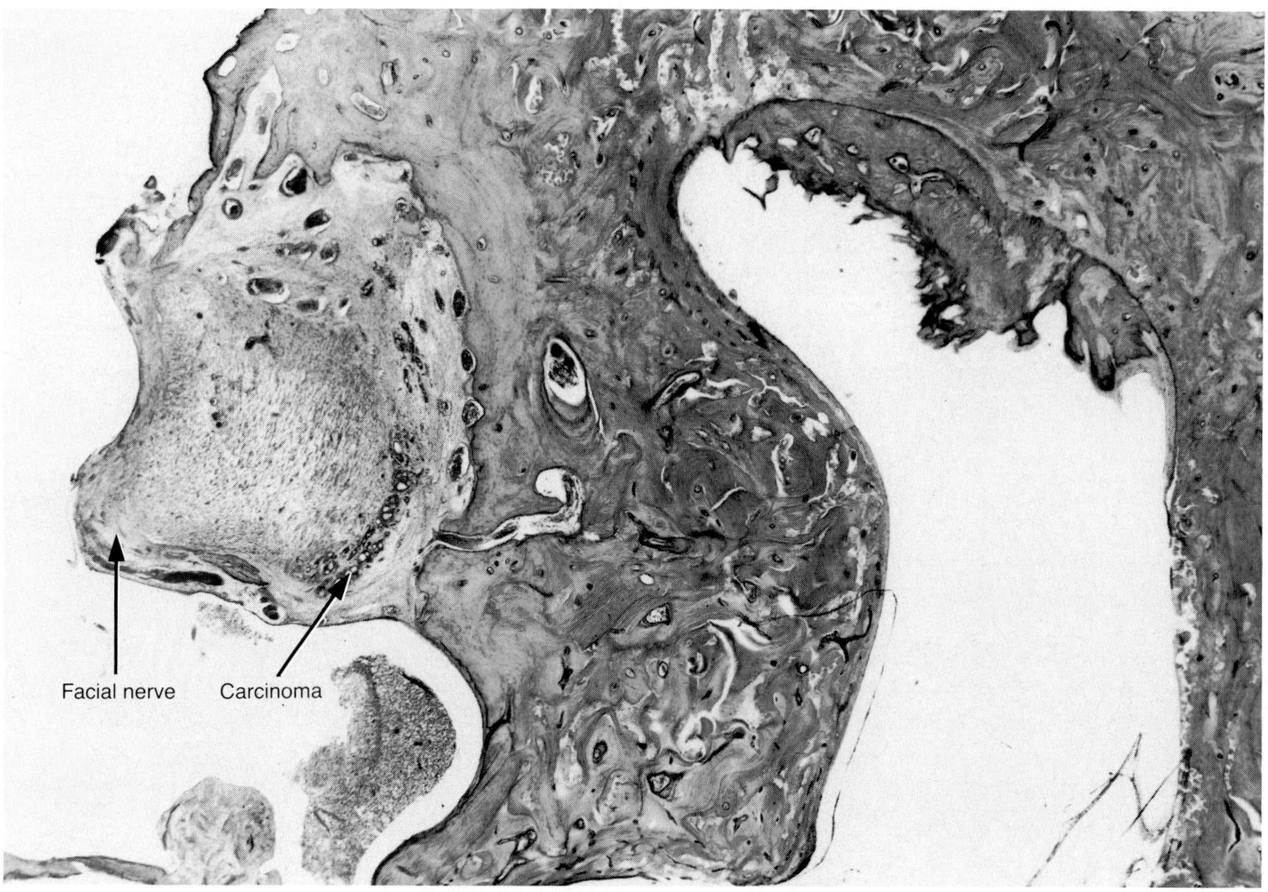

FIGURE 18–6.

CHAPTER 19

Tumors of the Middle and Inner Ear

Tumors of the middle and inner ear include glomus tumors and acoustic neuromas. Glomus tumors, or primary vascular tumors of the middle ear, are classified according to their location and size. Glomus tympanicum tumors are limited to the middle ear and mastoid; glomus jugulare tumors involve the jugular bulb, middle ear, and base of the skull. This chapter describes three surgical approaches to glomus tumors based on their size. Small and large glomus tympanicum tumors are discussed, as well as glomus jugulare tumors. The chapter also describes a translabyrinthine approach for acoustic neuromas.

Glomus Tympanicum Tumors

Highlights

1. Accurate preoperative assessment of the tumor is essential to ensure that the tumor is limited to the middle ear or mastoid.
2. If a glomus tumor is limited to the promontory and all of its borders can be seen by a transcanal approach, an exploratory tympanotomy or endaural approach may be used.
3. When the entire circumference of tumor cannot be visualized by a transcanal approach and preoperative assessment shows no involvement of the jugular bulb, an extended facial recess approach is used.

Small Glomus Tympanicum Tumors

An exploratory tympanotomy approach is used to expose this tumor, if all of its borders can be visualized through a transcanal approach (Fig. 19–1*A*). If needed, endural incisions also may be used to aid in exposure (see Chapter 7). Often it is useful to elevate the tympanic membrane off the malleus (using a sharp knife or pick) to increase exposure.

When adequate exposure is obtained, removal of the tumor is begun. It is important to realize that bleeding may be profuse and necessitates working quickly and effectively. Topical Adrenaline and Surgicel or a similar packing may also be used during the procedure as needed. An incision is made in the mucous membrane at the periphery of the tumor. The tumor is then elevated from the promontory, mobilizing all borders (Fig. 19–1*B*). Occasionally, a major feeding artery is seen; it may be fulgurated (care must be taken not to touch the promontory with the current). The tumor is then removed intact (Fig. 19–1*C*). Again, if bleeding is brisk the surgeon must work quickly (with large suction and packing as needed) to remove the tumor totally; the bleeding will be easy to control once the tumor has been removed. Closure and packing are the same as for the standard approaches.

Larger Glomus Tympanicum Tumors

If the entire border of the tumor cannot be visualized and radiologic studies show that it is limited to the middle ear, a posterior approach is used. This

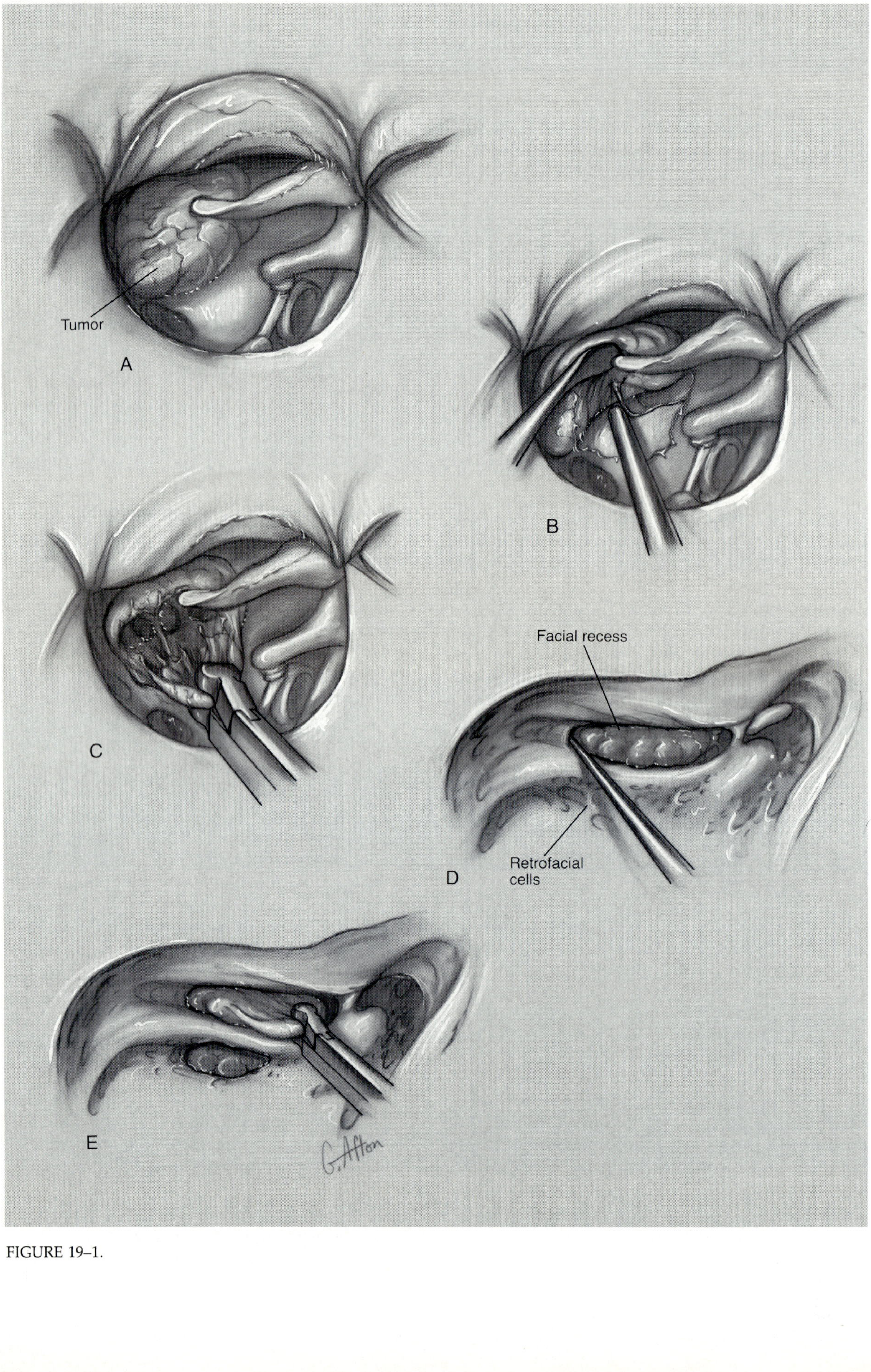

FIGURE 19–1.

allows visualization of the superior, posterior, and—most importantly, to ensure that there is no jugular bulb involvement—inferior borders. A transcanal tympanotomy for anterior border exposure may be used if there is any question of carotid artery involvement.

The posterior approach includes a postauricular incision, complete mastoidectomy, and opening of the facial recess. The facial recess is then extended inferiorly to expose the hypotympanum; this requires sacrificing the chorda tympani. The borders of the extended facial recess are the fibrous annulus laterally and the fallopian canal medially. The recess is carried inferiorly until it is flush with the floor of the middle ear. At this point, the inferior border of the tumor is seen in the hypotympanum. With a blunt probe, the bony wall of the hypotympanum may be palpated to ensure bone integrity and noninvolvement of the jugular bulb. The retrofacial air cells should also be opened since larger tumors often extend into this space (this approach allows good access to this area) (Fig. 19–1*D*). Superiorly, if the tumor involves the ossicles, the incudostapedial joint may need to be disconnected and the incus removed to allow safe removal of the tumor. An exploratory tympanotomy may be performed concurrently to help expose a superiorly located tumor. Again, elevating the tympanic membrane off the malleus will enhance exposure (and also allow delineation of the tumor's anterior border).

At this point, tumor removal may commence. Again, brisk bleeding necessitates rapid and efficient work. If possible, the tumor is freed in its entirety and removed (Fig. 19–1*E*). Usually the tumor is too large to permit this, and it is removed in pieces after freeing of its periphery. When brisk bleeding is encountered, this area may be packed and attention directed elsewhere. Care must be taken to look for dehiscence or involvement of the jugular bulb inferiorly and of the carotid artery anteriorly.

When complete removal is accomplished, ossicular reconstruction is performed (if needed). The incisions are closed in the usual manner.

Infralabyrinthine, Infratemporal Approach for Glomus Jugulare Tumors

Highlights

1. A complete mastoidectomy (mastoid tip removed) is performed with an extended facial recess.
2. The bony external auditory canal, tympanic membrane, incus, and malleus are removed.
3. The facial nerve is mobilized and transposed anteriorly.
4. The jugular vein is identified in the neck and controlled inferior to tumor.
5. The sigmoid sinus is controlled distal to tumor.
6. The tumor is removed in an anteroinferior-to-superior direction, with constant attention given to the internal carotid artery anteriorly.
7. A smaller intracranial extension may be handled with this approach.
8. The external auditory canal is sutured closed (creating a blind pouch); with a dural defect, the cavity is packed with fat or muscle.

Pitfalls

1. Injuring the internal carotid artery (most commonly infratemporally at the caroticotympanic branch).
2. Causing deficits or injuries to the ninth, tenth, eleventh, and twelfth cranial nerves, with associated postoperative problems.
3. Failing to recognize associated lesions (such as pheochromocytomas, carotid body tumors, and so on).
4. Cerebrospinal fluid leaks.

Procedure

After preoperative evaluation has established jugular bulb involvement, a more extensive approach to the skull base is indicated for total tumor removal with the smallest risk of morbidity or mortality.

The patient is placed in the supine position. The involved side is shaved, prepared, and draped in the usual sterile manner; the surgical field includes the ipsilateral neck. A postauricular incision is made in a curvilinear fashion following the postauricular crease (slightly more posterior than for a standard mastoidectomy) (Fig. 19–2*A*). The inferior limb of the incision is carried into the neck, extending along the anterior border of the sternocleidomastoid muscle.

A complete mastoidectomy is performed, delineating the tegmen, sigmoid sinus (exposure is extended posteriorly to the sinus), antrum, and bony labyrinth. The mastoid tip is completely opened and removed. The external auditory canal is transected with a scalpel at the level of the cartilaginous-bony junction and then brought forward with retractors.

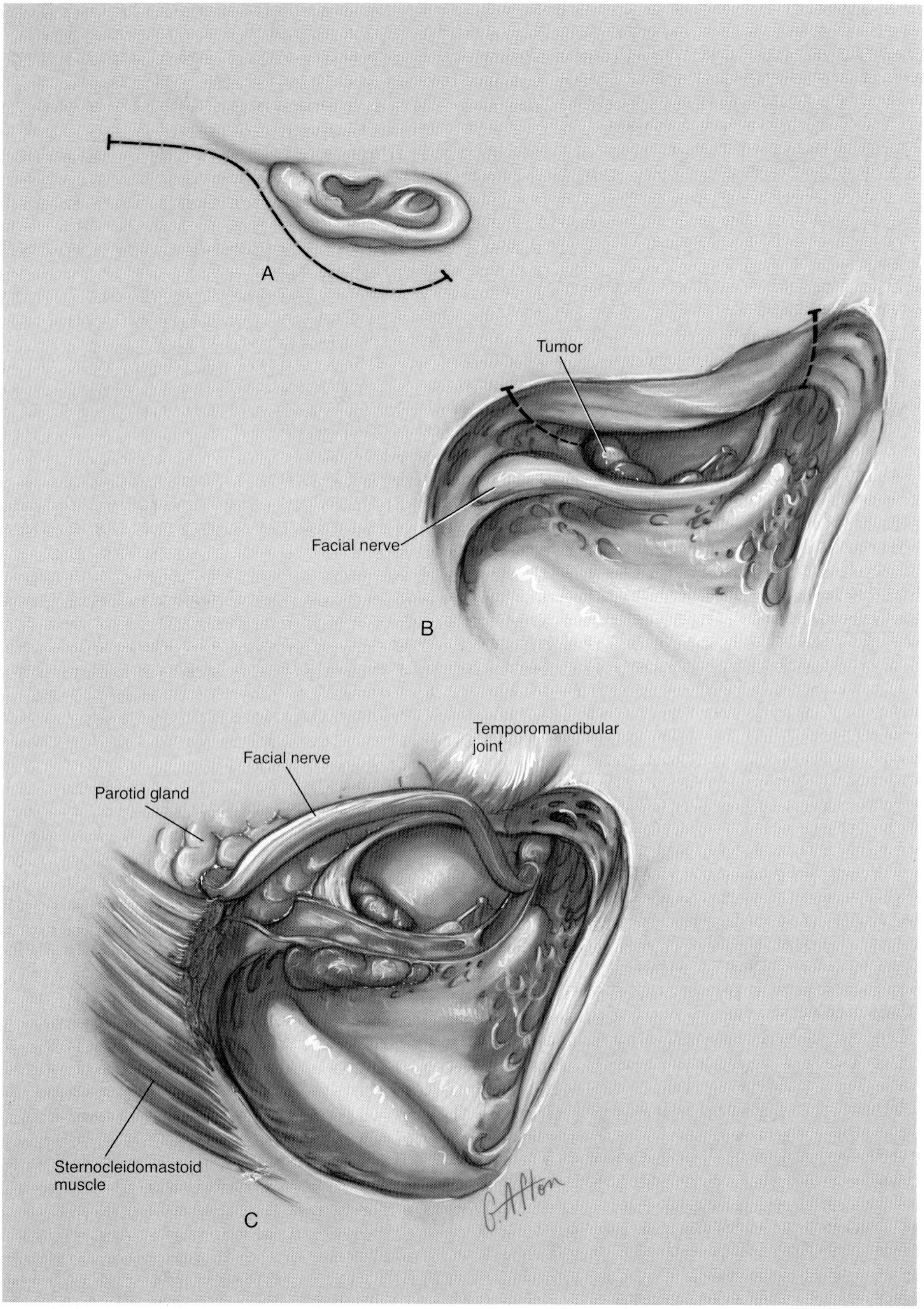
A
Tumor
Facial nerve
B
Temporomandibular joint
Facial nerve
Parotid gland
Sternocleidomastoid muscle
C

FIGURE 19–2.

The canal is thinned and an extended facial recess is opened to the floor of the hypotympanum.

The incudostapedial joint is dislocated with a joint knife and the incus is removed. The thinned posterior external auditory canal is then removed, as well as the tympanic membrane, malleus, and skin of the bony external auditory canal. The bony anterior and inferior canal is also removed with a diamond bur while preserving the periosteum (this aids anterior exposure and retraction). The stapes is left intact.

With a diamond bur, the bony fallopian canal is removed from the geniculate ganglion to the stylomastoid foramen. The facial nerve is mobilized and transposed anteriorly. A soft tissue sling may be created to help hold the nerve out of the field. With the facial nerve now located anteriorly, an obstructed view of the jugular bulb and tumor is possible (Fig. 19–2*B*, *C*). With large cerebellar retractors, the mandible condyle may be dislocated and retracted anteriorly for an additional 1- to 2-cm exposure to the infratemporal region. Care must be taken not to injure the transposed facial nerve with the retractors. If necessary, the mandible ramus may be transected.

Decompression of the sigmoid sinus must be completed to allow for distal control of venous bleeding. Bone decompression is performed from just below the sinodural angle and carried inferiorly to the jugular bulb (or tumor). Inferiorly, the bone over the posterior fossa also is removed. The tumor can now be clearly visualized from the jugular bulb, with its extension into the middle ear or mastoid.

The neck is now entered to obtain proximal exposure and control of the jugular vein and carotid artery. If not already accomplished, the mastoid process attachments of the sternocleidomastoid and digastric muscles are sharply dissected and reflected anteriorly. The lateral process of the first cervical vertebra is palpated. Just inferior to this process is the eleventh nerve. By following this nerve forward, the jugular vein is found. The relationship of the eleventh nerve to the vein varies; most commonly it runs laterally to the jugular vein, but occasionally it runs medially. The vein is isolated, ties are placed, and the vein is ligated medial to the tumor for proximal control. Distal control is accomplished at the decompressed sigmoid sinus. Usually packing is used either extraluminally or intraluminally after an opening is made in the lumen (Fig. 19–3*A*). The carotid artery is identified and isolated in case injury occurs, requiring control of bleeding.

With total exposure now accomplished, tumor removal is begun. The superior border is mobilized from against the bony labyrinth. Anteriorly the tumor is mobilized unless there is involvement with and adherence to the carotid artery. Removal begins inferiorly where the jugular vein was transected. Dissection begins here and continues superiorly, developing and following a plane between the tumor and carotid. Anteriorly the carotid artery often is involved with larger tumors and presents a formidable task to safely mobilize and separate the tumor. Infratemporally, where the carotid turns to its horizontal course, a small branch (caroticotympanic branch) often supplies the tumor and presents a particularly troublesome problem. Ideally it is dissected a short distance from the carotid lesion to afford an opportunity to safely control it; however, it may be avulsed, injuring the carotid lumen at a point where distal control of bleeding is difficult. If carotid injury occurs, repair of the lumen with a fine arterial suture (if proximal and distal control can be obtained) should be attempted. If this cannot be accomplished, packing of the area will control the bleeding (with its accompanying risk of severe morbidity or mortality).

As the tumor dissection continues superiorly, the ninth, tenth, eleventh, and twelfth cranial nerves will be encountered. An attempt should be made to identify these nerves and preserve them if possible. Often they are intimately involved with the tumor mass (or are difficult to identify), and are sacrificed or injured.

At the level of the jugular bulb and sigmoid sinus, the medial wall of the sinus is dissected from the tumor mass, leaving the dura intact (Fig. 19–3*B*). Profuse bleeding is encountered in the area of the bulb from the inferior petrosal sinus, which empties into the bulb on its medial side. Packing is needed to control this bleeding, since there is no way to obtain control of this sinus.

Following dissection anteriorly and posteriorly, the tumor mass is hinged in the hypotympanic, infralabyrinthine area and is removed carefully. If intracranial extension is present, a cerebrospinal fluid leak will be encountered upon tumor manipulation. Tumor bulk may be removed to improve visualization, and the dura may be opened wider to enhance posterior fossa exposure. A small intracranial extension may then be carefully removed, protecting and preserving intracranial structures (anteroinferior and posteroinferior cerebellar arteries, brainstem, cranial nerves, and so on).

After the tumor has been completely removed, the dural defect is closed with either free abdominal fat or a muscle plug. The transposed facial nerve is released and placed in a tension-free position. The transected external auditory canal is everted and closed with a permanent suture (resulting in a blind pouch). The postauricular incision is closed in layers and dressings are applied. Occasionally for large

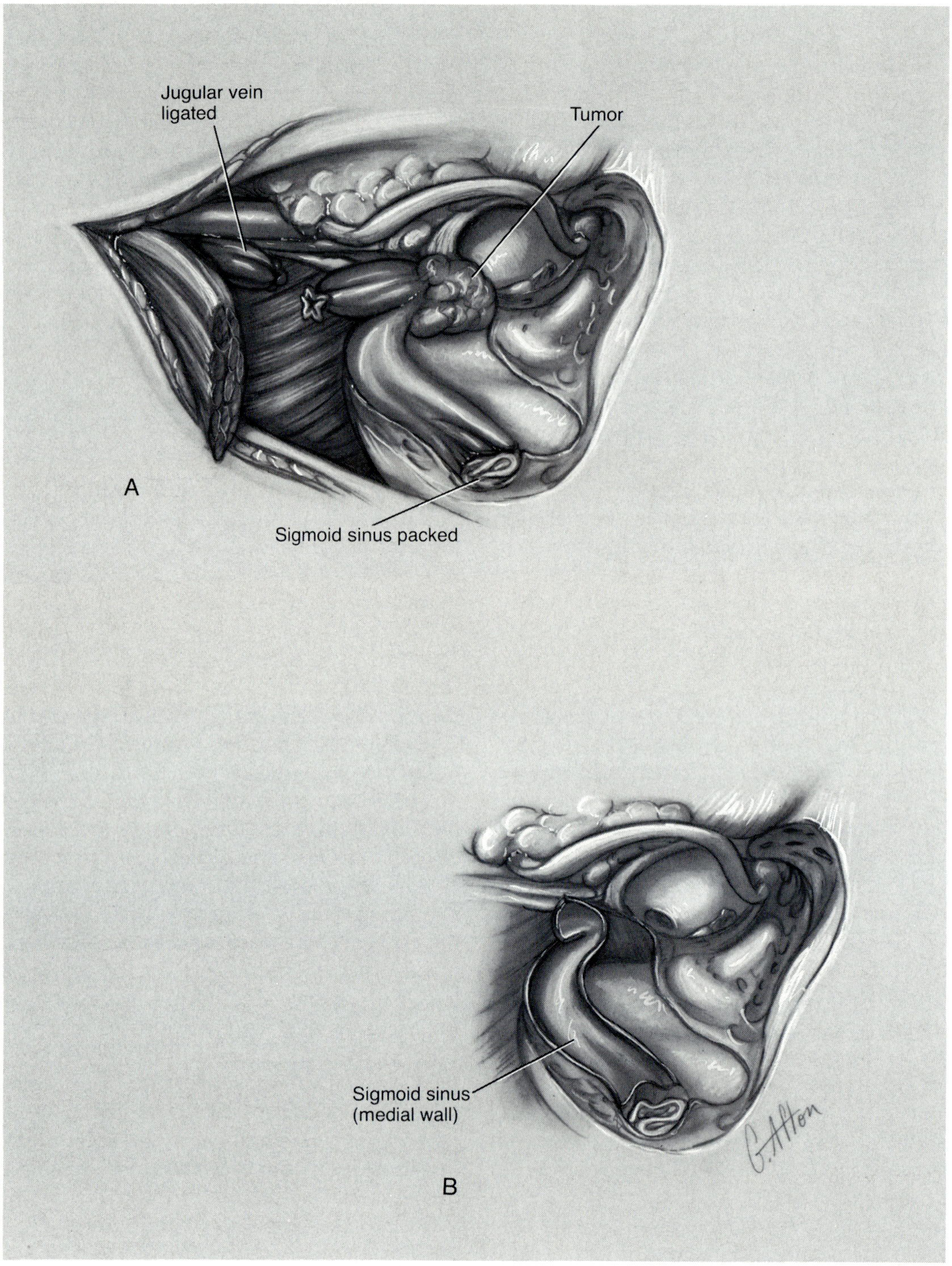
Jugular vein ligated
Tumor
A
Sigmoid sinus packed
Sigmoid sinus (medial wall)
G. Alton
B

FIGURE 19–3.

dural defects, lumbar drains are placed at the end of the procedure to help prevent cerebrospinal fluid leakage.

Translabyrinthine Approach for Acoustic Neuromas

Aim

Wide exposure of the tumor with early identification of the facial nerve, allowing for total excision of the tumor with preservation of the nerve.

Highlights

1. The incision is more posterior than the usual postauricular incision.
2. Drilling is done posterior to the sigmoid sinus in order to allow posterior decompression (retraction) of it.
3. The internal auditory canal is identified and the posterior half of the bone is removed.
4. The facial nerve is identified at Bill's bar as it begins its labyrinthine course.
5. The superior and inferior vestibular nerves and the cochlear nerve are avulsed.
6. The tumor is removed away from the facial nerve.

Pitfalls

1. Failing to adequately decompress the sigmoid sinus and to remove bone from the posterior fossa dura.
2. Failing to open the internal auditory canal widely for full exposure of the tumor.
3. Failing to positively identify the facial nerve before avulsing nerves.
4. Stretching (or completely transecting) the facial nerve during tumor removal.
5. Incompletely removing the tumor.

Procedure

For this approach the patient lies supine. Preparation and draping are the same as for a standard ear procedure with the exception of a larger head shave. By placing the patient's head at the foot of the table, the surgeon will have room for his or her legs under the table and be more comfortable. The patient must be securely strapped to the table, since frequent side-to-side rotation is needed.

The postauricular incision is designed as usual but located farther posteriorly, to allow drilling posterior to the sigmoid sinus (Fig. 19–4*A*). This is essential for complete decompression of the sigmoid sinus and optimal later visualization into the cerebellopontine angle; if an error is made, it should be made in making the incision too far posterior. The incision lies 1 to 1½ in (at its most posterior position) behind the auricle and runs in an extended C shape. It is carried through the periosteum of the mastoid cortex, avoiding the temporal muscle superiorly. The periosteum is then elevated and the ear held forward with cerebellar retractors. Retractors placed in the superior-to-inferior direction will hold the temporal muscle out of the surgical field.

Using the largest cutting bur and suction irrigation, drilling is begun. The mastoid cortex is removed as in a routine mastoidectomy. Care is taken to saucerize the edges and keep the lateralmost opening as wide as possible. In this procedure, it is important to extend the drilling posterior to the sigmoid sinus. This bone removal is completed down to the posterior fossa dura. For large tumors, the posterior dissection may extend 1 to 1½ in behind the sigmoid sinus. Final bone removal is accomplished later with the diamond bur to avoid tearing of the dura and subsequent cerebellar herniation. In this area emissary veins are found running from the sigmoid sinus to the cortex; occasionally quite large, they may be a source of troublesome bleeding and must be approached cautiously.

At this point the operating microscope is brought into the field. The mastoidectomy is completed as described in previous chapters, after which step the surgeon should be able to identify definitely the horizontal and posterior semicircular canals. With this basic landmark, the positions of the incus, facial nerve, and posterior semicircular canal are known even if they are not yet fully seen. Bone over the tegmen, sigmoid sinus, posterior fossa, sinodural angle, and external auditory canal is thinned to allow full exposure and deeper dissection. If the sigmoid sinus is displaced anteriorly, it may be decompressed at this stage; if it is possible to perform the labyrinthectomy now, it may be better to delay the actual decompression. This prevents the problem of cerebellar herniation if the dura is inadvertently opened or of vision being obstructed by packing if the sinus is injured.

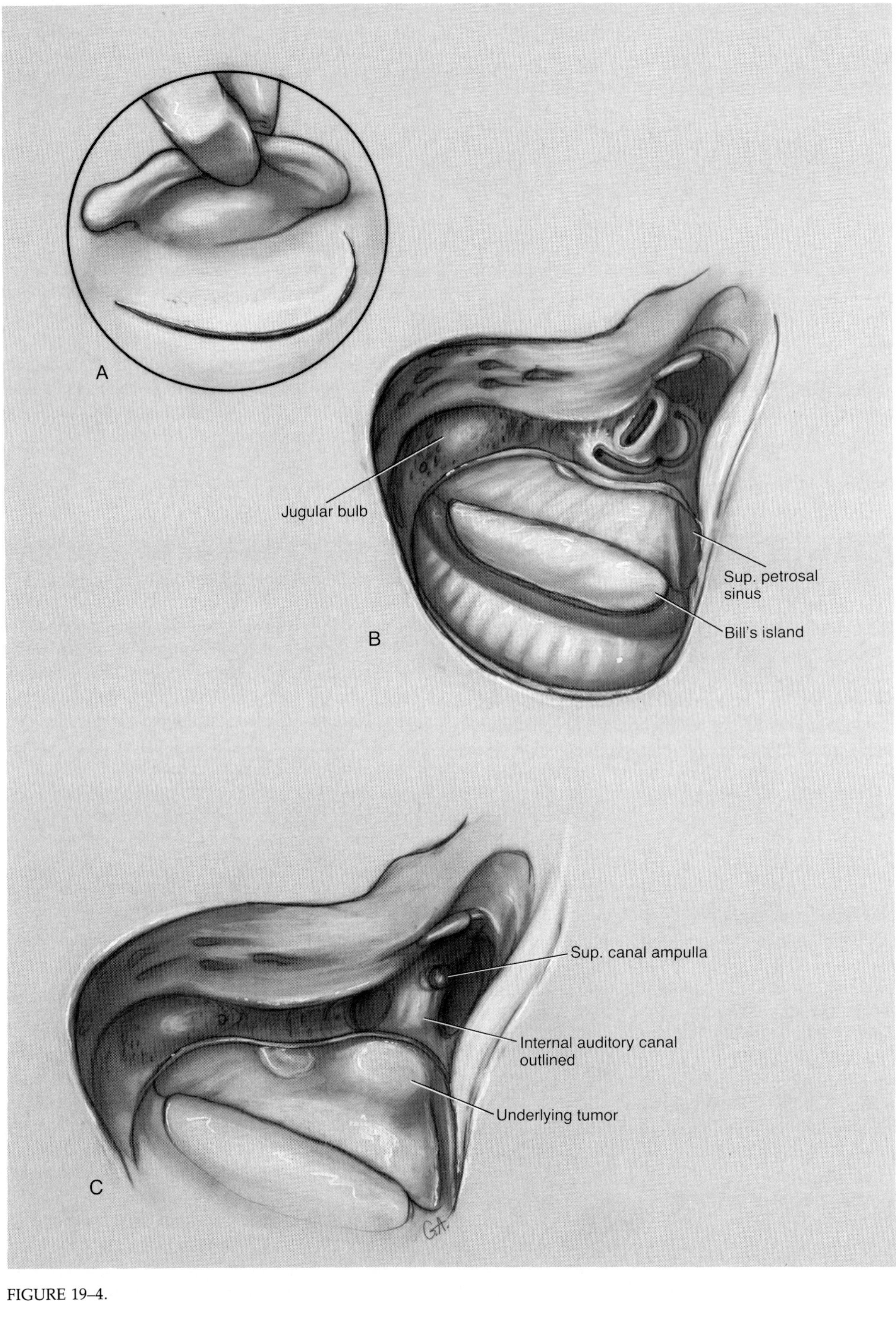
A
Jugular bulb
Sup. petrosal sinus
Bill's island
B
Sup. canal ampulla
Internal auditory canal outlined
Underlying tumor
C

FIGURE 19–4.

A full labyrinthectomy has been discussed in previous chapters. Dissection is started in the area of the common crus (just anterior to the sinodural angle); this is the safest place to begin, since the facial nerve is far anterior. Dissection is continued medially and inferiorly until each canal is found and completely "drilled out." Remember to keep the sinodural angle clean and widely open to allow for maximum exposure later. The bone here is thinned, and the superior petrosal sinus is seen as it runs from the sigmoid to the petrous apex (Fig. 19–4*B*). The posterior canal is encountered first and followed as it courses anteroinferiorly. In approaching the ampulla, be aware that the facial nerve is just lateral in order to avoid injury to it. The jugular bulb lies inferior to the posterior canal and rarely may be so high as to touch the posterior canal. By following the common crus medially, the superior semicircular canal can be entered and then followed in its anterosuperior course. Remember that this canal lies in a much deeper (medial) plane than the other two canals. As the ampulla of the superior canal is entered, it is left partially intact to provide a later landmark to the superior vestibular nerve and lateral-most end of the internal auditory canal. As the dissection continues anteriorly (forward), the lateral canal is opened completely; the side of the cutting bur (not the tip) is used, allowing for a safer approach with better visualization of the facial nerve. Using the diamond bur, the facial nerve is positively identified. This marks the anterior limit of the dissection. Carefully skeletonizing the facial nerve affords as much room as possible for full visualization of the vestibule and, later, the lateral end of the internal auditory canal.

The final steps are to fully open the vestibule and to completely thin the middle fossa tegmen, sinodural angle, and posterior fossa dura to the level that the dissection has reached. The dissection is carried inferiorly to identify the jugular bulb; seen as a bluish discoloration through the bone, it represents the inferior limit of dissection. As the dissection is called inferiorly, the retrofacial air cells often are opened to enhance exposure. Also found in this area is the vestibular aqueduct as it runs medially to the posterior canal from the endolymphatic sac. The labyrinthectomy has now been completed.

Immediately medial to the vestibule lies the internal auditory canal (remember that the medial wall of the superior canal ampulla is the lateral wall of this canal). At this point, the sigmoid sinus should be decompressed so that it can be retracted posteriorly; this provides more working area, especially posteriorly at the brainstem-tumor junction. A large diamond bur and constant irrigation is used to thin the bone over the entire sinus. Final bone removal is accomplished with the diamond bur or a blunt pick. A thin island of bone (Bill's island) is left over the exposed sinus to prevent injury from the shank of the bur when deeper dissection is resumed. Bone may be removed posterior to the sinus exposing the dura and allowing more retraction with increased visualization into the internal auditory canal and cerebellopontine angle. The thinned bone is then removed from the posterior fossa medial to the sigmoid sinus to the level that the dissection has reached; this is done with the diamond bur, suction, and blunt instruments. Care must be taken not to tear the dura (to prevent cerebellar herniation and avoid vessels that may lie immediately underneath) or to rupture the superior petrosal sinus behind the sinodural angle. With large tumors, the working area is improved by removing bone from the posterior end of the tegmen, allowing a better angle for instrumentation.

With the superior, inferior, and anterior limits now well defined, full attention is given to the internal auditory canal. The objective is to obtain 180-degree bone removal of the posterior half of the canal. This is necessary for full exposure and to prevent bony overhangs that hinder work within the canal. Two important points must be remembered. (1) The canal runs anterior to posterior as it becomes more medial; thus more bone will be removed near the posterior fossa dura, and only minimal bone removal will be needed at the superior canal ampulla landmark (which was left behind). The course it will run approximates a line from the second genu of the facial nerve to the sinodural angle. (2) The canal will be very expanded owing to the presence of the tumor (Fig. 19–4*C*).

Bony troughs are created around the superior and inferior borders of the internal auditory canal; they are deepened between the tegmen and the canal and between the jugular bulb and the canal, respectively, until the posterior half of the canal has been exposed and the bone has been thinned to eggshell thickness. Superiorly, caution is needed since occasionally the facial nerve crosses the superior aspect of the tumor and may be injured with the diamond bur. The bur bit should always rotate toward the tegmen, to prevent "jumping" into the canal if it catches on a bony ledge; this involves clockwise rotation in a left ear and counterclockwise rotation in a right ear. In developing the "trough" inferiorly, the cochlear aqueduct is found between the jugular bulb and the canal. It usually appears as a white spot, and inserting a pick into it often produces a cerebrospinal fluid leak. This is an important landmark, since the ninth nerve is just anteroinferior and medial to it as it exits the skull to proceed across the medial superior aspect of the jugular bulb. In order to protect this nerve, dissection should not proceed anteriorly to the cochlear aqueduct. Focusing on the superior canal ampulla, the superior vestibular nerve can be identified through the bone by careful dissection with a diamond bur. With continuous copious irrigation to prevent heat transfer from the bur, the facial nerve can be blue-lined and identified as it enters the labyrinthine portion of the fallopian canal, medial and slightly superior to where the superior vestibular nerve ends. (It may be followed for a short distance in its labyrinthine course for positive identification.) Inferior to the superior vestibular nerve is the transverse crest, which divides the lateralmost end of the internal auditory canal into superior and inferior compartments (Fig. 19–5*A*). If the bone remaining over the canal has been thinned properly, usually it can be cracked with pressure from a blunt instrument and removed in one piece, or drilled carefully with a diamond bur. It is important to completely remove the bone from the posterior half of the canal. The tumor itself is now exposed and bone overlying the posterior fossa dura has been removed completely, from the sigmoid sinus to the porus acusticus (lateral to medial) and from the tegmen to the jugular bulb (superior to inferior).

A dural flap incision is begun posterosuperiorly to the jugular bulb, and carried across the porus acusticus and then laterally up the posterior fossa dura parallel to the superior petrosal sinus. Its inferior limb may be carried laterally along the sigmoid sinus. The flap is pulled backward and the posterior surface of the tumor is visualized (Fig. 19–5*B*). The incisions must be made cautiously so that any underlying vessels and nerves are not injured. Rarely, the facial nerve traverses the superior aspect of the tumor (usually it is on the anterior surface); the petrosal vein is found along the posterior aspect, draining into the superior petrosal vein. At the tumor's inferior aspect, the cisterna magna usually can be visualized and gently probed to obtain a profuse cerebrospinal fluid leak. This will release pressure and allow the cerebellum to relax. The plane between the posterior aspect of the tumor and the arachnoid is developed, and the dural flap is laid in the plane to protect the cerebellum (if possible, include the petrosal vein under the flap). Long Cottonoid strips may also be laid to protect the cerebellum and help in developing the plane. Developing the proper plane will produce less bleeding.

At this point the lateral end of the tumor is mobilized from the facial nerve. By rotating the table away the area is brought into view. The superior vestibular and facial nerves are identified. Using a blunt right-angled hook, the ridge of bone (Bill's bar) that separates the superior vestibular and facial nerves is identified and palpated by finding the end of the superior vestibular nerve and following the bone backward until it ends (which is where the facial canal begins). This is crucial to preserving the facial nerve, since everything lateral to this ridge is vestibular nerve and may be avulsed safely (Fig. 19–5*C*). As the avulsed nerve is pulled back, the facial nerve is brought into full view behind. It is best not to probe into the facial canal in order to prevent trauma to and swelling of the facial nerve. The first few millimeters of the facial nerve are cleaned to identify it positively. Arachnoid that envelops the nerve on its superior and inferior edges is separated with the hook (Fig. 19–5*D*). Often this is difficult, since the nerve may thin considerably and make the nerve edges hard to distinguish. Inferior to the superior vestibular nerve is the transverse crest; as mentioned previously, it separates the superior and inferior compartments of the internal auditory canal. The inferior compartment is cleaned of tumor with the hook. A tongue of tumor often extends up between the transverse crest and inferior compartment and must be swept clean (Fig. 19–6*A*). The inferior vestibular nerve is avulsed, and usually the cochlear nerve as well. The anteroinferior cerebellar artery usually lies along the inferior border of the tumor, anterior to the cochlear nerve. This important vessel must always be watched for and protected from injury. The tumor is pulled toward the surgeon during this lateral mobilization.

The procedure from this point depends on the size of the tumor. Dissection may proceed as above; however, for a larger tumor debulking will be required, to prevent traction from being placed on the facial nerve as the tumor is rolled away from it. In debulking, the tumor is opened over its posterior surface and the contents are removed "intracapsularly," allowing it to collapse inward. This can be accomplished with an Urban dissector, laser (Fig. 19–6*B*), Cavitron, or cup forceps. Care is taken to remain inside the capsule in order to prevent injury to nerves or vessels that may traverse the tumor surface. With adequate debulking the tumor will collapse inward, allowing further mobilization from the facial nerve anteriorly (Fig. 19–6*C*) and the brainstem posteriorly (Fig. 19–6*D*). Bipolar cautery may be used to control bleeding within the tumor, which occasionally is abundant. With large tumors, the ninth nerve may traverse the capsule inferiorly. Usually the anteroinferior cerebellar artery has been pushed inferiorly by tumor growth. Superiorly the fifth nerve may cross the capsule in large tumors; occasionally, the seventh nerve may traverse the superior edge of the tumor.

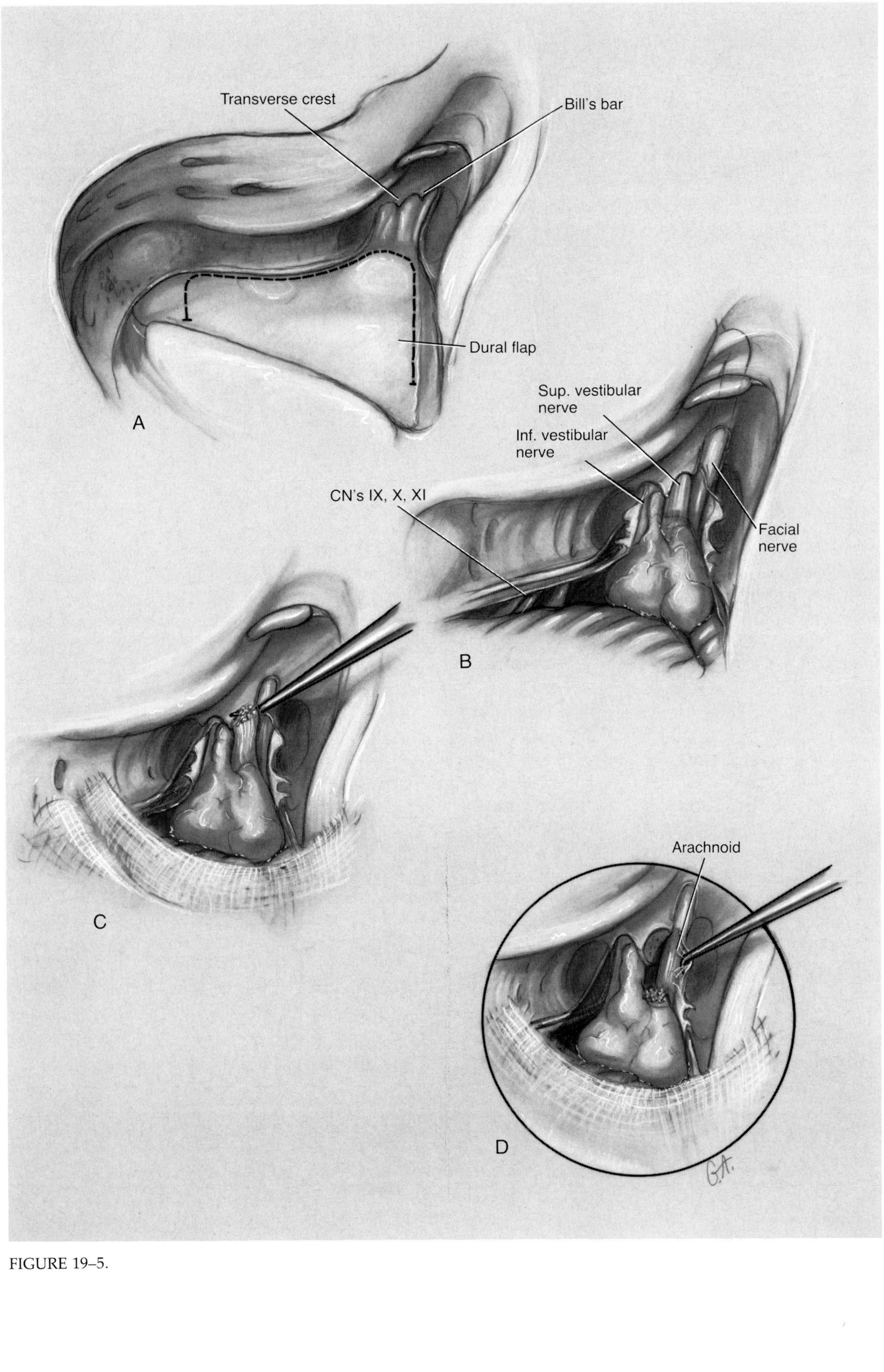
Transverse crest
Bill's bar
Dural flap
A
Sup. vestibular nerve
Inf. vestibular nerve
CN's IX, X, XI
Facial nerve
B
C
Arachnoid
D

FIGURE 19–5.

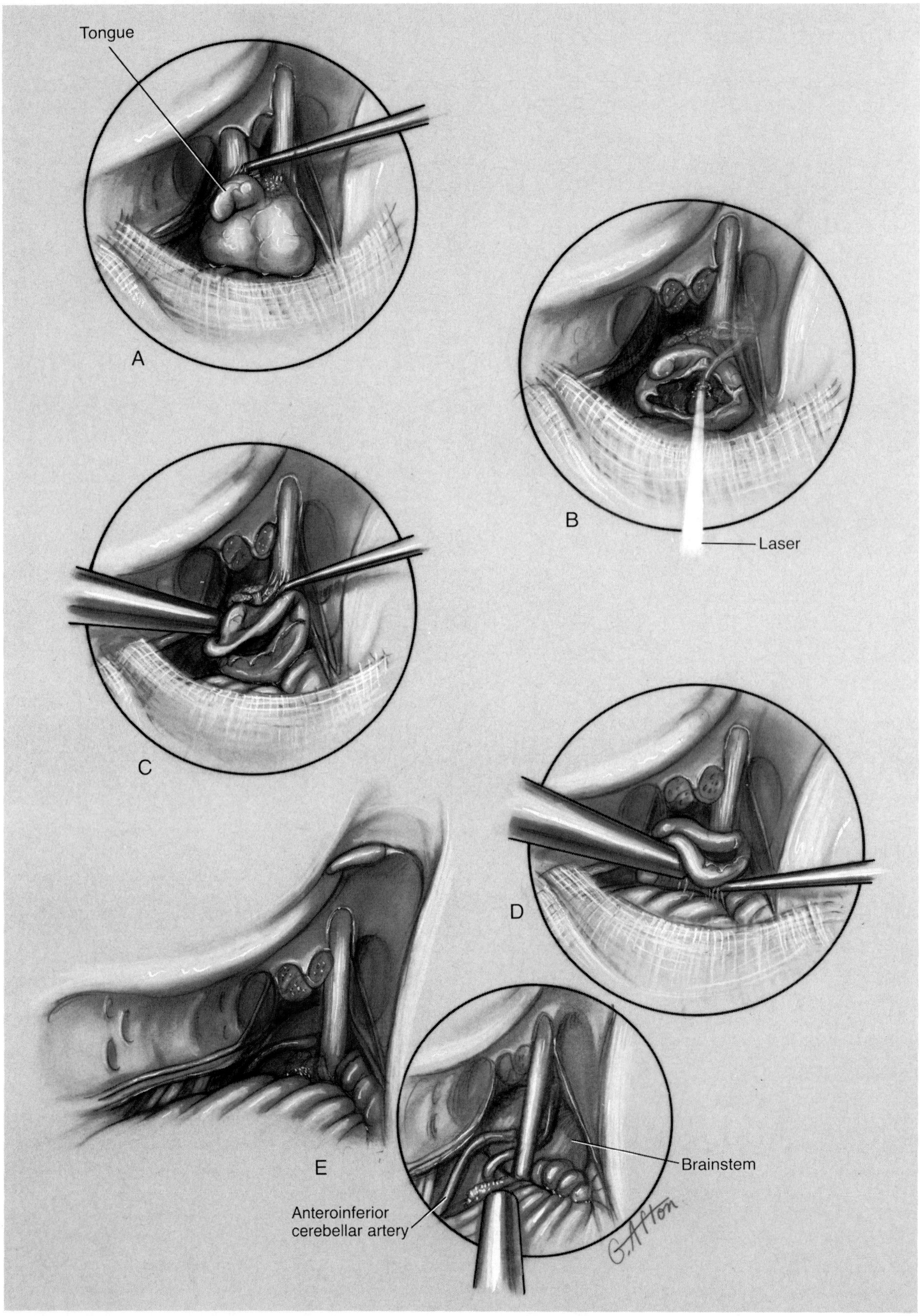
Tongue
A
B
Laser
C
D
E
Brainstem
Anteroinferior
cerebellar artery
G. Alton

FIGURE 19–6.

During mobilization and tumor removal, these structures must be watched for and protected.

After adequate debulking, the plane for the facial nerve is further developed and the tumor continues to be rolled toward the surgeon. It is important (although difficult) to avoid pushing the tumor mass inward, which may stretch the thinned nerve. It is best to follow the facial nerve to the brainstem, separating and removing the tumor as the plane continues to be developed. At the porus acusticus the facial nerve usually thins considerably, making the dissection difficult. Often it is necessary to return to the posterior, inferior, and superior borders of the tumor to develop this plane (if needed for maneuvering). Always try to avoid pushing the tumor anteriorly. Once the facial nerve has been freed from the tumor, the bulk of the tumor is removed to enhance visualization (Fig. 19–6*E*). The plane between the remaining tumor and the brainstem is developed and care is exercised superiorly for the fifth nerve and inferiorly for the anteroinferior cerebellar artery (Fig. 19–6*E*). Vessels that traverse the tumor surface are dissected away, if possible; if not, they are carefully clipped or cauterized. With careful dissection, total removal of the tumor can be accomplished in almost all cases.

Before closure, sufficient time must be taken to ensure that adequate hemostasis is obtained within the cerebellopontine angle. Fat is taken from the abdomen and placed in long strips just inside the dural opening; this has been found to provide a good seal against postoperative cerebrospinal fluid leakage. The long tails of the strips are then folded into the mastoid cavity and antrum, and the postauricular incision is closed.

Intraoperative Complications or Problems

1. Sigmoid and superior petrosal sinus bleeding.
2. Jugular bulb bleeding.
3. Facial nerve avulsion.
4. Vital sign changes.

Sinus Bleeding. Bleeding arising from injury to the sinus during bone removal may be profuse at times. Although alarming, with proper management it may be controlled without serious consequences. Sigmoid bleeding arising from emissary veins usually can be controlled by full exposure of the vein and bipolar cautery; packing with bone wax or Surgicel is another option. For tears within the sinus itself, packing with Surgicel will control the immediate problem of blood loss; however, if bone removal has been completed there are no bony ledges against which to wedge the packing. Large packs hinder dissection more medially; in addition, the packs may be caught in the drill, creating a whipping action with the Surgicel. One solution to this is to cover the packing with bone wax draped over Bill's island; a long strip of Cottonoid is then draped over the area and the entire complex is retracted with the suction irrigator or with a malleable retractor hooked to the cerebellar retractors. Again, bleeding usually can be controlled; the objective is to continue dissection farther medially without hindrance.

Jugular Bulb Bleeding. Inadvertent injury to the jugular bulb is signaled by profuse bleeding. Packing immediately will control the bleeding. Caution must be exercised since the ninth, tenth, and eleventh nerves are in this area and may be injured by injudicious packing. For small tears in the jugular bulb, packing may control the bleeding and allow the procedure to continue. Only large pieces of packing material are to be used here, in order to prevent displacement of material into the lumen of the vein and a resulting pulmonary embolus (this is also a concern with tears in the sigmoid). For large tears, it is often necessary and safer to tie the vein off in the neck by extending the postauricular incision inferiorly (for all neurologic procedures the upper neck is included in the draping). The jugular bulb is then packed intraluminally to prevent back-bleeding.

Facial Nerve Avulsion. If the facial nerve is lost or avulsed during tumor removal, a decision must be made whether to attempt immediate or delayed rehabilitation. Because the best and most consistent results are obtained from immediate rehabilitation, it should be attempted if possible. If the brainstem side of the avulsed nerve is found and is long enough, the infratemporal portion of the facial nerve may be mobilized in its entirety from its canal. With this maneuver, an additional 1-cm length of nerve is obtained (bypassing the labyrinthine and temporal course of the nerve) and an end-to-end anastomosis may be attempted. If possible, a suture is placed to hold the avulsed ends together (collagen [Avitene] has been placed around the two ends to hold them in apposition). If this is not feasible, a hypoglossal-facial nerve anastomosis is performed later.

Vital Sign Changes. Vital signs are constantly monitored throughout tumor removal surgery. Continuous cardiac monitoring is done, as well as monitoring of blood pressure with arterial lines. With any rise or change in blood pressure or pulse regularity, the surgeon is notified, traction is stopped, and large Cottonoid packing is removed in order to eliminate

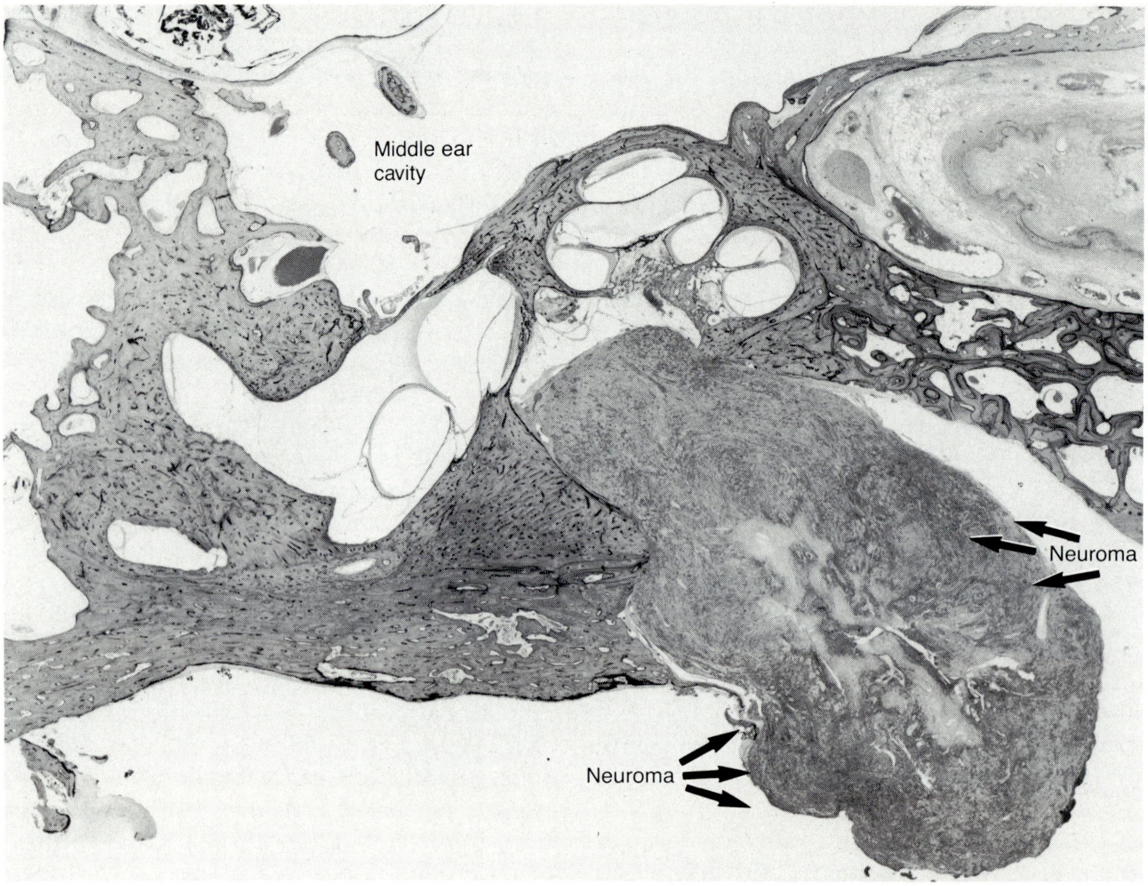

FIGURE 19–7.

pressure on vessels. Usually responses return to normal in a few minutes and surgery continues. If they recur, a decision is made whether to continue surgery but only perform a subtotal removal; if tumor is left behind, it may be removed electively in about six months. By that time the brainstem circulation has usually improved from tumor debulking and release of pressure, and total tumor removal can be performed safely. Constant monitoring and replacement of blood loss is important to prevent early signs of shock (increased pulse, decreased BP) from offsetting the effect of vessel traction or spasm (decreased pulse, increased BP).

Pertinent Histopathology

FIGURE 19–7

This horizontal section of a temporal bone shows the presence of an acoustic neuroma.

CHAPTER 20

Plastic Surgery of the Pinna

The pinna, or auricle, is the projecting part of the ear that lies outside the head; its basic anatomy is shown in Figure 20–1. It consists of two types of tissue: elastic (yellow) cartilage and, in the ear lobe, fibroareolar tissue. It is connected to the head and scalp by the superior, anterior, and posterior auricular muscles. Blood is supplied to the pinna by branches of the superficial temporal and posterior auricular arteries, and it is innervated by branches of the greater auricular and auriculotemporal nerves, the mastoid branch of the lesser occipital nerve, and a small branch of the vagus nerve in the concha bowl. This chapter describes several surgical procedures for repair and reconstruction of the pinna.

Treatment of the Cleft Ear Lobe

Patients are often seen in the clinic with cleft ear lobes secondary to trauma from piercing the ear for earrings. They most often present with a healed cleft, but occasionally with a "fresh" or incomplete cleft; very rarely a congenital cleft is seen. Regardless of the presentation, the treatment is the same.

Aim

To correct a cleft ear lobe defect.

Highlights

1. Make a Z-plasty or V-plasty at the free margin to prevent postoperative notching.
2. Do not use a post-type earring to maintain the earring hole after the repair; even a lightweight earring will enlarge the hole postoperatively.

Pitfalls

1. Failing to perform a Z-plasty often results in a notch at the free margin of the lobe and a depressed scar.
2. If the patient wears an earring too soon after the repair, an enlarged earring hole will result.

Instruments

No. 11 and No. 15 scalpel blades and handles.
Two skin hooks, either single or double hook type.
0.5-mm ophthalmic forceps.
Fine Storz "stitch" scissors.
Sutures: 5-0 Vicryl on a cutting needle, 6-0 chromic or 6-0 nylon on a small cutting needle, 0 prolene or nylon.

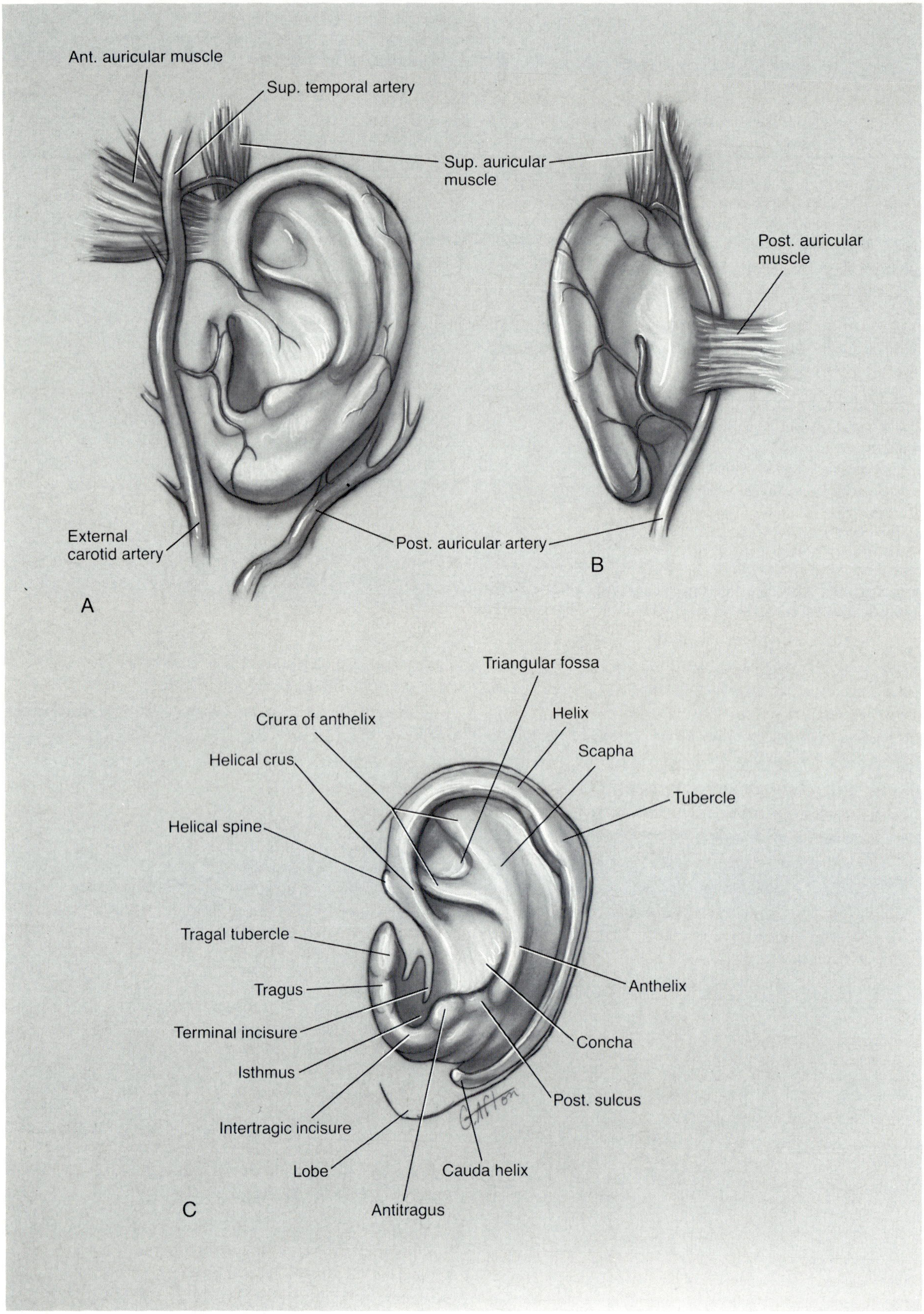
Ant. auricular muscle
Sup. temporal artery
Sup. auricular muscle
Post. auricular muscle
External carotid artery
Post. auricular artery
A
B
Triangular fossa
Crura of anthelix
Helix
Scapha
Helical crus
Tubercle
Helical spine
Tragal tubercle
Tragus
Anthelix
Terminal incisure
Concha
Isthmus
Post. sulcus
Intertragic incisure
Lobe
Cauda helix
C
Antitragus

FIGURE 20–1.

Procedure

Lidocaine 1 to 2% with 1:100,000 epinephrine is used. First the edges of the cleft are excised. If the cleft is not quite complete, the small bridge of skin also is excised. A Z-plasty is fashioned anteriorly (Fig. 20–2–*A*–C). One can also be made posteriorly, but this is not necessary. A Z-plasty should also be made at the free margin of the lobe to prevent a small notch from forming during the healing process. Alternatively, the free margin can be closed in a "V" tongue-and-groove fashion. If the patient still wishes to have a pierced ear, a length of 0 prolene suture is formed into a 1-in loop passing through the former earring site. Some patients, not wishing to have the loop of suture in their lobe for several weeks, may decide simply to have the ear repierced after the repair has healed. The fibroareolar tissue is closed with interrupted 5-0 Vicryl and the skin is closed with interrupted 6-0 nylon or 6-0 chromic sutures.

Bacitracin ointment is applied to the incision for a few days. 6-0 nylon sutures are removed at four to five days. If 6-0 chromic sutures are used, the patient can be seen at seven to 10 days, at which time the remaining wisps of suture can be gently wiped off. An earring may be worn after four weeks.

Treatment of Keloids

Keloids are a common problem of the ear lobe, especially in blacks. They usually involve the medial aspect of the lobe, and most often are the result of deep dermal injury to the lobe of the ear when the ears are pierced for earrings. Large lesions can be painful when holding a telephone receiver against the ear or when sleeping. Any keloid large enough to cause a cosmetic or functional defect should be excised.

Aim

To excise and prevent the recurrence of the ear lobe keloid.

Highlights

1. The key to treatment is to prevent recurrence after excision. This is accomplished with intralesional steroid injections and the use of pressure earrings.

2. Stay as close as possible to the stalk of the keloid during excision, in order to preserve as much normal skin of the ear lobe as possible.

Pitfalls

1. Repiercing of the lobe after successful treatment of a keloid is not recommended.

2. Failing to prevent a recurrence is the most common problem after excision of a keloid. Close follow-up and the use of intralesional steroids are the best methods of preventing a recurrence.

3. The patient with large keloids must be advised that the ear lobe may be less fleshy after excision of the keloid; that owing to the mass of the keloid, little fibrofatty tissue is available for advancement into the wound for closure; that the lobe may be smaller after excision of the keloid, owing to the excision of skin on both surfaces of the lobe; and that the lobe may be rotated slightly anteriorly after the excision of a lateral keloid and slightly posteriorly after the excision of a medial keloid.

Instruments

No. 1 and No. 15 scalpel blades and handles.
0.5-mm ophthalmic forceps.
A fine needle holder.
Storz "stitch" scissors.
Skin hooks, either single or double.
Sutures: 5-0 chromic or Vicryl, and 6-0 chromic or 6-0 nylon on a small cutting needle.

Procedure

The treatment of keloids involves three treatment modalities: steroid therapy, pressure therapy, and excision. These modalities are often used at different times in the treatment of the same keloid.

Small keloids can be treated with injections of 40 mg per ml of triamcinolone acetonide every four to six weeks. The steroid can either be delivered with a Dermajet apparatus or injected into the dermis with a 25- or 27-gauge needle. A Dermajet needleless injector dispenses 0.1 ml of the steroid solution in a fine droplet form uniformly into the tissues; this avoids the bolus injection of steroids that can result from direct needle injection into dense scar tissue.

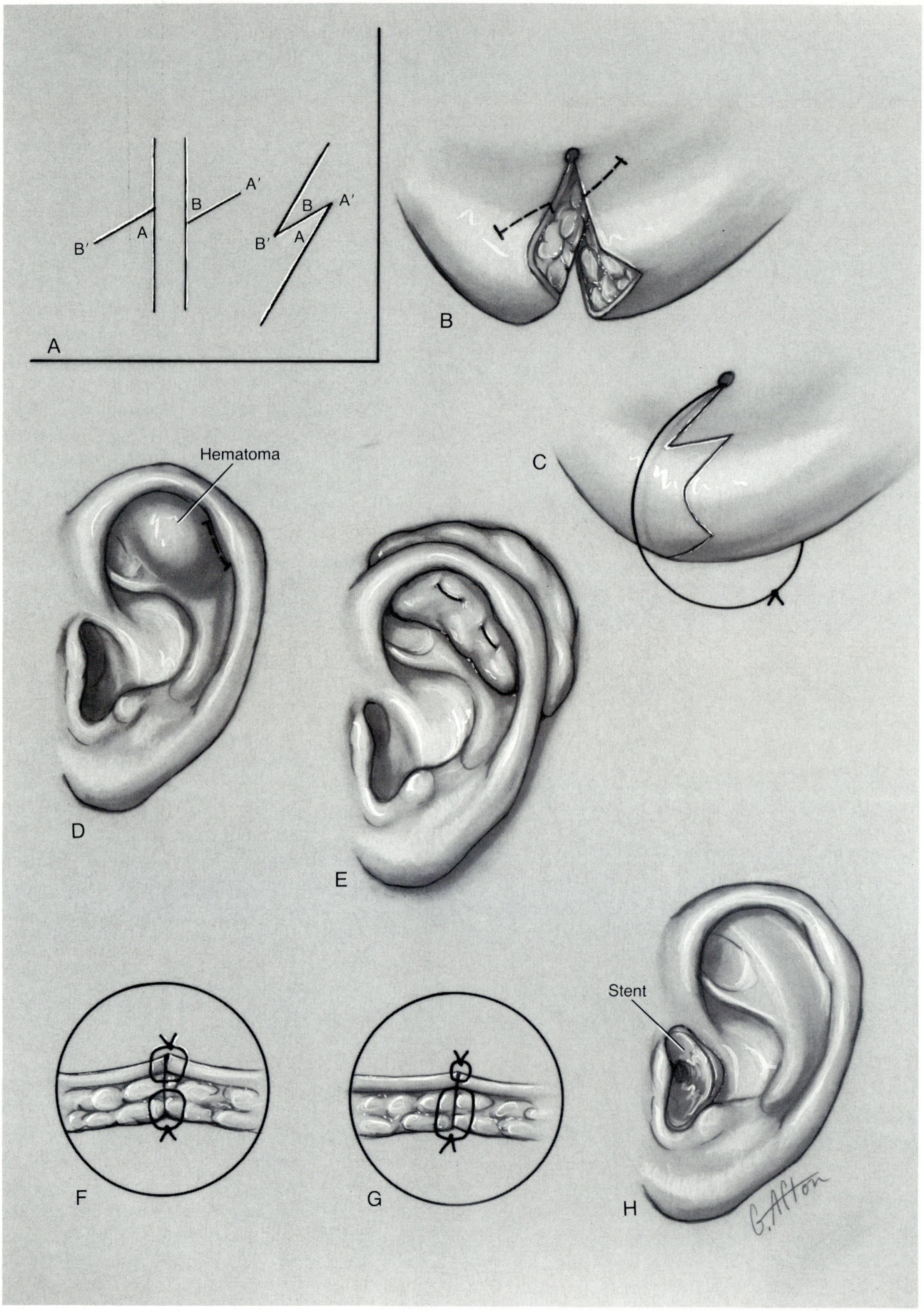

FIGURE 20–2.

Overzealous injection can cause skin atrophy, telangiectasis, and hypopigmentation. It may take six to 12 months to resolve the keloid.

It is also possible to treat small keloids with pressure therapy. A pressure-type clasp earring (Padgett Co, Kansas City, MO) may supply enough pressure to blanch the capillaries supplying the fibrous tissue and cause a regression of the lesion. It must be worn continuously for several months. When the earring is taken off the keloid can recur; therefore, it is probably best to combine use of the pressure earring with monthly steroid injections.

For keloids that are too large for pressure therapy or that do not respond to steroids, excision is indicated. The entire keloid should be excised. Delicate handling is necessary to prevent trauma to the surrounding tissues. If the keloid is especially large, it is important to free up surrounding fibrofatty tissue to fill in the soft tissue defect. A W-plasty or Z-plasty is used to camouflage the repair. Sometimes a small rotational flap must be used for closure. Steroids can be injected directly into the surgical site at the end of the procedure. 5-0 chromic or Vicryl is used for deep sutures and 6-0 chromic or nylon is used on the skin.

Bacitracin is applied for a few days. Nylon sutures can be removed after four to five days. When excision alone is used the recurrence rate is over 50%; therefore, the surgical site should be injected with steroids every month for approximately six months or until the scar is mature. To stabilize the ear lobe when using the Dermajet, it is helpful to place a tongue blade against the lateral surface of the lobe. At the first sign of recurrence, a pressure earring should be added to the treatment regimen.

Traumatic Injuries of the Pinna

Injuries of the pinna are classified as follows:

1. Traumatic hematoma with or without cellulitis or perichondritis.
2. Laceration without tissue loss.
3. Laceration with skin or cartilage loss, or both.
4. Total amputation of the pinna.

Hematoma of the Pinna

A hematoma of the pinna is caused by blunt trauma and most often affects the lateral surface (Fig. 20–2*D*). It should be drained as soon as possible before the clot organizes. An organized hematoma requires more extensive surgery.

Aim

To drain the hematoma, prevent reaccumulation, avoid secondary cellulitis or perichondritis, and prevent the deformity caused by organization of the hematoma (cauliflower ear).

Highlights

1. The most important step is the placement of a well-molded dressing to prevent a recurrence.
2. The incision should be hidden or should run favorably with the anatomy of the pinna.
3. A drain may be necessary when treating a large hematoma.

Pitfalls

1. Recurrence of the hematoma owing to an inadequate dressing.

Instruments and Supplies

No. 11 or No. 15 scalpel and handle.
Curved hemostat (mosquito).
0.25-in Penrose drain (optional).
Cotton balls.
Povidone-iodine (Betadine) ointment.
50-50 mixture of mineral oil and Betadine solution (optional).
4 × 4 "Fluffs."
2-in rolled bandages.
2-0 nylon or prolene on a large cutting needle.
Hibiclens or Betadine scrub.
Normal saline irrigating solution.

Procedure

Lidocaine 1% with 1:100,000 epinephrine can be used as a field block or injected locally. The ear is prepared with Hibiclens or Betadine scrub. A vertical curvilinear incision is made over or along the side of the hematoma (usually under either the helical or anthelical fold to camouflage it). It is better to make an incision large enough for good drainage and deal with the resultant scar later than to be faced with a persistent or recurrent hematoma and secondary perichondritis. A curved mosquito hemostat may be used to open up any loculations. A culture of the hematoma should be taken if cellulitis is present.

The hematoma can then be irrigated gently with sterile normal saline. A ¼-in Penrose drain or rubber band drain should be used for extensive hematomas. Skin sutures should then approximate the skin of large incisions but still allow adequate drainage. Next cotton balls saturated with Betadine ointment (or a 50-50 mixture of Betadine solution and mineral oil) are formed into shapes that precisely correspond to the folds of the pinna overlying the hematoma. An additional piece of cotton should be molded to fit into the postauricular crease (Fig. 20–2*E*). An exact fit is necessary to prevent reaccumulation of the hematomas. The pieces of cotton are held in place with through-and-through 2-0 nylon or prolene mattress sutures; usually two will suffice. A mastoid dressing of "Fluffs" and a 2-in rolled bandage are then applied.

Postoperative Care

The patient should be placed on an oral antibiotic that covers for skin flora, predominantly *Staphylococcus.* The mastoid dressing and cotton balls can be removed after two days and the pinna inspected. If there has been no reaccumulation, no further mastoid dressing is needed and the cotton bolsters are removed in two to three days. If reaccumulation has occurred, the hematoma must be drained again, and the same type of precise cotton packing with a mastoid dressing is reapplied. If there is evidence of perichondritis, cultures should be taken and parenteral antibiotics started. A Penrose drain or a through-and-through suction irrigation system may be necessary. If there is evidence of cartilage necrosis, wide debridement of necrotic soft tissue and cartilage is needed. The reconstruction of any defects resulting from perichondritis is similar to that performed after neoplasm resection (described below).

Laceration without Tissue Loss

The ear's prominent and exposed location on the head renders it vulnerable to lacerations. Complex lacerations should be carefully examined for foreign bodies and any evidence of soft tissue loss. The skin is densely adherent to the underlying cartilage, and any full-thickness injury of the dermis will expose the cartilage to the risk of infection. All full-thickness lacerations should be repaired.

Aim

To repair a laceration of the pinna.

Highlights

1. Intracartilaginous sutures are often necessary.
2. Apparently nonvital tissue should be saved whenever possible. If a cutaneous link of skin persists, the skin of the pinna has a remarkable ability to withstand vascular compromise. The nonvital tissue will demarcate several days later and can be debrided then.
3. Use of a stent with external auditory canal lacerations to prevent stenosis.

Pitfalls

1. Post-traumatic tattooing due to incomplete debridement.
2. Imprecise closure resulting in prominent scarring or irregularities in the cartilage formation.
3. Failing to recognize an external auditory canal laceration.

Instruments

A basic plastics pack.

Procedure

Usually 1% lidocaine with 1:100,000 epinephrine can be used. If there are flaps or regions with a compromised blood supply, 1% lidocaine without epinephrine should be used. Simple lacerations of the skin of the pinna should be meticulously cleaned. It is important to remove all debris to prevent post-traumatic tattooing. The laceration should be closed with 6-0 chromic or 6-0 nylon suture. If necessary, subcutaneous sutures also are used to reduce tension and evert the skin edges; 5-0 Vicryl or chromic sutures work best for this (Fig. 20–2*F, G*). Sutures of 6-0 chromic are placed through the skin differently from 6-0 nylon sutures. Chromic sutures usually are not removed and only serve to approximate the skin edges, rather than drawing through the subcutaneous tissue; they are indicated when there is no tension on the wound edges. Either running locked sutures or simple interrupted sutures can be used.

Lacerations involving cartilage can be closed by directly suturing the cartilage together with 5-0 Vicryl. Unless the cartilage is grossly contaminated it does not need debriding. Horizontal mattress sutures in the plane of the cartilage provide accurate reapproximation.

Lacerations through the external auditory canal are treated initially with a bacitracin gauze pack. The pack can be removed in five to seven days, at which time a stent much like that for a hearing aid can be placed to prevent post-traumatic stenosis of the canal (Fig. 20–2*H*). A central hole should be drilled to allow hearing. The stent should be worn for three to six weeks, depending on the severity of the injury.

Bacitracin is applied to the laceration to prevent crusting. If the laceration is extensive, a mastoid dressing with cotton molding (like that used for pinna hematomas but without the mattress stay sutures) should be applied and worn for two to three days.

Laceration with Skin or Cartilage Loss

Reconstruction of the pinna after lacerations with tissue loss is similar to that after the resection of a neoplasm (described below).

Total Amputation of the Pinna

Fortunately, total or subtotal amputation of the pinna is a rare occurrence. Cases in which the amputated piece is missing or grossly contaminated obviate the need for immediate reconstruction. Delayed total auricular reconstruction or prosthetic rehabilitation are outside the scope of this text. When less than 50% of the tissue of the pinna has been lost, and the amputated part has been saved, reconstruction of the remnant is similar to that performed after neoplasm resection.

Aim

To reattach the amputated portion of the pinna.

Highlights

1. If the amputated piece is available, reimplantation should be attempted unless the patient's medical condition contraindicates a lengthy general anesthetic.
2. Close postoperative follow-up is needed to watch for infection, venous congestion, and necrosis.

Pitfalls

1. The larger the amputated part, the greater is the likelihood of partial or total loss.
2. Venous congestion may not be preventable even with pie-crust incisions or leeches.
3. The cartilage skeleton will not be as sharp or well-defined when re-epithelialized with the thicker postauricular skin.

Instruments

A basic plastic pack plus a dermabrader.
Microvascular instruments.

Procedure

General anesthesia usually is indicated owing to the length of the repair. When the amputated part is available it should be rinsed in cold saline, wrapped in a moist cotton gauze, placed in a sealable plastic bag, and then packed in ice. When dealing with an amputated pinna, it is important to let the patient and family know the poor prognosis even in the best of circumstances.

In clean amputations without much crushing or avulsion of tissue, microvascular reattachment of an amputated pinna may be indicated. If this service is available it is probably a worthwhile effort.

If only a small piece (1 to 2 cm of tissue or the helical rim) has been amputated it can simply be reattached, but reattachment of a totally amputated pinna without re-establishment of the circulation by microvascular surgery often results in a total loss of the pinna secondary to vascular congestion. However, if there is a small cutaneous bridge linking the pinna to the head, simple reattachment is advantageous. Medicinal leeches have been used to reduce the venous congestion.

In some cases, when the pinna has been totally amputated and microvascular repair is not available or indicated, the cartilaginous framework may be salvaged by dermabrading all of the epidermis from the cartilaginous skeleton and burying the pinna in a postauricular pocket for three to four weeks. The cartilaginous skeleton can then be "released" from this pocket and allowed to slowly re-epithelialize.

If only a portion of the pinna has been amputated, all of the soft tissue overlying both surfaces of the amputated segment is removed, sparing the perichondrium; the cartilage segment is then reattached to the remaining pinna with mattress sutures to reapproximate the cartilage. The denuded cartilage segment is then buried in a postauricular pocket, which has been created by incising the postauricular skin, followed by wide undermining (Fig. 20–3).

Another method of salvaging the cartilaginous skeleton of the amputated ear is to remove the skin

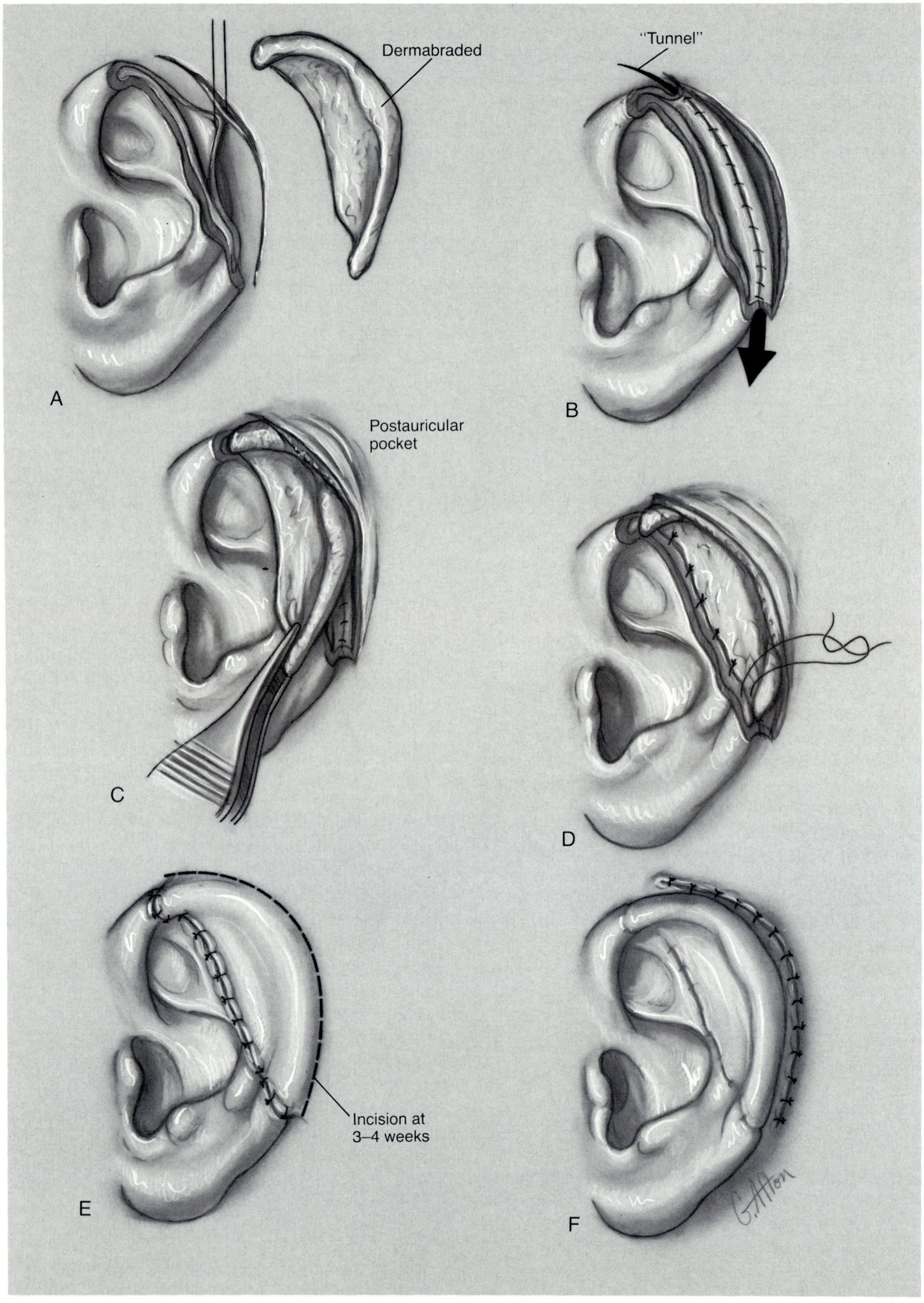
Dermabraded
A
"Tunnel"
B
Postauricular
pocket
C
D
Incision at
3–4 weeks
E
F

FIGURE 20–3.

from the medial surface of the pinna and perforate the cartilage. The postauricular skin is then removed and the ear is reattached by suturing the helical rim to the free margin of remaining postauricular skin (Fig. 20–4). "Pie-crust" incisions or medicinal leeches may be necessary if venous congestion is a problem.

The last two methods require that the helical rim be lifted after three to four weeks by incising the postauricular skin. The defect left in the postauricular area can sometimes be closed by primary closure. A split-thickness or full-thickness skin graft from the opposite postauricular region or from the supraclavicular area also can be used. Another method is to place a fossa tissue expander behind the ear, and to use this expanded skin to resurface the postauricular area.

If the postauricular area is badly injured and not suitable for one of the above methods of reconstruction, the pinna can be "banked" under cervical skin. This is done by removing the soft tissue from the cartilage, making a pocket under a cervical skin flap, and leaving it there until the postauricular skin has healed. A crescent-shaped tissue expander can then be placed in the postauricular/mastoid region and slowly expanded over four to six weeks until twice as much surface area is expanded (see Fig. 20–4*B*). The "banked" cartilage skeleton is removed from beneath the cervical flap and placed into the expanded pocket. High-vacuum suction is necessary to obtain good apposition of the skin to the interstices of the cartilage.

Postoperative Care

Steroids, heparin, antibiotics, pie-crust incisions and, lately, medicinal leeches have all been advocated in the care of the reimplanted pinna. Meticulous wound care with bacitracin and Adaptic gauze is necessary. Often there is de-epithelialization of the amputated part, but with gentle debridement the pinna usually can re-epithelialize. If the reimplantation is successful, the patient must be cautioned that the new circulation may not be resilient enough to be immediately exposed to extremes of temperature or injudiciously exposed to the sun.

Neoplasms of the Pinna

The pinna is a frequent site of basal cell and squamous cell carcinomas and, less frequently, malignant melanomas. All but shaved, punched, or curetted biopsies should be repaired. The techniques used to reconstruct defects of the pinna after resection of a neoplasm can also be used to reconstruct the pinna after a laceration with tissue loss.

Aim

To reconstruct the pinna after resection of a neoplasm.

Highlights

1. Gentle handling of the tissues is necessary to reduce operative trauma.
2. Small defects are repaired by primary closure or composite graft.
3. Larger defects most often are repaired with a postauricular pedicled graft.
4. The less complex the repair, the greater is the likelihood of good results.
5. All margins of resection should be histologically examined.

Pitfalls

1. Imprecise closure may lead to a cosmetic deformity.
2. A composite graft may be lost if it is too large (> 1.5 cm).
3. A pinna may "cup" after a wedge resection if wedges of skin and cartilage are not removed along the anthelical fold.

Instruments

The instruments listed below form the basics of a plastics tray used for most soft tissue surgery of the head and neck. These instruments will be used for the procedures described in the rest of this chapter.

No. 11 and No. 15 scalpel blades and handles.
Medium and fine needle holders.
0.5-mm ophthalmic forceps.
Brown-Adson forceps.
No. 3 single or double skin hooks.
No. 2 Senn retractors.
Storz "stitch" scissors.

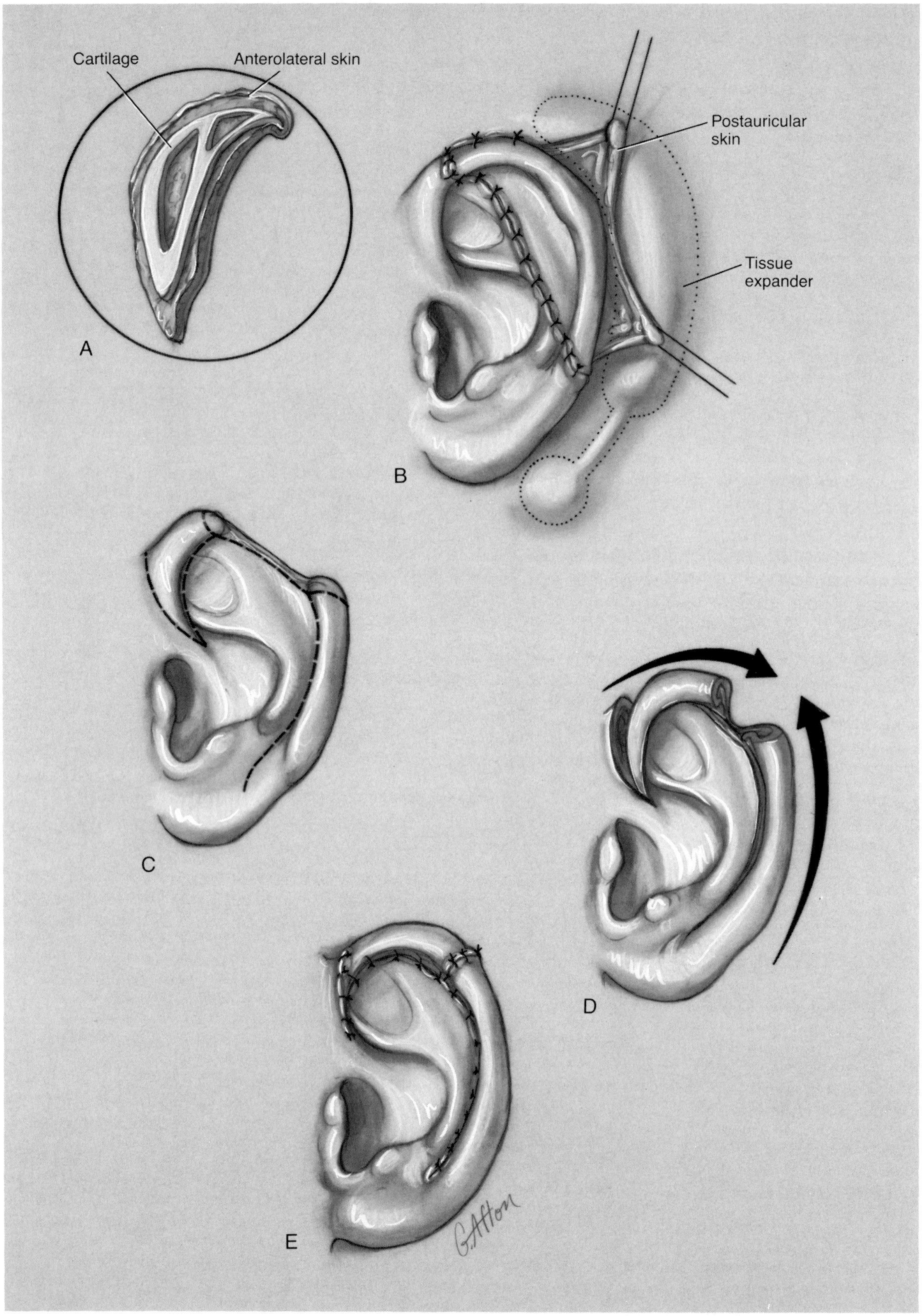
Cartilage
Anterolateral skin
A
Postauricular skin
Tissue expander
B
C
D
E

FIGURE 20–4.

Curved and straight iris scissors.
Small Metzenbaum scissors.
Tenotomy scissors.
Sutures: 4-0 and 5-0 Vicryl, 4-0 and 6-0 nylon, 6-0 chromic.
Marking pen.
Cotton-tipped applicators.
Dressing: Tincture of benzoin, Steri-Strips, 4 × 4 "Fluffs," 2-in rolled bandage, cotton balls, and Betadine ointment.

Procedure

Depending on the extent of the reconstruction, either local anethesia with 1% lidocaine and 1:100,000 epinephrine or general anesthesia can be used.

After the resection of a neoplasm, the pinna can be reconstructed by many methods, limited only by the surgeon's imagination and ingenuity. The following discussion, which is not intended to be encyclopedic, outlines methods that have worked well over the years and that are based on general principles of flap design.

After removing the neoplasm, all margins must be examined histologically.

The pinna can be reconstructed in three ways: (1) primary closure, (2) a composite graft from the other ear, and (3) a pedicled skin/cartilage flap.

Primary Closure. When less than 30% of the pinna has been excised, the defect often can be closed primarily, especially if it involves the upper and middle portions of the pinna (Fig. 20–5*A*, *B*). When closing a defect primarily, it is usually necessary to use any of a variety of releasing incisions along the anthelical fold and conchal bowl to allow for the advancement of adjacent tissue. The rigid cartilaginous framework of the pinna, the densely adherent skin, and the lack of subcutaneous tissue hinder the closure of even small defects. Without these incisions, closure of the defect may cause cupping of the pinna. Often, small wedges of conchal bowl cartilage must be removed so that proper closure can be obtained. Closure is accomplished with interrupted 5-0 Vicryl suture in the cartilage and a cutaneous layer of running locked 6-0 chromic or interrupted 6-0 nylon suture.

Composite Graft. Another satisfactory method of repairing small defects of the pinna (no greater than 3 cm) is to use a composite graft from the opposite ear. A through-and-through graft up to 1.5 cm in size can be harvested from the donor ear. The size of the graft is usually half the size of the defect—that is, for a 2-cm defect a 1-cm composite graft is harvested. The donor site is closed primarily as described above. The composite graft is then sutured in place with a minimal number of sutures, securing the cartilage with 5-0 Vicryl and closing the skin with 6-0 chromic or nylon suture. Too many sutures can compromise the viability of the graft. Composite grafts often undergo epidermolysis with discoloration and blister formation, but usually re-epithelialize if infection is avoided.

Pedicled Skin Flap. For larger defects, a skin flap based either anteriorly or posteriorly on the postauricular skin is elevated and sutured into the defect (Fig. 20–5*C*, *D*). If the defect has been created by resection of a neoplasm or a traumatic tissue loss, an anteriorly based flap is not feasible. The blood supply is better when the flap is based posteriorly, but anteriorly based flaps usually do not require a secondary takedown procedure. The length-to-width ratio is usually low (1:1 to 2:1) because of the close proximity of the donor site. A piece of contralateral conchal bowl cartilage or costal cartilage can be placed under the flap primarily, or secondarily when the flap is taken down (Fig. 20–5*E*). For small defects the use of cartilage is not necessary. The postauricular sulcus often can be preserved by leaving a strip of postauricular skin intact when developing the flap. The free margin of skin on the medial surface of the pinna is sutured to the free margin of the postauricular skin. The leading edge of the elevated flap is sutured to the free margin of the lateral skin of the pinna. After three or four weeks the pedicled flap can be separated from the postauricular skin and rolled around to make a new helical rim (Fig. 20–5*F*, *G*). If the helical fold is not well defined, small cotton bolsters can be placed on the lateral surface of the pinna and sutured in place with 4-0 nylon to help recreate this portion. Subcutaneous and cartilaginous sutures are 5-0 Vicryl, with 6-0 chromic or nylon used for the cutaneous layer. The donor site usually can be closed primarily with extensive undermining, but a skin graft may be necessary.

Defects of the conchal bowl can be closed primarily if they are small. For a larger defect, a full-thickness postauricular skin graft works well. Large defects also may be repaired with a postauricular pedicled skin flap, which is elevated and laid through a slit made through the conchal cartilage (Fig. 20–6*A*). The flap is sutured anteriorly, superiorly, and inferiorly, leaving the posterior through-and-through slit (Fig. 20–6*B*). After three or four weeks the flap is released along the posterior slit and the defect is closed primarily (Fig. 20–6*C*).

Loss of the ear lobe can be repaired by designing a bilobed flap based anteriorly, which is lifted and folded upon itself (Fig. 20–7*A*, *B*). The donor site is

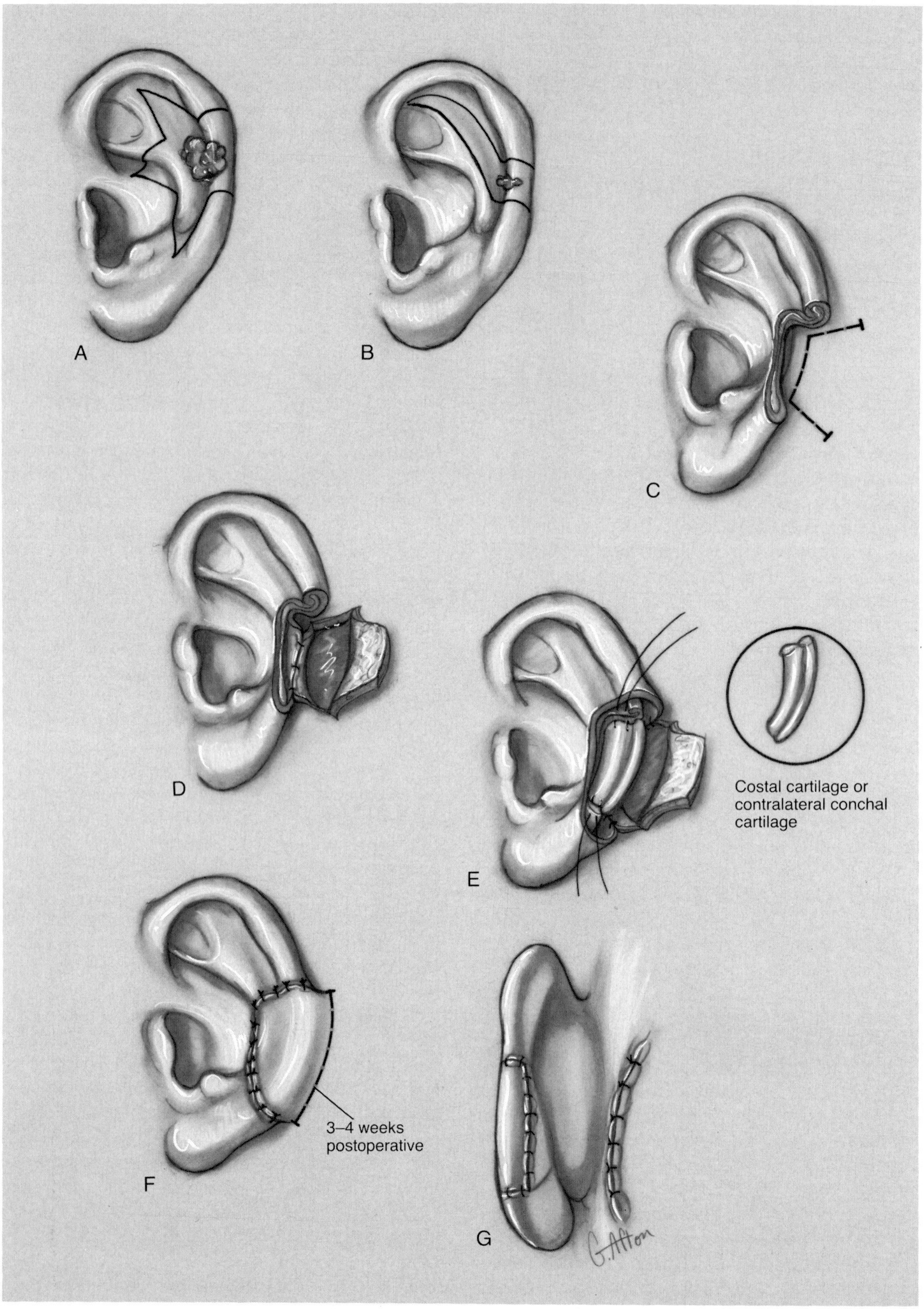
A
B
C
D
E
Costal cartilage or
contralateral conchal
cartilage
F
3–4 weeks
postoperative
G
G. Alton

FIGURE 20–5.

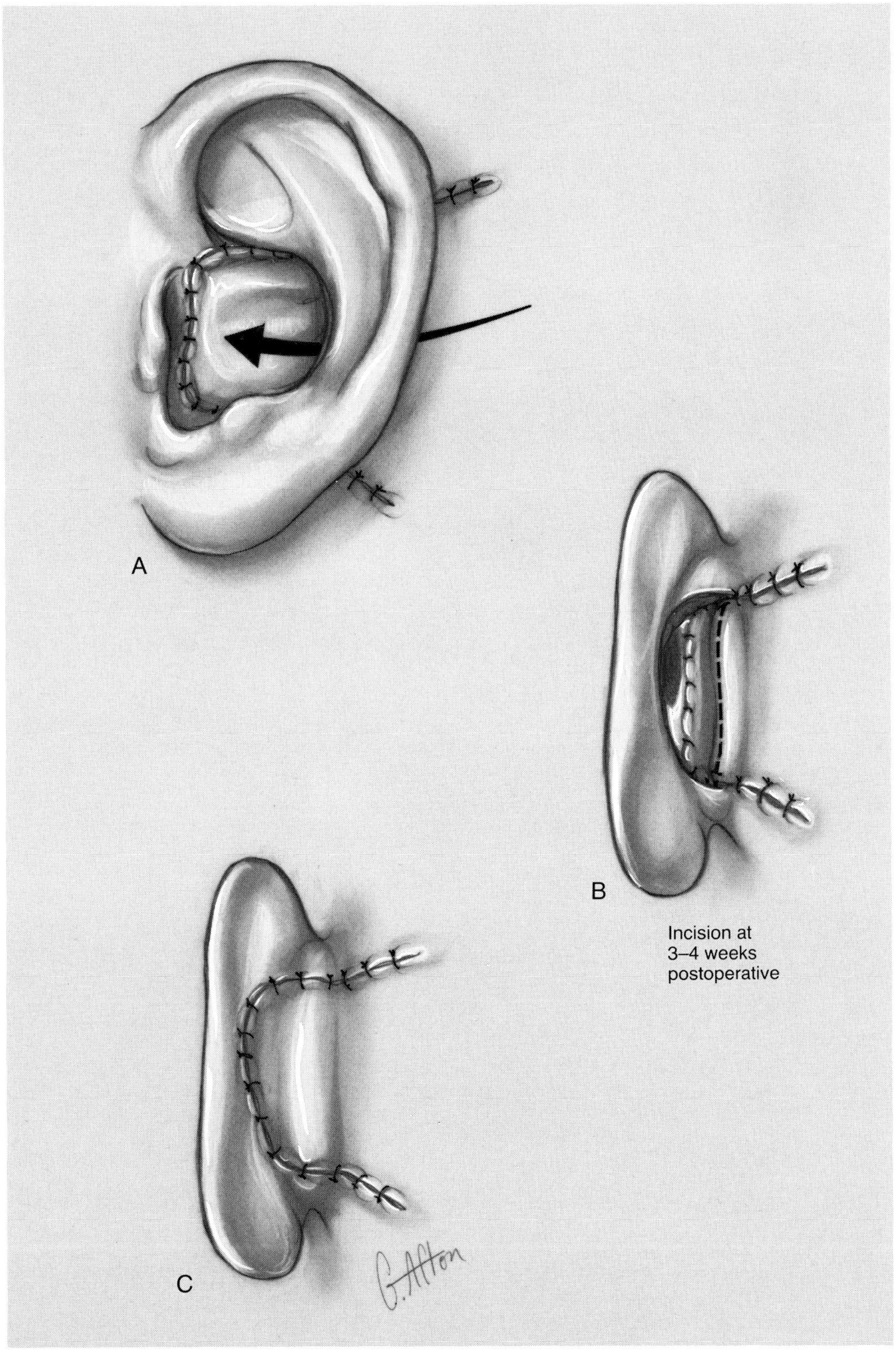

FIGURE 20–6.

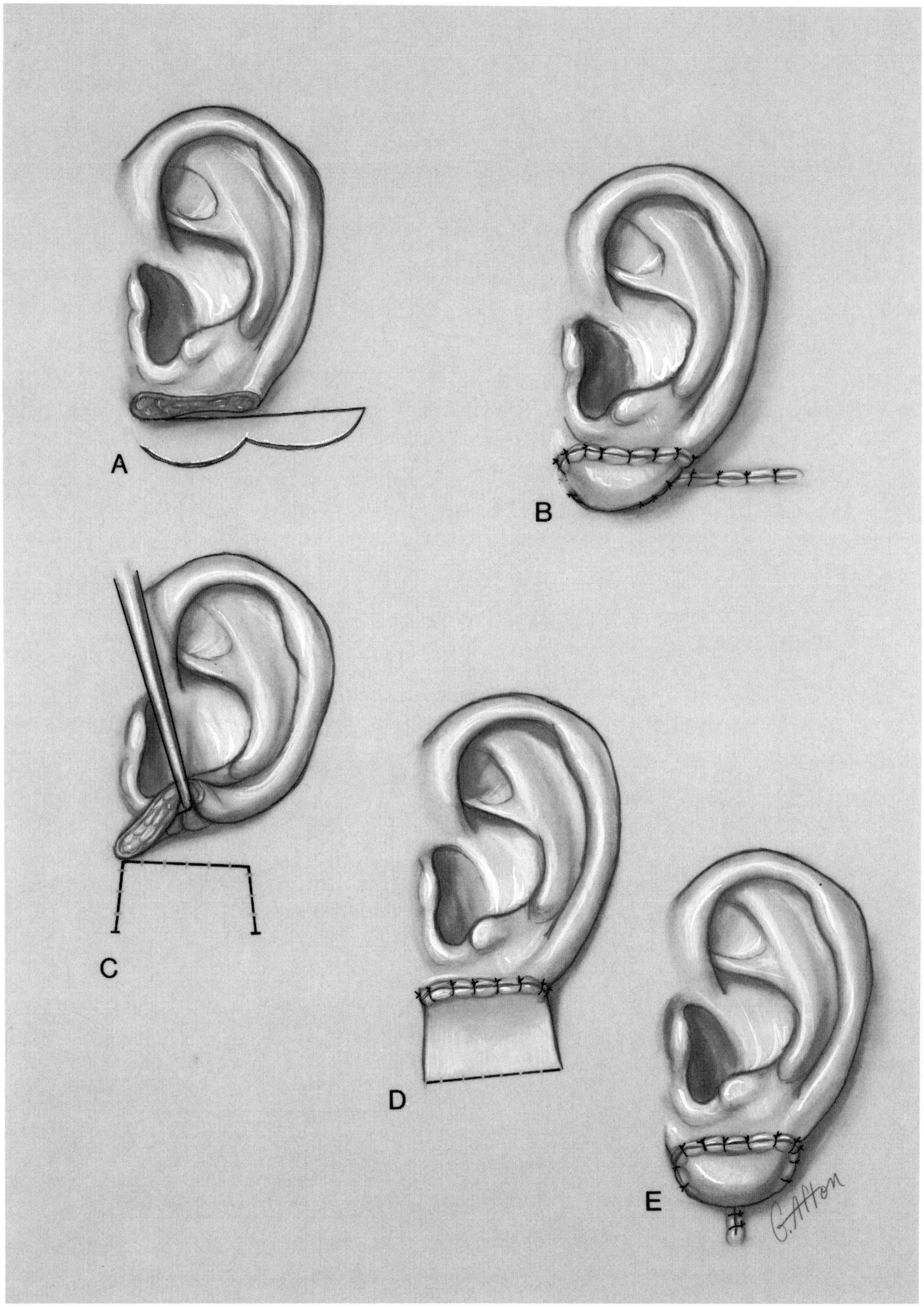

FIGURE 20–7.

closed primarily or with a skin graft. Alternatively, an inferiorly based flap is elevated and sutured to the inferior edge of the remaining pinna. After three to four weeks the flap is separated inferiorly and folded upon itself (Fig. 20–7*C–E*).

Postoperative Care

Bacitracin ointment is applied to the incisions. A light mastoid dressing is applied to prevent the patient from disturbing the repair. Too tight a dressing might compromise the blood supply. The dressing can be removed in a few days, and the bacitracin is continued for another day or two. If a takedown is necessary, it is performed after three to four weeks. After the second stage of a pedicled flap there is usually edema of the flap side of the flap/normal skin interface; this makes the repair more noticeable and may take several months to resolve. If, after six to nine months, a depressed scar has formed (this can be especially noticeable on the helical rim), a small Z-plasty can be performed under local anesthesia.

Otoplasty

Excluding microtia, the two general types of congenital malformations of the pinna are lop ears and prominent ears. A lop ear occurs when the superior portion of the helical rim is folded down like a hood over the rest of the pinna. The cartilage is folded on itself at an acute angle. A prominent ear can be due to either the lack of the anthelical fold or an overprojecting conchal bowl. The normal angle of the ears to the skull is 30 degrees, and a normal projection from the postauricular area to the middle one-third of the helix is 17 to 20 mm. Surgical correction is performed when a patient or parent, if the patient is a child, requests it and there are no medical contraindications. Children are usually operated on before starting school to avoid any ridicule their deformity might cause.

Aim

To correct the deformity present in either a lop or a prominent ear.

Highlights

1. A dumbbell-shaped postauricular incision is used.
2. Excess cauda helix is resected.
3. Excess conchal bowl cartilage is resected at the external auditory meatus.

Pitfalls

1. Collapse of the external auditory canal may occur if an insufficient amount of conchal bowl cartilage is removed when the conchal-mastoid sutures are placed.
2. Failing to resect excess cauda helix.
3. A sharp-edged anthelical fold may result from too deep crosshatching from the medial surface of the ear.
4. Imprecise measuring may result in asymmetry between the two ears.

Instruments

A basic plastics pack.
Methylene blue dye.
A 22-gauge needle.

Procedure

General anesthesia commonly is used since the operation is most often performed on children; however, local anesthesia can be used in adults. Generally, a patient with lop or prominent ears presents as a young child for corrective surgery. Occasionally, a newborn infant is seen within the first day or two of life with a prominent or lop ear, and it is possible to correct the defect nonsurgically. Immediately after birth maternal estrogens are still present in the infant, which makes the cartilage soft and malleable; stenting of these deformities in the neonatal period is successful until the drop in maternal estrogens causes the cartilage to become firm and resistant to structural change. Using Steri-Strips and cotton, the infant's ear is formed and taped into proper position. The ear must be taped in this manner for two to three months (Fig. 20–8*A*, *B*).

Text continued on page 358

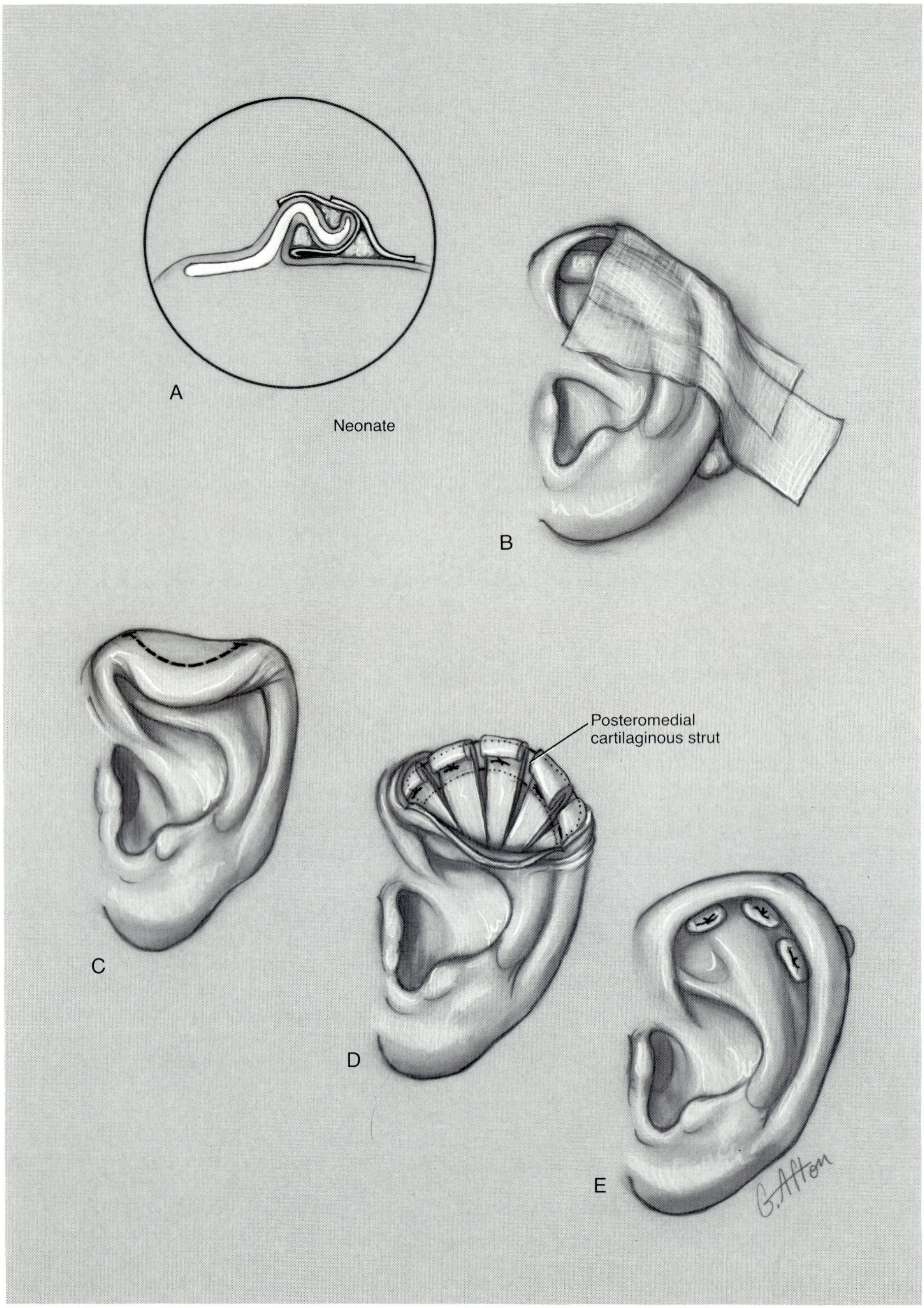

FIGURE 20–8.

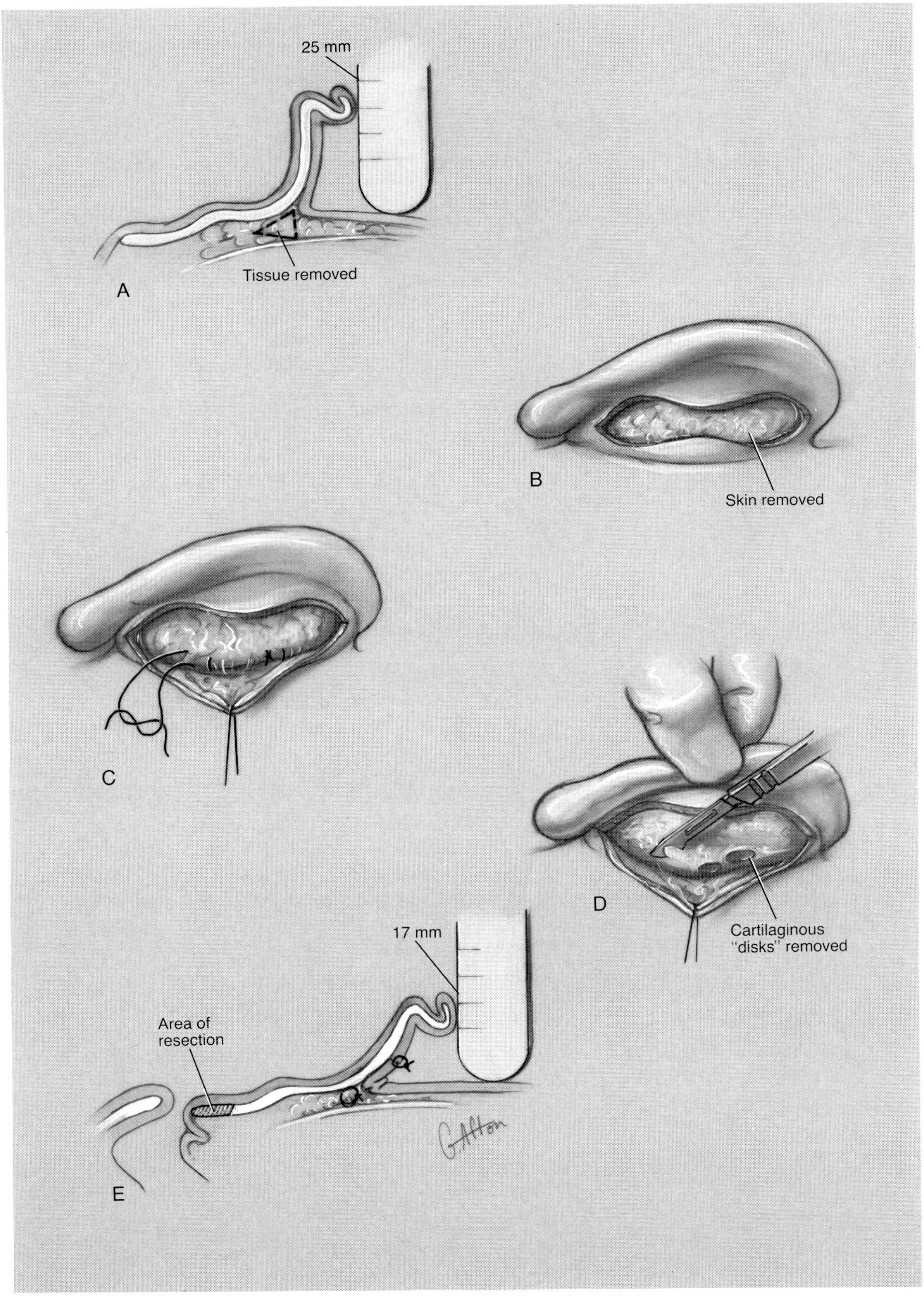
25 mm
Tissue removed
A
B
Skin removed
C
D
Cartilaginous "disks" removed
17 mm
Area of resection
E
G. Alton

FIGURE 20–9.

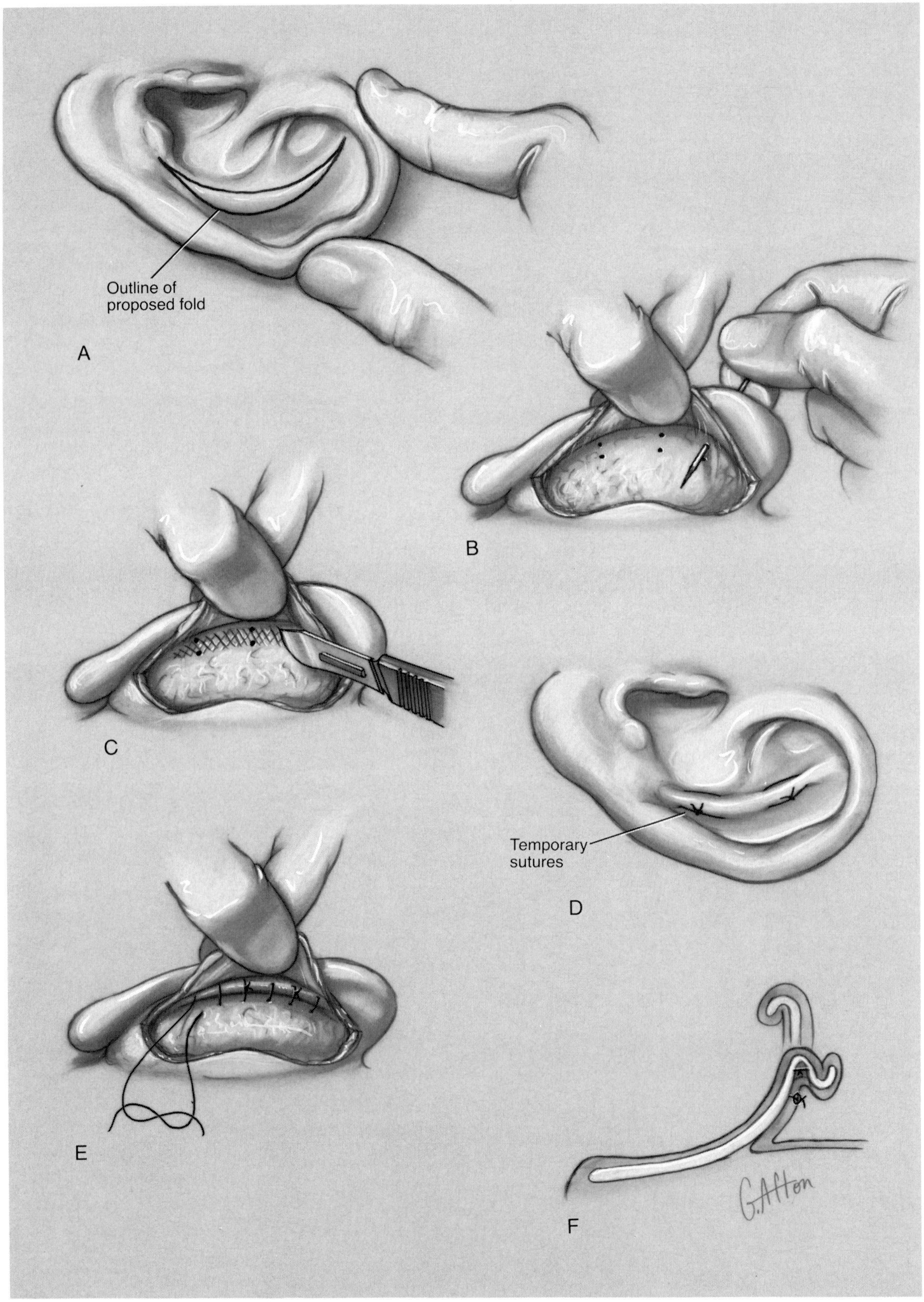

FIGURE 20–10.

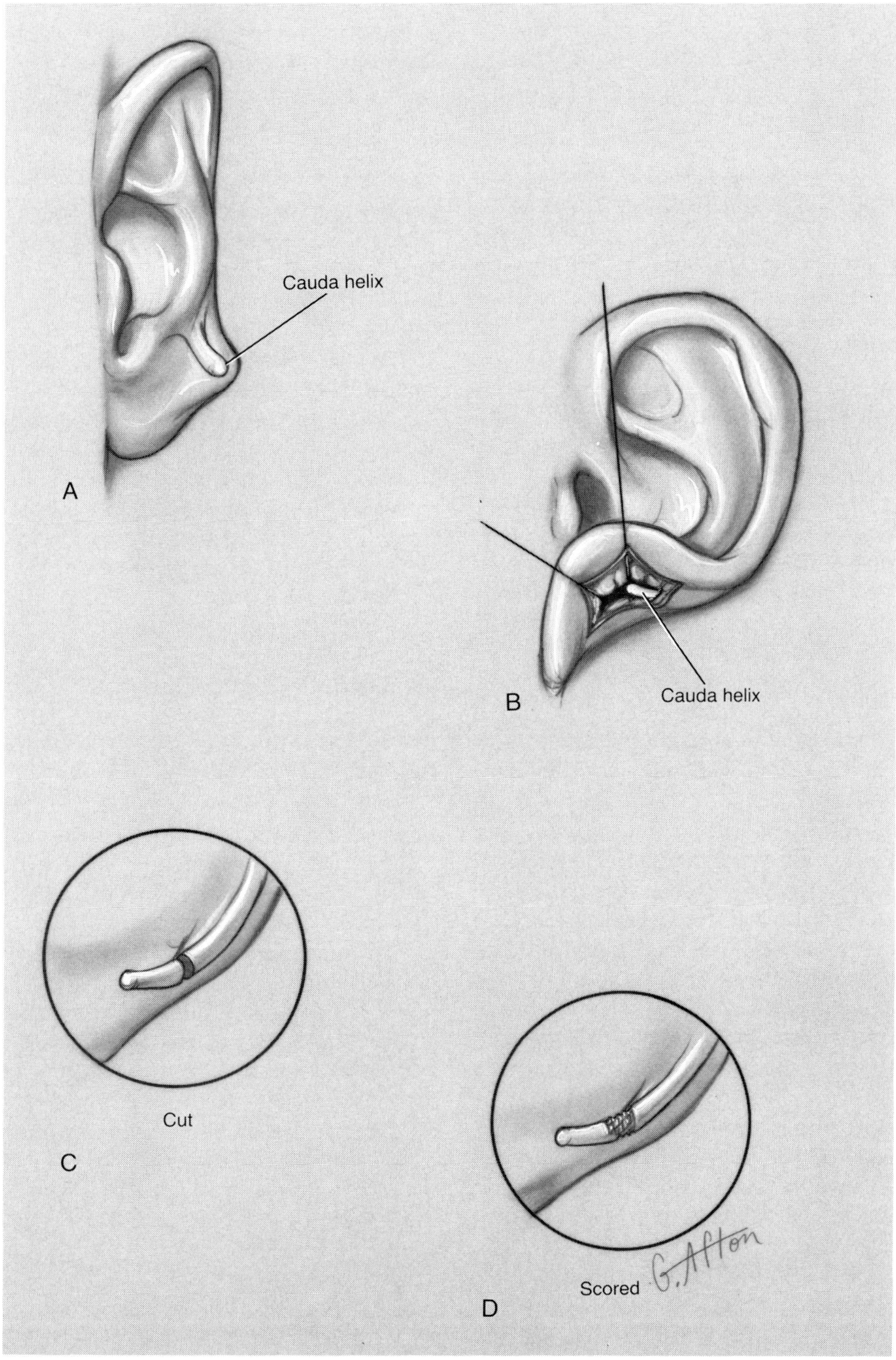

FIGURE 20–11.

To correct a lop ear surgically, an incision is made along the medial edge of the helical rim (Fig. 20–8C). The soft tissues on both sides of the "hooded" pinna are elevated, thus exposing the deformed cartilage. Vertical incisions are made down through the helix all the way to the conchal bowl, allowing the folded cartilage to unfold and flare out. A strut of conchal bowl cartilage is sutured to the medial surface of the new helical rim to give more support (Fig. 20–8*D*). If enough skin is present, primary closure is obtained with 5-0 Vicryl and either 6-0 chromic or nylon sutures; otherwise a postauricular flap like that used for repair of pinna defects is elevated and sutured into place. Small bolsters of cotton secured with 4-0 nylon suture help give definition to the helical rim (Fig. 20–8*E*).

The correction of prominent ears depends on whether the deformity is overprojection of the concha, lack of an anthelical fold, or a combination of the two. Most prominent ears have an element of both deformities.

A wooden tongue blade is used to measure the right and left ears at the start of the procedure so that symmetry can be obtained (Fig. 20–9*A*). After the first ear is finished, its projection is marked on the tongue blade and used as a guide for the second ear.

A dumbbell-shaped incision is made on the medial surface of the pinna and the ellipse of skin and soft tissues is removed (Fig. 20–9*B*). If there is only slight overprojection of the concha, conchal-mastoid sutures of 4-0 white Ethibond are placed in a mattress pattern from the mastoid periosteum to the conchal bowl perichondrium (Fig. 20–9C). Extra correction can be obtained by removing small disks of conchal bowl cartilage at the conchal-mastoid junction (Fig. 20–9*D*). A sharp No. 15 blade is used to shave the disks from the medial surface of the conchal bowl; care is taken to leave a layer of cartilage and perichondrium intact on the lateral surface. Caution should be exercised when the conchal bowl is brought back into proper position because the anterior conchal bowl cartilage can project into the external auditory canal and narrow it. If the canal is made too narrow, this excess cartilage should be excised.

The anthelical fold is corrected through the same incision. The proposed anthelical fold is outlined on the lateral surface of the pinna with a marking pen (Fig. 20–10*A*). The surgeon often can get a clear idea of where the anthelical fold should exist by gently pressing the helical rim toward the head; the unpronounced anthelical fold will appear over the formerly flat surface of the scaphoid region. A 22-gauge needle is passed through the lateral skin and cartilage and into the postauricular incision. Methylene blue dye is then applied to the needle tip and the needle is withdrawn (Fig. 20–10*B*). This marks the medial surface of the cartilage and serves as a guide for suture placement. The cartilage along the medial surface of the proposed anthelical fold is scored with a No. 15 blade through the cartilage, but not through the perichondrium on the lateral surface (Fig. 20–10C). If the incisions are through-and-through, an unattractive anthelical fold results. Next, temporary 4-0 silk horizontal mattress sutures are placed through the lateral surface of the pinna, through the cartilage, and back out the lateral surface, using the marks made as a guide. Temporary stay sutures allow the surgeon to "adjust" the anthelical fold to obtain symmetry with the opposite ear (Fig. 20–10*D*). White 4-0 Ethibond horizontal mattress sutures are then placed on the medial surface of the cartilage through the postauricular incision (Fig. 20–10*E*). Care must be taken not to exit through the lateral surface skin. When three to four sutures are in place the temporary silk sutures are removed. An anthelix has now been formed (Fig. 20–10*F*).

With the ear now in proper position, the appearance of the cauda helix must be assessed (Fig. 20–11*A*, *B*). Excess projection should be removed (by cutting the cauda helix) or morselized (by scoring) so that it lies flatter (Fig. 20–11*C*, *D*). The skin on the lateral surface of the pinna in the region of the cauda helix should also be undermined, so that after resection of the cauda helix the skin redrapes properly. The postauricular incision is closed with 4-0 Vicryl and 6-0 chromic or nylon sutures, and a bilateral mastoid dressing is applied. The dressing can be left on for one week to prevent trauma to the ears. If nylon sutures have been used, they can be removed when the dressing is removed. The patient must be cautioned against engaging in contact sports until six weeks after the surgery.

SECTION V

Selected References

Anson BJ and Donaldson JA: *Surgical Anatomy of the Temporal Bone,* 3rd ed. Philadelphia, WB Saunders Co, 1981.

Bailey BJ: Cochlear prosthesis implantation: Review of the issues (editorial). JAMA *251*:3282, 1984.

Brackman DE: *Neurological Surgery of Ear and Skull Base.* New York, Raven Press, 1982.

Brant-Zawadzki M and Norman D: *Magnetic Resonance Imaging of the Central Nervous System.* New York, Raven Press, 1985.

Chakeres EW and LaMasters DL: Paragangliomas of the temporal bone: High resolution CT studies. Radiology *150*:749–753, 1984.

Daniels DL, Millen SJ, Meyer GA, et al: MR detection of tumor in the internal auditory canal. AJNR *8*:249–252, 1987.

Doyle PJ: Indications for and technique of endaural and postauricular incisions. Otolaryngol *6*:262–266, 1977.

Farrior JB: Incisions in tympanoplasty: Anatomic considerations and indications. Laryngoscope *93*:75–86, 1983.

Fisch U: *Tympanoplasty and Stapedectomy.* New York, Thieme-Stratton, 1980.

Friedmann I: *Pathology of the Ear.* Oxford, Blackwell Scientific Publications, 1974.

Gacek RR: Transection of the posterior ampullary nerve for the relief of benign paroxysmal positional vertigo. Ann Otol Rhinol Laryngol *83*:596–605, 1974.

Gallagher JC: *Histology of the Human Temporal Bone.* American Registry of Pathology. Washington DC, Armed Forces Institute of Pathology, 1967.

Goodhill V: Sudden deafness and round window rupture. Laryngoscope *81*:1462–1474, 1971.

Griffin C, De La Paz R, and Enzmann D: MR and CT correlation of cholesterol cysts of petrous bone. AJNR *8*:825–829, 1987.

House WF: Surgical considerations in cochlear implantation. Ann Otol Rhinol Laryngol *91*(Suppl):15–20, 1982.

House WF and Luetje CM: *Acoustic Tumors,* Vols I and II. Baltimore, University Park Press, 1979.

Jansen C: Posterior tympanotomy: Experience and surgical details. Otolaryngol Clin North Am *5*:79–96, 1972.

Latack JT, Kartush JM, Kemink JL, et al: Epidermoidomas of the cerebellopontine angle and temporal bone: CT and MR aspects. Radiology *157*:361–366, 1985.

Lim DJ: Human tympanic membrane. Acta Otolaryngol *70*:176–186, 1970.

Lim DJ: Functional morphology of the lining membrane of the middle ear and eustachian tube. An overview. Ann Otol Rhinol Laryngol *83*(Suppl):5–26, 1974.

Marquet JFE (ed): *Surgery and Pathology of the Middle Ear.* Boston, Martinus Nijhoff, 1985.

Nager GT and Nager M: Arteries of the human middle ear, with particular regard to the blood supplies of the auditory ossicles. Ann Otol Rhinol Laryngol *62*:923–949, 1953.

Naumann HH: *Head and Neck Surgery. Vol 3: Ear.* Philadelphia, WB Saunders Co, 1982.

Naunton RF: Tympanostomy tubes: The conservative approach. Ann Otol Rhinol Laryngol *90*:529–532, 1981.

Paparella MM and Shumrick DA: *Otolaryngology* (Vols. 1 and 3). Philadelphia, WB Saunders Co, 1988.

Portmann M: *The Ear and Temporal Bone.* New York, Masson, 1979.

Proceedings of the second international symposium and workshops on surgery of the inner ear (Snowmass, Aspen, Colorado): Part 2. Am J Otol *8*:271–368, 1987.

Proctor B: The development of the middle ear spaces and their surgical significance. J Laryngol Otol *78*:631–648, 1964.

Proctor B and Nager GT: The facial canal: Normal anatomy, variations and anomalies. Trans Am Otol Soc *70*:49, 1982.

Schuknecht HF: *Stapedectomy.* Boston, Little, Brown & Co, 1971.

Schuknecht HF: *Pathology of the Ear.* Cambridge, Harvard University Press, 1974.

Schuknecht HF and Gulya JA: *Anatomy of the Temporal Bone with Surgical Implications.* Philadelphia, Lea and Febiger, 1986.

Shambaugh GE Jr and Glasscock ME III: *Surgery of the Ear,* 3rd ed. Philadelphia, WB Saunders Co, 1980.

Shea D, Chole R, and Paparella MM: The endolymphatic sac: Anatomical considerations. Laryngoscope *89*:88–94, 1979.

Surgical implantation technique for Xomed Audiant Bone Conductor (based on the technique of J. Hough) (pub. no. 50–1500). Jacksonville, Xomed Inc, 1986.

Swartz JD: *Imaging of the Temporal Bone: A Text-Atlas.* New York, Thieme, 1986.

Wolff D, Bellucci RJ, and Eggston AA: *Surgical and Microscopic Anatomy of the Temporal Bone.* New York, Hafner Publishing Co, 1971.

Index

Page numbers in *italics* indicate illustrations.

P

R

S

U

V

Z